Pharmacokinetics and Pharmacodynamics of Antimalarial Drugs Used in Combination Therapy

Authored By

Qigui Li

&

Mark R. Hickman

Walter Reed Army Institute of Research
USA

CONTENTS

CHAPTERS

FOREWORD

Prior to World War II, Department of Defense efforts to control malaria relied primarily on vector control measures, largely unchanged from those of COL William C. Gorgas in early 20th century Cuba and Panama. With the outbreak of the war, the US government greatly accelerated antimalarial drug research with limited access to quinine and the poor tolerability of atabrine. After the establishment of the Army's Malaria Drug Development Program, novel antimalarial drugs such as chloroquine, amodiaquine, proguanil, and pyrimethamine were developed. In 1944, the 8-aminoquinolines underwent testing by research teams under contract to the U.S. Army, ultimately resulting in the approval of primaquine as a radical cure for *P. vivax* malaria in U.S. troops returning from the Korean conflict. Subsequently, with the advent of chloroquine resistance during the Vietnam War, the U.S. Army established a long-term malaria drug research program under the direction of the Division of Experimental Therapeutics at the Walter Reed Army Institute of Research (WRAIR), leading to the FDA approval of mefloquine and halofantrine. With the subsequent evolution of mefloquine resistance and the recognition of its adverse effects, the WRAIR obtained FDA approval of doxycycline for prophylaxis against both *P. falciparum* and *P. vivax* malaria. The continued development of drug resistance, most recently against artemisinins as well as piperaquine in Southeast Asia, has renewed urgency for the development of both new ways to use existing drugs in addition to the development of new drug candidates.

The WRAIR's Dr. Qigui Li and Dr. Mark Hickman continue this tradition and have provided numerous insights in the pharmacology of antimalarial drugs for more than two decades, to include seminal work on the pharmacology of artemisinins. With the emergence of multi-drug resistant malaria, and in particular resistance to artemisinins, the cornerstone of current malaria treatment with artemisinin combination therapy (ACT) is now at risk. It is now time for the malaria field to apply the lessons of HIV and TB, where multiple drug therapy to avoid the development of drug resistance is standard practice. To this end, understanding the complex pharmacokinetic-pharmacodynamic relationships of current and future antimalarials used in combination therapy will be critical to curbing further resistance and continued progress towards malaria control and elimination. This monograph provides a detailed overview of these challenges and the experimental methods and tools needed to accelerate the clinical development of new antimalarial combination therapies.

Robert M. Paris

Colonel, Medical Corps
Director, Military Malaria Research Program
Walter Reed Army Institute of Research
Silver Spring, MD
USA

PREFACE

Antimalarial drug discovery and development is a lengthy process, and given the lack of resources available for development of antimalarial drugs, discovery and development of antimalarials as single entities or combinations can take much longer than development of drugs for treatment of diseases that affect patients from first world countries. Given the limited resources for development of drugs to treat a disease not found in first world countries, drug development processes must be as efficient as possible, and expensive clinical studies must be well-planned and geared toward yielding the maximum amount of information to get the best "bang for the buck".

Safety, comparative efficacy, and dose determination studies are all best conducted by thorough consideration of pharmacokinetic and pharmacodynamic variables that impact on how quickly all of the relevant questions can be answered to develop a drug for clinical use in man. Development of drugs to the standards to regulatory standards set by first world regulatory agencies like the FDA or EMA, in particular, imposes a high threshold that must be met with limited funds.

Well-planned clinical trials of comparative efficacy that have a sound foundation of safety and PK studies are more likely to be successful than clinical trials developed with minimal PK and safety data. The use of physiologic based pharmacokinetic/pharmacodynamic (PB PK/PD) studies, innovative population PK/PD studies, factorial study designs, and drug resistance models are all modern tools that can provide a faster path forward than simple empirical trial designs that do not utilize these techniques. The issue of malaria drug resistance in the modern era imposes yet another burden on drug developers as development of an antimalarial drug for treatment of a disease, which is difficult to begin with due to limited funds, is not a "one and done" activity. Every antimalarial drug developed to date eventually has come up against problems with drug resistance, and all of these drugs come with a limitation on their use in terms of the length of time on market until clinical resistance is encountered.

Drug combinations offer the potential to extend the life of existing antimalarial drugs, and drug combinations also have the potential to limit the development of drug resistance through disease treatment with two or more drugs whose different or synergistic mechanisms of action are mutually protective. The development and deployment of artemisinin combination therapies (ACTs), in particular, over the last decade has revolutionized malaria treatment in endemic areas. While ACTs have become the wonder drug antimalarial combination treatment of the new millennia, all ACTs on market will eventually run into drug resistance problems that preclude their use in various endemic areas. Accordingly, new and novel antimalarial drug combinations must be innovated to try and stay ahead of the growing tide of malaria drug resistance. Fundamentally, this is a contest between a parasite's ability to mutate and man's ability to innovate.

We believe that proper application of new, modern PK/PD tools can radically improve clinical trial design and execution which maximizes the "bang for the buck" and speeds the development of new antimalarial drug combinations.

Qigui Li & Mark R. Hickman
Walter Reed Army Institute of Research
USA
E-mail: qigui.li.civ@mail.mil

ACKNOWLEDGEMENTS

Some of the data cited in this book was derived from studies performed at Walter Reed Army Institute of Research (WRAIR) over the past 30 years, and these studies were supported by the United States Army Research and Materiel Command. The manuscript has been reviewed by the WRAIR. There is no objection to its presentation and/or publication. The opinions or assertions contained herein are the private views of the author and are not to be construed as official, or reflecting the views of the Department of the Army or the Department of Defense.

CONFLICT OF INTEREST

The author confirms that this ebook contents have no conflict of interest.

INTRODUCTION

The existing antimalarial drugs available for prophylaxis and treatment of malaria are limited due to drug resistance and cross-resistance among related drugs. The majority of drugs on market, however, have an ongoing role as antimalarials and their lifetimes could be extended if they were deployed in a rational planned manner by administering them in combination based on their pharmacodynamic and pharmacokinetic properties. WHO has defined combination therapy as the synergistic or additive potential of multiple drugs to enhance efficacy and deter emergence of drug resistant parasites to individual combination partners. Drug synergism has a number of outcomes that are favorable which include enhanced efficacy, cutting drug doses to avoid toxicity and still maintaining the same efficacy, deterring drug resistance and lastly providing selective target or efficacy synergism against the malaria parasite or decreasing individual drug toxicity. For these therapeutic benefits, combinations of drugs have been utilized for treatment of other infectious diseases such as HIV and tuberculosis, and combination therapy has become the leading choice to treat malaria [1, 2].

Antimalarial combination therapy (CT) is defined as the concurrent administration of multiple blood schizonticidal drugs each with an independent mechanism of action and each with a distinct and different biochemical parasite target. Accordingly, multiple-drug treatments including certain antimalarial drugs meet the criteria of a synergistic combination can be operationally thought of as single products as neither drug partner would be administered alone for anti-malarial treatment (ex. sulfadoxine-pyrimethamine). Artemisinin-based combination treatments (ACTs) have been demonstrated to enhance efficacy for treatment of malaria where they have been deployed around the world, and these combination drugs have been shown to contain drug resistance in Southeast Asia.

Parasite resistance to antimalarial drugs is a major threat to global public health. Artemisinin therapies are the only currently available mainstream drugs where *P. falciparum* drug resistance is limited to a discrete geographical region, has a regional impact, and has a confirmed molecular marker (K13-propeller polymorphism) for tracking the emergence and spread of artemisinin resistance [1-6]. For traditional drugs (chloroquine, amodiaquine, mefloquine, sulfadoxine-pyrimethamine, and quinine), the degree of resistance varies from drug to drug and from region to region. Artemisinin and artemisinin analogues have been shown to be quick acting, highly efficacious antimalarials. These compounds are very potent extremely fast-acting antimalarials with a broad therapeutic index. Artemisinins, however, as a group, have shown high rates of recrudescence for malaria cures when administered as monotherapy. In 2005, the World Health Organization described reduced drug susceptibility of *P. falciparum* to artemisinin drugs, which specifically warned against the possible introduction of artemisinin resistance, and the danger that such resistance would pose to global health [2]. In 2006, the WHO recommended monotherapy with artemisinin be dropped altogether and endorsed artemisinin combination therapies as a "policy standard" and first-line treatment for treatment of malaria in regions where *P. falciparum* is the dominant species of malaria [1]. While many countries have enforced a ban on artemisinin monotherapy sales [3], some pharmaceutical firms have continued to manufacture and distribute artemisinin monotherapy drugs in malaria-endemic countries [4].

The frequent failures of artemisinin monotherapy has been overcome by using oral ACTs where artemisinin compounds are co-administered with long-acting antimalarial drugs which facilitate the killing of residual parasites not killed by the artemisinin component. ACTs can improve the efficacy of failing individual component drugs, lower the incidence of malaria, and provide some protection for individual component drugs against the development of higher levels of resistance.

In the past decade, evidence of increased falciparum drug resistance to artemisinin and artemisinin analogues has been observed along the border between Cambodia and Thailand. Monitoring the extent and spread of artemisinin resistance has been very challenging due to the lack of a molecular marker of resistance, however, recent publications of a polymorphism in the propeller region of a kelch protein in *P. falciparum*, the K-13 mutations, may aid in monitoring artemisinin-resistant *P. falciparum* [5, 6]. Reduced parasite susceptibility to artemisinin drugs makes ACT partner drugs, in turn, more vulnerable to drug resistance. This new artemisinin drug resistance phenomenon coupled with previously noted development of parasite drug resistance to all of the partner drugs currently in use suggests that current ACT combination drug treatments will fail. This failure will result in recrudescent malaria infections after failed therapy for an initial infection, decreased efficacy of severe malaria treatment using artemisinin-derived drugs, and the failure of ACTs to eliminate parasites from infected populations treated for malaria eradication [7]. Despite the delays in parasite clearance noted in patients infected with malaria in the Cambodia-Thailand border region, ACTs are still the best therapy for uncomplicated *falciparum* malaria, and the majority of patients in this region with delays in ACT response are eventually cured as long as the partner drug is still efficacious. Patients with delays in parasite clearance from artemisinin resistance coupled with mutations associated with drug resistance to partner drugs, however, will be at high risk for recrudescent infections [2, 8].

The World Health Organization (WHO) has implemented a Global Plan to contain resistance to artemisinin, which should be put into operation by all countries with endemic malaria. There is, a brief window of time to contain artemisinin resistance until it spreads to areas with high malaria transmission, which will endanger recent malaria control achievements. The problem of emerging artemisinin resistance must be confronted quickly as there are no other drugs that exist providing similar efficacy and tolerability as the ACTs, and no drugs in the pipeline to replace them in the near term. To enhance artemisinin drug efficacy and protect these compounds from emerging drug resistance, WHO has called for combination treatment with other partner drugs having different modes of action and extended half-lives [1-4, 8]. Artemisinin analogues rapidly decrease the parasite biomass, which leaves a small population of residual parasites alive to be killed by a partner drug. An efficacious partner drug typically has no problem eliminating the few parasites that remain. In addition, the likelihood of a simultaneous series of mutations against an artemisinin drug and a partner drug with a different parasite target is very small [9]. Therefore, for *P. falciparum* treatment, combining multiple drugs with different targets together is the best method to insure malaria infections are cured and resistance is deterred [8, 9].

ACTs are based on combining fast acting artemisinin-based compounds with drugs from a different class. Companion drugs commonly used for ACT treatment include mefloquine, lumefantrine, sulfadoxine-pyrimethamine, amodiaquine, chlorproguanil-dapsone, and piperaquine. Artemisinin analogues that are in use in ACTs include artesunate, dihydroartemisinin, and artemether. Carrying out the WHO's recommendation has required rapid introduction of a limited array of combination drugs that are affordable and co-formulated. With attractive pricing by a number of vendors, many countries have actually implemented this recommendation. A co-formulated drug is defined as a combination of multiple drugs in one fixed dose formulation, either a tablet or granule and the use of fixed dose combinations in one form helps ensure both drugs are administered. Artemether-lumefantrine was the first combination treatment formulated as a fixed-dose ACT to treat uncomplicated *falciparum* malaria. AL has been shown to be efficacious in both sub-Saharan Africa and in regions of Southeast Asia with multi-drug resistant falciparum malaria. A second fixed-dose combination comprised of amodiaquine and-artesunate was introduced in February 2007. The benefits of ACTs include their rapid action, efficacy, and a decreased probability of the development of parasite drug resistance to either partner drug. To maximize these benefits, issues of cost, delivery and, access must be addressed.

When compared to the other three major artemisinin compounds (artemisinin, dihydroartemisinin and artemether), artesunate (AS) is the only artemisinin analogue available formulated for IV injection to provide peak concentrations necessary for rapid parasite killing required for treatment of severe malaria. Injectable AS is pharmacokinetically and pharmacodynamically superior compared to other artemisinins, which do not have this fundamental property. Studies of drug disposition (pharmacokinetics or PK) and studies of compound efficacy (pharmacodynamics or PD) of the artemisinin compounds have shown the astonishing speed of artemisinin killing is associated with the peak drug concentrations achieved as measured by the C_{max} (maximum concentration). Among the five-artemisinin compounds, peak drug concentration is the only PK variable that correlates with parasite killing which reinforces the finding that AS has superior PK and PD properties after IV or oral administration. Assessment of other PK parameters like overall drug exposure (AUC) or drug exposure time (half-life) tends to be less significant [10].

PK/PD evaluations have also shown that malaria efficacy associated with the long acting drugs from the quinoline and antifolate classes, for example, is a property of the minimum inhibitory concentration (MIC) and biological half-life ($t_{1/2}$) while the overall exposure shown by the AUC or peak drug concentrations illustrated by the C_{max}, tend to be less important. Further PK/PD evaluations have also revealed that of all of the quinoline compounds, piperaquine has superior PK/PD parameters following oral administration when compared to the other standard partner drugs. PK studies of standard antimalarials provide the basis for picking appropriate partner drugs for an ACT.

Studies of drug disposition and drug efficacy (PK/PD evaluations) are essential for understanding why drugs work as antimalarials. PK/PD studies increase our knowledge of drug disposition and efficacy, and they illustrate issues with drug resistance, drug safety, and drug toxicity that are critical for finding the appropriate drug dose that is efficacious but avoids toxicity. One example of drug toxicity found in antimalarial drugs is that of halofantrine. Halofantrine was shown to induce marked QT prolongation on an electrocardiogram test at therapeutic concentrations after it came on market in the 1990s, and treatment with halofantrine above the recommended dose (which was conducted to cope with drug resistance observed in Southeast Asia) was linked to sudden death likely from ventricular tachyarrhythmia. Halofantrine has also been shown to prolong the PR interval on an electrocardiogram test, and this drug has been shown to cause *Torsade de pointes* or cardiac blockade at elevated plasma levels. The absorption of halofantrine, a highly lipophilic antimalarial drug, is extremely variable and depends on the amount of co-administered fats. Thus, plasma drug concentrations of halofantrine are quite variable in a population of individuals. As cardiotoxicity is concentration dependent, the probability of an individual experiencing cardiotoxicity is very hard to predict [11].

Unfortunately, many of the tools for evaluating cardiotoxicity risk that are common today, particularly *in vitro* testing of compounds for their propensity to have cardiotoxicity risks, were not available when halofantrine was developed as a drug. Today, *in vitro* testing for the propensity of novel compounds to block the hERG channel is readily available, which would have shown this risk during development, and halofantrine as a drug might never have been developed. Highly expensive animal testing of cardiotoxic potential was available in the 1980s and 1990s that could also have been used to rule out halofantrine's development as an antimalarial drug based on a positive *in vitro* test result, which unfortunately was not available as a drug development tool at that time. This episode also highlights the value of broader Phase 1 studies that test a larger range of doses in a diverse population, which also would have helped assess the propensity of this antimalarial drug for cardiotoxicity.

Toxicokinetic studies in laboratory animals have been used to highlight issues with antimalarial drugs that may cause problems when these drugs are developed and finally tested in man. One example of toxicokinetic studies (TK) that is pertinent is neurotoxicity associated with administration of artemisinin drugs. Animal assessment of the oil-soluble artemisinin derivatives arteether and artemether administered intramuscularly or the water-soluble artemisinin artelinic acid administered orally demonstrated the potential for serious and fatal neurotoxicity. Toxicokinetic (TK) assessments have shown oil-soluble artemisinin derivitives can form depots at the sites of intramuscular injection, and these depots have been linked to muscle inflammation at those sites. Oral administration of artelinic acid has been shown to induce GI toxicity associated with delays in gastric empyting.

All of this data supports the hypothesis that the duration of drug exposure beyond threshold levels leads to accumulation of artemisinin derivitives in the blood and ultimately to neurotoxicity. A variety of toxicokinetic (TK) studies of artemisinin compounds have been conducted in different animal models and the duration of drug exposure beyond threshold levels has been shown to be the most important TK factor associated with induction of neurotoxicity. Additional neurotoxicity studies have shown significant differences in toxicodynamic (TD) observation of neurotoxicity between different animal species which suggests the exposure time necessary for artemisinin-induced neurotoxicity has been shown to be much longer in man than in lower species [12, 13]. These studies were very useful in deciding which artemisinin was worthy of further development. At Walter Reed Army Institute of Research, where we work, these toxicity studies led our development group to abandon arteether, artemether, and artelinic acid in favor of developing water-soluble artesunate for treatment of severe malaria. This TK/TD example shows the successful use of animal studies to help guide antimalarial drug development [14].

Early animal studies in pregnant rodents have shown artemisinin compounds, particularly injectable artesunate, have reprotoxicity effects resulting in fetal death and embryo malformations when administered at low doses. Animal studies of reprotoxicity have shown injectable AS has the propensity in animal models to induce severe embryolethality after both IV and IM injections. TK studies of this phenomenon demonstrated that the root cause of embryotoxicity is due to the high peak drug concentrations achieved after AS administration in pregnant animals. Fortunately, further TD studies showed that this artemisinin-induced neurotoxicity occurs within a limited period in early fetal life. Based on this data, the WHO has suggested avoiding administration of artemisinin compounds early in pregnancy. Studies of this phenomenon in 1,837 pregnant women administered combination therapy using ACTs for treatment of uncomplicated malaria including 176 patients in their first trimester has not shown this embryotoxicity in this population. This demonstrates the value of TK/TD studies to reveal toxicity issues that require further studies in animal models and caution when prescribing drugs in man [15].

In rodents, TK/TD analysis has shown that sensitive early red blood cells exposed to artemisinin drugs administered through either single or through multiple exposures can result in a high proportion of these cells lost to cell death. This finding helps explain why artemisinin-induced embryotoxicity occurs. Further studies in primates showed a longer period of 12 days of drug exposure was required for induction of embryo loss. In man, there is little information published regarding red blood cell development in early embryogenesis, but this phase of development is known to occur throughout a longer period. It is possible that treatment with an ACT for 3 days will not affect RBC development to a toxic extent. In addition, ACT administration *via* orally administered artemisinins will lead to lower drug levels and decreased exposure times, and accordingly, it is unlikely that such a concentration–course profile could be achieved by oral ACTs that actually induces embryotoxicity in man [16]. This example shows the relevance of TK/TD studies and drug toxicity mechanism studies to explain animal findings, highlight drug risks, and develop data to guide drug administration policies to achieve antimalarial efficacy and avoid toxicity.

Antimalarial drugs used for treatment of malaria have shifted from monotherapy to the use of drug combination therapy, particularly after the introduction of ACTs. There is, however, no proper rationale for the choice of dose or duration of combination therapy. Few attempts have been made to utilize PK/PD mathematical models to describe the time-course of parasitemia in malaria-infected individuals before or after treatment with various antimalarial drugs, used either as monotherapy or in combination [17]. New comprehensive mathematical models to describe malaria transmission and the spread of drug resistance have been developed to model data reported empirically in various comparative efficacy studies. These models can be a useful tool to inform the design of treatment policies, particularly when deciding which combination therapy to introduce and why one combination therapy may be superior in one geographic region and unsuitable in another [17, 18].

Historically, combination treatments such as sulfadoxine-pyrimethamine have been used for malaria treatment; however, this combination has problems associated with toxicity (development of Stevens-Johnson syndrome, a form of toxic epidermal necrolysis) and high-grade resistance in many parts of the world. ACTs have been quite successful antimalarial drug combinations due to a variety of factors: 1) Safe and fast-acting artemisinins are still largely free from resistance; 2) ACTs were created focused on ease of administration to gather commercial interest in development; 3) ACTs have been formulated based on suitable matching PK and PD profiles both to deter resistance and to improve efficacy; 4) *In vitro* tests suggest that ACTs may reverse the previous rise in mefloquine resistance; 5) The therapeutic indices of partner drugs both fast- and long-acting are wide with low toxicity.

To protect existing ACTs and novel drug combinations devised in the future, new efforts are needed to assess artemisinin resistance and come up with new strategies to cope with this phenomenon. PK/PD evaluations and other TK/TD studies that we will discuss in depth in this book will outline the advantages and disadvantages of leading prospective drug combinations that are the most effective and most sustainable in the populations of malaria endemic countries. We will also discuss the pros and cons of developing novel CT drugs with new mechanisms of action not based on current ACTs, and the strategies by which it may be possible to optimize the use of currently available combination therapy drugs for years to come.

CHAPTER 1

Current Issues in Antimalarial Drug Resistance

Abstract: Artemisinins are the only currently available mainstream drugs that do not have widespread issues with *P. falciparum* drug resistance outside of Southeast Asia. Initial reports of artemisinin resistance were noted in western Cambodia near the border with Thailand in 2009 and a possible molecular marker was identified in 2014. For other traditional antimalarial therapies, malaria resistance has been observed to be highly variable and the geographical distribution of resistance and rate of spread have varied significantly. The times for resistance to appear have varied from 278 years for quinine, 35 years for the artemisinins, 12 years for chloroquine, 5 years for mefloquine, 1 year for proguanil, and less than 1 year for sulfadoxine-pyrimethamine and atovaquone. Given the emergence of artemisinin resistance and the possibilities of the spread of resistance out of the border regions of Cambodia, it is essential to prevent the loss of artemisinin combination therapies (ACTs) which are the current first-line treatments for malaria. The use of drugs in combination for treatment of malaria is the best tool to decrease the incidence and spread of malaria drug resistance. The rationale for this approach is threefold: 1) drug combinations are often more effective than monotherapy with one drug; 2) artemisinins substantially reduce gametocyte carriage and thus reduce transmission; and 3) if a mutation arises in a malaria parasite during treatment with one drug, this parasite should still be killed by the partner drug. As each drug protects the other, resistance should be discouraged from occurring. An antimalarial drug combination must provide partners which are each independently capable of treating the disease. In addition, drug combinations used to treat malaria such as the ACTs often provide radical cures of malaria when administered in a 3-day treatment regimen, which also provides protection against emergence of artemisinin resistance.

Keywords: Artemisinin-based combination therapy (ACT), artemisinins, chloroquine, drug combination, malaria, malaria infection, malaria parasite, malaria transmission, mefloquine, proguanil, resistance, resistant spread.

1.1. ANTIMALARIAL DRUG RESISTANCE

The artemisinin therapies are the only currently available mainstream drugs that do not have widespread problems with *P. falciparum* drug resistance. Initial reports of resistance to artemisinin on the border between Cambodia and Thailand have been published and follow-on studies have confirmed these findings [5]. Other reports of artemisinin resistance have been noted in the Greater Mekong sub region formed by six countries to include Cambodia, Laos, Myanmar, Thailand, Vietnam, and China [8].

For other antimalarial medications (amodiaquine, chloroquine, mefloquine, quinine and sulfadoxine-pyrimethamine), the level of resistance, spread of resistance, and

Qigui Li and Mark R. Hickman

distribution of resistance geographically has historically varied (Fig. **1**). Chloroquine resistant *P. falciparum* has been noted in virtually every country endemic for malaria except Central America and the island of Hispaniola. SP resistance is widely prevalent in Africa, South America, and in Southeast Asia. Mefloquine resistance in *P. falciparum* has been reported in Southeast Asia and in areas of Africa and South America where mefloquine has been used as a single agent. As previously mentioned, the time required for malaria drug resistance to appear upon introduction of a new antimalarial drug is quite variable from 278 years for quinine to less than 1 year for atovaquone (Table **1**) [2, 5-8, 19].

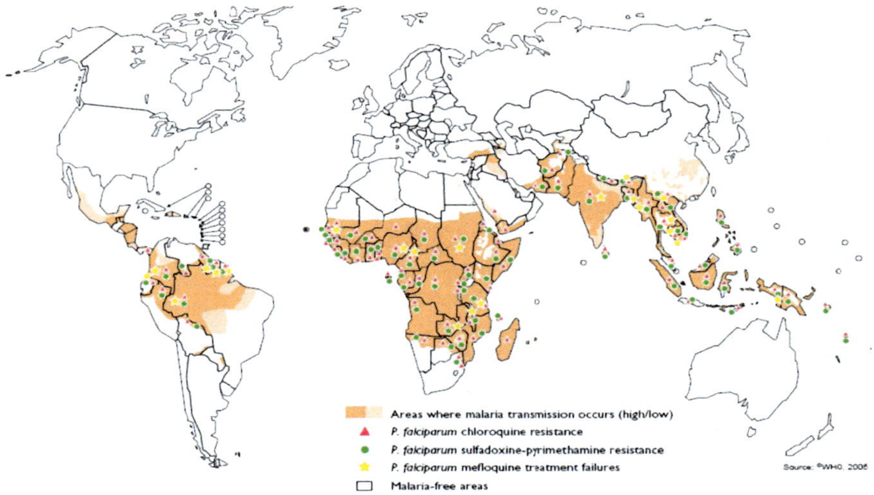

Figure 1: Malaria transmission areas and reported *P. falciparum* resistance. The designations employed and the presentation of material on this map do not imply the expression of any opinion whatsoever on the part of the World Health Organization concerning the legal status of any country, territory, city or area or of its authorities, or concerning the delimitation of its frontiers or boundaries. Source: Adapted from Global Plan for Insecticide Resistance Management in malaria vectors, WHO, Geneva, 2012.

Table 1: Dates of drug introduction and first reports of antimalarial drug resistance

Antimalarial Drug	Introduced	First Reported Resistance	Difference (Years)	Refs.*
Quinine	1632	1910	278	[19]
Artemisinins	1971	2006	35	[2, 7]
Chloroquine	1945	1957	12	[19]
Mefloquine	1977	1982	5	[19]
Proguanil	1948	1949	1	[19]
Sulfadoxine-pyrimethamine	1967	1967	0	[19]
Atovaquone	1996	1996	0	[19]

*Data were from Wongsrichanalai *et al.*, 2002 [19] and WHO 2010-2012 [2, 7].

Resistance to chloroquine has been noted in patients infected with *P. vivax* in a number of areas. Cases of prophylactic and therapeutic failures have been reported in several regions (Fig. **2**). *P. vivax* resistance to chloroquine is difficult to confirm and additional evidence may be required, in particular, chloroquine blood concentrations. Malaria treatment guidelines developed and published in 2006 include a protocol for assessing chloroquine efficacy for *P. vivax* treatment [1]. Some of the best evidence for chloroquine resistance to *P. vivax* has been shown in Papua New Guinea, East Timor, Indonesia, and other areas of Oceania, and there are reports of chloroquine-resistant *P. vivax* in Peru. In other areas of the world such as Southeast Asia, India, the Middle East, Korea, north-east Africa and most of South and Central America, *P. vivax* remains chloroquine sensitive [1, 2]. The increase in antimalarial drug resistance observed over time for most of the antimalarials on market can be reviewed from a historical perspective to appreciate potential future antimalarial drug resistance.

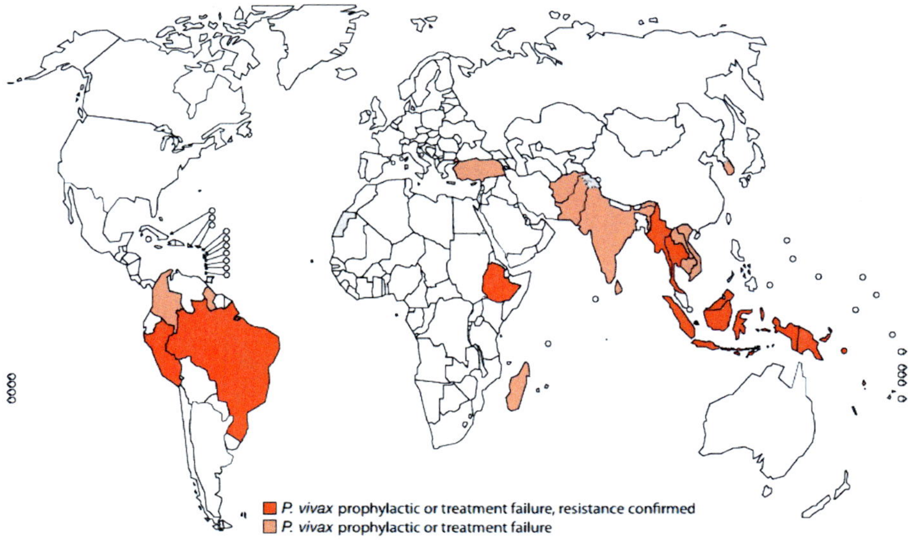

Figure 2: Prophylactic and treatment failure and confirmed resistance of *P. vivax* to chloroquine. Parasites carrying the Tyr976Phe mutation of *Pvmdr1* showed reduced susceptibility to chloroquine *in vitro* when compared with wild-type parasites from Indonesia and Thailand; however, this marker was not found to be useful for monitoring chloroquine resistance in Madagascar [1].

Artemisinins

WHO recently provided an update on artemisinin resistance (Fig. **3**), and the WHO initiated a Global Plan for Artemisinin Resistance Containment (GPARC) after reports of artemisinin resistance in Cambodia in patients and follow-on data showing a molecular marker of artemisinin resistance, polymorphisms in a *falciparum* protein, the kelch propeller domain, (PF3D7_1343700 kelch propeller domain), were confirmed [6, 20]. The goal of GPARC is to insure that artemisinin based combination therapies (ACTs) are protected and remained as an effective therapy for *falciparum* malaria. WHO has characterized artemisinin drug resistance as a clinically observed delay in parasite clearance, and this document summarizes a number of studies characterizing artemisinin resistance as follows [8].

- Given this definition, artemisinin resistance has been definitively demonstrated at Pailin, Cambodia and Mae Sot, Thailand [5].

- Studies to define the molecular mechanism and a genetic marker for artemisinin resistance are underway world-wide, and candidate marker genes that have been examined include single mutations and copy number mutations in *pfmdr1*, alteration in the sarco-endoplasmic reticulum calcium ATPase6 gene, *pfserca*, mutations in mitochondrial genes, and mutations in a de-ubiquitination enzyme, *pfubp1* [8].

- More recently, reports of artemisinin *in vitro* and *in vivo* resistance have been published in Nature in 2014 associated with mutations in the PF3D7_1343700 kelch propeller domain. This study-involved whole-genome sequencing of an artemisinin-resistant parasite from Africa and whole genome sequencing of parasites isolated from Cambodia from patients demonstrating delays in parasite clearance after artemisinin treatment [5, 6].

- The presence of all of these markers in artemisinin resistant strains has been shown to correlate significantly with clinical manifestation of artemisinin resistance in Southeast Asia. There is no good correlation, however, for *in vitro* IC_{50} determinations of artemisinin antimalarial potency to delays in parasite clearance. The measurements of artemisinin drug levels in the blood or inside the erythrocyte may be a better, more effective assessment of drug resistance than drug concentrations measured in the plasma of treated patients.

- The rate of parasite clearance is a marker of infection *in vivo* that is a better assessment tool than the fraction of parasitemia positive cases by day 3. Parasite clearance is calculated by measuring the slope of parasite clearance on a log-linear curve, and this metric is not dependent on the initial parasitemia noted.

- There are ongoing efforts to monitor ACT efficacy in many countries around the world, and thus far, there are no confirmed reports of delays in parasite clearance in African patients treated with artemisinins.

The rise in *P. falciparum* resistance to artemisinin drugs is a significant global health issue, and there is a limited opportunity to contain this problem before it spreads to other locations outside of Southeast Asia assuming this phenomenon spreads geographically as opposed to arising *de novo* in a new location. ACTs are recommended as the first choice for treatment of uncomplicated malaria and the implementation of ACTs worldwide has been an essential component for treatment of malaria given the rise of resistance to other drugs. There are no other alternatives at present to ACTs that are similarly efficacious and well tolerated.

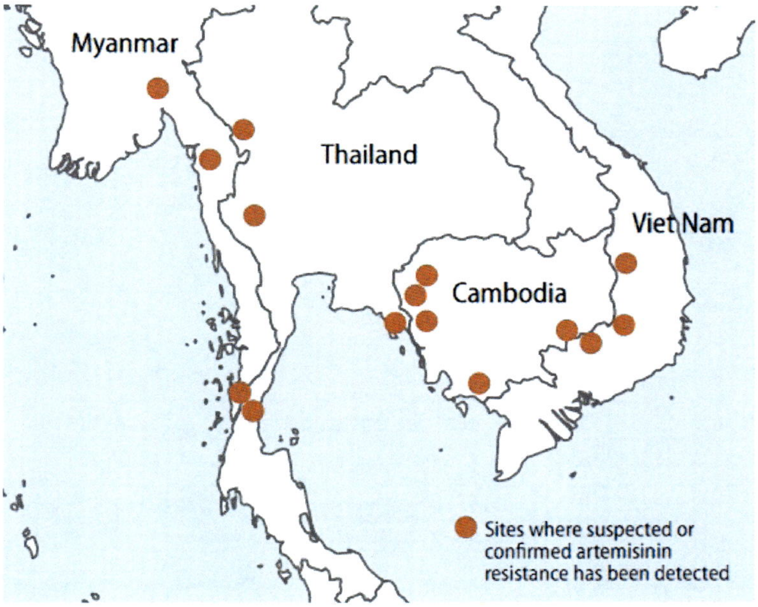

Figure 3: Sites where suspected or confirmed artemisinin resistance has been detected in therapeutic efficacy studies, Mekong subregion, 2007-2012: Map production: Global Malaria Programme (GMP), World Health Organization; Source of data: WHO Global Database on Antimalarial Drug Efficacy, as of November, 2012 [20].

Chloroquine

Chloroquine resistant *P. falciparum* was noted in Columbia and in the border region between Thailand and Cambodia in the 1950s. Chloroquine resistance was originally observed in Indochina until the 1970s when chloroquine resistance was noted in neighboring geographic regions. Chloroquine resistance in Africa was observed later, and 10 years was required for chloroquine resistance to spread throughout the continent. Today, chloroquine remains effective only on the island of Hispaniola and in countries north of the Panama Canal. While chloroquine is cross-resistant with amodiaquine, a chloroquine analogue, amodiaquine is still a more effective drug than chloroquine in areas of chloroquine resistance. As reported by WHO, the incidence of chloroquine treatment failure by day 14 after treatment is initiated has been shown to be >10% in 93% of African countries and 100% in Asian countries and the Americas (Table **2**) [1].

Table 2: Clinical failure rates on day 14 after treatment with chloroquine or pyrimethamine-sulfadoxine by region [1]

Drugs **Region**	**Day 14 Clinical Failure (%)***			**No. of Countries**
	< 10	**10-25**	**> 25**	
Chloroquine				
Africa	7	38	55	42
Asia	0	11	89	19
Americas	0	0	100	5
Sulfadoxine-pyrimethamine-				
Africa	71	24	6	34
Asia	20	53	27	15
Americas	20	80	0	5

* Data are % of countries.

Amodiaquine

Given the enhanced efficacy of amodiaquine in areas of chloroquine resistance, amodiaquine was chosen as a partner drug for combination with artesunate. Amodiaquine has been shown to lose efficacy after induction of parasite mutations associated with chloroquine resistance, and drug resistance is increased in areas in areas where authorities have chosen to use amodiaquine extensively. Between 2000 and 2007, there were 59 studies of amodiaquine efficacy conducted in 23 countries. Evaluation of these data in total have shown that amodiaquine median treatment failure rates are lower in western Africa than in other regions while the Middle East and South America show amodiaquine treatment failure rates from 28.8% to 53.1% [21].

Sulfadoxine-Pyrimethamine

The combination of sulfadoxine-pyrimethamine (SP) was created to replace chloroquine, however, this combination became useless in Thailand in the early 1980s and resistance spread quickly in South America. Malawi was the first

African country to initiate replacement of SP with chloroquine in 1993, and other African countries began using SP in the late 1990s. The median SP drug failure rate of 52.8% in eastern Africa is higher than the 18.7% drug failure rate noted in western African countries, while the central and southern African regions show drug failure rates of 23.0% and 23.2% respectively. Molecular studies of SP resistant parasites in a variety of nations have shown resistance rapidly develops after SP use was initiated country-wide [22]. SP resistance has been shown in 30% of African regions while resistance in Asia and the Americas is as high as 80%. In addition, this combination is associated with risk of Stevens-Johnson syndrome, a form of toxic epidermal necrolysis, which has also limited its use.

Mefloquine

Mefloquine resistance was initially observed in areas near the border of Thailand and Cambodia in the late 1980s only a few years after this drug was introduced. Mefloquine resistance may have been initiated by existing use of chloroquine and quinine in these areas. As a single agent, mefloquine is not effective today in regions of Cambodia near the Thai and Myanmar borders despite, or perhaps because of, widespread use of mefloquine as a single agent in the early to mid-1990s where mefloquine was shown to be efficacious in >75% of cases. A number of *in vitro* tests provide a quantitative metric of *P. falciparum* drug resistance. This is usually expressed as the IC_{50}, the concentration of drug that inhibits parasite growth by 50% which is shown by quantitating parasite DNA replication by the incorporation of tritiated hypoxanthine or fluorescent dyes, or by quantitating the level of a parasite protein, typically the *P. falciparum* histidine rich protein 2 (HRP2). A number of reports have shown increases in malaria IC_{50} determinations of potency *in vitro*, and studies in West Africa noted increased IC_{50} values for mefloquine even before it was used therapeutically in this region.

Quinine

With the introduction of ACTs as first-line therapy, quinine treatment has been relegated to second-line use but it remains the drug of choice for pregnant women. Quinine also remains the drug of choice for treatment of severe malaria in many countries despite evidence of the superiority of artesunate for treatment of severe malaria in children and adults [23]. While resistance to quinine has been noted, these reports are likely an overestimate of the risk of resistance as the recommended dose of 24 mg/kg for 7 days is often exceeded and *in vitro* assessment of quinine resistance through IC_{50} determination is not well defined.

Atovaquone-Proguanil

Atovaquone administered experimentally as a single agent in Thailand resulted in treatment failures associated with rapid selection of resistant parasites, and a synergistic combination of atovaquone with proguanil was developed to avoid treatment failures and drug resistance. This combination is expensive, and the use of atovaquone-proguanil is limited to travelers from high-income countries. Atovaquone-proguanil efficacy remains high in most areas of the world, although treatment failures in Cambodia have recently been reported. Parasites recovered from treatment failures of atovaquone have been analyzed at the genetic level to determine the molecular mechanism of resistance, and this mechanism and its marker are associated with a single point mutation in the cytochrome b gene. Treatment failures have also been associated with the variable absorption of atovaquone, which is heavily dependent on fat intake concomitant with drug administration [2, 23].

In summary, antimalarial drug resistance has not only caused increases in morbidity and mortality, but also has led to increases in costs for malaria control. Patients who have failed therapy must be treated as inpatients and repeat infections lead to lost work productivity and school absence. Treatment failures have also been associated with diagnoses of anemia in children. In Central Africa, hospital admission rates were shown to increase due to chloroquine resistance and increases in mortality were noted in Senegal. *P. falciparum* drug resistance has also lead to changes in the proportion of *falciparum* malaria to other malarias; previously in India, *falciparum* malaria added up to 23% of cases while today *falciparum* malaria is noted in 50% of all malaria cases [2].

Malaria drug resistance occurs due to mutations in genes coding for the actual drug target or in genes such as transporters associated with access to the drug target. Drug resistance parasites are selected if drug concentrations are high enough to inhibit sensitive parasites but insufficient to inhibit the growth of resistant parasites. Drug selection is increased by exposure of parasites to sub-therapeutic doses of drugs and may be influenced by factors that include: 1) long drug half-life; 2) mutations arising from single mutations; 3) poor patient compliance; 4) immune response and 5) how widely a drug is prescribed in a particular region. In general, it is likely that parasite, vector, and human variables play relevant roles [24].

Antimalarial drug resistance leads to a burden on public health due to extended illness particularly associated with recrudescence of disease and progression of disease from uncomplicated to severe malaria. Low levels of resistance have been shown to result in anemia, increases in gametocyte transmission, extended illness, and a higher probability of treatment failure for recurrent infections. In low transmission areas, the impact of drug resistance is particularly acute due to the lack of infrastructure and resources for diagnosis and treatment. The influences of drug resistance on public health include [24, 25]:

1. Prolonged or recurrent illness,
2. Increased number of outpatient cases,
3. Increased progression to severe malaria,
4. Increased cerebral neurological sequelae associated with malaria infection,
5. Prolonged or worsening anemia and chronic effects of anemia,
6. Increased hospital admissions and death,
7. Increased gametocyte carriage and increased spread of drug resistant parasites,
8. Increased demand on diagnosis, and
9. Higher cost and lower cost-effectiveness of combination treatment.

Drug resistance noted at low levels in areas of low transmission does not present in a readily observable pattern. Patients resolve their initial infections, symptoms vanish, and patients may feel better for weeks. Recurrence of disease weeks later is often associated with anemia and an enhanced probability of gametocyte carriage resulting in further spread of drug resistant malaria. This recurrence, however, may be interpreted by the patient and by providers as a new infection rather than a recrudescence of infection, absent any testing for parasite drug resistance, which is not common in clinical settings. As drug resistant parasites become more common in a geographic area, the time between the primary infection and a recrudescent infection will shorten, and eventually, symptoms of disease will not disappear after therapy. At this point, the incidence of malaria may rise in a low transmission setting, and rates of mortality will increase.

In addition to vector control, other measures will be needed to eradicate malaria including drug resistance surveillance and implementation of malaria drug policies based on valid epidemiology data, implementation of simple malaria rapid diagnostic tests, new malaria drugs and drug combinations coupled with operational research on all aspects of malaria treatment.

1.2. EARLY EVIDENCE OF RESISTANCE OF *P. FALCIPARUM* TO ARTEMISININ

The history of antimalarial drug resistance has demonstrated a number of newly introduced antimalarial drugs such as sulfadoxine-pyrimethamine, and atovaquone, show induced resistance soon after coming on market. While other drugs have retained effectiveness longer (Table **1**), *e.g.*, sulfadoxine-pyrimethamine, less than 1 year; mefloquine, approximately 5 years (1977-1982); chloroquine, approximately 12 years (1945-1957); artemisinins, approximately 35 years (1971-2006), and quinine, approximately 278 years (1632-1910) [19]. With experimental studies showing that genetically stable reduced artemisinin sensitivity can be induced and transmitted by mosquitoes in a rodent model, and that a single amino acid substitution in *P. falciparum* confers reduced artemisinin sensitivity [26], the relevant question appears to be when and whether, artemisinin will become less effective. The greatest incidence of artemisinin resistance has been found in areas where artemisinin sale and use are poorly controlled, and this finding is similar to what can be expected for other antimalarials [27].

Previous indicators of malaria drug resistance to artemisinin in the Greater Mekong sub-region and the border regions between Cambodia- and Thailand and Cambodia and Myanmar are critically important as drug resistance against virtually all other antimalarials has been documented in this region and there are few effective therapies left. The WHO published a recent report entitled "Susceptibility of *P. falciparum* to Antimalarial Drugs", and in this document the WHO has reinforced the absolute necessity of conducting *in vitro* drug resistance surveillance in the Greater Mekong sub region and the border regions of Cambodia [2].

In Vitro Studies

In 2005, when this WHO report was released [28], a number of publications were released showing data from *in vitro* monitoring over time in China and Vietnam that revealed increased IC_{50}, IC_{90} or IC_{99} values for artemisinins [29, 30]. In a further publication, *in vitro* drug resistance data was released comparing samples from Bangladesh, western Cambodia, and Western and Eastern Thailand where increases in artemisinin IC_{50} values were observed [31]. In a different publication on a study in Cambodia, the highest IC_{50} value to date was reported from western Cambodia [32].

In Vivo Studies

Recently, artemisinin resistance in *P. falciparum* parasites has been associated with polymorphisms in the kelch propeller domain of a *falciparum* protein (PF3D7_1343700 kelch propeller domain), and this gene appears to be a useful molecular marker for tracking the emergence and spread of artemisinin resistant *P. falciparum* [6]. This is more complicated in the modern era due to the effects of readily available travel options for infected patients that may take them from one region endemic for artemisinin resistant malaria to another that is not. The 2005 WHO report demonstrated that artemisinin clinical studies showed a decline in artemisinin efficacy *in vivo* where artemisinin was used in 5- or 7-day monotherapy regimens. There are a number of reports in the literature on artemisinin "resistance", but these case reports are suspect due to poor documentation. These reports included treatment failures associated with short term therapy, and unexpected early deaths from cerebral malaria. The lack of PCR data to demonstrate these infections were caused by a new infection rather than the recrudescence of an existing infection makes these reports suspect along with their lack of drug quality control data. Given the fact that widespread distribution of drugs that are adulterated or not per the label is quite common in malarious regions, unfortunately, and an assessment of drug quality is essential to confirm a treatment failure due to resistance [2, 8, 22]. The majority of the treatment failures discussed in these reports came late in the course of drug treatment; however, two case reports have been published on patients who failed therapy with 7-day artemisinin monotherapy in Thailand [33].

Clinical Trials on the Cambodia-Thailand Border

One of the best studies showing artemisinin resistance in man was conducted by the Armed Forces Research Institute of Medical Sciences in a study assessing the efficacy of artemisinin monotherapy on the Cambodia-Thailand border region [25, 34]. The nature and extent of artemisinin resistance in *P. falciparum* parasites is not well understood, and studies are ongoing to define the geographic distribution [35, 36].

The Armed Forces Research Institute of Medical Sciences (AFRIMS) study involved treatment of patients in Tasanh in Battambang Province to the south of Pailin. The patients were admitted to the hospital for 28 days. They were treated with either oral artesunate monotherapy at a dose of 4 mg/kg body weight per day for 7 days or they were treated with quinine at a dose of 30 mg/kg body weight per day plus tetracycline at a dose of 25 mg/kg body weight per day. In those patients, quinine/tetracycline dosing was split and patients were treated every 8 hours for 7 days. Four treatment failures were noted in the 60 patients treated with artesunate. Subsequent drug levels taken from these patients showed two of the four patients had adequate drug plasma levels, and this determination lead to their classification as being infected with artemisinin-resistant *P. falciparum* malaria. One of these patients presented with a parasite clearance time of 133 hours while the other presented with a parasite clearance time of 95 hours, which is substantially longer than the normal parasite clearance time of 52 hours [36].

The IC_{50} values obtained for dihydroartemisinin against parasites obtained from these patients were 4 times the geometric mean for patients who were cured and 10 times the IC_{50} for DHA noted against the reference Southeast Asian parasite W2. Convincing proof supporting this hypothesis of the emergence of artemisinin resistant parasites was shown through additional findings of delayed parasite clearance times in Pailin in western Cambodia, which were substantially longer than those noted in Wang Pha in northwestern Thailand after monotherapy with artesunate or treatment with the combination of artesunate and mefloquine [5].

The median parasite clearance times observed in Wang Pha and Pailin were extended from 48 to 72 hours in cases where patients were administered artesunate monotherapy at a dose of 2 mg/kg body weight and from 72 to 84 hours in patients treated with artesunate at 4 mg/kg body weight combined with mefloquine. There were obvious pharmacokinetic or age related explanations for the prolongation of parasite clearance times observed in these two patient groups. The cure rates for patients in this study, however, exceeded 90%, so while the parasite clearance times observed were longer than the norm, artesunate still remained efficacious for treatment. Some of the known causal reasons that have been put forth to explain the rise of artesunate resistance in this region include 30 years of artemisinin monotherapy in western Cambodia (a practice that is now officially not permitted). Use of drugs of poor quality or administered incorrectly, and the likely existence of unknown parasite factors favor rapid induction of drug resistance. Given this same geographic region gave rise to chloroquine resistance and mefloquine resistance, it is reasonable to conclude that Cambodian parasites have an inherent propensity for resistance to any antimalarial drug administered [37-39].

Resistance to Partner Drugs in ACTs

Another potential factor in development of artemisinin resistance is resistance to the partner drugs in ACTs, which effectively results in artemisinin monotherapy in cases of complete resistance to the partner drug. A meta-analysis of clinical trials that examined the efficacy of artesunate combined with a partner drug compared to the efficacy of the partner drug alone showed, overall, that adding artesunate makes standard regimens more effective [40]. Failure rates in the ACT groups, however, were shown to remain unacceptably high with less-effective partner drugs. For example, sulfadoxine-pyrimethamine plus artesunate was shown to be more efficacious than sulfadoxine-pyrimethamine alone in East Africa where sulfadoxine-pyrimethamine resistance is common, but the ACT groups still experienced high 28-day failure rates (approximately 30%-45%) [40].

1.3. DEFINING ARTEMISININ RESISTANCE: A WORK IN PROGRESS

The Bill and Melinda Gates Foundation funded WHO's Global Malaria program to conduct a series of studies entitled "Artemisinin resistance: pilot studies to confirm, characterize, and plan for containment (ARC3)" in 2007. The project studies included four clinical studies, which encompassed *in vitro* drug resistance surveillance, molecular studies to examine the genetic basis for potential artemisinin resistance, and a drug quality control study. The ARC3 project objectives included:

1) Confirming clinically significant artemisinin resistance,

2) If clinical resistance was shown, the ARC3 project called for the *in vitro* definition of the resistance phenotype coupled with identification of a genetic marker of artemisinin resistance,

3) In addition, ARC3 project objectives included examining how prevalent counterfeit drugs were in regions of the Cambodia-Thai border, and

4) Lastly, the WHO was tasked with coming up with a strategy to limit the spread of artemisinin resistance in the Greater Mekong sub-region.

The investigators conducting ARC3 studies suggested that early indicators of artemisinin resistance be shown initially in clinical trials of the efficacy of artemisinin combination therapy and artemisinin monotherapy. The studies of oral artesunate monotherapy were conducted to examine treatment failures by day 28 or by day 42, the fraction of patients showing parasitemia on day 3, the parasite reduction ratio at 48 hours, the drug levels of artesunate noted at discrete time intervals and examination of the slope shown for the parasite clearance curve. The investigators in the ARC3 study set thresholds of 10% parasitemia by day 3 to demonstrate artemisinin resistance while parasitemia positive patients showing values between 3% and 10% were considered to be in a zone where artemisinin resistance was deemed possible [2, 8].

Artemisinin resistance was difficult to confirm during routine testing given the absence of definitive markers at that time as most clinical studies conducted during this period and since are designed to test the efficacy of an artemisinin combination therapy not artemisinin monotherapy. Artemisinin monotherapy is the only reliable method *in vivo* to determine artemisinin resistance, and such studies must be accompanied by drug level determinations to assess patient compliance with dosing. New studies suggest a potential artemisinin genetic marker, the PF3D7_1343700 kelch propeller domain, and if this marker is shown over time to be definitively predictive of artemisinin resistance, conducting surveillance of artemisinin resistance will become much easier [6]. Given that a precise definition of artemisinin resistance is ongoing, claims of observed artemisinin resistance must be judged carefully and considered with caution; such studies must show clear review of all possible variables associated with efficacy failures including patient compliance [7].

The WHO working definition of artemisinin resistance involves determination of resistance based on patient outcomes and associated parasite clearance times observed in clinical studies. It is not yet clear if the delayed clearance of parasites in patients treated with artemisinins has a further consequence in terms of gametocyte carriage rates or enhanced propensity of such patients to spread their resistant parasites to biting mosquitoes. One study from the border region between Thailand and Myanmar showed that patients treated with the combination of artesunate and mefloquine presented with delays in parasite clearance, which were, in turn, associated with an elevated risk of gametocytemia [41].

Increases in gametocytemia that can be attributed to artemisinins would suggest that quantitation of gametocytes after treatment may be a useful tool to assess artemisinin resistance, and such data can be obtained through thick smears acquired on Day 7 and Day 14 after treatment begins. The rationale for assessment on Day 7 is to detect sequestered gametocytes that are immature, and the reason for collection on Day 14 after treatment begins is to detect early ring forms which require 14 days to develop into mature gametocytes.

In vitro assays to distinguish between parasites that clear quickly *versus* those clearing more slowly is ongoing [5, 8, 35]. Given a particular artemisinin dose and duration of therapy, a small number of parasites survive artemisinin treatment and multiply to detectable levels. Those parasites likely have an intrinsically higher proportion of slow clearing parasites that arise from dormancy after artemisinin treatment compared to other parasite lines that are cleared more quickly. Hopefully, research into artemisinin resistance biomarkers will provide a reliable marker of drug resistance that can be used in artemisinin combination therapy studies to avoid the need to conduct artemisinin monotherapy studies to study artemisinin resistance [42]. Identification of a reliable artemisinin resistance marker may also inform the molecular basis for artemisinin resistance, which could guide follow-on development of new artemisinin analogues that are not prone to artemisinin resistance [6]. Other studies have focused on the expression of parasite genes after high dose artesunate exposure, which has suggested increased expression of a protein called P-Art that has been used *in vitro* to define artemisinin drug resistance [43, 44].

In vitro data has suggested a number of possible genes involved in artemisinin resistance; however, the true relevance of these genetic markers will involve correlation of gene expression with delays in parasite clearance. This data has not been forthcoming in studies of candidate gene correlation to parasite clearance rates in Western Cambodia with the exception of the recent study showing the association of the K-13 propeller polymorphisms with delays in parasite clearance [6, 45]. Genome wide association studies may help identify reliable genetic markers of artemisinin drug resistance in patients with malaria who demonstrate slow parasite clearance. One study of highly similar parasite clones observed in a number of patients in western Cambodia showed the clones possessed similar fast or slow clearance rates, which would support the hypothesis of a genetic basis for artemisinin resistance [7, 45].

Molecular studies of artemisinin drug resistance have identified a number of candidate genes to include changes in the copy number of the drug transporter *pfmdr1*; however, a clear association of a gene with parasite clearance rates in drug treated patients is needed. Recently, a Nature publication reported mutation associations in the PF3D7_1343700 kelch propeller domain with artemisinin resistance [6]. Mutations in the K13-propeller alleles from parasites in Cambodia were shown to cluster in areas of Cambodia where resistance to artemisinin is common. The authors noted strong correlations between the mutant K13 alleles, the survival of parasites *in vitro* after drug exposure, and elongated clearance rates *in vivo*. Additional studies will be needed on a broader scale to see if the K13 propeller mutations identified in this publication are associated consistently with artemisinin resistance, and clearly, a molecular basis for artemisinin resistance that provides a cause and effect relationship with the K13 propeller mutant will be needed assuming one exists [6, 46, 47]. Recent studies on the mechanism of artemisinin resistance have suggested that *P. falciparum* parasites may enter a dormant state after exposure to artemisinin drugs. Such a state of dormancy would reduce the hemoglobin degradation rate in early ring parasites which in turn would reduce the quantity of hemoglobin degradation products present for artemisinin to affect leading to enhanced survival over a limited period of time [48].

The phenomenon of parasite dormancy is not related to the delays in parasite clearance observed after ACT or artesunate monotherapy; however, it is believed this phenomenon could readily explain the elevated rate of recrudescence noted after patient treatment with artemisinins [49]. Modeling of treatment responses by parasites in patients infected in Cambodia and Thailand suggests that extended parasite clearance times may also reflect drug resistance in ring stage parasites [50].

1.4. A STRATEGY TO CONTAIN THE SPREAD OF ARTEMISININ RESISTANT MALARIA PARASITES

A strategy has been developed by a panel of experts who met in 2008 to devise a means of containing artemisinin resistance and set research goals to achieve this objective. Their strategy included case management changes to enhance diagnosis, insure rapid and effective treatment, and measures to control insect vectors. The focus of the containment strategy of artemisinin resistance included targeting efforts to both fixed and mobile populations. This strategy also includes measures to counteract distribution of counterfeit drugs and a public education program to promote proper use of antimalarial drugs. Operational research elements were also incorporated to quantify the spread of artemisinin resistance and to elucidate causal factors [2].

1.4.1. Artemisinin Resistance Containment Project on the Cambodia-Thailand Border

One of the elements of this containment strategy is vector control, and one of the most effective tools for malaria vector control has been the insecticide treated bed net. In excess of 500,000 insecticide treated bednets have been given to the populace in these afflicted regions, and 200,000 existing bed nets have been re-treated with insecticide to prolong their use. In order to improve case management, village health workers were trained to provide better diagnosis and treatment, and these health workers were also provided the reagents and equipment necessary for free screening tests to be conducted. Patients who present with positive malaria diagnostic test results in turn also receive free treatment and follow-up care.

An additional element of enhanced case management includes follow-up care. In Thailand, patients are followed for up to 28 days post treatment and in Cambodia, patients are assessed during the first 3 days of treatment. Patients who are parasitemia positive after the third day of treatment are followed to day 28 as well. By providing free diagnosis services and free antimalarial drugs, patients are assured of receiving valid malaria diagnostic test kits and valid drugs at no cost. Over time, these measures will decrease the sale of counterfeit drugs, which are a clear danger not only to patient health but also to the health of the public as a whole.

The objectives of this artemisinin resistance containment strategy includes killing artemisinin resistant parasites by successfully treating all infected patients in the areas of greatest concern to prevent spread of artemisinin resistant gametocytes. By insuring the regional governments ban artemisinin monotherapy, the pressures of drug resistance, which selects for resistant parasites, are diminished. Additional objectives include vector control, personal protective measures, public education on proper malaria diagnosis and treatment, and a full program of operational research on best practices. The educational campaign planned includes posters, brochures, street theater, village meetings, and radio and television advertisements. A special educational campaign was launched to target migrant workers in the border regions of Cambodia and Thailand. Migrants come to the Cambodia-Thailand border area to work on agricultural, forest, and construction projects, working in gem mines, and as soldiers sent to patrol the border. In order to insure comprehension on both sides of the border, the educational program written materials will be written in both Thai and Khmer with similar presentation in both languages. To insure diagnosis and treatment of migrant workers, health clinics will be established in construction camps and in quarters assigned to military families, and mobile malaria health clinics will be established at border crossings

One of the most significant factors in the development of artemisinin resistance is the private sector sale of counterfeit or substandard drugs. The Government of Cambodia banned the sale of oral artesunate monotherapy drugs, and police routinely enforce this ban by inspections of pharmacies and markets where these products have been sold. The 20 villages in Cambodia that are the most at risk from artemisinin resistance due to treatment failures have been targeted for intensive investigation into the prevalence and spread of artemisinin resistance.

Malaria screening, treatment, and follow-up provide important epidemiological information to understand the spread of artemisinin resistant parasites. All of the outcome data on these interventions will inform plans for future activities. One likely outcome is to extend this program to the areas outside the Thailand-Cambodia border and to other areas in the Greater Mekong sub-region. As no other effective therapy is at hand, these containment strategies are essential to preserve the use of artemisinin combination therapy for first-line treatment. Some of the challenges of defining artemisinin resistance (which hopefully will be surmounted by identifying a reliable genetic marker, such as the K13 propeller mutation) are not reasons to delay initiating containment strategies in areas where artemisinin resistance and treatment failures are well documented [6].

1.4.2. WHO Recommendations to Contain or Eliminate Artemisinin Resistance

With the well-documented spread of artemisinin resistance in the Greater Mekong sub-region, WHO created a set of recommendations to limit the spread of artemisinin resistance. These recommendations were based on the containment strategy previously discussed in the last section. These recommendations are targeted for implementation in any area where artemisinin resistance to *P. falciparum* has been documented [8].

The first recommendation revolves around stopping the spread of artemisinin resistant parasites. In areas with artemisinin resistance, malaria control and eradication measures are essential. In areas where no artemisinin resistance has been documented, malaria control can reduce the rate of malaria transmission that in turn reduces the probability of spreading artemisinin resistant parasites. The second recommendation revolves around vector control, which must be a top priority. The third recommendation is directed toward national malaria control programs which must include both targeted malaria screening of patients to detect active cases, and may entail mass drug administration consistent with the best evidence under the WHO guidelines. WHO has recommended endemic nations routinely monitor the efficacy of antimalarial drugs at sentinel sites every 2 years to inform decisions on which drug regimens remain efficacious [2]. The most important recommendation revolves around access to effective, inexpensive diagnostics and drugs which will improve patient survival and diminishes the possibility for drug resistant parasites to spread particularly those that are resistant to the artemisinin component and the partner drug [23].

WHO also recommends research in five related areas to support containment of artemisinin resistance. These disciplines include laboratory research to identify a molecular marker of artemisinin resistance, research and development into non-artemisinin based drug combination therapy. Field researches undertake pilot studies of tools for transmission reduction particularly mass patient screening and drug administration, operational research into intervention programs for mobile populations, and mathematic modeling to predict the impact of artemisinin resistance on the burden of malaria on the populace. The WHO's GPARC containment plan will be successfully implemented if the various stakeholders at local, regional, national, and global levels are invested in actually completing the list of activities recommended. Given the dollars required to conduct this list of activities, leadership from the malaria community and from political leaders will be needed.

1.4.3. Improved and Increased Monitoring and Surveillance of Drug Efficacy

WHO has recommended monitoring of the efficacy of antimalarial drugs on a routine basis to inform treatment policies [23]. As oral artesunate monotherapy is no longer a recommended treatment for uncomplicated malaria, this monitoring should be targeted toward evaluating ACT efficacy. In the absence of molecular marker(s) of artemisinin resistance that are uniformly predictive and correlate well with phenotypic resistance (which hopefully has been alleviated if the recent association of mutations in the K-13 propeller gene with artemisinin resistance pans out) [6], monitoring efforts must be focused on prolongations in parasite clearance in treated patients. As many countries utilizing ACTs for treatment of uncomplicated malaria do not conduct routine efficacy studies on a 24-month basis as recommended by WHO, a complete understand of the geographic spread of artemisinin resistance is not possible. Routine efficacy monitoring is therefore essential to informing a decision to implement comprehensive containment strategies and artemisinin resistant parasites may survive, thrive, and spread [51].

The data gained in Thailand and Cambodia on artemisinin containment has suggested that if more than 10% of treated patients have parasites detected on the third day of treatment, artemisinin resistance confirmation studies should be initiated which include efficacy testing using artesunate monotherapy for 7 days. Where patients present with parasites in <10% but greater than 3% of cases after ACT treatment, it may be appropriate to start containment activities. There are 106 malaria endemic countries, and 92 of the 106 are endemic for *falciparum* malaria. 75 of these countries have a high enough malaria burden to warrant ACT efficacy monitoring on a routine basis. As of August 2010, 44 of the 75 countries with endemic *falciparum* malaria had not undertaken efficacy testing as the WHO has recommended due to a variety of reasons to include lack of funding, political, and social unrest, natural disasters, or unfortunately due to complacency [2]. Consequently, we do not fully understand where artemisinin resistance exists [52].

Efficacy monitoring studies have logistical challenges in some settings, and may not be doable in others due to low rates of malaria transmission, which translates into low numbers of infected patients, and may not necessarily inform an artemisinin resistance finding given host factors such as immunity or pas drug intake that can be study confounders. Another issue for efficacy monitoring studies is prompt publication of results; data that is not published is not actionable.

1) Clinical Trials for Monitoring Drug Efficacy

Efficacy trials provide fundamental data on the effects of the drug on the malaria parasite and clinical utility of a drug. Comparison of aggregate data such as a meta-analysis study is sufficient to estimate the efficacy of an antimalarial drug where studies have been done in different locations at different times. To avoid these problems a number of strategies are suggested to compare clinical trials more effectively: 1) The Worldwide Antimalarial Resistance Networks (WWARN) is focused on using individual resistance data of patient drug to provide direct comparisons among studies to create a full assessment of antimalarial drug resistance; 2) The primary outcome of such trials will also be the first reappearance of parasites, unless an early treatment failure has occurred; 3) Another innovation is the use of parasite survival analysis that assesses the time between patient treatment and the reappearance of parasites; 4) The WWARN proposes to reach an agreement on how to distinguish between the first malaria infection and a recrudescent infection, which will make data comparisons between studies much more meaningful [53]. An in-depth discussion on how to use the WWARN database can be found in Price *et al.* [54]. The WWARN database is a work in progress than can be accessed at www.malariadrugresistance.net/warn/clinical. The malaria community members are encouraged to comment on the WWARN effort and utilize the existing data in the database.

2) In Vitro Surveillance of Drug Sensitivity of Clinical Isolates

The WWARN has proposed to create a database of comparable *in vitro* drug resistance data from current patient isolates to assess the efficacy of ACT drugs in use. The WWARN effort is focused on harmonizing differences between testing centers by agreeing on four simple parameters associated with *in vitro* malaria culture and testing: the culture conditions used, the duration of drug-parasite incubation, the starting parasite density, and the hematocrit of red blood cells used for testing. By standardizing these parameters, the WWARN group believes the data produced will be far more comparable and useful taken together rather than only being useful in the particular. Quality control is a key feature to their proposed harmonization plan along with the use of standard reference strains.

Culture adaptation of currently circulating parasites will be essential along with proper cryopreservation of resistant strains so that any interesting results noted can be confirmed in other laboratories. In addition, common sources of antimalarial drugs and their metabolites will be required to insure consistency in testing. By using these common features, an *in vitro* testing network can be created which provides data that is comparable between geographically distinct areas and across time. *In vitro* testing provides data on the antimalarial potency of both the artemisinin component and the partner drug in an ACT as each element is tested individually. This is an advantage over *in vivo* testing of ACTs, where efficacy failures could be attributed to either the artemisinin component or the partner drug. Early identification of drug resistance to either drug will provide prompt notice of the rise of drug resistance in a particular region that merits changes in malaria drug policy or initiation of a resistance containment strategy. The details of the *in vitro* component of the WWARN database have been published by Bacon *et al.* [55].

3) Pharmacological Surveillance

Pharmacokinetic drug surveillance is an essential element of a drug efficacy study. Patient treatment failures may involve the influence of drug resistance to either the artemisinin drug or the partner drug or they may simply be the result of problems with patient compliance, a common occurrence, or a number of other problems leading to inadequate drug levels in the blood. Treatment failures can arise due to the use of counterfeit drug products of poor quality, inadequate dosing, poor patient compliance, poor drug absorption, or accelerated drug clearance [56]. The vast array of new antimalarial drug combinations and the speed of their introduction frequently results in a lack of available information on the proper drug dose required for treatment. This lack of information is most commonly noted in populations at high-risk to include infants, poorly nourished patients, pregnant women, and HIV-infected patients. These high-risk groups are the most likely to present significant differences in the four most important pharmacological drug disposition processes, absorption, distribution, metabolism, and excretion. PK/PD studies in these groups are urgently required.

In addition, drug levels in individual patients must be assessed when patients are participating in drug efficacy studies, which will provide essential information on pharmacokinetic properties of each drug, which may affect the therapeutic response. A blood sample taken on day 7 may provide enough information in and of itself to inform an assessment of drug exposure for the artemisinin partner drugs in an ACT assuming the proper foundation studies were in place. Quantitation of malaria drug levels can be challenging work; however, there are laboratories in endemic areas that can provide accurate blood levels to support such studies. In order to standardize the quantitation of drug levels, the WWARN has instituted a quality control program to provide assistance with testing protocols, reference drugs, SOPs, and a quality improvement proficiency testing program to assist regional laboratories in achieving the most scientifically accurate drug quantitation data possible. Without a system of harmonized methods and rigorous quality control, the drug level data derived from individual laboratories will be no more comparable than the *in vitro* drug potency data we have previously discussed. The details of this pharmacokinetic component of the WWARN database can be found in a publication by Barnes *et al.* [57].

4) Identification and Monitoring Genetic Correlates of Drug Resistance

Molecular markers of drug resistance have been defined for some of the older antimalarial drugs used in ACTs and identifying and validating these markers will be necessary to provide tools for field studies of ACT drug resistance. Previously identified markers include both single nucleotide polymorphisms such as those found in the *pfcrt* gene, which mediates chloroquine resistance, and copy number changes such as the increase in copy numbers of *pfmdr1*, the transporter associated with mefloquine resistance. The recent studies identifying mutations in the K-13 propeller region associated with artemisinin resistance [6] will be another useful tool assuming initial reports of this gene association are reproduced [58]. The identification of the K-13 propeller mutations was conducted using genome wide association of drug resistant isolate that is the best method possible for identifying loci associated with drug resistance. This method has proven itself for identifying loci associated with resistance to older antimalarial drugs and will likely prove useful in the future for identifying genomic markers of resistance to new malaria drugs. There are a number of centers involved in comparative genomic analyses, and these groups are sharing data on both reference and field strains of *P. falciparum* [59]. A comparative genomics approach will establish the baseline genomic data on parasite diversity necessary to provide comparisons on the genomes of potentially resistant strains and sensitive strains. The molecular component of the WWARN database is detailed in a publication by Plowe *et al.* [60].

Malaria control efforts worldwide are challenged by the rising tide of drug resistance, which has made previously used antimalarials such as chloroquine and sulfadoxine-pyrimethamine ineffective. The rise of drug resistance to older drugs is no doubt related to their overuse and misuse over time. With the introduction of ACT drugs, which are the mainstay of malaria treatment today, these lessons of drug failure from the past should guide our practice in the present and in the future. Careful monitoring of drug resistance with all available phenotypic *in vitro* assays and genomic assays will be essential tools for keeping both the artemisinin component drug and the partner drug effective in the future. There are three tools developed recently that are available for monitoring antimalarial drug efficacy and detecting early signs of drug resistance for standardized and coordinated use [52].

Improving drug resistance surveillance requires first monitoring therapeutic efficacy *in vivo* where repeated assessments are conducted of both the parasitology outcome and the clinical outcomes after malaria drug treatment during a fixed follow-up period to detect any signs of clinical recrudescence shown by resumption of malaria symptoms and appearance of blood parasitemia. Other available methods of monitoring resistance include *in vitro* drug resistance assays of parasites in culture and molecular marker studies of gene mutations or increases in copy number associated with parasite drug resistance [17, 35]. Containment strategies focused on limiting the spread of malaria drug resistance must be carefully coordinated with an organizational structure established to insure a timely response of vector control, public education, and mobilization of the malaria community for assistance. Any current use of artemisinin monotherapy should be strongly discouraged, and co-blistered ACT drugs should be replaced with co-formulated drugs to enhance patient compliance. Dosing patients with co-blistered drugs increases problems with compliance, which increases the probability of underdosing either drug leading to drug resistance.

1.5. PREVENTING OR DECREASING THE RATE OF SPREAD OF DRUG RESISTANCE THROUGH THE USE OF ANTIMALARIAL COMBINATION THERAPIES

1.5.1. Consequences of Artemisinin Resistance

The spread of artemisinin resistance has raised new challenges to patient care, as resolution of disease will likely take longer period. Prolonged parasite clearance may affect treatment outcomes for severe and complicated malaria, which is currently treated with injected artesunate. In the ARC3 oral artesunate monotherapy study, some of the patients who had fever and blood parasitemia on day 3 were noted to have resolved their symptoms and their parasites without any rescue treatment [5]. Accordingly, providers should be cognizant of the fact that early treatment "failures" may be noted in patients treated with oral artesunate monotherapy in artemisinin resistant areas that may lead to an overestimation of the true rate of treatment failure. Oral artemisinin monotherapy and ACT treatment has been associated with increases in parasite clearance time which are also known to be associated with increases in gametocyte carriage [41].

The implications for transmission of gametocytes are not yet clearly understood in areas of artemisinin resistance. Data on transmission of artemisinin resistant parasites and data on how infective the resulting sporozoites may be are not yet available. The loss of artemisinin efficacy raises concerns as this phenomenon may lead to failure of the artemisinin component to fulfill its role in reduction of the parasite biomass and its role in protecting the partner drug. Longer parasite clearance times could lead to increases in parasite biomass for an extended period leading to higher probabilities of *de novo* drug resistance mutations occurring against the partner drug. Once such a *de novo* mutation arises, parasites would be favored to survive under partner drug pressure. With known concomitant increases in resistance to existing partner drugs such as mefloquine, lumefantrine, and amodiaquine in many parts of the world, ACT treatment failures caused by parasites with resistance to both drugs will rise. This raises the need for continued research into long lived, efficacious malaria partner drugs to replace existing partner drugs facing drug resistance pressure. Given the long timeline for malaria drug development and the high risk of drug development failure, development research of partner drug is of paramount importance [23].

Currently, the WHO has recommended parenteral treatment with intravenous artesunate for severe, complicated malaria. In the future, this practice may not be appropriate. Clinical trials should be conducted in areas of artemisinin resistance to examine the questions regarding efficacy of intravenous artesunate and the fatality rates observed in patients with severe malaria who are treated with intravenous artesunate. Routinely, patients with severe malaria treated with injected artesunate are administered oral treatment as soon as they can tolerate it, which translates into an inability to assess systematically the efficacy of a 7-day artemisinin treatment regimen or the consequence of parasitemia appearing on the third day after initiation of treatment. In these circumstances, the parasite reduction ratio observed in the first 48 hours is a useful piece of information and should be recorded for future reference and comparison to other treatment outcomes noted in patients with severe malaria treated with injected artesunate [2, 8, 23].

1.5.2. Prevention or Delay of Resistance by Antimalarial Combination Therapy

Prevention of resistance to malaria drug treatment involves complete drug coverage and, as seen with tuberculosis treatment, involves the use of drug combinations instead of drug monotherapy. Resistance to older malaria drugs triggered changes in antimalarial treatment through experiences gained with treatment of tuberculosis and HIV/AIDS where successful patient outcomes required combination drug treatment where each drug acts on separate targets. It is common in tropical areas of the world to encounter drugs of poor quality widely available through the private sector, and it is common to run into problems with patient compliance. Artemisinin resistance will most likely arise in patients with elevated parasitemia who receives substandard or inadequate artemisinin monotherapy treatment rather than treatment with a high quality ACT regimen. Insuring patients receive a complete dose of artemisinin combination drugs is essential to limiting the spread of artemisinin drug resistance.

By 2003, various expert committees such as the WHO, the Roll Back Malaria Partnership, and the Global Fund to Fight Aids, TB and Malaria had all recommended malaria treatment with artemisinin combination therapy which has now become first-line therapy in all endemic areas. The artemisinin component of this combination is derived from Chinese herbal treatment for fever going back thousands of years. Artemisinin analogues are highly potent, rapid acting drugs capable of killing immature, ring-stage parasites to insure rapid reduction of the parasite biomass [1]. The rationale for artemisinin combination therapy or combination therapy in general is twofold. 1) The combination of drugs is frequently more effective than monotherapy with one drug. 2) Given the low probability that a parasite develops a *de novo* mutation to one of the combination drugs during the infection, the now drug resistant parasite can still be killed by a partner antimalarial drug. Accordingly, drug combinations provide mutual protection that is believed to delay or prevent emergence of drug resistance. In order to obtain these two advantages of a combination therapy, the partner drugs in a combination must be independently efficacious when used to treat malaria [23].

Drug combinations can accelerate response to therapy, increase cure rates and insure component drugs are protected against resistance. The theory underlying the combination of two drugs for therapy relies on the fact that treatment with two drugs with different mechanisms of action and therefore different mechanisms of resistance have a probability of developing resistance to both drugs based on the product of their individual per parasite drug resistance probabilities. If the probability of a *de novo* mutation to drugs A and B is one in a million then the probability of developing resistance to both is one in one trillion [24]. Stable parasite resistance to artemisinin compounds has not been induced in the laboratory, which may support the hypothesis that such resistance is rare. In order to preserve the artemisinin compounds from development of drug resistance; they should only be used as a drug combination with another antimalarial. Artemisinin derivatives demonstrate desirable key performance parameters as combination partners given their very high rates of parasite killing, their lack of significant drug resistance outside of the Cambodia border region and they are generally well-tolerated clinically [61].

Many debates have been had regarding the best pharmacokinetic properties of a prospective antimalarial compound. From a perspective oriented toward preventing resistance, combination drug partners should ideally possess similar pharmacokinetic properties. Rapid drug clearance ensures residual drug does not act as a selective filter to insure survival of resistant parasites. Artemisinin drugs, if used as monotherapy, which is banned in Cambodia and not recommended anywhere else in the world, must be administered for 7 days, and having patients adhere to a 7-day drug treatment regimens is difficult. Even 7-day monotherapy with artemisinin drugs is associated with failure rates approximating 10%. In order for an artemisinin combination treatment to be highly effective over a 3-day period it is essential that the elimination half-life of one drug component be longer than 24 hours.

As artemisinin derivatives are eliminated rapidly from the body, drug combinations including artemisinin derivatives given for 3 days must be co-administered with a slowly eliminated partner drug. These drugs are commonly older antimalarial drugs such as mefloquine, piperaquine, or amodiaquine, which provide protection for the artemisinin component generation of *de novo* mutation as long as drug adherence is maintained. Accordingly, parasites cannot be exposed to the artemisinin component alone during one asexual cycle without having the partner drug present. One drawback to the pharmacokinetically imbalanced artemisinin combination drug is this does leave the “tail” of the partner drug, which is more slowly eliminated unprotected by the artemisinin compound. The remaining number of parasites exposed to the partner drug by itself after two asexual cycles, is a small fraction, below 0.00001%, of the total parasites present during the acute infection.

In addition, these few remaining parasites are exposed to high levels of the partner drug, and, even if drug resistance to the partner drug is present, the drug levels onboard are generally capable of killing the remaining parasites. The extended "tail" of the elimination phase of partner drug, however, provides a filter to select for resistant parasites newly acquired, and these parasites contribute to antimalarial drug resistance. Having said that, in a region on the northwestern border of Thailand, which is a low malaria transmission area where mefloquine resistance is already present, use of the artesunate-mefloquine drug combination, was shown to be very effective to deter the emergence of resistance and reduce malaria infection rates. This approach might be expected to be more capable of precluding development of *de novo* resistance at increased transmission levels, where infections with malaria parasites yields a higher biomass of parasites constituting a significant source of *de novo* resistance [24].

Given the problems associated with administration of quinine, particularly poor patient compliance because of unpleasant side effects such as tinnitus, artemisinin compounds are more commonly being used for *falciparum* therapy. Artemisinin compounds are derived from originated from artemisinin, which is naturally found in the sweet wormwood plant. Most of these artemisinin derivatives have dihydroartemisinin as their active metabolite. Artemisinin compounds are not only capable of quickly killing parasites in the blood; they are also capable of preventing generation of gametocytes. Both of these properties assist in decreasing development of antimalarial drug-resistance, and given the rapid elimination of artemisinin compounds, necessitate the use in combination with a partner drug. Some of these drugs used in combination with an artemisinin derivative include pyronaridine, piperaquine, mefloquine, amodiaquine, lumefantrine, and chlorproguanil-dapsone, and all these combinations have been tested in field trials, some of which involved treatment of thousands of patients. Artesunate is on market in Asia and Africa for both intravenous and oral administration. Intravenous artesunate has been shown to be superior to quinine for treatment of severe malaria, and the clinical field trials that proved this in Asia and Africa will be discussed later in this book.

1.5.3. The Use of ACTs to Prevent the Emergence of Artemisinin Resistance

Antimalarial drug resistance results from a change in drug accumulation, an increase in drug efflux, or diminished affinity to a drug target. Examples of changes in drug accumulation or efflux due to mutation can readily be seen in resistance to quinine, mefloquine, halofantrine, chloroquine, or amodiaquine. Examples of drugs where resistance manifests by reduced affinity of the drug to a drug target because of point mutations include cycloguanil, pyrimethamine, the sulphonamide, and atovaquone. Other known mechanisms of resistance for antibacterial drugs including transferable resistance genes, drug destroying enzymes, or activation of an accessory metabolic pathway, do not appear to play a role in antimalarial drug resistance [62].

The hypothesis that drug resistance could be prevented or delayed through drug combinations with different targets was first tested treating patients with tuberculosis, and drug combinations have been used for treatment of HIV infection and cancer. The use of antimalarial drug combinations is not new, and neither is the hypothesis that using drugs with different antimalarial targets in combination will delay development of malaria drug resistance. The data shown from combination of artemisinins with partner drugs particularly mefloquine, illustrate accelerated patient recovery, increased rates of cure, decreased malaria transmission, and drug combinations appear to have aided in delaying development of drug resistance and reducing the incidence of malaria [54]. Artemisinin derivatives on market have been combined with a number of partner drugs including lumefantrine (paired with artemether - this drug combination is the most commonly used ACT globally), amodiaquine (typically combined with artesunate), mefloquine (paired with artesunate), sulfadoxine-pyrimethamine (paired with artesunate), piperaquine (paired with DHA), and pyronaridine (commonly combined with artesunate) [23]. These combinations typically provide radical cures of malaria infections after administration of 3-day treatment regimens, which aid in protecting the emergence of drug resistance to the artemisinin derivative [63, 64].

CHAPTER 2

Currently Used Antimalarial Drug Combination Therapies

Abstract: Drug combination therapy is derived from the premise that administering two or more drugs at the same time that have synergism or additive effects with independent efficacy and different targets will lead to enhanced efficacy and diminished drug resistance. As medicinal chemistry and biological knowledge of the malaria parasite advances, drug combinations for treatment of malaria have become the standard of care. A number of efforts have been made over the years to quantitate the relationship between dose and effect of each drug partner alone and the dose effect relationship of the drugs in combination and to assess whether a drug combination provides a synergistic effect. Antimalarial drug combination therapy (CT) involves the administration of two or more blood schizonticidal drugs each with a separate and different mechanism of action and each targeted to a different parasite protein or process. As described here, drug combinations for antimalarial treatment that include a non-antimalarial drug provided to enhance antimalarial efficacy of a blood schizonticidal drug do not qualify as combination therapy. Artemisinin based combination therapies (ACTs) have been adopted in Asia since 1992 and in Africa since 2000, and these drug combinations have been shown to improve vastly antimalarial treatment efficacy. ACTs are now first-line treatment for *P. falciparum* malaria globally; they are more effective than non-artemisinins combinations or monotherapies, and ACTs reduce the chances of development of parasite drug resistance. ACTs demonstrate certain key performance parameters associated all of which are related to the unique activities of the artemisinin component, and these features include:1) rapid reduction of the biomass of the parasite; 2) swift clearance of parasites; 3) prompt resolution of patient symptoms; 4) successful treatment against multidrug-resistant *P. falciparum* and 5) decrease in incidence of gametocyte carriage, which, in theory, will result in turn in reduction of transmission of drug resistant parasites bearing drug resistance alleles.

Keywords: Additive, artemisinin derivatives, combination therapy, first line, monotherapy, non-artemisinin drug combination, standard of care, synergism, therapeutic efficacy.

Antimalarial combination therapy, like other forms of combination therapy, is the simultaneous administration of two or more drugs with independent targets and separate mechanisms of action. The elements of a drug combination, antimalarial, antiviral, or anti-tubercular, have either drug synergism or additive effects that provides improved treatment efficacy and delays induction of resistance to each partner drug.

As previously described, antimalarial combination therapies are derived from administering two drugs with antimalarial activity with separate targets and

Qigui Li and Mark R. Hickman

mechanisms of action. Administration of a drug that enhances an antimalarial drug's activity does not constitute a drug combination under this definition. Accordingly, some antimalarial drugs, for example antifolate drugs, do meet the criteria of a synergistic drug combination that operationally cannot be administered separately for antimalarial therapy due to concerns about drug resistance to each drug partner if administered alone (ex. sulfadoxine-pyrimethamine). Sulfadoxine-pyrimethamine (SP) is always prescribed as a combination rather than as two individual drugs, and another example is atovaquone-proguanil, which is always prescribed as a combination rather than as individual drugs.

Approximate 90% of malaria infections in man and 90% of mortality attributed to malaria occurs in sub-Saharan Africa. Malaria control efforts in this area have been significantly impacted by the emergence of chloroquine resistance and its spread worldwide. Chloroquine resistance in sub-Saharan Africa was first noted in 1979 in East Africa; however, chloroquine resistance has now been reported in virtually all malaria endemic countries in Africa. SP was implemented as a follow-on drug to address problems of chloroquine resistance, however, resistance to SP is developing rapidly in many malaria endemic countries, and the longevity of this drug as an antimalarial even as part of an ACT is questionable [23].

Artemisinin-based combination therapies (ACTs) have revolutionized treatment of malaria in drug resistant areas in Southeast Asia leading to their implementation in Africa [35-39]. Major challenges, however, exist when deploying antimalarial drug combination therapies such as the ACTs in Africa. These challenges include:

- The proper choice of drug combination that is most suited for a given epidemiological area.
- The costs of combination therapy are higher than the cost greater than the cost of individual monotherapies.
- The timing of a decision is to introduce combination therapy in an area where malaria monotherapy is still effective.
- The operational issues impeding effective implementation particularly those associated with patient drug compliance.

2.1. ANTIMALARIAL COMBINATION THERAPY (CT) WITHOUT ARTEMISININS

Non-artemisinin based combination treatments have been used over the years with varying degrees of efficacy. These non-artemisinin based combination therapies include sulfadoxine-pyrimethamine plus chloroquine (SP-CQ), mefloquine plus sulfadoxine-pyrimethamine (SP-MQ), and sulfadoxine-pyrimethamine plus amodiaquine (SP-AQ). The rationale behind these combination therapies lies in the existing high levels of drug resistance to each of these drugs when administered as monotherapy that have also led to reductions in efficacy even when these drugs are administered as partners in combination. There is no body of proof that administration of chloroquine plus sulfadoxine-pyrimethamine has any benefit over administration of SP, and thus, this combination is not a recommended drug combination for malaria treatment. The combination of amodiaquine plus SP has been shown to be more effective than either partner drug by itself, however, this combination has been shown to be less efficacious than ACTs, and thus, the combination of amodiaquine plus SP is not recommended for malaria treatment [23].

Drug combinations of non-artemisinin based drugs such as the combination of SP, proguanil-dapsone, sulfalene-pyrimethamine, atovaquone-proguanil, or chlorproguanil-dapsone are based on synergy between each partner drug. Efficacy of the AQ-SP combination have been studied in clinical trials compared to recommended ACTs, and the efficacy of the AQ-SP combination has been shown to be highly variable. Rates of treatment failure by day 28 (after adjustment by polymerase chain reaction testing) have ranged as high as 16% in Uganda and as high as 24% in Rwanda. AQ-SP has also been shown to be less effective for reduction of gametocyte carriage than artemisinin based-combination. Studies of the efficacy of AQ-SP were conducted in Senegal in 2003, Burkina Faso in 2005, and Madagascar in 2006, and in these trials, the efficacy of AQ-SP was shown to be adequate but not exceptional. The ongoing spread of parasites with resistance to amodiaquine and SP will likely reduce the efficacy of this combination in many African countries and, accordingly, the use of these individual drugs as partners in an ACT combination will be reduced.

Chloroquine Plus Sulfadoxine-Pyrimethamine (CQ-SP)

Chloroquine (CQ) and SP are two older antimalarial drugs used commonly in Africa as first-line or second-line treatments for *falciparum* malaria. CQ is a 4-aminoquinoline while both sulfadoxine and pyrimethamine are antifolate compounds commonly administered in a fixed dose combination. These drugs are all active against blood stage schizonts of *P. falciparum*, and while resistance to each drug partner has been noted in individual parasites, these drugs are not cross resistant (resistance to CQ, for example, does not induce resistance to SP). In Africa, the spread of chloroquine-resistant *P. falciparum* parasites has increased since CQ-resistant parasites were first shown to occur in Africa in 1979. Similarly, the incidence of *P. falciparum* parasites with resistance to SP has increased since the late 1980s. The spread of SP-resistant parasites has been particularly swift and broad in East Africa where SP was used on a larger scale as a first-line antimalarial treatment. Resistance to SP has also been shown in parts of West Africa. The combination of CQ-SP has been increasingly prescribed for treatment of *falciparum* malaria for treatment of individuals, and national health authorities have implemented the CQ-SP combination in some countries such as Ethiopia where infections with both *falciparum* and *vivax* malaria are common.

CQ and SP have different biological targets in the malaria parasite, however, they do both possess similar pharmacokinetic profiles, and therefore, these drugs are suitable for inclusion as partners in a combination therapy. There are no published reports on pharmacodynamic synergism of CQ and SP, and their activities are likely additive in nature. In areas with high levels of circulating *falciparum* parasites that are highly CQ resistant and moderately SP resistant, the combination of CQ-SP is not expected to be any more efficacious than SP alone. In addition, the use of CQ-SP is not likely to diminish the induction and spread of parasites with resistance to SP. Despite issues with CQ-parasite resistance, chloroquine possesses substantial anti-inflammatory activity achieved through cytokine pathway modulation, and one could expect treatment with CQ-SP would lead to quicker resolution of patient symptoms than SP treatment alone.

The anti-inflammatory activity of chloroquine has also lead to its widespread use for treatment of autoimmune diseases such as lupus in developed nations. Studies conduct to compare safety and efficacy of the CQ-SP combination to that of SP by it have shown that CQ-SP efficacy is highly dependent on levels of parasite resistance to individual partner drugs. The CQ-SP combination was used in Vanuatu since 1994, and no reports of malaria-associated mortality have been reported since 1996, although the reduction in patient mortality rates cannot be attributed in whole to use of this combination of CQ-SP. The CQ-SP combination has also been used for treatment of malaria in Papua New Guinea since 2000 and on the Malaysian peninsular since 1997. All of the efficacy trial data has shown that CQ-SP is unlikely to be more efficacious than SP by itself in regions with *falciparum* malaria where parasites have high levels of resistance to CQ. This situation is representative for most of sub-Saharan Africa, and utilizing CQ-SP as first-line treatment will not likely provide long-term effective use [65].

Amodiaquine Plus Sulfadoxine-Pyrimethamine (AQ-SP)

Amodiaquine (AQ) is a 4-aminoquinoline analogue of chloroquine with similar structure and activity. AQ also has anti-inflammatory and antipyretic activities. Over the past ten years, efficacy studies of amodiaquine treatment of *falciparum* malaria have been conducted in Africa, and the results of those studies have shown that amodiaquine has an increased efficacy and faster clinical recovery than treatment with chloroquine. This difference in efficacy and recovery time was seen in geographic areas exhibiting drug resistance to chloroquine ranging from mild to moderate. The overall use of amodiaquine has decreased due to issues of adverse events associated with its use for a prophylactic indication that include agranulocytosis and hepatitis. AQ continues to be used in some countries, for treatment of uncomplicated malaria with few reports of adverse events.

Three published studies on efficacy and safety of the AQ-SP combination *versus* AQ alone were conducted in the 1980s to test the efficacy and safety of AQ-SP compared to AQ alone. One of these three studies was conducted in China, and the other two studies were conducted in Mozambique. A meta-analysis was conducted using data from all three studies, and the rates of parasite clearance at day 28 favored the AQ-SP combination *versus* AQ. A recent trial of the AQ-SP combination in Uganda also noted higher rates of parasitological cure with AQ-SP than with SP monotherapy. The efficacy rates for the AQ-SP combination, however, were similar to SP as a single agent, which showed efficacy of 95% when utilized as a sole agent. The safety data derived from these clinical trials did not demonstrate adverse reactions due to the co-administration of SP along with AQ. In some countries in Central and West Africa, drug resistance against AQ is less than drug resistance to CQ, and a change to a combination of AQ-SP could be more effective and cheaper option than a change to SP monotherapy given the longer half-life of the AQ component with reduced costs associated with treating recrudescence against SP. Some concerns remain regarding safety of AQ when it is utilized for broad, largely unsupervised treatment of *falciparum* malaria particularly when treatment of recrudescence is required. Additional safety data for AQ particularly when used for intermittent prophylaxis during pregnancy or for repeat malaria treatment during a short interval is needed [65].

Atovaquone-Proguanil

Atovaquone-proguanil is administered as a fixed-dose combination of the two partner drugs, atovaquone and proguanil, which is marketed by GSK as Malarone™. Atovaquone-proguanil is available as film-coated tablets (which aids in absorption) for both adult and pediatric treatment. While atovaquone has independent activity against *falciparum* malaria as a sole agent, parasite recrudescence occurs in one-third of *falciparum* treated patients. The combination of atovaquone with proguanil hydrochloride, however, delivers a synergistic effect, which reduces the propensity for parasite recrudescence. The combination of atovaquone-proguanil can be used for *falciparum* malaria treatment, and cure rates of 94-100% against chloroquine and mefloquine resistant strains have been observed.

Considerable data on the pharmacokinetics and toxicology of Malarone™ are available from various studies, and while the absorption of this drug combination is highly variable with elimination half-lives varying from 2-4 days, this combination is well tolerated with few side effects even when used long term for malaria prophylaxis. While the data on the efficacy and safety for Malarone™ as a treatment regimen are very good, this drug combination is expensive, more so than other ACT treatment options, and this cost has largely restricted the use of Malarone™ to prophylaxis of travelers from high-income countries. Glaxo Smith Kline does not contemplate selling this drug broadly in malaria endemic nations. Instead, a Malarone™ Donation Program was initiated by GSK, and this program has a goal of contributing one million courses for treatment of uncomplicated *falciparum* malaria where treatment with other agents has been unsuccessful. The Malarone™ Donation Program was initiated at a number of locations in Uganda and Kenya. The guidelines of the Malarone™ Donation Program restrict use of this combination to patients with confirmed *falciparum* malaria who fail therapy with existing first and second-line treatments.

The use of Malarone™ for treatment of *falciparum* malaria in anemic children is under study in Zambia. The use of Malarone™ co-administered with artesunate is under evaluation in Cambodia and Thailand. Assessment of the safety and efficacy of Malarone™ for treatment of uncomplicated malaria in pregnant populations is an area of current research. Known contra-indications for Malarone™ include renal problems precluding clearance or drug sensitivity to proguanil or atovaquone. While pediatric data exists for the administration of Malarone, no data on administration of this drug to pregnant or breastfeeding women exists, and the administration of this drug to pregnant women must be balanced against potential risks [65].

Mefloquine-Sulfadoxine-Pyrimethamine

The drug combination of mefloquine combined with SP (MSP) was innovated for treatment of uncomplicated malaria based on the hypothesis that each individual partner drug is capable of additive activity against the malaria parasite. Furthermore, the developers hypothesized that the drug combination of these three drugs might be capable of delaying parasite drug resistance. There are unknown drug-drug interactions between the partner drugs, and the elimination kinetics of SP and mefloquine are similar to those obtained from patients administered equivalent doses of each partner drug alone. Mefloquine has significant advantages from a pharmacokinetic perspective with a long elimination half-life of 20 days for treatment of uncomplicated malaria, however, the residual sub-therapeutic drug remaining in patients is a disadvantage in high-transmission areas where the remaining sub-therapeutic drug concentrations in treated patients exerts selection pressure on parasites.

While many have theorized about the "selective filter" that sub-therapeutic drug levels may impose to select drug resistant parasites, the use of MSP has actual data to show why this is a concern. Along the border between Thailand and Cambodia, the use of MSP for first-line therapy of uncomplicated *falciparum* malaria was related to a rapid rise in parasite drug resistance to mefloquine. The most likely hypothesis to explain this phenomenon is the presence of sub-therapeutic drug levels of mefloquine in the blood of treated patients who remained in these areas of intensive endemic malaria as opposed to an effect caused by the relatively low dose of mefloquine (15 mg/kg) used in the drug combination. Other contributory factors for poor efficacy include the presence of drug resistance to SP in this geographic area as well as simultaneous use of mefloquine as monotherapy in this region. There are additional factors relating to the pharmacokinetic mismatch between the elimination half-lives of mefloquine and SP; mefloquine has a long half-life of 20 days while the half-life of SP is much shorter (7-10 days).

Accordingly, SP would only provide protection during the period of treatment leaving the remaining 10 days or more of the mefloquine half-life with only mefloquine present. Consequently, the combination of MSP is no longer recommended for treatment of malaria or for use as a malaria prophylactic drug [1, 23].

Quinine-Tetracycline and Quinine-Doxycycline

Tetracycline has been co-administered with quinine for treatment of *falciparum* malaria in endemic regions with quinine resistant parasites where a 7-day treatment regimen with quinine alone is not efficacious. The combination of quinine plus tetracycline was innovated in the 1970s for treatment of uncomplicated *falciparum* malaria. Doxycycline, a tetracycline analogue, has similar efficacy against *Plasmodium*, and the combination of quinine and doxycycline is now being used for malaria treatment. Doxycycline demonstrates better drug absorption, enhanced stability, greater lipid solubility, and a longer half-life than tetracycline, and doxycycline has a lower probability of metabolic transformation to a toxic product. As the cost of doxycycline is equivalent to tetracycline, a daily treatment with doxycycline is easier to administer than tetracycline, as tetracycline must be dosed 4 times per day rather than once.

The combination of quinine and tetracycline has challenges operationally given concerns over safety and patient compliance. Quinine requires administration every 8 hours and tetracycline requires administration every 4 hours, which is a particularly unwieldy regimen of 37 to 49 drug doses over a 7-day period. Patient adherence to such a schedule is difficult to enforce, and adverse reactions to quinine (also known as cinchonism) include tinnitus, blurred vision, impaired hearing, confusion, reversible high-frequency hearing loss, headache, abdominal pain, rashes, drug-induced photosensitivity, vertigo, dizziness, dysphoria, nausea, vomiting, and diarrhea. This drug combination can be made much simpler by substituting a daily dose of doxycycline in place of tetracycline. Administration of either doxycycline or tetracycline is not recommended for children under 8 years of age, breastfeeding women, or pregnant women. Given the limitations mentioned, administration of the quinine plus tetracycline combination is not a popular drug combination for treatment of *falciparum* malaria, however, the combination of quinine plus doxycycline may be considered as a secondary or tertiary treatment option assuming the patient is capable of taking oral drugs.

Quinine-Clindamycin

The combination of quinine-clindamycin is not widely used; however, clinical trials of this drug combination have shown it to be safe and efficacious for treatment of uncomplicated malaria in pregnant women, adults, and children. Outcomes of treatment studies of both resident patients and non-immune travelers in Southeast Asia, Africa, and South America have shown this combination is efficacious. As quinine and clindamycin are both examples of drugs with short half-lives (the half-life of clindamycin is 2-4 hours), the combination may have advantages for decreasing selection of drug resistant parasites. However, clearly, this drug combination has a number of issues associated with both the side effects of quinine treatment and the frequency of drug administration particularly where clindamycin must be administered at a minimum of every 6 hours. Clindamycin treatment is associated with development of colitis in 5% of hospitalized patients, and the risk of developing colitis is increased with co-administration of quinine. The risk of developing colitis is minimized in non-hospitalized outpatients while the risk of colitis is increased in patients who are older; endure longer malaria therapy, or who are infected with other disease [66].

Sulfadoxine-Pyrimethamine-Quinine

Monotherapy with quinine requires 7 days of treatment that can be difficult to endure given the side effects of treatment combined with the unpleasant, bitter taste of quinine, which certainly affects patient compliance. For treatment of severe malaria, injected quinine is the only other recommended treatment beyond injected artesunate. The combination of quinine plus clindamycin or a tetracycline antibiotic has been shown to be efficacious for treatment of malaria infections. The combination of quinine-sulfadoxine-pyrimethamine (SP) has been assessed in a number of clinical studies, however, this drug combination demonstrated poor efficacy in studies conducted in in Bangladesh and Brazil, and the efficacy failures were linked to parasite resistance against the SP partner, which is endemic in the local parasite population. In a study in South Africa conducted in an area where parasites are still sensitive to SP, the combination of SP and 3-day treatment with quinine was shown to be more effective than treatment with either quinine or SP alone. The adverse effects of this combination therapy were reported to be similar to those observed in patients treated with SP and quinine individually.

Chlorproguanil-Dapsone

Dapsone is an anti-folate sulfa drug that has been combined with chlorproguanil, another antifolate drug, as a malaria drug treatment in combination. The half-life of dapsone is 30 hours while the half-life of chlorproguanil is 20 hours, so pharmacokinetically this drug combination is well matched. This drug combination was developed by a public-private partnership as an inexpensive treatment option for African children infected with *falciparum* malaria. This combination was shown to be well tolerated and efficacious in a Phase 3 multicenter study.

There was an increased risk of hematological adverse events noted in the chlorproguanil-dapsone combination, however, a lower incidence of adverse events was observed in patients treated with sulfadoxine-pyrimethamine. The incidence of hematological adverse events such as hemolysis and methemoglobinemia is highest in patients with glucose-6 phosphate dehydrogenase deficiency (G6PD deficiency). Testing for G6PD deficiency on a routine basis among patients in endemic areas prior to administering treatment for malaria is an operational concern given the expense involved. Induction of parasite drug resistance is another concern given both drugs are antifolate drugs and any use of this combination is problematic in areas where SP has already been used and resistance to antifolate drugs may well be already established.

Chloroquine-Proguanil

Studies have been conducted on fixed dose combination treatment with chloroquine and proguanil. Efficacy and tolerability of this drug combination was assessed in a study of 194 French travelers travelling to areas with endemic malaria. Adverse gastrointestinal symptoms were most commonly reported in 10% of patients and in 2% of the volunteers with the neuropsychiatric side effects in this study, however, the side effects were not deemed serious in nature. The incidence of neuropsychiatric side effects in this study is much lower than the rates of neuropsychiatric side effects noted in populations taking mefloquine where neuropsychiatric side effects have been reported in 11.5% of individuals treated.

Proguanil as a sole agent has been used on occasion for malaria prophylaxis, and the tolerability and efficacy of this prophylactic regimen were assessed in two studies. In one study of 470 British soldiers in Belize, patients reported development of mouth ulcers associated with treatment which affected 24% of soldiers treated with proguanil monotherapy for prophylaxis and 37% of soldiers treated with the combination of CQ-proguanil reported problems with mouth ulcers as well (relative risk = 1.56). A telephone survey was conducted to obtain tolerability data from returning British travelers treated with the combination of CQ-proguanil, and reports of adverse effects from this drug combination were noted to be similar to those taking mefloquine. 0.09% of respondents taking CQ-proguanil noted neuropsychiatric symptoms while 0.7% of respondents administered mefloquine demonstrated neuropsychiatric side effects ($p = 0.021$). Side effects associated with mild gastrointestinal upset were noted in 16.3% of respondents administered CQ-proguanil while 12.5% of respondents reported GI upset in the mefloquine group ($p = 0.009$).

Fosmidomycin-Clindamycin

The combination of fosmidomycin and clindamycin has been assessed for treatment of uncomplicated malaria. Both fosmidomycin and clindamycin affect the replication of the apicoplast organelle, which is required for parasite propagation. In initial clinical trials, fosmidomycin was shown to kill rapidly parasites, however, monotherapy with fosmidomycin did not show a higher cure rate compared to treatment with either fosmidomycin or clindamycin as sole agents. The combination of fosmidomycin and clindamycin was shown to result in drug synergy. In a study of Gabonese children treated with the combination of fosmidomycin and clindamycin, rapid clearance of the malaria parasites was noted and cure rates of 100% were observed 28 days after treatment [65].

2.2. ANTIMALARIAL PROFILES OF ARTEMISININ AND ITS DERIVATIVES

2.2.1. Artemisinins Show a Superior PK/PD Profile as an Antimalarial Drug

Crude extracts derived from the sweet wormwood plant (*Artemisia annua* or qinghao) were used historically 2,000 years ago for patient treatment of fevers in China, and records of this herbal remedy were first recorded in the "Handbook of Prescriptions for Emergency Treatment" edited by Ge Hong (281-340 B.C.). In this text, the author prescribed treatment of fever and chills with tea-brewed from *Artemisia* leaves. The use of *Artemisia* tea extracts for treatment of malaria was discussed in the 16th century reference "Compendium of Materia Medica" authored by Li Shizen who referenced Ge Hong's prescription. In the 1970s, the active component of the sweet wormwood plant extract was shown to be artemisinin or qinghaosu [65]. After this discovery, a variety of semi-synthetic lipid and water-soluble artemisinin analogues were innovated, and a number of different artemisinin formulations have been tested clinically for treatment of malaria. Artemisinin compounds have been shown to have potent antiparasitic activity *in vitro* with rapid killing of parasites at nanomolar concentrations. Artemisinin compounds have been shown to act on ring stage *falciparum* parasites, which is a unique property not shared by other antimalarials.

Artemisinin is a sesquiterpene lactone, and its unique structure contains an endoperoxide bridge (C-O-O-C). Originally, artemisinin was shown to be effective clinically for treatment of *falciparum* malaria in the 1980s, and lipid and water-soluble semi-synthetic analogues were created to enhance artemisinin's potency and pharmacologic properties. Analogues of artemisinin are derived from the reduced lactol derivative of artemisinin, dihydroartemisinin, or DHA, which is also the principle active metabolite [65]. There are three semisynthetic analogues of artemisinin that have been widely used in treatment of malaria; the lipophilic artemisinins, arteether and artemether, and the water-soluble analogue, artesunate (Fig. **4**). Artemisinin compounds possess unique properties not found in other antimalarial drugs, and they are an irreplaceable treatment against otherwise multidrug-resistant *P. falciparum*. Evaluation of the clinical and pharmacologic properties of the artemisinin class of compounds have been ongoing for many years, and there are four clear advantages of this class of drugs over other antimalarials [65] as listed below.

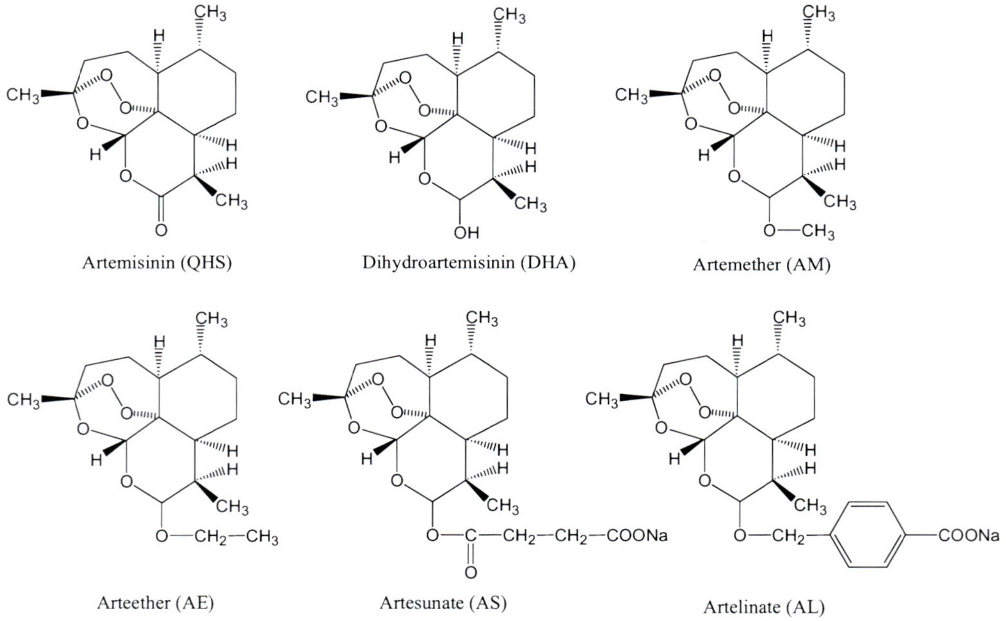

Figure 4: Chemical structures of artemisinin (QHS) and its five derivatives, dihydroartemisinin (DHA), artemether (AM), arteether (AE), artesunate (AS) and artelinic acid (AL).

1) Rapid Action and Strong Efficacy Against Multi-Drug Resistant P. falciparum

Artemisinin derivatives have been shown to be efficacious for treatment of asexual parasites from all four species of *Plasmodium* that infect man. Of all the antimalarial drugs, the artemisinins have been shown to have the most rapid initial reduction of parasite biomass. The half-lives of the artemisinins are very short compared to the half-lives of other antimalarial drugs yet the effect noted clinically on parasite clearance persists beyond the half-life of the compound. This phenomenon does suggest an effect similar to that observed in bacteria after administration of antibiotics where persistent inhibition of bacterial growth is noted following even short exposure to an antibiotic. Of the available artemisinin analogues, artesunate has been shown to have the best pharmacological profile to act as part of drug combination treatment of malaria [10].

Artesunate possesses a hemisuccinate group as part of its structure, and this group provides increased oral bioavailability and elevated solubility in water. Artesunate is rapidly converted *in vivo* to dihydroartemisinin, which is a potent metabolite. Artemether, arteether, artemisinin, and dihydroartemisinin are all less soluble in water, and that, in turn, affects compound absorption, which is slower and less efficient than artesunate. Plasma concentrations noted after oral dosing of all of the artemisinins provides a high enough plasma concentration beyond what is required to kill malaria parasites [65].

2) P. falciparum Artemisinin Drug Resistance Just Initially Identified on Patient Outcomes

Artemisinin resistant *P. falciparum* parasites have been identified in the border regions of Thailand-Myanmar and Thailand-Cambodia in 2009 [5]. In 2014, the K13-propeller polymorphism was found to be a useful molecular marker for tracking the emergence and spread of artemisinin resistant *P. falciparum* [6]. As resistance previously emerged in this region to chloroquine in the 1950s and mefloquine in the 1990s, this is hardly a surprise. Drug resistance to all antimalarial medicines has been shown in various parts of the world (particularly Southeast Asia where resistance has been documented to virtually all antimalarials available), and drug resistance is a significant barrier to controlling malaria. The indiscriminate use of antimalarial drugs puts high pressure to select drug resistant *P. falciparum* parasites for survival. Drug resistance can be averted or delayed through implementation of treatment regimens composed of drug combinations where each partner drug has a different parasite target and mechanism of action. Drug resistance can also be averted by focusing on achievement of high rates of clinical cures; this is very much dependent on achieving full patient compliance.

In the last five years, increased attention has been focused on the discovery of emerging *P. falciparum* drug resistance to artemisinin compounds, which has been demonstrated clinically in the border regions of western Cambodia and eastern Thailand and in areas of the Thai-Myanmar border. This resistance to artemisinin is characterized clinically by an extended delay in parasite clearance after artemisinin treatment [5, 6]. The emergence of artemisinin-resistant parasites in regions of the Thai-Cambodian border is a phenomenon of increasing concern particularly as the caseload of *falciparum* malaria has been radically reduced in recent years. Diminished parasite susceptibility to artemisinins, in turn, renders the ACT partner drugs more vulnerable to the development of resistance. Despite the delays in parasite clearance in patients treated with artemisinins in areas of the Cambodia-Thailand border region, ACTs are still the best treatment option for patients infected with uncomplicated *falciparum* malaria, and the majority of patients who present with delays in parasite clearance are still cured as long as the antimalarial partner drug is still effective [2, 8].

Many believe there is a limited window of time to contain or eliminate artemisinin resistance in afflicted areas before parasite drug resistance spreads to areas of high malaria transmission, which endangers recent gains in malaria control. Accordingly, it is essential to understand the presence of drug resistant parasites in a particular area so that robust containment measures can be implemented. Surveillance of drug resistance through *in vitro* phenotypic resistance testing and assessment of molecular markers of drug resistance will be critical tools to monitor emergence and spread of resistance. While artemisinin analogues are capable of reducing most of the parasite biomass initially, effective partner drugs can be relied on to eliminate the few remaining parasites present. Furthermore, the odd of a parasite emerging with multiple spontaneous mutations to both the artemisinin component and an unrelated partner drug at the same time is very low [9]. Therefore, for *P. falciparum* treatment, the use of multiple drugs in combination with different parasite targets and mechanisms of action is essential to insure high cure rates and minimize the spread of drug resistance.

The fly in the ointment, however, is the dearth of new antimalarial partner drugs with no established drug resistance present in circulating parasites in endemic areas such as Southeast Asia. All of the partner drugs combined with artemisinins currently in use such as mefloquine, amodiaquine, sulfadoxine-pyrimethamine, or piperaquine are older drugs with known problems with established parasite drug resistance, or in the case of lumefantrine, known cross-resistance with mefloquine. The absence of new partner drugs for malaria combination therapy is as large a problem as the presence of artemisinin resistance. Having new partner drugs to combine with an artemisinin analogue would help compensate for the delays in parasite clearance noted in regions with artemisinin resistance [8, 9].

3) Low Toxicity and an Excellent Safety Profile

Artemisinin compounds have been very well tolerated. Adverse events that are most commonly reported include vomiting, nausea, headache, dizziness, bowel disturbance, and abdominal pain, which also include symptoms noted because of malaria infection itself. Symptoms of reversible and mild EKG and hematological abnormalities to include first degree heart block and neutropenia have been observed less frequently.

Artemisinin-associated neurotoxicity resulting in drug-induced brainstem lesions were first shown in animals receiving high doses of artemisinins over long periods of time, especially with oil-soluble artemether and arteether. In contrast, few neurotoxic effects have been induced by water-soluble artesunate (AS) or experimental analogues such as artelinic acid (ALA), which have never produced any CNS side effects in animal species after intravenous injection. Pharmacokinetic profiles of the artemisinin derivatives demonstrate that drug exposure time plays a more important role in producing neurotoxicity than drug exposure level, production of the more active metabolite, dihydroartemisinin, or drug location in the CNS system. There have been limited reports of neurological side effects in man to include hearing loss, slurred speech, or ataxia; however, these side effects are not likely to be clinically important particularly as the artemisinins demonstrate limited penetration into the cerebrospinal fluid [66]. In addition, it has been demonstrated that at sub-clinical doses, injectable artesunate can cause fetal death due to an accumulation of high concentrations of artesunate during the sensitive period of early gestation in animals. To date, however, the neurotoxicity and reproductive toxicity observed in animal toxicity studies have not been convincingly established in humans treated with any of the artemisinins. Fatal neurotoxicity can be avoided by reducing the drug exposure time that varies greatly between the different artemisinin compounds. Reproductive toxicity can be avoided by limiting the exposure of artemisinins during this sensitive period in fetal development with combination therapy [67].

4) Gametocidal Effect Which Reduces Parasite Transmission

Artemisinin derivatives have been shown to be indirectly active against the sexual gametocyte stage of the malaria parasite. Gametocytes are subsequently passed on to mosquitoes, which feed on infected humans. These gametocytes undergo sexual reproduction in the mid-gut of the mosquito and form the sporozoite stage, which infects the liver cells of man. Accordingly, artemisinin treatment can therefore reduce malaria transmission rates in the population as a whole. The exact mechanism of anti-gametocyte activity is not known. The endoperoxide bridge of the artemisinins may generate destructive free radicals capable of damaging the malaria parasite when the endoperoxide bond is broken. Alternative explanations of artemisinin efficacy include formation of covalent bonds, or alteration of the parasite proteins such as critical membrane transporters.

The artemisinin analogues are not capable of killing mature *P. falciparum* directly; however, these drugs prevent development of gametocytes because of artemisinin activity against more mature and younger asexual parasites, which are the predecessors of the more mature forms of the gametocyte. Antimalarial drugs that act later in the asexual life cycle, such as the quinoline antimalarials, are not as effective at blocking development of mature sexual forms of the malaria parasite. Artemisinin drugs have other benefits, and they should be used for treatment of all malaria infections not simply those infections in areas with established presence of drug resistant parasites. In clinical studies of patients who were treated with an artemisinin compound successfully for malaria with rapid parasite clearance, artemisinin treatment resulted in a five-fold reduction in gametocyte carriage compared with treatment by quinine, mefloquine, or halofantrine [68].

2.2.2. Artemisinins Have an Inferior Antimalarial Profile as Monotherapeutic Agents

Despite the limited evidence for clinically relevant resistance to artemisinin drugs *in vivo* when artemisinin drugs are used as partners in a drug combination regimen, artemisinin monotherapy has long been known to limit efficacy. Consequently, WHO has suggested artemisinin monotherapy is banned as part of a containment strategy to limit the spread of artemisinin resistance [69]. Recrudescence after artemisinin monotherapy appears late in the course of clinical therapy, and studies of recrudescence where patients were followed for periods up to day 42 have shown a higher degree of recrudescence than studies where assessment of recrudescence was halted at day 28. Recrudescent infections after artemisinin monotherapy assessed by day 28 day are estimated to be 20-40% of cases in Africa and approximately 20% of cases in Southeast Asia. The length of artemisinin monotherapy has been shown to be of prime importance in achieving antimalarial efficacy, and extension of artemisinin monotherapy treatment to 7 days has been shown to improve cure rates significantly [70].

The therapeutic potentials of all artemisinin drugs as monotherapeutic agents with various dose regimens for treatment of malaria in 54 different clinical trials have been summarized in Table **3**. Successful treatment, defined as a 100% cure rate, is found in neither the 3-5 day monotherapy treatments nor the high dose (4.8 mg/kg) monotherapy regimens [65]. The curative rate, parasite clearance time

(PCT), and the fever clearance time (FCT) are traditional measurements of antimalarial drug efficacy in man. The cure rate, the FCT, and the PCT are three parameters that can be used to evaluate the therapeutic potential of intravenous, intramuscular, and oral agents in various regimens. Reviewing the data shown in Table **3** for various artemisinin analogues demonstrates differences in efficacy for artemisinin monotherapy simply by changing vehicles. Administration of arteether (AE) formulated in sesame oil vehicle, for example, is inferior to treatment with intramuscular artemether (AM), oral dihydroartemisinin (DHA), oral or intravenous artesunate (AS), or even injection of intramuscular α/ß-arteether (AE) dissolved in peanut oil.

Table 3: Summary of the outcomes of monotherapy using artemisinin derivatives in patients with uncomplicated, severe, and complicated malarias in 54 clinical trials [65]

Drug and Regimen	PCT (hr)	FCT (hr)	% of Recrudescence	Clinical Trials No.
AE in sesame oil (Artemotil)				
(IM 3.2 mg/kg-1.6 mg/kg x 4)	70.2	81.0	40.0	1
(IM 4.8 mg/kg-1.6 mg/kg x 5)	59.2	61.5	22.2	1
AM				
(IM 3.2 mg/kg-1.6 mg/kg x 4)	28.3 ± 13.0	38.8 ± 4.4	8.6 ± 6.2	8
(oral 200 mg-100 mg/kg x 5)	39.7 ± 2.2	34.8 ± 6.9	5.2 ± 2.2	9
AS				
(IV & oral in various regimens)	30.3 ± 10.7	35.9 ± 11.1	7.5 ± 3.1	23
DHA				
(oral in various regimens)	49.1 ± 7.5	33.8 ± 7.7	6.0 ± 1.8	7
AE in peanut oil				
(IM 150 mg daily for 3 days)	37.8 ± 12.2	49.9 ± 16.2	9.4 ± 4.1	5

Values are given mean ± SD.
DHA = Dihydroartemisinin, AM = Artemether, AE = Arteether, AS = Artesunate,
IM = intramuscular, IV = intravenous, PCT = parasite clearance time, FCT = Fever clearance time.

Given this data, and the well-known speed of artemisinin action, the artemisinins are viewed to be very effective agents when compared to other traditional malaria treatments. Short treatments of artemisinin as monotherapy over a period of 3 to 5 days have been shown to be associated with high rates of recrudescence [6]. Data derived from clinical studies conducted with all of the existing artemisinin analogues administered as monotherapy has shown that in patients administered a dose of an artemisinin analogue sufficient for induction of initial clearance of parasites and clinical recovery, the length of monotherapy is the best indicator for recrudescence. After 3 days of artemisinin monotherapy, recrudescence is observed in 30-50% of patients, after 5 days, 6-15% of patients recrudesce, and after 7 days of monotherapy, 2-6% of patients recrudesce which demonstrate the significant problems associated with monotherapy for all artemisinin derivatives

[71]. Some authors have suggested that preventing recrudescence is not the highest priority compared to initial malaria treatment, and some authors have advocated that recrudescent infections should be treated again with the same therapy used initially rather than switching drug regimens. This point of view, however, enhances the risk of developing drug resistant parasites, which will lead to continued recrudescent infections. The best treatment regimen for artemisinins clearly exists when they are combined with partner drugs in a combination regimen that offers the best possibility of a first-time cure rather than monotherapeutic artemisinin treatment, which may result in multiple rounds of recrudescence and requirements for additional antimalarial therapy.

2.3. ARTEMISININ-BASED COMBINATION THERAPY (ACT)

Artemisinin-based combination therapies (ACTs) are now recommended first-line treatment for *falciparum* malaria globally, and artemisinin combination treatments are clearly more effective than non-artemisinin-based combinations or monotherapies. A welcome side benefit of artemisinin therapy is the reduction in the probability of development of drug resistance in *P. falciparum* parasites [40, 69]. ACTs show many of beneficial features related to their unique mode of action that include the follows:

- Rapid and substantial reduction of the parasite biomass,
- Rapid parasite clearance,
- Rapid resolution of clinical symptoms,
- Effective action against multidrug-resistant *P. falciparum*, and
- Reduction of gametocyte carriage, which potentially reduces transmission of resistant alleles.

There are few reports of adverse clinical effects associated with artemisinin treatment of humans [72]. Due to the short half-lives of artemisinin analogues, monotherapy treatment must be conducted for 7 days with treatment every day. By combining an artemisinin analogue with a partner antimalarial drug with a long half-life, the duration of malaria treatment can be dropped from 7 days for artemisinin monotherapy to a 3-day combination regimen that provides increased efficacy and reduces the possibility of induction of drug resistance. The initial effect of the artemisinin component is reduction of the parasite biomass. The few remaining parasites are exposed to a long half-life of partner drug, well above the minimum inhibitory concentration required for parasite killing, which results in a decreased probability of development of drug resistance.

The data derived from human testing of artemisinin combination therapy regimens clearly show that artemisinins have an amazing degree of activity as antimalarial drugs showing reductions in parasite number by a factor of approximately 10,000 fold per asexual cycle while other antimalarials are only capable of reducing parasite numbers by a factor of 100 to 1,000 fold per asexual cycle. Furthermore, artemisinins have activity against early and later stage parasites and thus they are capable of being used for treatment of uncomplicated and severe malaria. Artemisinins are capable of inhibiting gametocyte carriage, which also aids in limiting transmission [23]. To date, there is very early evidence of stable resistance to artemisinin compounds in therapeutic use or in experimental systems [5, 6].

Treatment of uncomplicated malaria can be achieved through a 3-day regimen of artemisinins combined with partner drugs such as one or more of the quinoline or antifolate drugs. Artemisinin combination therapy has been shown to be efficacious, enhances patient compliance, and leads to decreased spread of parasite resistance [23]. The majority of artemisinin combination therapies in use today rely on a slowly eliminated partner drug such as mefloquine. The partner drug is left unprotected after the artemisinin analogue has been cleared leading to exertion of selective pressure on the partner drug for existing and new infections. The impact of using "pharmacokinetic mismatched" drugs is not clear [73] at present, and questions exist regarding the potential for induction of drug resistance in areas of Africa with elevated parasite transmission. The best solution to this "mismatch" is to combine the artemisinin compound with a partner drug that has a short residual half-life while still ensuring clearance of parasites with a 3-day drug regimen; this goal may be difficult to attain with the limited array of partner drugs available.

There are a number of factors that affect the choices of antimalarial drug combination partners to inhibit parasite resistance; two or more drugs with antimalarial efficacy, different parasite targets and mechanisms of action, at least additive and hopefully synergistic properties in combination, and a good match on pharmacokinetic parameters. As reported by Hastings and Watkins [73], drug combinations that are not matched pharmacokinetically do not have an impact on limiting the emergence and extent of drug resistance, and mismatched partners may enhance the probability of diminished component drug efficacy against parasites where resistance is still nascent such as the artemisinins. Therefore, combination drug partners should have comparable elimination half-lives to provide constant pressure of two drugs on existing and new parasites. In an ideal world, antimalarial drugs possessing short half-lives would be best to decrease the probability of exposing a re-invading parasite to sub-therapeutic concentrations of drug that may induce selection for resistance [74].

The principal artemisinin drug combinations that have been implemented to date consist of a quinoline paired with an artemisinin or an antifolate drug paired with an artemisinin. Other combinations have been evaluated, but these new combinations are not yet being used broadly. The artemisinin-quinoline combinations have shown mixed results when tested in clinical trials. The different mechanisms of action of the two drugs should provide an additive or synergistic effect. The differences in the elimination half-life between the an artemisinin whose half-life lasts no more than 1 day for artemether (for DHA and artesunate, the half-life in man is 1 hour) and quinoline compounds whose half-life ranges from 2-4 weeks is reason for concern from the perspective of drug resistance. Artemisinin analogues have been most frequently used in combination with quinolines such as mefloquine, lumefantrine, and amodiaquine.

The combination of artesunate and mefloquine has been shown to be very efficacious in clinical trials; however, the combination of artemisinin and mefloquine is expensive. This combination clearly shows a mismatch in elimination half-lives as mefloquine has a half-life between 14-21 days while artesunate is eliminated in 1 hour, which may lead to increased levels of mefloquine drug resistance and concomitant risks to artesunate long-term. In addition, studies have shown elevated clinical failure rates in locations with elevated resistance to mefloquine. From a pharmacokinetic perspective, the combination of lumefantrine with artemether (half-life 3-6 days) is a better match as lumefantrine has a half-life of 3-6 days, however, artemether-lumefantrine is expensive and a number of studies have shown this combination is less effective than AS-mefloquine when utilized in locations where multidrug resistant parasites are prevalent [75, 76]. The combination of artesunate with amodiaquine (AS-AQ) was recently introduced in sub-Saharan Africa as a cheap artemisinin combination therapeutic. The combination of artesunate and amodiaquine also has a pharmacokinetic mismatch as the principal active metabolite of amodiaquine, desethylamodiaquine, has an extended half-life of 9-18 days while artesunate, as stated previously, is cleared in 1 hour [77]. Studies in Africa have shown significant rates of clinical failure associated with amodiaquine resistance. Drug resistance to amodiaquine is likely to spread quickly as the AS-AQ combination has been implemented as first-line treatment in a number of African countries [74]. The list of currently implemented antimalarial combination therapies with a review of their advantages and disadvantages are summarized in Table **4**.

Table 4: Currently used antimalarial combination therapies with their advantages and disadvantages [updated from 74]

Drug Combinations	Advantages	Disadvantages
Sulfadoxine + Pyrimethamine (SP)	Synergistic activity, inexpensive	Widespread resistance, medium-long half-lives, moderate PK mismatch
Chlorproguanil + Dapsone	Synergistic activity, good PK match, short half-lives	Cross-resistance with SP
SP + Amodiaquine	Similar pharmacokinetic profiles	Resistance to both components spreading, medium-long half-lives
SP + Artesunate	Efficacious	Significant PK mismatch, efficacy dependent on level of SP resistance
Proguanil/Dapsone + Artesunate	Efficacious, similar PK profiles, short half-lives	Cross-resistance with SP may limit its application
Artesunate + Mefloquine	Efficacious	PK mismatch, resistance to mefloquine spreading
Artesunate + Amodiaquine	Efficacious	PK mismatch, resistance to amodiaquine spreading
Artesunate + Fosmidomycin	Efficacious, excellent PK match, Short-half-lives	Not suitable for prophylaxis
Artesunate + Clindamycin	Efficacious, similar PK match, Short-half-lives	Not suitable for prophylaxis, treatment failure observed
Proguanil + Atovaquone	Synergistic activity, efficacious	Moderate PK mismatch, resistance easy to acquire
Dihydroartemisinin-Piperaquine	Highly efficacious, Reduction of transmission with better gametocyte clearance	PK mismatch

PK = pharmacokinetic.

The combination of artesunate and mefloquine, while pharmacokinetically mismatched, has led to some interesting findings after implementation on the border between Thailand and Myanmar [35]. After AS-MQ was introduced, four epidemiological and clinical outcomes were observed:

1) Efficacy of AS-MQ was shown to exceed 95% while high-dose mefloquine treatment showed failure rates of 25%,

2) The 95% efficacy level for AS-MQ has been sustained for 12 years,

3) Transmission of *falciparum* parasites has been shown to be reduced with corresponding decreases in gametocyte carriage believed to be due treatment with the artesunate component,

4) An *in vitro* potency assessment of the IC_{50}s of mefloquine against parasites in this area has declined, which suggests the AS-MQ combination may have had an effect on mefloquine drug resistance in the region.

These studies were conducted in locations where medical services are readily available and the transmission of malaria is low. It is not known if these results are attainable in Africa or other regions of high malaria transmission. In addition, clinical studies evaluating the utility of ACTs in delaying the induction and spread of parasite drug resistance in Africa are still needed to provide operational research toward answering this important question. Field trials using combinations of artesunate partnered with mefloquine, chloroquine, sulfadoxine-pyrimethamine, and amodiaquine, for treatment of uncomplicated *falciparum* malaria are being conducted to answer questions regarding comparative efficacy and impact of ACTs on emergence and spread of drug resistance in South America, Asia, and Africa.

The advantages and disadvantages of ACTs are shown in Table **5**. ACTs should be evaluated in different settings. In locations where an ACT combination shows increased efficacy *versus* monotherapy, the use of an ACT is well justified *versus* monotherapy despite the added expense. In regions where monotherapy remains efficacious but concerns exist regarding how long monotherapy may remain efficacious given trends of parasite resistance, ACT implementation is harder to justify. While the concept of the value of implementing ACTs is broadly accepted at the operational level, questions remain concerning the actual impact ACT implementation may have on the ground. Ministries of health may be reluctant to implement Acts due to expense given the value of such implementation is not yet clear and barriers to successful implementation may remain.

2.4. ADOPTION AND DEPLOYMENT OF ACTS IN ASIA SINCE 1992

One of the first ACT combinations introduced, artemether plus lumefantrine, has been shown to have drug synergy *in vitro* against *P. falciparum*, and this oral artemisinin combination treatment has been shown to reduce rapidly parasite biomass due to the activity of the artemether component. The reduction in parasite numbers enhances efficacy, and the combination is believed to decrease selective pressure on both artemether and lumefantrine for development of parasite drug resistance [62]. Nonclinical *in vivo* toxicology studies conducted with artemether and lumefantrine in rats and dogs showed that a fixed dose combination at 1:6 ratios of artemether to lumefantrine was well tolerated by both species who received doses 10 times higher than the equivalent dose in man used subsequently in field studies. Data derived *in vitro* and through clinical trials conducted in several hundred patients led to the further conclusion that the 1:6 ratio of artemether to lumefantrine was not only well tolerated but also efficacious. No serious adverse events were noted in these studies, and the artemether-lumefantrine combination was shown to be very effective. This combination of artemether-lumefantrine was originally registered 1992 in China. Subsequent development of this combination by Novartis led to approval of artemether-lumefantrine (CoArtem) in 2008, and at this time, this is the only fixed dose ACT combination drug approved for use in the US for treatment of uncomplicated *falciparum* malaria [61].

Table 5: Factors for and against the introduction of artemisinin-based combination therapy

Factors for	Against
• The need to replace inadequate drug regimens that are leading to increased malaria-related morbidity and mortality. • Potential avoidance of the loss of available effective and affordable antimalarial drugs, especially in Africa. • Excellent efficacy (both clinical and parasitological clearance) of artemisinin derivatives despite extensive use with resistance reported only in discrete areas of Southeast Asia. • Potential reduction in transmission (especially of resistant mutants) due to the gametocytocidal effect of artemisinin derivatives.	• Highest cost • Problems of adherence to non-fixed combinations and their rational use, particularly in the home. • Lack of extensive clinical experience with most of the combinations currently under investigation. • Lack of evidence so far in Africa of its effectiveness in delaying the development of resistance. • Importance of not misusing artemisinin derivatives in view of their role in the treatment of severe malaria.

In Southeast Asia, increased parasite drug resistance to sulfadoxine-pyrimethamine led to the use of mefloquine for treatment of *falciparum* malaria in 1984. Mefloquine (MQ) was used first as a drug combination with sulfadoxine-pyrimethamine, in time, MQ was administered as monotherapy at a higher dose, and ultimately, mefloquine is now used as a drug combination with artesunate (AS) beginning in 1994. Since the drug combination of AS-MQ was implemented in 1994, the overall *falciparum* malaria cure rate increased to almost 100% by 1998 despite the fact that MQ resistant *falciparum* malaria was highly prevalent in Southeast Asia when the AS-MQ combination was implemented. A steady decline in *falciparum* malaria cases has also been shown in regions of Southeast Asia where the drug combination was implemented. *In-vitro* IC_{50} potency testing MQ against *P. falciparum* circulating parasites has demonstrated a significant drop ($p = 0.003$). In areas of where transmission of malaria is low, prompt diagnosis and initiation of treatment with the AS-MQ combination has been shown to reduce the number of *P. falciparum* infections and diminished the spread of MQ resistance [78].

Reductions in transmission of *falciparum* malaria have also been observed in regions where AS-MQ has been used supporting the hypothesis, that artemisinin combination therapy leads to decreases in gametocyte carriage. Subsequent research beginning in 1998 by the WHO Special Program in Research and Training in Tropical Diseases (WHO/TDR) was initiated to examine questions of efficacy and safety of artemisinin combination treatments focusing on studying the use of antimalarial partner drugs used such as chloroquine, amodiaquine, and sulfadoxine-pyrimethamine [79].

With the successful introduction of the AS-MQ combination therapy in Southeast Asia, four ACTs were developed by a WHO Expert Consultative Group in 2001 to include artesunate-amodiaquine, artesunate-sulfadoxine-pyrimethamine, artesunate-mefloquine, and artemether-lumefantrine [69]. Despite the recommendations by WHO in 2001, deployment of ACTs in regions endemic for *falciparum* malaria has been slow. The limiting factors for adoption of ACT therapies include expense, lack of public awareness and knowledge about combination therapy (CT) and ACTs. Operational limitations involve appropriate drug use, limited knowledge involving ACT safety profiles when used to treat pregnant women, lack of appropriate formulations for ACTs, an imbalance between supply and demand, and a lack of surveillance activities to assess efficacy after implementation.

Through a focused effort by multilateral organizations and consultation by policy makers with the local scientific community, slow progress is being made on several fronts leading to recent increased use of ACTs worldwide [78]. Similar to the success noted in Thailand after implementation of the AS-MQ drug combination discussed previously, decreases in transmission of malaria were noted in South Africa and Vietnam after ACT treatments were introduced [80].

These benefits to public health are a direct consequence of the action of artemisinin drugs to kill gametocytes, which reduces transmission, and drastic and rapid reduction in parasite biomass in infected patients. The role of artemisinin drugs in reducing transmission has been studied in areas with low to medium levels of malaria transmission, and it is not clear if a similar outcome would be observed in high transmission areas. While artemisinin analogues are capable of radical reductions in parasite biomass leading to reduced infectivity in treated patients, these drugs are not capable of killing all of the malaria parasites by themselves. Accordingly, research will need to be conducted to determine how reduced gametocyte carriage can be implemented in high transmission areas as well as other areas of reduced transmission.

WHO and the Roll Back Malaria (RBM) Partnership have played an important role along with local scientists to facilitate drug selection with national malaria control program by providing technical guidance and input on drug policy decisions. Despite the recognized urgency in implementing new combination therapies, the implementation of ACTs in malarious regions was so slow in the period from 2001 to 2003 that concerns were raised by public health experts in the malaria community regarding the sluggish pace of change [81]. Accordingly, the remainder of this chapter is focused on the opportunities and challenges that remain as barriers to rapid implementation of ACTs in Southeast Asia and Africa.

Areas in Southeast Asia endemic for multi-drug resistant *falciparum* malaria began using artemisinins for malaria treatment in the early 1990s [78]. In Vietnam and China artemisinins were deployed as monotherapy initially, except for the use of a combination drug composed of multiple partner drugs, DHA-piperaquine-trimethoprim plus primaquine, a drug combination identified as CV8; this multidrug combination regimen was deployed in Vietnam on a limited basis. In Cambodia and Thailand, AS and mefloquine combination therapy was initiated in certain l regions. By the year 2000, however, no country had yet adopted ACTs as first-line treatment regimens defined in their malaria treatment policy.

Since 2001, more countries have implemented ACTs as first-line treatment regimens for uncomplicated malaria (Fig. **5**). Given a lag of 12-18 months between the original decision to implement and actual implementation on the ground, the fraction of countries that have actually deployed ACTs has increased as well. Most countries initially limited deploying ACTs to certain regions where they were used to treat children under five who are most vulnerable or to regions with a well-defined diagnostic capability to insure ACTs were most appropriately used to treat a real case of malaria as opposed to a fever of unknown origin. ACTs have not been distributed to home-based treatment programs in any country other than Cambodia.

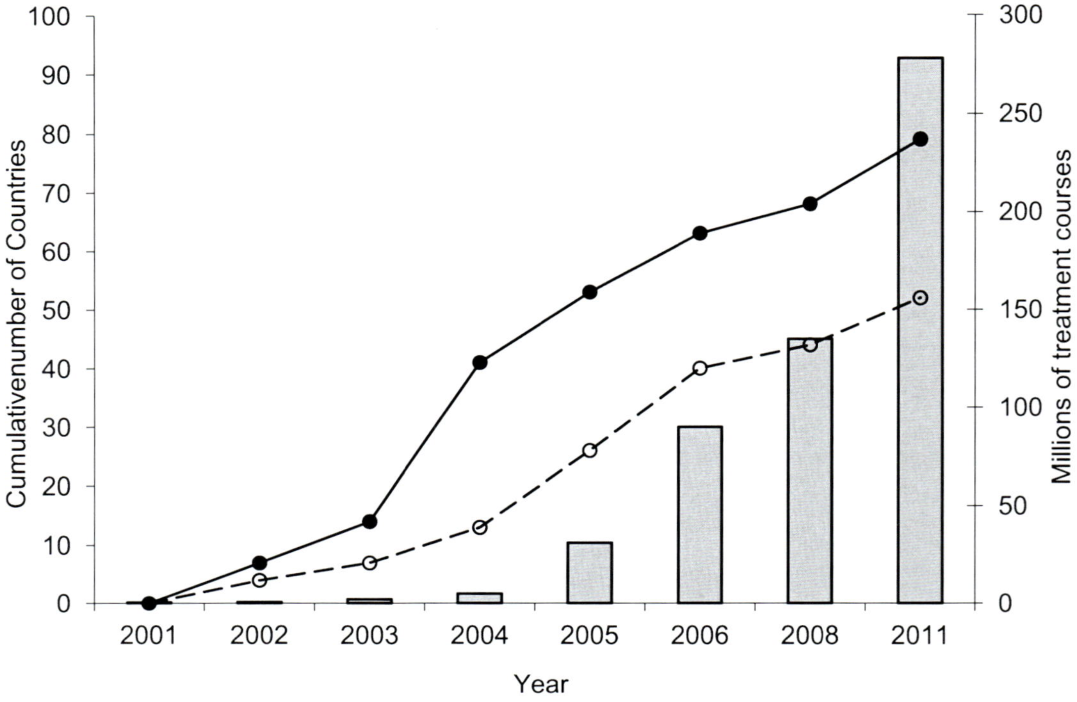

Figure 5: Cumulative number of countries adopting (continuous line) and deploying (interrupted line) ACTs as first-line treatment of malaria from January 2001 to July 2011. The annual ACT orders for the public sector in period 2001-2011 (solid bars) and the demand forecast (hatched bar) for 2012. By the end of 2011, ACTs had been adopted as national policy for first-line treatment in 79 of 88 countries where *P. falciparum* is endemic [82, 123].

By 2010, 70 endemic countries (24 in Asia and 46 in Africa) were deploying ACTs for treatment of *falciparum* malaria, and by 2011, ACTs have been implemented for first-line treatment of *falciparum* malaria in 79 of 88 countries with endemic disease [82]. Only two countries have implemented ACTs as second-line treatment only. Nine endemic countries to include China, Botswana, Swaziland, Columbia, Nepal, Eritrea, Pakistan, Vanuatu, and Sri Lanka have shown malaria treatment failure rates >10% with non-ACT based first-line drugs, and per the WHO guidance [23], these countries should implement ACTs. Artemether-lumefantrine was the most popular ACT, and this ACT was implemented in 32 countries while the combination of artesunate-amodiaquine

(AS-AQ) was implemented in 19 countries. The combination of artesunate and sulfadoxine-pyrimethamine (AS-SP) was implemented in 12 countries, artesunate-mefloquine (AS-MQ) was implemented in seven countries, and the combination of dihydroartemisinin-piperaquine (DHA-PPQ) was implemented in 1 country [23, 82].

2.5. ADOPTION AND DEPLOYMENT OF ACTS IN AFRICA SINCE 2000

As 90% of global malaria mortality is seen in Africa, drug resistance against antimalarials is a significant issue in this region. With the onset of chloroquine resistance in 1979 in East Africa, alternate therapies have been required for treatment of uncomplicated malaria. SP and mefloquine were implemented in place of chloroquine for treatment of chloroquine-resistant parasites, but these drugs are now less efficacious as monotherapy given the emergence and spread of mefloquine and SP resistant parasites. There are a number of different strategies being developed to halt these trends to include the use of ACT regimens [83, 84].

African leaders at a Roll Back Malaria meeting called the Abuja Summit held in April 2000 approved the goal of providing, at a minimum, 60% of malaria patients in Africa rapid access to appropriate and inexpensive treatment within 24 hours of diagnosis by 2005. Systematic implementation of ACTs are widely believed to be one of the few means by which endemic countries can actually "roll back malaria" per the Abuja Summit goals and actually cut the morbidity and mortality rates in half by 2010 [1, 23]. Currently four ACTs have been registered for use in sub-Saharan Africa with either fixed dose or co-administered formulations produced to globally recognized standards. These four ACTs include; artesunate-mefloquine, artesunate-SP, artemether-lumefantrine, and artesunate-amodiaquine. Despite the importance of implementing ACTs for treating uncomplicated *falciparum* malaria in sub-Saharan Africa, a comprehensive, up to date review of the public health impact of ACT deployment worldwide is needed to assess progress and outcomes.

The International Artemisinin Study Group [40] has shown in a number of studies that ACT implementation leads to higher rates of cure, quicker clearance of parasites and reductions in gametocyte carriage compared with artemisinin administered by itself as monotherapy. WHO has determined that artemether-lumefantrine has shown rates of cure >95%, even when this drug combination has been administered in regions with multi-drug resistant parasites [69]. The drug combinations of artesunate-amodiaquine and artesunate-SP have been shown in Africa to be very effective, with the caveat that rates of cure may decline due to emergence and spread of SP drug resistance. The combination of artesunate-amodiaquine has been shown to be more effective than artesunate-SP, and this combination may remain more efficacious for a longer period given the rise and spread of SP resistant parasites. The combination of artesunate-amodiaquine has been implemented as a first-line treatment in 15 African countries [85]. Studies in sub-Saharan Africa have demonstrated that artesunate combined with amodiaquine has a 28-day PCR corrected efficacy >90%, however, one study did show efficacy of AS-AQ <90%. Further results of studies of the AS-AQ combination have shown that it is safe, demonstrating rapid reduction of fever, clinical efficacy >90% and also reduced gametocyte formation during follow-up over a 14-day period beyond the 28 day efficacy assessment [84, 86].

The most important consideration when considering the implementation of ACT therapy is that the primary aim of malaria treatment is saving lives. Prompt and effective treatment in the early stages of *falciparum* malaria reduces the risk of death as much as 50-fold, while effective treatment after progression to severe illness produces only 5-fold reduction of mortality [9]. Malaria treatment can also reduce transmission of malaria in endemic areas, and this portion of the chapter will review the role of treatment as a control measure for reducing malaria transmission and past and present chemoprevention strategies implemented for residents of malaria-endemic areas.

The Ingwavuma district in northern KwaZulu Natal had the highest malaria burden in South Africa until 2000. This unfortunate status changed after improvements in vector control in KwaZulu Natal and neighboring southern Mozambique during 2000, and the implementation of an artemisinin combination therapy (ACT), artemether-lumefantrine (AL), in January 2001. These interventions were followed by a 78 percent decrease in malaria case notifications in the province within 1 year. There was a further 75 percent decrease in notifications in 2002 [80], and this decrease was sustained throughout 2003.

To aid in controlling malaria, the government of Rwanda gave out insecticide-treated bed nets (ITN) and distributed ACT drugs widely starting in 2005. The public health impact of these different interventions on the burden of malaria, hospital admissions, and malaria deaths was studied using data from household surveys and from 30 district hospitals. Case trends, number of admissions and malaria associated deaths from the study period between 2000 to 2010 were evaluated by segmented log-linear regression, where the effect size was adjusted for time trends observed during the pre-intervention period from 2000-2005 with the post-intervention period from 2006-2010. Deaths all causes in children under five in Rwanda were assessed in household surveys conducted in 2005 and 2010 to correlate this data with the hospital data on deaths. The hospital and survey reports confirmed the number of malaria cases increased in 2009, which occurred at the same time ITN coverage was decreased and the numbers of cases declined again in 2010 after completion of an ITN distribution campaign. All age groups showed declines of 72% in the numbers of microscopically confirmed cases of malaria observed in the post-intervention period from 2005 onward. In 2010, the last studied time in this Rwandan study, the rate of malaria slide-positive cases declined by 58%, the number of malaria inpatient cases declined by 76% and overall the number of malaria deaths decreased by 47%. In children under five years of age, the number of malaria inpatient cases decreased by 82% and malaria hospital deaths decreased by 77% [80].

The success of this dual intervention is further reflected by the 89% decrease in both malaria-related hospital admissions (decrease in admissions ranged from 81-92%), and deaths (decreases in deaths ranged from 78-93%) across the three rural district hospitals that serve the Ingwavuma community. Even though KwaZulu Natal also has the highest burden of HIV/AIDS in South Africa, the total number of "all cause" hospital admissions was reduced following improved malaria control. Dr. Hervey V. Williams, medical superintendent of Mosvold hospital, a rural district hospital in Ingwavuma, reported, "During the peak of the 2000 malaria epidemic, hospital admissions were averaging three patients per bed." Following the reduction in the overall number of hospital admissions, it is expected that the standard of care for all patients could be improved given the reduced burden of malaria inpatients to care for.

The use of multi-drug combinations is a chemotherapeutic strategy implemented to improve outcomes and retard development of drug resistance to individual partner drugs. The benefits of ACT implementation are clear for improvement of therapeutic outcomes and reduction in the emergence of drug resistance, which has been shown in Southeast Asian areas of low to moderate malaria transmission. Experience in Africa with antimalarial drug combination treatment in regions of intense malaria transmission in, however, is very limited despite ACTs are now the recommended treatment regimen for uncomplicated malaria. Table **6** shows a comparison of factors favoring and limiting implementation of artemisinin combination therapy in Africa.

Table 6: ACT use in Africa

Factors in Favor of
• Current inadequacy of first-line treatments in many countries, including possible hidden burdens of disease and death from malaria and chronic anemia,
• Potential for protecting effective and affordable antimalarial drugs currently available for future use,
• High clinical and parasitological cure rates,
• Absence of documented parasite resistance, and
• Potential for reducing transmission in areas of low to moderate transmission due to a reduction in gametocyte carriage,
Limiting Factors
• Potential misuse of artemisinin derivatives in view of their value in the treatment of severe malaria,
• Problems of compliance with non-co-formulated combinations, particularly at the household level,
• Higher cost of artemisinin derivatives,
• Lack of evidence for ACT delaying resistance in areas of high transmission, and
• Effort and cost of policy change.

The number of ACT treatments provided by governments of endemic countries for treatment of patients with uncomplicated *falciparum* malaria increased from approximately half a million treatment courses in 2001 to 31.3 million courses in 2005, 76 million courses in 2006, and reached a grant total of 278 million treatment courses in 2011 (Fig. **4**) [82]. Artemether-lumefantrine (AL) was the most frequently prescribed ACT with 77% share of the market in 2011. The second most commonly prescribed ACT by volume of treatment courses delivered was the combination of artesunate and amodiaquine which increased from less than 1 million treatment courses in 2007 to 63 million treatment courses in 2011 [82]. While most countries have implemented one ACT, a few have implemented different ACTs for different geographical regions, which can be seen in South Africa, Sudan, Peru, and Tanzania. Some countries like Uganda and Nigeria have implemented two ACTs for first-line treatment, however, only one ACT is provided by the Nigerian government.

2.6. WHO IMPLEMENTATION OF ACTS AS FIRST LINE "STANDARD OF CARE" IN 2001

ACTs have been proposed as the preferred first-line treatment option, and these drug combinations are the most frequently used treatment regimen in nations who have changed their antimalarial drug policies over the last ten years. Recently, WHO has endorsed ACTs as a "policy standard" for all countries with endemic *falciparum* malaria infections in their 2006 treatment recommendations [1], and this policy was updated in 2010 [23]. Given data on efficacy, the ACTs recommended for treatment of uncomplicated *falciparum* malaria include:

- Artemether-lumefantrine (AL),
- Artesunate-sulfadoxine-pyrimethamine (AS-SP)
- Artesunate-amodiaquine (AS-AQ),
- Artesunate-mefloquine (AS-MQ), and
- Dihydroartemisinin-piperaquine (DHA-PPQ)

While there are modest differences in bioavailability and absorption between the artemisinin analogues, there is no data suggesting a clinically significant difference when patients are treated with different artemisinin compounds. Ultimately, the pharmacokinetic and pharmacodynamic properties of partner drugs have a greater impact on ACT treatment efficacy, and data driven decisions should be made on which ACT combination is the best choice for a particular region. The rise and spread of drug resistance to partner drugs has a significant impact on ACT efficacy particularly given the increased incidence of artemisinin resistant parasites who present clinically with delays in parasite clearance. In addition to the four initial ACT combinations previously discussed that were recommended treatment of malaria infections with *P. falciparum*, there is a growing body of data on the efficacy and safety of dihydroartemisinin plus piperaquine (DHA-PPQ) which was added to the list of ACT drug combination alternatives listed by the WHO for malaria treatment in 2010 [23].

For the next decade, no alternative drugs to the artemisinin analogues are available, which have similar properties of rapid killing across multiple stages of parasite development. Accordingly, the WHO has focused its energies on maximizing use of ACTs. The ACT combinations have been shown to help contain drug resistance in *P. falciparum* parasites to both artemisinin and collaborate drugs. Sadly, however, the indiscriminate use of artemisinin and partner drug monotherapies has led to the emergence and spread of resistant to both drug partners [1, 23].

In January 2006, the WHO made a major appeal to drug manufacturers to stop making and marketing artemisinin monotherapy drugs and work on producing and marketing quality ACT drug combinations consistent with whose policies [4].

This campaign was broadly promoted *via* WHO Offices and through WHO briefings of national health ministry staff at national and regional meetings. The vast majority of suppliers and funding agencies have been willing to cease making or funding oral artemisinin monotherapy drugs. In April 2006, the Global Malaria Program of the WHO gave a presentation to 25 drug companies producing and selling artemisinin monotherapy drugs. Of these 25 firms, 15 firms openly stated they would be willing stop producing and selling artemisinin monotherapy drugs, however, 10 companies were not willing to make the same commitment (meeting report available at: www.who.int/malaria/docs/Meeting_briefing19April.pdf). Furthermore, nations hosting significant pharmaceutical companies making artemisinin monotherapy drugs, such as Pakistan and China, have been targeted for visits by WHO to further discuss what can be done at the national level to limit production by domestic manufacturers in both countries of artemisinin monotherapy drugs sold in areas with endemic *falciparum* malaria.

In May 2007, the 60th World Health Assembly committed to strong measures to limit the production and sale of oral artemisinin monotherapy drugs, and they agreed to resolution WHA60.18, which states:

- Countries were urged to stop providing oral artemisinin monotherapies in both the public and private sectors, commit to promoting implementation of artemisinin-combination therapy drugs, and work to implement national guidelines prohibiting manufacture, distribution, advertising, and sale of counterfeit antimalarial drugs;

- International funders, and non-government organizations were requested to stop funding the manufacture and sale of oral artemisinin monotherapy drugs, and to support public health campaigns to outlaw manufacture and sale of counterfeit antimalarial drugs;

The benefits associated with ACT treatment have made them an essential component of modern efforts to decrease morbidity and mortality associated with *falciparum* malaria infections, and the preservation of these drugs for future generations is the challenge of this generation [82].

CHAPTER 3

Clinical Significance of Antimalarial Combinations

Abstract: Combination therapies composed of new antimalarial therapeutics with distinctly different parasite targets and mechanisms of action are the best tools to enhance treatment of uncomplicated *falciparum* malaria and delay the appearance and expansion of drug resistant malaria. The efficacy of artemisinin combination therapies is the most relevant criteria for evaluating drug combinations. The demonstrated values of an ACT to improve clinical outcomes and delay emergence and spread of parasite drug resistance were all factors in the decision by the WHO to recommend that ACTs be used as the best treatment for treating uncomplicated infections with *P. falciparum* malaria in Asia and Africa. As discussed in the last chapter, the list of recommended ACTs includes dihydroartemisinin-piperaquine, artemether-lumefantrine, artesunate-mefloquine, artesunate-sulfadoxine-pyrimethamine, and artesunate-amodiaquine. All of these combinations have been shown to be efficacious; however, efficacy of an ACT is affected by resistance to either drug partner. The cost of artemisinin analogues derivatives is a significant contributor to the increased cost of ACT treatment courses. A research project called the artemisinin project was initiated to develop an inexpensive method of semi-synthetic production of artemisinins through fermentation rather than deriving artemisinin analogues by extracting artemisinin from the sweet wormwood plant. A cheaper manufacturing method will make ACTs more affordable, and it will be possible to increase distribution to patients in need. Innovations that facilitate production of cheaper ACTs will enhance the odds of a full recovery from *falciparum* malaria infections with decreased side effects and limit the emergence and spread of drug resistant parasites. Through vigorous efforts to enhance manufacture of inexpensive artemisinins coupled with improved prescription and enhanced patient compliance, the artemisinin drug combinations may still be effective for decades to come.

Keywords: Action mode, adverse effects, Artemether- lumefantrine, artesunate-amodiaquine, artesunate-mefloquine, clinical recovery, dihydroartemisinin-piperaquine, low cost, parasitological cure, therapeutic efficacy.

3.1. SYNERGISM OF ANTIMALARIAL DRUG COMBINATIONS

The utilization of antimalarial combinations to treat malaria may affect multiple targets within a single parasite, multiple subpopulations of a number of parasites, or multiple diseases simultaneously as many antimalarial drugs have activity against other diseases of related parasites. One example of treatment of multiple diseases from related parasites is the use of atovaquone-proguanil, which is commonly prescribed for treatment of toxoplasmosis and babesiosis. Combinations of drugs with distinct mechanisms are believed to enhance efficacy leading to reduced morbidity and mortality. The possible outcomes that may be noted for drug

Qigui Li and Mark R. Hickman

combinations with additive or synergistic effects include: 1) enhanced efficacy, decreased drug dose for each partner drug while achieving similar or better treatment efficacy and avoiding toxicity; 2) decreasing the emergence and spread parasite drug resistance; and 3) and achieving drug synergy against a particular target or actually providing toxicity antagonism against a partner drug to protect the patient. To achieve these treatment benefits, the combination of drugs have been broadly used. It has become first-line treatment options for life-threatening diseases such as malaria, HIV, and TB. If a combination of drugs is synergistic, it is favorable because the doses of the partner drugs may be reduced which maintains antimalarial efficacy while minimizing side effects [87]. Interactions between antimalarial drugs of various classes have been known for many years, and partner dose reduction is a significant benefit of antimalarial combination therapy that can address this issue.

Antimalarial drugs are believed to interact when the potency of two or more drugs combined in an assay of antimalarial activity is either higher giving a synergistic effect (also known as potentiation) or a similar effect (also known as an additive effect) or a decreased effect (also known as antagonism). The effects would not be expected from the individual activities of each drug. Interaction in this sense does not usually, but might, imply actual physical contact between the different drugs in question. More often, the activity of drug A is affected by drug B and/or *vice versa* because of the molecular interactions of the drugs with components of the target parasites and the biochemical/physiological consequences of these interactions. It follows, therefore, that the existence and strength of drug interactions may tell us something about what the individual drugs do to parasites. Studies of drug interactions *in vitro* using cultured parasites are therefore commonly used as an adjunct to mechanistic studies on antimalarial drugs. From the point of view of controlling infectious disease, the effects of drug interactions on combination therapy or prophylaxis with antimalarial agents are important. It is common to use two or more antimalarial agents in combination in order to avoid treatment failure with a single agent. Conversely, combination therapy with two drugs known to be antagonistic is generally avoided. It is therefore essential to understand the nature of the interactions between drugs in clinical use and this information is used in the choice of new drug combinations.

Malaria in man is triggered by infection with four different *Plasmodium* species (human infections with a fifth species, *Plasmodium knowlesi*, which primarily infects primates is on the rise), and *P. falciparum* produces the majority of morbidity and mortality [65]. The complex developmental cycle of the parasite takes it through an Anopheline mosquito vector and into the human host *via* the saliva of the insect. Sporozoites injected during a blood meal invade hepatocytes, and after intracellular growth and multiplication, new parasites are released as merozoites. Drugs that kill liver-stage parasites are often called tissue schizonticides. Merozoites, in turn, invade erythrocytes, in which they can follow one of two developmental pathways. The majority of parasites undergo asexual replication, and these parasites are then released as new merozoites. This cycle, which lasts approximately 48 hours in *P. falciparum*, is associated with clinical disease. Drugs acting on asexual, intra-erythrocytic stages are often called blood schizonticides, and blood schizonts are the target stage of most antimalarial drugs. The alternative pathway of development in erythrocytes leads (after approximately 14 days in *P. falciparum*) to the formation of male and female gametocytes, which are responsible for sexual reproduction and transmission through mosquitoes. Some drugs have activity on gametocytes, but this is not a common property of most antimalarial compounds [88].

3.1.1. *In Vitro* Drug Interactions between Antimalarial Agents

Drug interaction studies using cultured, asexual intraerythrocytic human or rodent parasites are easy to set up once the culture techniques have been mastered. A number of *in vitro* drug combination studies have been reported on the potency and pharmacokinetic interactions of artemisinin analogues with other antimalarial compounds [14, 88] (Table **7a & b**). Combinations of artemisinin analogues have shown synergism, for example, with tetracycline and mefloquine, additive effects with chloroquine, primaquine, and doxycycline, and antagonistic effects with pyrimethamine [89, 90]. The combination of artemether-lumefantrine has been shown to result in synergism while the combination of artesunate-pyronaridine has been shown to result in antagonism [91, 92]. Azithromycin has been shown to achieve synergistic to additive effects when combined to quinine or artemisinin compounds and it has been shown to have no cross-resistance with traditional antimalarials [93]. Some individual *in vitro* studies of combination synergism are described below.

Table 7a: Selected publications of *in vitro* drug interaction studies of non-artemisinin derivatives with other drugs [88]

Parasite Strains*	Compound A	Compound B	Drug Interaction Effect
F-32	Amodiaquine	Quinine	Synergism
K39, 1B-B5, QC-13, FCB, PKDSII	Sulphadoxine	Pyrimethamine	Synergism
	Dapsone	WR99210	Synergism
K39	Dapsone	WR158122	Synergism
K39	Dapsone	WR158122	Synergism
K39	Sulphisoxazole	WR99210	Synergism
K39	Sulphisoxazole	WR158122	Synergism
K39	Sulphisoxazole	WR159412	Synergism

Table 7a: contd...

D6	Quinine	WR 148999	Synergism
W2	Mefloquine	WR 148999	Synergism
W-2, C2B	Cycloguanil	Atovaquone	Synergism
K1, FCR3, K1, LS25, T996, K1, NGATV01, W-2, D6, C2B	Proguanil	Atovaquone	Synergism
Dd2	Proguanil	Atovaquone	Synergism

*Unless otherwise stated, inhibition of growth/development of blood-stage parasites was tested. antagonism; antagonism in the strains listed but not in one or more other strain(s); synergism; synergism in the strains listed but not in one or more other strain(s).

Table 7b: Selected publications of *in vitro* drug interaction studies of artemisinin derivatives with other drugs [14, 88]

Parasite Strains*	Compound A	Compound B	Drug Interaction Effect
W2, D6	Artemisinin	WR148999	Synergism
K1, NF54	Artemisinin	Chloroquine	Antagonist to additive
FCR-3, K-1	Artemisinin	Quinine	Synergism
FCR-3	Artemisinin	Mefloquine	Synergism
D6, W2	Artemisinin	Erythromycin	Synergism
(Most of 31 isolates)	Artemisinin	Doxycycline	Synergism
T-996, LS-21	Artemether	Lumefantrine	Synergism
RSA11	Artesunate (AS)	Chloroquine	Antagonist to additive
7G8, S007	Dihydroartemisinin	Clindamycin	Synergism
(8 Strains)	Dihydroartemisinin	Atovaquone	Antagonist to additive
NF54, K1, D10, RSA11	Artemisinin, AS	Mefloquine	Synergism
NF54, K1	Artemisinin	Tetracycline	Synergism
31 Isolates (Thailand)	Artemisinin, AS	Doxycycline	Synergism/additive
D10, RSA11	Artesunate	Quinine	Synergism
D10, RSA11	Dihydroartemisinin, AS	Chloroquine	Antagonist to additive
D10, RSA11	Artesunate	Pyrimethamine	Antagonism
T996, LS-21	Artemether	Lumefantrine	Synergism
3D7, NF54	Artesunate	Pyronaridine	Antagonism
73 fresh isolates	Artesunate	Azithromycin	Additive to synergism
F-32, FCR-3, K1	Artemisinin	Atovaquone	Synergism
37 fresh isolates	Artemisinin	Atovaquone-proguanil	Synergism
FCB, 3D7	Artemisinin	Riboflavin	Additive
3D7	Artemisinin	Triclosan	Mild Synergism
3D7	Artemisinin	Ketoconazole	Antagonism
FC27, T996, 3D7, 106/1, K1, RSA11, 7G8-m dr, 34-1/E	Dihydroartemisinin	Piperaquine	Antagonism
	Dihydroartemisinin	Amodiaquine	Antagonism
	Artemisinin	Retinol	Synergism

*Unless otherwise stated, efficacy against blood-stage infections in mice was tested.
Antagonism; antagonism in the species/strains listed but not in one or more other species/strain(s); synergism; synergism in species/strains listed but not in one or more other species/strain(s).

The interactions of artemisinin with quinine, atovaquone, mefloquine, and quinine were tested using three different strains of *P. falciparum* using an *in vitro* potency test [94]. The *falciparum* parasites were cultured for 48 hours in the presence of two different drugs at one time in different concentrations and proportions. The atovaquone-artemisinin combination showed a range of effects from additive to synergistic at proportions of atovaquone/artemisinin considered relevant to doses achieved in patients *in vivo*, and synergism was noted with combinations of artemisinin and mefloquine or quinine. Synergism of atovaquone and artemisinin was further enhanced by adding proguanil to make a three-drug combination [95]. Existing *in vitro* data has long shown the combination of atovaquone-proguanil is efficacious; however, the efficacy of the atovaquone-proguanil drug combination can be further enhanced by artesunate, a water-soluble derivative of artemisinin (Table **7a**).

The combination of riboflavin with artemisinin was shown to be additive, and the combination was shown to provide markedly increased activity against *falciparum* schizonts *in vitro* when compared to the activity of each agent by itself [96]. The interactions of artemisinin with triclosan or ketoconazole were tested against *P. falciparum* parasites using a fixed-ratio isobologram method, and artemisinin was shown to have a mild synergism when combined with triclosan, and an antagonistic effect *in vitro* ranging from modest to pronounce when combined with ketoconazole [97]. In a drug interaction test, artemisinin did not demonstrate synergism or antagonism when combined with a new orally bioavailable antimalarial, pafuramidine, or pafuramidine's active metabolite, DB75 [98]. These antiplasmodial drug interactions, however, require *in vivo* confirmation to insure the synergistic or antagonistic interactions shown *in vitro* are real.

Piperaquine, which was developed in the 1970s, has been resurrected as an antimalarial drug acting as the long-lived antimalarial partner to dihydroartemisinin. The combination of DHA-piperaquine demonstrates strong potency *in vitro*, and drug interaction assays have shown that piperaquine combined with dihydroartemisinin, chloroquine, and amodiaquine demonstrated results that ranged from indifferent activity tending towards antagonism [99]. A new combination using retinol appears to have promise as an antimalarial treatment when combined with artemisinin analogues, and the combination of retinol with an artemisinin derivative demonstrates significant synergistic antimalarial activity [100]. The results of these studies demonstrated that a novel artemisinin analogue, artemisone, shows increased potency *in vitro* over artesunate against multidrug-resistant *P. falciparum*. When artemisone was combined with chloroquine, atovaquone, or pyrimethamine *in vitro*, the combination showed a slightly antagonistic trend, while the *in vitro* assessment of the combination of artemisone-mefloquine or artemisone-lumefantrine demonstrated antimalarial synergism. These findings are consistent with prior study data obtained with other artemisinin derivatives [101].

Drug interaction data *in vitro* provides the basis for continued research of drug combinations in animal models to confirm the synergistic, additive, or antagonistic effects observed. The *in vivo* animal efficacy data, in turn, provides the basis for selecting potential combination partners to be tested in the field against *falciparum* malaria in man. There are several reports of synergism between the artemisinins and quinine or mefloquine, and these findings could result from the different but related actions of the two groups on heme in the digestive vacuole. Mefloquine has demonstrated synergy with artemisinin compounds, and clinically, mefloquine is being used as a combination drug with the artemisinins for treatment of uncomplicated malaria especially in Southeast Asia where drug resistance is particularly prevalent. By contrast, there are reports of strain-specific antagonism between the artemisinins and chloroquine, which may preclude their combination for clinical treatment [99] (Table **7b**).

The combination of azithromycin with fast artemisinin derivatives was shown to be efficacious for uncomplicated *falciparum* malaria treatment in Phase 2 clinical trials. One particular study was aimed at establishing the best ratios of drugs to be combined for azithromycin with quinine or dihydroartemisinin. The study was conducted, to determine whether the *in vitro* synergisms noted translated into enhanced efficacy *versus* each drug alone. The parasites in this study were assessed using *in vitro* potency to determine IC_{50} values against quinine, chloroquine, and mefloquine, and the values determined showed an IC_{50} of 11.4 ng/ml against mefloquine, while IC_{50s} against quinine of 64.4 ng/ml and 54.5 against chloroquine suggested resistance against the latter two drugs. A correlation between the *in vitro* results for quinine and parasite clearance suggests sensitivity to this drug combination ($R = 0.53$; $P = 0.001$). The combination of azithromycin and DHA showed a weaker correlation ($R = 0.34$; $P = 0.038$), while no significant correlation was seen for azithromycin as a single agent [102]. The *in vitro* data suggests artemisinin analogues combined with azithromycin or azithromycin combined with quinine provides interactions that range from additive to synergistic, no azithromycin cross-resistance was observed against traditional antimalarials, and other studies have observed substantial antimalarial activity of azithromycin as a single agent [102].

The sensitivity of *P. falciparum* parasites to the combination of artemether and lumefantrine, alone, and in combination, was tested *in vitro* using a multi-drug resistant Thai strain (T-996) and an Indian chloroquine-resistant strain (LS-21). Both strains were sensitive to artemether alone or lumefantrine alone. The combination of artemether and lumefantrine examined on an equimolar basis tested in different ratios between 100:1 and 1:100 showed significant synergism against both malaria strains, particularly at the IC_{90} and IC_{99} levels. This synergistic phenomenon is similar to the synergy observed between artemisinin analogues and mefloquine. This synergism was, first seen in laboratory models and later studies confirmed this synergism in clinical treatment in the field. Preliminary pharmacokinetic information suggests that the intended oral dose regimen of an artemether: lumefantrine drug combination would provide coverage for artemether (t½ of 1-2 hours) in the early phase of dosing and coverage with lumefantrine (t½ of 60 hours) over 3-5 days. Dosing with lumefantrine was shown to result in concentration increases until day 2 or day 4, respectively, and a relatively slow reduction until day 7. Recent experience with the simultaneous therapeutic administration of mefloquine and artemether or artesunate in areas with mefloquine-resistant *P. falciparum* indicates that the earlier laboratory-based observation of synergism between mefloquine and artemisinin derivatives actually does translate into clinical treatment [25]. Such synergism has also been confirmed in a *P. falciparum in vitro* model simulating the interaction of artemisinin and mefloquine *in vivo* [103].

3.1.2. *In vivo* Drug Interactions Between Antimalarial Agents

The additive and synergistic effects of artesunate with other antimalarial drugs were tested *in vitro* against *falciparum* strains resistant and sensitive to both mefloquine and chloroquine. The initial findings from this study have demonstrated that the combination of artesunate and mefloquine has an additive inhibitory effect against *falciparum* parasites that are both mefloquine-sensitive and resistant, and a synergistic effect was observed against chloroquine-sensitive or resistant *falciparum* strains [104]. Today, it is generally accepted that the phenomenon of synergism and additivity noted with the combination of artesunate and mefloquine actually increases the clinical efficacy of both drugs, and this combination has proven of value in delaying the emergence of resistance to either drug [105]. The combination of artemisone, a novel artemisinin analogue, with chloroquine and with clindamycin has been shown to have a synergistic effect when tested *in vivo* in animal efficacy studies using the chloroquine-resistant NS strain of *P. yoelii* [106]. An additive antimalarial effect was shown in an efficacy model with rodent malaria for the combination of dihydroartemisinin and doxycycline as well as the combination of pyronaridine and artesunate [92, 107]. Based on these and other data, the WHO has recommended an array of artemisinin combination treatments for uncomplicated malaria as shown in Table **8**.

Table 8: *In vivo* synergistic and antagonistic interactions between antimalarial agents in animal models [88, 92, 106, 107]

Test System*	Compound A	Compound B	Drug Interaction Effect
P. yoelii HAL	Tafenoquine	Halofantrine	Antagonist to additive
P. berghei N	Fenozan B07	Artesunate	Synergism
P. berghei ANKA	Chloroquine	Arteflene	Synergism
P. berghei ANKA	Quinine	Arteflene	Synergism
P. yoelii NS	Halofantrine	Fenozan	Synergism
P. yoelii NS	Pyronaridine	Fenozan	Antagonist to additive
P. yoelii nigeriensis N-67	Pyrimethamine	Azithromycin	Synergism
P. yoelii nigeriensis N-67 (sporozoite-induced)	Pyrimethamine	Azithromycin	Synergism
P. vinckei petteri 106WH	Artemether	Mn-TPPSc	Antagonist to additive
P. berghei NY	Pyronaridine	Artesunate	Synergism
P. berghei, P. yoelii	Mefloquine	Artemisone	Synergism
P. berghei ANKA	Doxycycline	Dihydroartemisinin	Additive

*Unless otherwise stated, efficacy against blood-stage infections in mice was tested.
Antagonism; antagonism in the species/strains listed but not in one or more other species/strain(s); synergism; synergism in species/strains listed but not in one or more other species/strain(s); TPPS, meso-tetrakis(4-sulphonatophenylporphyrin).

The artemisinin series of compounds are all expected to interact with the malaria parasite in a similar manner, and as one might expect, no synergism or antagonism between artemisinin compounds has been reported. This not true, however, of other endoperoxides such as the trioxanes. Fenozan B07, a trioxane compound, was found to be synergistic with artesunate against *P. berghei* in a murine infection model [108], and the combination of the tetraoxane WR148999 with artemisinin was shown to be synergistic in drug combination studies conducted *in vitro* against *P. falciparum* [109]. The mechanism by which these combinations of endoperoxide drugs achieve synergism is unclear, and there has been little discussion of combining an artemisinin with another endoperoxide for treatment purposes.

The synergy observed *in vitro* of artemisone combined with lumefantrine or mefloquine was comparable to the reports of drug synergy reported for the combination of artesunate with mefloquine, and this *in vitro* finding was reproduced *in vivo* [106]. The combination of piperaquine with the experimental endoperoxide OZ277 or artemether (AM) was evaluated *in vitro* against *falciparum* malaria and *in vivo* using *P. berghei* parasites [110]. The *in vitro falciparum* test data showed that the combination of piperaquine with OZ277 and the combination of piperaquine with artemether show a small degree of antagonism and, *in vivo*, artemether and piperaquine were shown to demonstrate borderline drug antagonism. Additive activity was observed, however, during the *in vivo* assessment of the combination of OZ277 and piperaquine suggesting that each molecule would demonstrate its individual full effect when dosed in malaria-infected patients. Artemisone and artesunate have also been shown to display a similar interaction pattern when these drugs were combined with standard antimalarials [106].

The sesquiterpene peroxide Ro 42-1611, arteflene, was tested against a variety of drug-resistant and drug-sensitive *in vitro* against *falciparum* malaria, and against *P. berghei* infected mice *in vivo*, and *in vitro*. Experimentally, the novel chemical entity, arteflene, has been shown to be a highly effective antimalarial drug, and *in vivo*, it is active at low doses against blood stages of *P. berghei* in mice after oral or parenteral administration. Drug interaction studies in *in vivo* and *in vitro* of arteflene combined with mefloquine, chloroquine, and quinine showed an additive to synergistic effect while antagonism with these drugs was not observed. Compared with standard antimalarials, the activity of arteflene *in vitro* is lower than would be expected from the *in vivo* results. This may be due to pharmacokinetic properties of the compound and the formation of an active metabolite, which sustains the activity of arteflene *in vivo* [111].

Tafenoquine, a novel 3-phenoxy-substituted 8-aminoquinoline, has been shown to have causal prophylactic, blood schizonticidal, and gametocytocidal efficacy against rodent malaria parasites. When tafenoquine was tested against blood stage parasites of the *P. berghei* N strain (known to be drug sensitive), tafenoquine is approximately nine times as active as primaquine (PQ). It is from four to 100 times as active *in vivo* as PQ against *P. berghei* or *P. yoelii* parasites that are resistant to currently used antimalarials. Tafenoquine is three times as active as PQ against the pre-erythrocytic stages of *P. yoelii nigeriensis*, but it has very poor gametocytocidal action and no sporonticidal activity against this parasite. In combination with chloroquine (CQ), tafenoquine and PQ have been shown to display a synergistic or 'resistance-reversing' action against CQ-resistant *P. yoelii* NS parasites. No such effects were seen when tafenoquine was combined with mefloquine against a mefloquine-resistant parasite or when tafenoquine was combined with artemisinin against an artemisinin-resistant parasite, and tafenoquine appears to be antagonistic to halofantrine when the combination was tested against a halofantrine-resistant parasite [112].

A difluorinated 3, 3'-spirocyclopentane called Fenozan B07 is a new antimalarial endoperoxide analogue with potent blood schizonticidal activity against rodent malaria parasites that are very resistant to a broad array of classic antimalarials. Similar to the artemisinins, the activity of Fenozan B07 is limited to the intra-erythrocytic stages, both asexual and sexual, and it is devoid of causal prophylactic activity. The combination of Fenozan B07 plus artesunate was tested against *P. varix*, and this drug combination was shown to be additive only in nature. A high degree of synergism was shown when the combination of Fenozan B07 plus artemisinin was tested *in vivo* against the rodent strain *P. yoelii* sp. NS. The conclusions drawn from these and other data support the hypothesis that there are significant differences between the blood schizonticidal actions of Fenozan B07 and the artemisinins [108].

The efficacy of sulfadoxine or pyrimethamine given together with azithromycin was assessed in a rodent model of malaria. Mice were initially inoculated with blood-stage rodent *Plasmodium* parasites, and the mice were administered azithromycin with and without sulfadoxine pyrimethamine starting at day 0 and ending on day 3. The efficacy of a variety of combinations of antifolates with azithromycin was tested with end-points defined ranging from a delay in patency to reach a parasitemia of 2% or a treatment cure. The results of this study showed the combination of azithromycin with sulfadoxine was shown to be curative. Similarly, in a test of causal prophylaxis conducted in mice infected with *P. yoelii*, a combination of one-sixteenth the dose of pyrimethamine and one-third the dose of azithromycin required for cure was administered, and this combination was shown to prevent liver stage infection. These results support the hypothesis that azithromycin combined with sulfadoxine-pyrimethamine may enhance treatment efficacy as opposed to treatment with sulfadoxine-pyrimethamine as a single treatment [113].

3.1.3. Drug Interactions Between Antimalarial Agents in Clinical Trials

Atovaquone-proguanil (Malarone^{TM}) has been shown to be efficacious for both malaria prophylaxis and treatment of uncomplicated *falciparum* malaria. The protective mechanism of this combination is believed to act *via* the mitochondrial cytochrome bc complex of *Plasmodium* which is a very different drug mechanism from other antimalarial drugs. For this reason, cross-resistance with other malaria drugs is not anticipated. Atovaquone monotherapy has been shown to result in treatment failure in 30% of patients, and monotherapy with proguanil has been shown to result in treatment failures in 90% of patients, while treatment failures are rare when a combination of these two drugs is used (<2%). The treatment failures for atovaquone monotherapy have been associated with rapid induction of drug resistance caused by a single point mutation in the target gene, cytb, which is mitigated by the synergism provided by proguanil. When used as a chemoprophylactic drug against *falciparum* malaria infections, Malarone™ has been shown to have efficacy greater than 95%. The safety and efficacy of Malarone™ as a malaria prophylaxis drug make it a suitable alternative to mefloquine and doxycycline where prophylaxis with either drug is contraindicated. Malarone™ is effective for treatment of uncomplicated malaria, and it may be used as an alternative to mefloquine for prophylaxis dosed on a daily basis rather than a weekly basis [114].

Emerging resistance of *P. falciparum* parasites to ACTs has been shown in western Cambodia, and this emerging resistance reinforces the ongoing need to develop new combinations of antimalarials. With reports from Malawi of the emergence of *falciparum* parasites that are chloroquine-sensitive because of a rigorously enforced ban on chloroquine sales, and a new report of synergism between chloroquine with azithromycin, a study was conducted to understand the *in vivo* efficacy of the combination of chloroquine and azithromycin. *In vivo* murine studies were performed at Walter Reed Army Institute of Research (WRAIR), and the results of these studies showed 99.9% suppression of *P. berghei* parasitemia after treatment with the combination of chloroquine and azithromycin added to the R-enantiomer of the calcium channel blocker, amlodipine. Pharmacokinetic and pharmacodynamic analyses conducted using a *P. berghei* rodent model and extrapolation of the dose to a 65-kg adult provided an estimate of the dose of R-amlodipine (1.8 g/day) needed to achieve efficacy in man. While these data suggest that amlodipine is not practical to be added to the combination of chloroquine- azithromycin, these studies support the hypothesis that azithromycin is an effective and safe partner drug for antimalarial combination treatment [115].

Pyronaridine was initially innovated in 1970 in China at the National Institute of Parasitic Diseases, and this drug has been used as a treatment agent for malaria in that country since that time. Pyronaridine has been shown to be very potent against *P. falciparum* parasites, including chloroquine-resistant strains. Conflicting data have been published regarding *in vitro* activity of pyronaridine when it is combined with other antimalarials. In one study, synergy was demonstrated between primaquine and pyronaridine, an additive effect was shown when pyronaridine was combined with drugs of the 4-aminoquinoline class, and weak antagonism was noted when pyronaridine was combined with antifolates, amino alcohols and dihydroartemisinin. Both synergistic and additive activity data have been published regarding the combination of pyronaridine and artemisinin. These differences are likely due to the method used for testing, and *in vivo* analysis have shown artemisinin and pyronaridine have a synergistic effect against *falciparum* parasites with native resistance to both of these drugs. Parasite drug resistance to pyronaridine has been noted appear slowly in the field, and this drug resistance is slowed when pyronaridine is administered in combination with antimalarials such as artesunate. Clinical studies conducted to treat patients infected with blood stage *falciparum* or *vivax* malaria using pyronaridine monotherapy or combination therapy have shown pyronaridine is efficacious for treatment of both blood stage infections. Pyronaridine has been combined with artesunate in a fixed dose combination comprised of 3 parts pyronaridine to 1 part artesunate to treat patients infected with uncomplicated cases of *falciparum* malaria and blood stage *vivax* malaria under the trade name Pyramax®, and this synergistic combination has received a positive review by the European Medicines Agency (EMA) [116].

3.2. ANTIMALARIAL DRUG COMBINATION EFFICACY MATCHING AND MISMATCHING

The efficacy of a combined drug treatment is the most relevant criteria for evaluating drug combinations. Accordingly, comparisons of efficacy of a drug combination can be shown by both clinical and parasitological cure combined with the speed of patient recovery. Clinical efficacy has been proposed as the best tool to evaluate questions of changing antimalarial treatment policies in the regions of Asia and Africa [23]. This metric could be used to evaluate the efficacy of antimalarial combination drugs. The parasitological cure rate is another important criterion as declines in cure rates have been linked to development of malaria drug resistance. The level of resistance of a parasite to a single drug is not considered useful as an evaluation parameter of a combination therapy, and *in vitro* resistance criteria have not yet been defined for combination therapies. The lower the IC_{50} observed for a particular drug the higher the probability that a combination drug will last longer for clinical use. Accordingly, the best partner drugs for a combination treatment are novel drugs not yet used for malaria monotherapy with no evidence of existing parasite drug resistance, which will not be used for malaria monotherapy.

3.2.1. Drug Combination Mode of Action Matching

The antimalarial efficacy of artemisinins is dependent upon alterations to its peroxide bridge. While the precise mode of action of the artemisinins has not yet been identified, it is believed that when the endoperoxide bridge is broken, artemisinin drugs cause alkylation of malaria proteins and free radical damage to various malaria organelles. The free radical release is catalyzed by intraparasitic iron and/or heme that may explain the selectivity of artemisinin drugs for the malaria parasite. Although the endoperoxide bridge of the artemisinins appears to be essential for antimalarial efficacy, the intrinsic antimalarial efficacy of the artemisinins appears to be too high to be explained by general oxidative damage. These drugs appear to have a number of specific parasite targets affected by generation of carbon-centered free radicals created by artemisinin breakdown while classic oxidants produce only oxygen-free radicals. By contrast, one mechanism by which quinoline and related compounds are believed to act is by chemical inhibition of heme polymerization, a critical detoxifying step required the malaria parasite to survive [61].

Two factors are relevant when choosing drug combinations with the aim of increasing antimalarial efficacy and containing the emergence and spread of drug resistant parasites - distinct but synergistic mechanisms of action, and an effective pharmacokinetic match. Quinolines, antifolates, and artemisinins have been deployed in a variety of combination treatments with each other to meet the two goals of enhancing antimalarial efficacy and delaying the emergence of drug resistance. For the majority of artemisinin combination therapies on market, such as artesunate- mefloquine, the non-artemisinin partner drug is slowly eliminated providing efficacy against parasites left alive after the artemisinin component drug has been cleared.

The minimum parasiticidal concentration (MPC) is defined as the minimum blood or plasma concentration capable of producing the maximum inhibitory activity of a drug, and this value can be approximated by the *in vitro* IC_{99} value [61]. Given a reduction in parasite biomass of 1,000-fold per cycle, which is common for many classic antimalarials, the minimum parasiticidal concentration (MPC) must be maintained for a period beyond four replication cycles to provide high malaria cure rates. Therefore, as artemisinin analogues reduce the majority of the parasite biomass during the rapid initial action, an effective drug partner with a long elimination half-life can usually eliminate the few remaining parasites. In addition, the probability of spontaneous mutation in a malaria parasite to two drugs each with distinct mechanisms of action is very low [9]. Consequently, ACTs provide the best combination with an excellent antimalarial efficacy match.

Many factors that might influence efficacy with antimalarial chemotherapy include the duration of the prescribed drug regimen. When treating patients in infected with uncomplicated malaria, the goal of treatment is to cut the parasite biomass to zero, or to a level so low host defenses can deal with the few remaining parasites, while the aim of severe malaria treatment is to save the patient's life. ACT treatment regimens that have a rapidly eliminated drug component must generally cover four asexual life cycles to insure all blood stage parasites have been killed. The concentration of slowly eliminated drugs must be higher than the minimum inhibitory concentration for that parasite, and preferably, the concentration should exceed the minimum parasiticidal concentration until all parasites are dead. Ring stage and mature schizonts are the two stages that are the most drug-resistant in a blood infection.

The majority of antimalarial drugs on market are primarily active against sequestered *falciparum* parasites not visible to the microscopist. The impact of this includes drug inhibition of trophozoite development and a considerable reduction in the rate of parasite multiplication. As drug susceptibility is dependent on the stage of development, timing of drugs to be administered to kill the dominant stage may determine the therapeutic response. The timing of dosing by stage to achieve maximum efficacy is called chronotherapy. Antimalarial treatment with quinolines and antifolates, and possibly other compounds can be maximized if peak drug levels are administered at the same time of development of the most sensitive mature stage of parasite development. This is quite difficult to in practice. In early Chinese studies of the artemisinins, treatment was initiated only when the majority of parasites were at the tiny-ring stage of development which, in theory, maximized the effect of the artemisinin drugs [65; unpublished data derived at WRAIR]. The advantages of chronotherapy must be established, and this is a research area that requires more data. The frequency of antimalarial drug administration is commonly determined by pharmacokinetic considerations, not efficacy considerations [117].

The quinoline and antifolate antimalarial drugs, by contrast, are long acting, and these drugs act by only killing mature parasites while the artemisinins are fast acting and eliminate immature ring stage parasites. The combination of these two classes of drugs provide low risks of drug resistance and recrudescence, and artemisinin based combination therapy can be conducted in a shorter treatment period, with better patient compliance [14]. Similar to infections of HIV and tuberculosis, malaria may not respond to treatment with drugs possessing matching modes of action. It is easy to understand why malaria parasites might not be killed by an antimalarial treatment if the partner drugs were not taken as prescribed, or the parasites were intrinsically resistant to the drugs given [5, 35].

3.2.2. Compatible Half-Life Matching of Drug Combination Compounds

The fever clearance time noted in patients administered artemisinin is only 32 hours as compared with a fever clearance time of 2-60 days noted in patients treated with older drugs. To delay the emergence of drug resistant parasites, artemisinins are administered in combination with one of a limited array of partner drugs with long half-lives such as amodiaquine, lumefantrine, mefloquine, piperaquine, and sulfadoxine-pyrimethamine, which provide coverage for residual parasites left alive after the artemisinin partner treatment. The pharmacokinetics of artemisinin combination drugs is quite complex. The artemisinins have very short half-lives, and their longer- lived partner drugs are dependent on achieving high drug concentrations in the plasma of patients to achieve efficacy [14, 61].

Conventionally, a drug should be administered at intervals roughly corresponding to its biological half-life, and the biological half-life of an antimalarial drug should be estimated in patients infected with malaria and not extrapolated from studies conducted on healthy volunteers. If the antimalarial drug provides efficacy only during the period where its concentration remains above a therapeutic level, then the biological half-life of that drug corresponds to the drug elimination half-life. If concentration-dependent killing and biological effects are observed well after the drug concentration has decreased below the therapeutic level, however, then the drug can be administered less often than one might predict given the elimination half-life of the drug shown by pharmacokinetic studies. The drug dose and interval of dosing should be coordinated to provide concentrations of antimalarial drugs sufficient for clinical and parasitological cure in non-immune patients. The rationale for this is antimalarial drug-treatment regimens are consistently more effective in patients who are semi-immune than in non-immunes, and, in some instances, shorter courses of treatment with lower doses of antimalarial treatment can be given to semi-immunes which are well below what is needed for non-immune patients [118].

The existing studies suggest that while artesunate is rapidly absorbed and the half-life of artesunate and dihydroartemisinin, the active metabolite of artesunate, is less than 1 hour, oral artesunate is equally efficacious if it is given once or twice daily [78]. This finding suggests that the biological effect of the artemisinins extends beyond their physical presence at therapeutic concentrations. The activity of artemisinins against a broad array of different developmental stages in the blood ensures that administration of drug once daily for a few hours in each asexual life cycle is sufficient to achieve efficacy. This challenges the idea that antimalarial drugs must be present in the blood at parasiticidal levels through the entire dosing interval [61].

Cures of uncomplicated malaria are assured if drug concentrations of antimalarials provide efficacy until all of the malaria parasites are killed. For slowly eliminated drugs, the AUC or integral of the concentration-time curve is a very useful predictor of efficacy as the AUC encompasses both drug concentration and exposure [118]. Provided the parasite reduction ratios of greater than 1,000 fold are achieved by the antimalarial drug per replication cycle, *P. falciparum* infections in man can be reliably cured [17, 118]. For slowly eliminated antimalarials like the quinoline or antifolate drugs whose elimination half-life is greater than 24 hours, the concentration of drug in the blood or plasma on day 7 has been shown to correlate well with the AUC and treatment response [118].

The principle of combining artemisinin derivatives with quinolines or antifolates drugs to create a combination therapy is based on the presence of the longer half-life partner drug which acts to kill residual parasites left over after artemisinin, a drug with a very short half-life, is no longer present [3, 86]. Combination of a long-lived antimalarial partner drug allows a reduction in the length of antimalarial treatment, which enhances efficacy and reduces the likelihood of the development of parasite drug resistance. The principal immediate effect of artemisinin drugs is to decrease the parasite biomass. The residual biomass will then be exposed to a maximum concentration of the long-lived partner drug at levels well above the minimum inhibitory concentration, providing a decreased likelihood of the survival of parasites with resistant mutations.

3.2.3. Matching Lead Quality Attributes of Combination Drugs for Malaria Treatment and Prevention

While rapid clinical improvement is the primary goal of patient treatment for uncomplicated malaria infections, the prevention of malaria transmission is an important secondary objective. Treatment with either counterfeit drug in sub-therapeutic drug levels or with compromised by incomplete patient compliance increases the treatment failure risk and provides pressure to select drug resistant parasites. Drug resistant parasites are equipped with a survival advantage as they are often associated with increased rates of gametocyte carriage in both primary and recrudescent infections [105]. Given the increased rate of gametocyte carriage of resistant parasites compared with decreased incidence of gametocyte carriage of drug sensitive parasites, there is a greater probability of transmission of resistant parasites, which thereby explains the spread of malaria drug resistance.

Artemisinin analogues are indirectly active against gametocytes, the sexual parasite stage that is taken up by the mosquito, and therefore artemisinins can reduce the rates of transmission. The artemisinin analogues do not kill the mature *P. falciparum* gametocytes, however, they do prevent the development of gametocytes by killing the early, and the more mature asexual-stage parasites and artemisinins are active against early gametocytes (stage I-III). Antimalarial drugs with efficacy against late stage asexual parasites like the quinolines are not as effective at interrupting gametocyte development.

An efficacy study conducted on the border of Thailand and Myanmar showed that patients treated with the combination of artesunate and mefloquine demonstrated a delayed clearance of parasites, and this delay in parasite clearance was associated with a higher probability of producing mature gametocytes [119]. Given the association of delays in parasite clearance with artemisinin resistance, quantitation of gametocytes after treatment may be a measure to assess artemisinin resistance and such increases in gametocytemia might suggest a higher transmission of artemisinin-resistant parasites. Initial screening studies of this phenomenon might only require microscopy on blood smears obtained on day 7 and on day 14 after the initiation of treatment. This data may be useful in informing investigators if sequestered immature gametocytes that are observed on Day 7 are actual mature gametocytes or ring stage parasites developing resistance to the artemisinins (ring stage parasites require 14 days to become mature gametocytes).

Some reports have shown that in areas of low malaria transmission on the borders of Thailand, accurate diagnosis and malaria treatment with a combination of mefloquine and artesunate has decreased the occurrence of malaria from *P. falciparum* and, in turn, stopped the spread of resistance to mefloquine [78]. Additional evidence of the benefits of this combination and other ACTs has been shown in other clinical trials in Southeast Asia. Mefloquine resistance was reversed in one study by the addition of artesunate, and the combination of AS-MQ showed a cure rate of over 95% in patients without hyperparasitemia [79]. Similar decreases in transmission of malaria have been observed following broad use of ACTs in South Africa and Vietnam [80]. The benefits of the artemisinin derivatives in patient treatment and in public health are not simply restricted to regions where drug resistant parasites are present.

Artemisinin combination therapies have been shown to reduce gametocyte carriage by a factor of five-fold compared to treatments with other quinoline drugs administered as monotherapy such as halofantrine, mefloquine, or quinine. Broad introduction of artemisinin analogues for malaria treatment has been shown to prevent the appearance and proliferation of parasites with drug resistance [68]. Therefore, artemisinin combination therapy has been shown to have significant benefits beyond enhanced efficacy for treatment of malaria and thus aids in the achievement of public health goals such as reduction in the transmission of malaria and preventing the spread of drug resistance [65].

3.3. IMPROVED CHEMOTHERAPY OF UNCOMPLICATED *FALCIPARUM* MALARIA WITH ACTS

3.3.1. Treatment of Uncomplicated Malaria

Uncomplicated malaria is characterized by development of malaria symptoms where the percentage of parasitized RBC is <5% and patients do not demonstrate symptoms associated with severe malaria such as organ failure. In patients infected with *falciparum* malaria, there is a range of disease observed from minor to serious. Young children under five and adults with no prior immunity infected with malaria can demonstrate rapid progression from mild to severe malaria. Any patient whom the physician suspects may have severe malaria based on symptoms and laboratory data should be treated promptly treated for severe malaria. The risks of having a patient expire for under-treated severe malaria are much higher than the risks associated with providing treatment of severe malaria to a patient who does not need it. There are two critical concepts when discussing the different treatment modes of malaria, which include both suppressive treatments and radical cures.

Concerning suppressive treatment, malaria symptoms are diminished by suppressing the growth of erythrocytic stage parasites. Suppressive therapy involves treatment with a blood schizonticidal drug to kill all of the parasites. In all cases of *vivax* malaria and some cases of *falciparum* malaria, suppressive therapy has been achieved by treatment with chloroquine. In areas with elevated transmission of malaria, it is wise to administer presumptive malaria treatment, which suggests in high transmission areas, one might presume that the majority of fever cases are caused by malaria. Initial therapy with an ACT should be conducted while a blood sample is drawn for diagnosis, and ACT treatment should be administered without waiting for a diagnostic result. If the diagnosis is indeed malaria, administration of ACT treatment allows for prompt treatment of disease and symptoms and avoids downstream problems due to severe malaria. If the fever symptoms are related to malaria infection, administration of an ACT also inhibits spread of drug resistant parasites, as the artemisinin component will act to destroy gametocytes and thus limit gametocyte carriage.

If the diagnosis of a potential fever turns out to be not caused by malaria, there are no adverse consequences associated with ACT administration, as administration of an ACT at a treatment dose is safe and there are no known consequences of toxicity associated with administration of an ACT treatment dose. To achieve reductions in parasite transmission, presumptive treatment in areas of high malaria transmission must be universally applied. This type of regimen is highly effective and it prevents the spread of *vivax* malaria.

Administration of ACTs to all individuals with confirmed malaria diagnoses ensures radical cure and inhibition of gametocyte carriage. About treatment of *vivax* malaria, treatment with primaquine for two weeks is necessary to eliminate dormant liver stage hypnozoites and prevent relapse infections. In patients with *falciparum* malaria treatment, including a single dose of primaquine will insure the destruction of all gametocytes, which will inhibit gametocyte carriage and spread of drug resistant parasites. Therefore, primaquine administration is necessary for preventing malaria cases, and two weeks of PQ treatment while inhibit gametocyte carriage for *vivax* malaria and a single dose of primaquine will inhibit gametocyte carriage in patients infected with *falciparum* malaria.

3.3.2. The Use of Currently Available ACTs for Treatment of Uncomplicated Malaria

Combination therapy is defined as the administration of two blood schizonticidal drugs with different mechanisms of action and dissimilar parasite targets. The component drugs of any antimalarial combination may be co-administered or co-formulated. Multiple drug therapies where neither drug has schizonticidal activity in blood stage as a single agent (*e.g.,* sulfadoxine-pyrimethamine) are not classified as combination therapy. Administration of a blood schizonticidal drug with a tissue schizonticidal drug is not considered combination therapy, nor is administration of a schizonticidal compound in blood stage together with a drug that has no antimalarial activity but merely enhances the activity of the blood stage drug. The value of artemisinin combination therapies lies in the ability of the drug combination to enhance treatment efficacy and delay development and spread of drug resistant parasites. These are all factors in the decision by the WHO to recommend that ACTs be recommended as the first-line therapy in Asia and Africa to treat uncomplicated *falciparum* malaria [69]. The choice of which ACT to use in a particular country is primarily based on the known level of partner drug resistance.

In Southeast Asia, artemether-lumefantrine and artesunate-mefloquine are recommended, while in Africa artesunate combined with lumefantrine, artesunate combined with sulfadoxine-pyrimethamine, and artesunate combined with amodiaquine are recommended. The artemisinin analogue of the combination must be administered for a period of 3 days, and artemether-lumefantrine should be administered in a regimen of 6 doses. Dihydroartemisinin-piperaquine is now suggested for worldwide treatment of *falciparum* malaria as a first line drug therapy. The drug combination of amodiaquine-sulfadoxine-pyrimethamine is an interim solution that may be employed in areas with rising resistance to monotherapy where ACTs cannot be provided.

Artemether-lumefantrine (AL)

The combination of artemether-lumefantrine (AL) is the first fixed dose co-formulated artemisinin combination therapy comprised of an artemisinin analogue with a second antimalarial drug. Artemether-lumefantrine tablets contain 20 mg of artemether and 120 mg of lumefantrine. The best course of treatment that has been shown to be most efficacious is a dosing regimen of six doses of the co-formulated tablet of artemether-lumefantrine administered two times a day over a 3-day period (Table **9**). When used to treat patients with drug resistant *falciparum* malaria, the regimen of six doses of AL has been shown to be efficacious, and this ACT has been shown to well tolerated, more so than the combination of artesunate-mefloquine. AL is becoming increasingly available in a number of endemic countries. The combination of these two drugs is, as mentioned, well tolerated, and the cost of this treatment is now down to $1.0 per treatment regimen for adults. There is a growing body of safety evidence for the use this

Use of artemisinin compounds in the first trimester is not recommended. One advantage to this artemisinin combination treatment is lumefantrine is not on market as a monotherapeutic treatment, and it has not been used as monotherapy in the field. This advantage is countered, to some extent, by the known cross-resistance of lumefantrine with mefloquine. Like many antimalarials, the absorption of lumefantrine is increased by co-administration with fat. Accordingly, providers must remind patients to take artemether-lumefantrine after a meal or after consuming a drink containing 1.2 grams of fat such as whole milk. A pediatric formulation of artemether-lumefantrine has been created for use in children, and this tablet is a dispersible formulation that is easily absorbed.

combination in pregnant patients in their second and third trimesters.

Table 9: Dosing schedule for artemether-lumefantrine (AL)

Body weight in kg (age in years)	Number of tablets at approximate timing of dosing* 0 h	8 h	24 h	36 h	48 h	60 h
5 - 14 (<3)	1	1	1	1	1	1
15 - 24 (≥ 3 - 8)	2	2	2	2	2	2
25 - 34 (≥ 9 - 14)	3	3	3	3	3	3
>34 (>14)	4	4	4	4	4	4

* The regimen can be expressed more simply for ease of use at the program level as follows: the second dose on the first day should be given any time between 8 h and 12 h after the first dose. Dosage on the second and third days is twice a day (morning and evening) [1].

Artesunate Plus Amodiaquine (AS-AQ)

In recent years, resistance of *P. falciparum* to amodiaquine has increased substantially in parts of Southern and East Africa. After administration orally, amodiaquine is subsequently metabolized to desethylamodiaquine, which provides the majority of antimalarial activity of this compound. Amodiaquine has been well tolerated, and patients have been shown to have marginally better tolerability for amodiaquine than chloroquine. The combination of artesunate-amodiaquine is marketed as two individual tablets. One tablet contains 50 mg of artesunate and the other tablet contains 153 mg of amodiaquine. Amodiaquine-artesunate tablets that are co- formulated are being developed. The recommended course of AQ-AS therapy is 4 mg/kg of artesunate and 10 mg base/kg of amodiaquine administered daily for 3 days (Table **10**). This combination has been shown to be efficacious only in areas where the cure rates at 28-days for amodiaquine administered as monotherapy are greater than 80%. Parasite drug resistance is predicted to increase in areas where chloroquine and amodiaquine are administered as monotherapy. Prospective information on safety of this combination through pharmacovigilance programs in endemic areas is needed.

One of the first clinical comparative efficacy trials between AS-AQ and AL conducted by Martensson *et al.* in 2005 utilized a 42-day period of follow-up PCR adjusted cure rates, and analysis of genetic polymorphisms associated with resistance to quinoline drugs [120]. 408 children in Zanzibar, Tanzania with uncomplicated *falciparum* malaria were in this study. Children ranging from 6-8 months old weighing 6-8 kg was given AS-AQ over a 3-day period. Children ranging from 9-59 months old and weighing more than 9 kg were given either AS-AQ or AL over a 3-day treatment period. The data showed a 91% efficacy rate adjusted by PCR to measure efficacy at day in patients treated with AS-AQ while efficacy rates of 94% were observed in the AL treatment group [120]. In the AS-AQ group, 5 recrudescent infections were noted while 7 recrudescent infections were noted in the AL groups after day 28.

Table 10: Dosing schedule for artesunate + amodiaquine (AS+AQ)

Age	Dose in mg (Number of Tablets)					
	Artesunate (50 mg)			Amodiaquine (153 mg)		
	Day 1	Day 2	Day 3	Day 1	Day 2	Day 3
5 - 11 months	25 (1/2)	25	25	76 (1/2)	76	76
≥ 1 - 6 years	50 (1)	50	50	153 (1)	153	153
≥ 7 - 13 years	100 (2)	100	100	306 (2)	306	306
>13 years	200 (4)	200	200	612 (4)	612	612

The data was cited from a WHO Guideline [1].

Assuming 10 malaria episodes with equivocal PCR results were actually recrudescent infections, the PCR adjusted cure rated for AS-AQ decreased to 88% while the AL group showed a 92% cure rate by day 28. By day 42, unadjusted cure rates were 56% in the AS- AQ group while the unadjusted cure rates in the AL group were 77% (P <0.001). 36% of patients in the AS-AQ group were re-infected by day 42, while 17% of patients in the AL arm were re-infected by day 42 (P <0.001). A number of isolated parasites from patients with reinfections after AL treatment showed a 2.2 fold increase in the multidrug resistance gene allele 1-86N compared with isolates acquired after *falciparum* infection was initially diagnosed. Both AS-AQ and AL were shown to be very efficacious; however, AL was shown to provide better protection against malaria re-infection. The percentage of patients who showed recrudescence by day 28 along with the appearance of genetic polymorphisms associated with drug resistance to the AQ partner drug does reinforce the practice of conducting extended follow-up when performing clinical efficacy studies. A long period of follow-up and PCR testing for both parasite presence and drug resistance genetic markers should be a part of all clinical efficacy trials of antimalarial drugs [120].

A multi-center study was conducted from 2006 to 2007 to compare the fixed dose combination of AS-AQ against the fixed-dose combination of AL. Three patient treatment groups were assessed in this study. Two groups of patients were treated with AS-AQ administered either once or twice per day, and one patient group was administered with AL two times per day using standard doses. The goal of this study was to show at day 28 post treatment, that AS-AQ was non-inferior to AL.

The other objectives of this study involved comparing parasitological and clinical efficacy of AS-AQ and AL by day 28 in children fewer than 5 years of age along with evaluating the efficacy of AS-AQ administered either once or twice per day. Overall, total 3,153 patients were enrolled in this study, and the following outcomes were observed. By Day 28, 95.2-97.1% of patients treated with AS-AQ given once per day, and 95.5-98.2% of patients treated with AL showed both parasitological and clinical cures. Thus, AS-AQ was shown to be non-inferior in all groups treated, including children less than 5 years of age. Both treatment arms were well tolerated and the side effects observed were all those expected from other studies.

AS-AQ and AL were shown to be equally efficacious to treat African children with uncomplicated malaria, and few adverse effects associated with drug treatment were noted during the one-year follow-up period. One question remains regarding AS-AQ treatment, and that question revolves around the frequent isolation of parasites resistant to amodiaquine in Africa, which may jeopardize the utility of amodiaquine as an ACT drug partner. Answering this question in Africa is a decision that will require continuous monitoring and evaluation. This data also reinforces the idea of a minimum follow-up period of 28 days to assess ACT efficacy, the utilization of PCR genotyping of drug resistance polymorphisms in all parasites isolated from patients who failed therapy, and the use of Kaplan-Meier statistics to estimate treatment efficacy [121-123].

Artesunate Plus Sulfadoxine-Pyrimethamine (AS-SP)

Sulfadoxine-pyrimethamine is on market as a fixed dose combination of two antifolate drugs, sulfadoxine, a sulfonamide, and pyrimethamine. Artesunate-SP is marketed as two tablets, one tablet contains 50 mg of artesunate, and the second tablet contains a combination of 500 mg of sulfadoxine and 25 mg of pyrimethamine. The total recommended course of treatment is 4 mg/kg bodyweight of artesunate given daily for 3 days and a single dose of SP administered on day 1 of treatment (Table **11**). While a single tablet of sulfadoxine-pyrimethamine on day 1 is adequate for treatment, administration of artesunate is required daily for 3 days to ensure cures. This artemisinin combination therapy is efficacious only in areas where cure rates with SP administered as monotherapy have been shown to be greater than 80%. Drug resistance to SP will increase with ongoing use of sulfalene-pyrimethamine, sulfadoxine-pyrimethamine, sulfadoxine-pyrimethamine, and cotrimoxazole (trimethoprim-sulfamethoxazole) when used for malaria monotherapy. The combination of AS-SP is currently being used in South Asia, the Middle East, and regions of South America where drug resistance to SP is low.

Table 11: Dosing schedule for artesunate + sulfadoxine-pyrimethamine (AS-SP)

Age	Dose in mg (Number of Tablets)					
	Artesunate (50 mg)			Sulfadoxine-pyrimethamine (500/25 mg)		
	Day 1	Day 2	Day 3	Day 1	Day 2	Day 3
5 - 11 months	25 (1/2)	25	25	250/12.5 (1/2)	-	-
≥ 1 - 6 years	50 (1)	50	50	500/25 (1)	-	-
≥ 7 - 13 years	100 (2)	100	100	1000/50 (2)	-	-
>13 years	200 (4)	200	200	1500/75 (4)	-	-

The data was cited from a WHO guideline [1].

Artesunate Plus Mefloquine (AS-MQ)

The combination of artesunate with mefloquine for a 2- or 3-day treatment regimen of uncomplicated *falciparum* malaria has benefits for both efficacy and diminishing the spread of drug resistant parasites. This combination can be dosed with separate tablets of artesunate and mefloquine (4 mg/kg/day of artesunate and 25 mg base/kg/day mefloquine) or with a more recently developed fixed dose combination tablet (50 mg artesunate and 250 mg base mefloquine). Administration with scored tablets split in half to diminish the side effects of mefloquine, particularly gastrointestinal, is commonly performed (Table **12**).

Table 12: Dosing schedule for artesunate + mefloquine (AS+MQ)

Age	Dose in mg (Number of Tablets)					
	Artesunate (50 mg)			Sulfadoxine-pyrimethamine (500/25 mg)		
	Day 1	Day 2	Day 3	Day 1	Day 2	Day 3
5 - 11 months	25 (1/2)	25	25	-	125 (1/2)	-
≥ 1 - 6 years	50 (1)	50	50	-	250 (1)	-
≥ 7 - 13 years	100 (2)	100	100	-	500 (2)	-
>13 years	200 (4)	200	200	-	1000 (4)	-

The data was cited from a WHO guideline [1].

Mefloquine dosing has been evaluated experimentally by examining antimalarial efficacy at 15 mg base/kg/day and 25 mg base/kg/day. The 15 mg base/kg/day dose does not have adequate efficacy, and this dose is not recommended. To reduce the gastrointestinal effects of mefloquine and enhance absorption, the 25 mg base/kg dose is typically split and administered as 15 mg base/kg/day on day 2 and then 10 mg base/kg/day is administered on day 3 or administered as 8.3 mg base/kg/day over a 3-day period. Mefloquine is known to have a number of side effects to include vomiting, nausea, sleep disturbances, dysphoria, and dizziness, however, in field trials these symptoms are generally tolerated well by patients.

Dihydroartemisinin Plus Piperaquine (DHA-PPQ)

The combination of dihydroartemisinin and piperaquine (Artekin) was innovated in China, and it is registered in both Cambodia and China. Artekin is inexpensive costing $1.00 US for an adult treatment, and this low cost, efficacious drug is a good candidate for use in African and Asian countries endemic for malaria. Non-GMP Artekin has been tested in clinical trials in Cambodia and China [124, 125], Vietnam [126] and Thailand [127], and this combination has been shown to be well tolerated and efficacious even against multi-drug resistant strains [128]. GMP-Artekin being manufactured by Sigma-Tau Farmaceutiche Riunite ApA in Italy marketed as Eurartesim™, and this combination has been registered with the EU and is now recommended by the WHO.

The combination of DHA-PPQ is on market as a fixed-dose tablet comprised of 40 mg of DHA and 320 mg of PPQ. The dosing of DHA-PPQ for treatment of uncomplicated malaria is 4 mg/kg/day DHA and 18 mg/kg/day PPQ administered daily for 3 days. The therapeutic dose range for DHA ranges from 2-10 mg/kg/day and for PPQ the therapeutic dose range is from 16-26 mg/kg/day. In DHA-PPQ treatment groups of patients with uncomplicated malaria, the parasitological cure rates defined by PCR, both corrected and uncorrected, on day 42 were 96.3% (uncorrected PCR) and 97.3% (PCR corrected parasitological cure rate). Efficacy studies of DHA-piperaquine have shown very few adverse events that were mild in nature. Any abnormalities in hematology and blood chemistry values had no corresponding effect clinically. The combination of DHA-PPQ has been shown to be very efficacious, well tolerated, and safe for treatment of malaria. The combination of these two drugs is promising for first- line treatment for a number of countries and is under review for use in Indonesia [129].

Artesunate Plus Tetracycline or Clindamycin or Doxycycline

Artesunate and antibiotics such as tetracycline, clindamycin, or doxycycline are available as co-packaged blister forms. These combinations have been held in reserve for treatment of patients who have failed therapy with mainstream ACTs, and for use in special populations such as pregnant women with malaria who have failed ACT treatment. These combinations are separately dosed, and this combination should be reserved for use in an inpatient settings. The treatment dose for artesunate plus tetracycline or doxycycline or clindamycin is as follows:

artesunate dosed at 2 mg/kg/day once daily plus tetracycline dosed at 4 mg/kg administered four times per day or doxycycline dosed at 3.5 mg/kg dosed once daily or clindamycin dosed at 10 mg/kg administered twice per day. All of these combinations must be administered over a 7-day period given the short half-life of these partner drugs.

3.3.3. Efficacy of Current Recommended ACTs

The International Artemisinin Study Group [40] has concluded that ACTs provide better cure rates, more rapid parasite clearance and decreased carriage of gametocytes when compared to monotherapy. The WHO has also concluded that artemether-lumefantrine (AL) has shown parasitological cures >95%, despite its use in areas with multidrug resistant parasites [69, 86]. Results from trials in Africa have shown that the combinations of AS-AQ and AS-SP are highly efficacious, although the efficacy of AS-SP has been adversely affected due to growing SP resistance [130]. Accordingly, the AS-AQ combination is believed to have a longer useful life than AS-SP, and AS-AQ will likely be an effective tool far longer than AS-SP [131, 132]. A number of studies [133, 134] in sub-Saharan Africa have demonstrated that AS-AQ has efficacy >90% at 28- days (PCR corrected) however, another study showed efficacy of AS-AQ to be <90% [135].

The efficacy and safety of AQ-SP, AS-SP, and AS-AQ were assessed in the Congo in children ranging in age from 6-59 months who presented with uncomplicated malaria [136]. The results of this study showed that all three of these combinations were efficacious with rapid reductions in fever, showed few adverse effects, and all three treatments showed 100% efficacy clinically with reduced gametocyte carriage during the follow-up period of 14 days. In another location in the Congo, Swarthout *et al.* [137] demonstrated that AS-AQ administered to 90 children aged 0 -59 months infected with uncomplicated malaria, who were given 3 days treatment with AS-AQ, were no differences to in children with malaria treated for 3 days with AS-SP. AS-AQ was shown to be more efficacious, however, than the AS-SP combination.

Children with uncomplicated *falciparum* malaria who were administered a six-dose regimen of AL were shown to have reduced prevalence of gametocytes, a shorter period of gametocyte carriage, and reduced transmission of gametocytes to mosquitoes compared to children treated with a CQ-SP combination. At day 7 after treatment was initiated, none of the AL treated children were observed to have circulating parasites in contrast to children treated with CQ-SP where 37% of the children still presented with circulating parasites. There was no significant difference in clinical or parasitological treatment failures for the two treatments [138]. In Senegal, the tolerability and efficacy of AS-MQ, AS-AQ, AL (both 4 dose and 6 dose regimens) and AQ-SP were assessed for treatment of uncomplicated *falciparum* malaria in a multicenter study. The results of this study showed excellent parasitological and clinical responses of 100% with one exception, the four-dose AL regimen, which showed clinical efficacy rates of 96.4% [139]. Data derived from a similar set of studies in Sudan [140] and Ghana [141] demonstrated this ACT therapy is highly effective.

More recently, one clinical trial in Ghana showed AL and AS-AQ demonstrated cure rates in children infected with uncomplicated *falciparum* malaria ranging from 94.2-98.2% with few adverse events noted. Long term, however, the widespread prevalence of AQ resistant malaria parasites does raise the question of how long AQ can be used as an ACT partner drug in Ghana. Given this question, monitoring and evaluation of AS-AQ treatment efficacy rates will require ongoing monitoring [121].

A number of clinical trials have demonstrated repeatedly that the combination of DHA-PPQ is both efficacious and safe for use as an ACT treatment for uncomplicated *falciparum* malaria and *vivax* malaria in blood stage. DHA-PPQ has shown cure rates >95% with one exception in Papua New Guinea where a high number of treatment failures were observed. The possibilities of treatment failure in this study due to either cross-resistance between other quinolones and piperaquine or issues with increased resistance to artemisinin were examined critically and both possibilities have been ruled out which may implicate patient compliance as a causal factor. There is an abundance of data demonstrating the safety and efficacy of DHA-PPQ combination therapy. Given this data, DHA-PPQ was approved in 2011 by the European Medicines Agency for treatment of *falciparum* malaria. In addition, the DHA-PPQ combination treatment is now recognized as a first-line treatment option by WHO for treatment of uncomplicated *falciparum* malaria [142].

3.4. MINIMIZING OR SLOWING THE DEVELOPMENT OF DRUG RESISTANCE

Combining antimalarial drugs to minimize the potential for inducing parasite drug resistance has been shown to be effective in animal models to delay parasite resistance; however, delays in parasite resistance in human malaria by using combination therapy have not yet been demonstrated formally. A clear demonstration of formal proof is not easy to show experimentally. A growing body of circumstantial evidence exists, however, that supports the hypothesis that that malaria drug resistance can be delayed. Accordingly, the rationale for combining a fast acting artemisinin analogue with a slower acting antimalarial with a different mechanism of action makes sense particularly in regions showing minimal or mid-range malaria transmission which tend to be the areas where drug resistance emerges. Antimalarial drugs prone to resistance due to a single or double point mutation should not be used as monotherapy, and these drugs should be consistently administered with an artemisinin analogue [62]. More discussions that are detailed are available in Section 1.5 on the use of antimalarial drug combinations to delay the onset of resistance (**Chapter 1**).

3.5. DECREASING THE DRUG EXPOSURE LEVEL OR TIME TO AVOID TOXICITY

There is no data showing adverse drug interactions between any of the artemisinin derivatives and other long-lasting antimalarials that may be used for combination treatment. Quinoline drugs such as halofantrine have been shown to induce significant prolongation in the QT interval shown on an EKG exam when administered at therapeutic levels, however, and one of these drugs, halofantrine, has been associated with sudden death that may be attributable to malignant ventricular arrhythmias. Quinoline compounds have also been shown to prolong the PR interval on an EKG, and this prolongation has been shown to be associated with transient heart block at elevated plasma drug levels concentrations. Earlier studies of artemisinins in animals had raised concerns about toxicity, particularly the studies showing embryotoxicity or malformation of infant animals in early gestation. A number of studies conducted in rats, dogs, and monkeys have shown that artemisinins can cause occult brainstem neurotoxicity.

Given this data, the WHO does not suggest using ACT therapy to treat pregnant women in their first trimester or children whose body weight is less than 5 kg. A variety of studies, however, have shown ACT treatment is safe in children weighing 5 kg or less and also for treating pregnant women in their second and third trimesters. In a study of 500 pregnant women with *falciparum* malaria, artemisinins were well tolerated throughout pregnancy even during the first trimester. The outcomes of births from pregnant women treated with ACTs during pregnancy were not different from the community rates of stillbirth, congenital abnormality, abortion, or the average gestation at delivery [23]. In another study of 50 pregnant women with *falciparum* malaria treated with DHA-PPQ, no toxicity to fetus or mother was noted and no serious adverse events were observed [143]. Other studies should be done to gather data prospectively to understand the safety profile of both artemisinins and ACTs used in clinical treatment [144]. Further discussion of these issues in detail can be found in **Chapter 9**.

3.6. DECREASING THE COST OF CURRENT ACTS AND THE POSSIBILITIES OF FUTURE ACTS

3.6.1. Lower Cost for the Combination of Artesunate-Amodiaquine (AS-AQ)

In a recent announcement by the pharmaceutical company and non-profit organization that developed it, the first affordable antimalarial combination treatment tailored for children, artesunate combined with amodiaquine (AS-AQ), will be provided across Africa at a reduced price that will potentially lead to millions of lives saved. AS-AQ was developed for clinical use as the outcome of a two-year effort costing $21 million conducted by the Drugs for Neglected Diseases Initiative and Sanofi-Aventis, the pharmaceutical manufacturer. To increase drug availability, this combination has not been patented and it will be available for anyone who chooses to manufacture it. "This drug will save lives," said Dr. Bernard Pecoul, executive director of the Drugs for Neglected Diseases Initiative. "The aim of this project was to develop a product as adapted as possible to the malaria situation in Africa" [145].

AS-AQ has been approved in a number of African countries. A fixed dose co-formulated tablet of AS-AQ has been created for young children. AS-AQ comes in three other formulations for older children and adults. All of these formulations are fixed dose co-formulated tablets that enhance patient compliance for the duration of AS-AQ treatment over 3 days. In addition, the probability of development of parasite resistance should be decreased with the advent of a single combination pill for treatment. Patient compliance with malaria drug therapy is an ongoing concern particularly about patients provided multiple pills in blister packs. Failure to take all of the malaria drugs prescribed will likely lead to parasite drug resistance. With a fixed dose combination of AS-AQ, there are fewer concerns about patient compliance.

AS-AQ costs $0.50 US for children and less than $1 for adults, which makes this drug combination an affordable alternative to more expensive antimalarial drugs, and AS-AQ will be provided at cost to malaria endemic countries and non-governmental organizations. While this cost seems very inexpensive by the standards of a developed country, this price may still be too expensive for Africa.

3.6.2. Cheaper Versions of Artemether-Lumefantrine (AL)

Artemether plus lumefantrine (AL) was first introduced in South Africa for first-line therapy for uncomplicated *falciparum* malaria in regions where chloroquine and sulfadoxine-pyrimethamine (SP) have become resistant. In September 2006, Novartis, a Swiss multinational pharmaceutical company, reduced the average price (children and adults) of CoArtem from US $ 1.57 to $1.00 US per treatment to help expand access to this combination therapy. Even at US $1.00, CoArtem is a more expensive malaria treatment compared to the much cheaper price paid for chloroquine or SP monotherapy.

Novartis subsequently announced a reduction of 20% for CoArtem from US $ 1.00 to US $ 0.80 to further enhance access to affordable malaria drugs (Basel, April 23, 2008, at: http://www.mmv.org/IMG/pdf/CoArtem_press_release_April_2008.pdf). Price reductions previously discussed have become possible through gains in efficiency in producing CoArtem. Novartis has provided 160 million treatments of CoArtem at no profit since 2001. With new, more efficient production of CoArtem, an even lower price of $ 0.37 US for children's doses was introduced in 2012, which will result in even greater access to drug and increases in the number of children who will be treated for malaria.

3.6.3. Opportunities for Further Use of ACTs

Additional funds for malaria drugs, drug research, and policy implementation have been provided over the last decade, and significant increases in funding have been made available by a variety of international agencies to include the UK Department for International Development, the Global Fund, the US Agency for International Development, the Bill & Melinda Gates Foundation, WHO/TDR, MMV, and other foundations. The best malaria control tools available today include insecticides, treated bed nets, and antimalarial combination therapies. Additional funding provided should be used to identify methods of deploying these tools most effectively to control malaria. Funds should also be invested in local capacity building to provide developing countries with necessary expertise. Appropriate expenditure of grants accompanied by clear policy implementation by both funder and host country are essential elements required for success. Incidents of misappropriated funds or unclear policies will lead to problems with ongoing support of large donors.

The Global Fund is the largest funder for ACT distribution for malaria treatment. Prior to providing funds, WHO and Roll Back Malaria (RBM) partners provide technical reviews for submitted applications to the Global Fund through the Country Coordinating Mechanism (CCM).

Failure to scrutinize some poorly thought out grant applications is considered to be a root cause for the Fund paying for some ineffective antimalarial drug policies (AMDPs) prior to 2003 [146]. Today, the operating role for CCMs is clearer; WHO/RBM and the WHO Country Offices provide very good technical advice to CCMs, and the Technical Review Panel of the Global Fund has improved by focusing on composition of expert member panel and reforms of its process to make decisions. With improved oversight and advice coupled with enhanced funding, significant increases in the number of countries who have received funding to deploy ACTs have been observed since 2004 [147].

Over the last decade, interest in antimalarial drug development of antimalarial compounds among some drug companies has increased accompanied by additional funding from Medicines from Malaria Venture (MMV) and the Bill and Melinda Gates Foundation (BMGF). At the same time, collaborative efforts between private and public sectors has resulted in development of cheaper drugs that are more affordable to developing countries. For example, the combination of chlorproguanil/dapsone (LapDap) was developed by research conducted by GlaxoSmithKline (GSK), the WHO, UK researchers, and the UK Department for International Development (DFID). LapDap was registered in the UK in 2003, and a number of other African countries have registered this drug combination. GSK has will be providing LapDap at preferred prices [148] to countries in sub-Saharan Africa.

The cost of LapDap to governments and NGOs has been projected to be $0.29 US for an adult treatment regimen and $0.15 US for children (http://bmj.com/cgi/content/full/327/741/360-b). To help meet the need for combination therapy, LapDap is being developed as an ACT by combining it with artesunate. Age-based blister packs of artesunate-sulfadoxine/pyrimethamine (AS-SP) and artesunate- amodiaquine (AS-AQ) have been created and tested in trials in Africa; however, there have been rapid increases in parasite drug resistance to both SP and amodiaquine in Africa, which creates a significant limitation for future use of both combinations [149].

Despite considerable efforts by non-governmental and governmental organizations to increase access to ACTs, antimalarial drugs are largely unaffordable in many of the world's countries with endemic malaria. The cost of derivatives of artemisinin, which are crucial elements of the ACT combination, is a large part of the higher cost of an ACT *versus* older antimalarial drugs used as monotherapy. With a grant from the Bill and Melinda Gates Foundation, a partnership was developed to synthesize artemisinin rather than extract artemisinin from Artemesia annua plants. This collaboration between Amyris Biotechnologies, the Institute for One World Health, and the University of California, Berkeley focused on creating yeast strains with *Artemesia annua* genes capable of producing artemisinic acid, a precursor of artemisinin through fermentation. In 2013, these new yeast strains were being used to produce low levels of artemisinin, and by 2014, artemisinin for 150 million treatment regimens is produced through this process [150, 151].

CHAPTER 4

Pharmacokinetics (PK) and Pharmacodynamics (PD) of Antimalarial Drugs

Abstract: Most of the antimalarial drugs available on market were introduced in an era prior to the introduction of more modern practices of dose design based on principles of pharmacodynamics (PD) and pharmacokinetics (PK). Antimalarial dose regimens have been derived by empirical means rather than based on PK/PD models to maximize efficacy. These analyses factor in a wide variety of PK/PD parameters to include drug half-life, drug exposure levels, and times, drug metabolism, drug tissue volume of distribution and clearance, and PK inter-individual variations derived from animal model experiments and clinical trials in man. The relationships of drug half-life to antimalarial efficacy and resistance, dosing regimens to antimalarial efficacy and toxicity, and drug peak concentration to rapid antimalarial effects are defined in this chapter. There are significant advantages associated with defining the PK and PD characteristics of novel antimalarial drugs precisely which includes devising better methods of assessing therapeutic response. A clear definition of required PK and PD properties will also help with the design of drug regimens for dosing antimalarial drugs. The dose to be administered, the duration of dosing, and the frequency of dosing, can be modeled to help predict treatment cures and failures. Ultimately, a well-planned dose regimen of an antimalarial combination therapy will aid in slowing the emergence of parasite drug resistance. Antimalarial drugs are administered therapeutically in doses that result in patient blood concentrations far beyond the levels required for maximum effect. To evaluate a usable antimalarial drug, the maximum antimalarial effect observed differs when examining the varied responses between individuals. Thus, defining *in vivo* therapeutic levels requires analyzing associations between drug levels (PK inputs) and the risk of recurrent parasitemia, recrudescence, and re-infection (PD inputs) which provides important data to both develop and refine antimalarial monotherapy and combination therapies.

Keywords: Artemisinins, drug exposure level, drug exposure time, drug peak concentration, drug therapy, half-life, pharmacodynamics (PD), pharmacokinetics (PK), pharmacokinetics and pharmacodynamics (PK/PD), rapid action, toxicity.

Most of the antimalarial drugs available on market now in use were introduced in an era prior to the introduction of more modern practices of dose design based on principles of pharmacodynamics (PD) and pharmacokinetics (PK). Antimalarial dose regimens have been derived by empirical means rather than based on PK/PD models to maximize efficacy. These analyses factor in a wide variety of PK/PD parameters to include drug half-life, PK inter-individual variation, drug exposure levels, and parasite clearance and fever clearance times derived from animal model experiments and through clinical trials.

4.1. CONCERNS REGARDING THE IMPACT OF DRUG HALF-LIFE ON ANTIMALARIAL EFFICACY AND RESISTANCE

4.1.1. Induction of Drug Resistance Through Use of Long Elimination Half-Life Drugs

High malaria transmission areas are defined as regions where patients are bitten by infectious mosquitoes three times per day. Patients with malaria in these regions who are prescribed antimalarial drugs expose the first infecting parasites to an antimalarial drug and also expose any newly acquired parasites to an antimalarial drug that may be encountered during the elimination phase of the drug administered. The exposure of newly acquired parasites to sub therapeutic doses of antimalarial drugs is directly correlated to the length of the elimination phase, and the longer the elimination half-life, the more exposure a newly acquired parasite will undergo. Accordingly, the duration of the drug elimination half-life determines the potential risk for an antimalarial drug to select for drug resistant parasites [152, 153]. Malaria is an infection of the blood, and responses to drug treatment correlate with the concentration of antimalarial drugs achieved in the blood over the course of therapy.

One of the questions that remain unresolved regarding artemisinin combination therapies is the precise definition of where combination therapy drugs should be used if the partner drugs in the combination have very different pharmacokinetic properties. Long-duration drugs provide extended protection against re-infection with another malaria parasite. This protection can last up to two months for drugs like piperaquine or sulfadoxine-pyrimethamine (assuming use in areas without antifolate drug resistance). This extended protection, particularly in areas of moderate to high transmission, provides a patient with post-treatment prophylactic benefits while they recover from anemia, which is a substantial driver of malaria morbidity and mortality. In areas with endemic malaria of short duration and low frequency, with susceptible populations and high clinical attack rates [154], drugs with longer elimination half-lives provide a similar benefit. In addition, drugs with extended elimination half-lives require only a few doses, which helps eliminate risks associated with compliance and under-dosage. Slowly eliminated drugs, however, linger in patients beyond the treatment period, and sub-therapeutic levels of drugs that remain select for survival of drug resistant parasites [152].

There are also two related reasons for the expansion of resistance. The first reason revolves around the enhanced probability in areas of moderate and high malaria transmission that a new infection will be encountered during the period when the concentration of antimalarial drugs persisting after treatment of the first infection has decreased below levels capable of protecting against the growth of a newly acquired parasite. The risk of this occurring is dependent on infection frequency and the half-life of the antimalarial drug. Mefloquine, for example, has a half-life ranging from 14 days in cases of patients with malaria to 21 days in uninfected patients, and the concentration of drug declines slowly and mono-exponentially. The mefloquine concentrations a parasite may encounter during the elimination phase range from 20-80% of intermediate drug levels associated with inhibition of *falciparum* growth. This contrasts with chloroquine, which has a half-life ranging between 1 to 2 months, and the elimination phase of chloroquine occurs at drug levels that are more than likely below the level where significant inhibitory effects are effective. Accordingly, although mefloquine has an extended elimination half-life, relatively little pressure may be exerted throughout its terminal elimination phase. The more drug resistant the parasite, the less pressure exerted during the terminal elimination phase. This phenomenon may help explain why resistance to chloroquine took longer to develop than other antimalarial drugs despite the fact that the pharmacokinetic properties of chloroquine would seem to place this drug in jeopardy for rapid induction of parasite drug resistance.

An additional factor associated with induction of parasite drug resistance against drugs with extended half-lives is the selective pressure that takes place inside of every patient when malaria infection is not completely eradicated. Repeated cycles of asexual replication are thus exposed to lower and lower concentrations of antimalarial drugs. If a high fraction of patients with malaria infections are actually treated and any resulting mutations that arise confer drug resistance without affecting parasite fitness, then drug resistance will rapidly develop. The role of the half-life as an important element in induction of resistance against antimalarial drugs has been examined in detail in Kenya by Watkins and other colleagues [152]. This group has published extensive work comparing drug resistance arising from treatment of patients with DHFR inhibitors that are either short-lived or long-lived. Their data shows DHFR inhibitors with short half-lives like chlorproguanil and dapsone elicit less drug resistance than drugs with a longer half-life such as sulfadoxine-pyrimethamine [154].

While longer-lived antimalarial drugs are quite beneficial to patients, they are not beneficial to the population. A number of models have been created to predict mathematically the emergence and spread of drug resistance [155]. These models are capable of illustrating antimalarial drug resistance, however, there are two elements not captured in these models [156]. The first feature lacking in these models involves the effects of drug half-life, which is assumed to have no effect. These assumptions can lead to a significant underestimation of the potential for induction of resistance. The second element lacking from these models of drug resistance is they assume there are only two parasite populations, either fully sensitive or fully resistant. A variety of published articles suggests this is not a valid assumption with one exception involving atovaquone. Atovaquone resistance involves a single mutation in one nucleotide in the *cyt b* gene, which results in clinical resistance. Drug resistance to malaria parasites has been shown to increase gradually (*e.g.,* resistance to mefloquine) or in a systematic fashion. The stepwise increase in drug resistance occurs by progression from completely sensitive parasites to less sensitive parasites and ultimately to fully resistant parasites (*e.g.,* resistance to pyrimethamine). Accordingly, three different classes of drug resistance can be hypothesized to make a mathematical model solvable and to identify intermediate resistant parasites, which matches field conditions.

These definitions of three classes of drug resistance have been used in all of the modern models of malaria drug resistance [156]. The three classes of drug resistance for *P. falciparum* include: *Res0*, wild type parasites susceptible to drug treatment; *Res1*, parasites with intermediary susceptibility levels that are tolerant of drug treatment but are still killed by it; and *Res2*, parasites which are entirely resistant to drug treatment. *Res1* and *Res2* resistance have been shown to evolve more quickly if antimalarial drugs in use have long half-lives. This revised model clearly shows other previous models have problems underestimating *Res2* parasite evolution because of parasite exposure to drugs with a long half-life. This model has been extended to examine other questions to include: 1) modeling resistance where antimalarial drugs are used in combination, in particular in cases where the two partners have different half-lives and 2) modeling resistance to sulfadoxine-pyrimethamine as a drug combination [153].

One of the most important details of this model is development of drug resistance in two distinct phases. In the first phase, phase A, *Res1* parasites are spreading, *Res 0* parasites are being replaced and *Res2* parasites exist at a lower level. The second phase, Phase B, begins when *Res1* and *Res2* parasites are selected that are capable of surviving drug treatment, and these parasites are subsequently quickly selected which leads to broad treatment failures in patients. Treatment of malaria infected patients is possible during Phase A, and providers may well be not aware of changes in the phenotype and genotype of parasite populations that are associated with the onset of the second phase, phase B, of resistance. In phase B resistance, treatment will become much more difficult, and the probability of treatment failure will skyrocket. Multiple mutations at one genetic locus may actually occur in both Phase A and Phase B. In phase A, the drug is tolerated by parasites, but they are ultimately cleared by treatment, while in phase B, treatment failures are observed. The time course for Phase B is generally quite rapid which reinforces the need for active drug resistance surveillance. In areas with high malaria transmission, phase A may actually occur more rapidly than phase B. These findings have been supported by a variety of field trials for the antimalarial combination drug sulfadoxine-pyrimethamine (SP).

Combination therapy has been shown to slow down induction of resistance, but combination therapy must actually be implemented prior to induction of resistance to either of the combination partner drugs [157-159]. It is essential to conduct surveillance of parasites by region to detect progression of drug resistance into Phase B particularly after a new antimalarial drug is introduced. This practice of active monitoring will provide data in advance on changes in drug efficacy and the potential for drug failure. This mathematical model is not just used for malaria infection but it has also been used for monitoring development of resistance to antibacterial drugs [153].

4.1.2. Avoidance of Drug Resistance with Short Drug Elimination Half-Lives

Rapidly eliminated drugs like the artemisinins do not present sub-therapeutic drug concentrations to malaria parasites as these drugs are eliminated rapidly and entirely within the two-day period encompassing the asexual parasite life cycle. By contrast, more slowly eliminated drugs have half-lives ranging from weeks to months (ex. chloroquine, piperaquine, mefloquine), and these drugs can provide long-term selective pressures capable of inducing drug resistance. While artemisinin derivatives are capable of rapid killing with kill rates over 10,000 fold per asexual replication cycle, standard antimalarials partner drugs are not capable of kill rates more than 1,000 fold per replication cycle [160]. After liver stage development, exposures of, at a minimum, two asexual cycles over a period of 4 days to antimalarial drugs at treatment concentrations are needed to kill emerging blood stage parasites. Even with the best possible kill rates against drug sensitive parasites and the best possible growth of resistant parasites, a resistant parasite takes three asexual cycles to "overtake" a drug sensitive parasite. Rapidly cleared drugs like quinine or the artemisinin analogues are not capable of drug selection during drug elimination given the short timeframe involved. Clearly, the degree of resistance provided by mutation of the resistant parasite correlates with the window for drug selection to take place; the more resistant the parasite the longer the drug selection window will be. Measurement of drug resistance can be conducted through malaria drug potency testing on cultured parasites which be measures the amount of drug required to inhibit either 50% (the IC_{50}) or 90% (the IC_{90}) of parasite growth.

In addition, patent gametocytemia is more commonly found in infections that are recrudescent than in initial infections. Accordingly, if *de novo* resistance emerges in a treated infection, the probability of transmission from recrudescent parasites with a newly acquired resistance mutation is increased compared to transmission of parasites derived from new infections of parasites. The patients infected during a period of sub-therapeutic exposure at the end of the drug elimination phase of an antimalarial drug administered for a past infection; even if that infection resulted in a similar density of parasites [160].

The artemisinin compounds and quinine are quickly eliminated with short half-lives and after treatment ends, the drug concentrations in the blood quickly fall to sub-inhibitory levels. After quinine treatment is halted, residual drug in the blood may inhibit parasites for a period of 48 hours (3-4 half-lives, given a half-life of 16 hours) however, artemisinin compounds and DHA, their metabolite, are eliminated within hours. If parasites survive exposure to sub-therapeutic drug levels in the blood, parasite growth is inhibited only by post-antimalarial drug effects or through immune responses, which may delay new parasite population expansion. Recrudescent infections tend to occur earlier than new infections following long-lasting drug treatment. For example, recrudescence in patients taking mefloquine often occurs approximately two weeks after therapy is discontinued. Accordingly, selective pressure resulting in drug resistance from the use of artemisinin derivatives or quinine is limited in nature [161, 162]. Resistance to these compounds will therefore develop slowly or it will not develop at all. It is also clear that recrudescence infections occurring one month after antimalarial drug treatment with a rapidly eliminated antimalarial are very unlikely, and this result is in accordance with clinical observations.

4.1.3. The Effects of Drug Half-Lives on Drug Regimens

The concentrations of antimalarial drugs in the blood are most relevant to treatment of a malaria infection as the pathology of the disease occurs during blood stage infection. Consequently, extravascular distribution or penetration of a drug to the tissues is less relevant for antimalarial drugs used for treatment (use of antimalarial drugs for prophylaxis imposes different requirements). Many malaria drugs with long half-lives are extensively distributed in the human body, which leads to an elevated apparent volume of distribution and extended clearance times. The residence times of malaria drug are extended and antimalarial drug concentrations in the blood often exceed the level necessary to inhibit parasite growth persisting for periods of weeks or even months after treatment is initiated. The elimination half-lives of antimalarial drugs are varied and can be summarized as follows: chloroquine: 1-2 months, mefloquine: 2-3 weeks, lumefantrine: 3-4 days, pyrimethamine: 3 days, sulphadoxine: 10 days, and atovaquone 1-3 days.

Given these half-lives, a single dose or a three day course of therapy is adequate to provide antimalarial treatment, while the much shorter half-lives of quinine (16 hours) and the artemisinin derivatives (1 hour) insures that these drugs must be administered daily for seven days for effective treatment [160, 161]. Despite the fact that malaria parasites reside inside red blood cells, parasites are exposed to drugs at a concentration quite similar to the free or unbound concentration of antimalarial drug in the plasma rather than the concentration of drug found in red cells of uninfected red blood cells. The effects of malaria on the human body may affect drug absorption because of vomiting, decreased visceral perfusion, and decreases in food intake. Malaria infection can also lead to changes in the volume of distribution through changes in tissue and plasma binding, and alterations in clearance may be noted by diminished liver and renal function.

4.2. THE RELATIONSHIP BETWEEN DRUG DOSING REGIMEN AND ANTIMALARIAL EFFICACY

4.2.1. Drug Dosing Regimens Drive Antimalarial Efficacy

The relationship between under dosing of antimalarial drugs to treatment failure is not well understood. Most recommended treatment regimens were derived from trials conducted with non-pregnant adults. Special populations such as children or pregnant women who have the most significant consequences from malaria infection have been shown to have the highest rates of treatment failure [163]. One hypothesis to explain this phenomenon has revolved around a diminished immune response in both populations; however, it is also well known that many antimalarial drugs show decreased concentrations in the blood of children and pregnant women when compared to non-pregnant adults. Accordingly, inappropriate treatment regimens may well explain some of the treatment failures observed in both pregnant women and young children.

Despite this concern, there are few studies of higher antimalarial doses in these vulnerable populations. Concentrations of antimalarial drugs that are sub-therapeutic will likely lead to poor responses to drug treatment and will likely lead to induction of antimalarial drug resistance in the malaria parasite. In addition, in uncomplicated malaria the degree of drug absorption as opposed to the rate of drug absorption is very important to achieve maximal clinical efficacy. In severe malaria, where the goal of treatment is to provide a timely, life-saving therapeutic intervention, the rate at which drugs are absorbed from an extra-vascular site is more important than the degree of absorption. The absorption rate can be an important element in the outcome of patient treatment. This is most relevant to traditional drug regimens with long half-lives, which work well for inhibiting parasites completely in cases of uncomplicated malaria, *versus* the artemisinin compounds, which act rapidly with life-saving efficacy against severe malaria.

Mature blood schizonts and less mature, early ring stage parasites are the most drug-resistant stages of blood-stage malaria infection [164]. The majority of antimalarial drugs on market are largely active on sequestered parasites not visible to microscopists. Accordingly, the principle effects of treatment are focused on inhibiting the growth of trophozoites and a considerable decrease in the multiplication rate of parasites. As drug susceptibility is stage dependent, synchronizing drug administration with parasite development stage, also known as chronotherapy, may provide an enhanced therapeutic response. Treatment of malaria with chloroquine and, possibly, other antimalarial compounds can be improved if the maximum levels of drug occur at the same time as the most drug sensitive stage of parasite development; however, this type of therapy is difficult to achieve in clinical settings [165]. Artemisinin and analogues of artemisinin are active against ring stage parasites. In initial studies of artemisinin conducted in China, drug treatment was synchronized when the majority of parasites were at the initial ring stage of development [166]. While the theory behind chronotherapy seems sound, more clinical trials will have to be conducted to demonstrate this approach has an advantage *versus* non-synchronized drug treatment.

In general, drugs are administered at intervals corresponding to the biological half-life as estimated in patients with malaria who are undergoing treatment, not extrapolated from trials conducted with healthy patients. If a drug provides efficacy only during the period when drug concentrations are beyond a therapeutic level, then the observed biological half-life will correspond with the drug half-life. If the killing effects of a particular antimalarial are based on concentration and the biological effects of the drug persist after the concentration of the drug has decreased below the therapeutic level, then the drug can be administered less frequently than might be predicted based on the elimination half-life shown through PK studies. The drug dose and interval of dosing should be focused on providing antimalarial drug concentrations that are sufficient to affect both a parasitological and clinical cure in a patient who is non-immune. This is necessary due to the fact that antimalarial drug-treatment regimens are always more efficacious in patients who are semi-immune rather than in non-immune patients and in some instances, lower doses or shorter courses of antimalarial treatment may be given than those provided to non-immunes [118].

4.2.2. Relationship Between Drug Dosing Regimens and Antimalarial Drug Resistance

Prevention of malaria transmission is an important secondary objective of uncomplicated malaria treatment. Sub-therapeutic levels of antimalarial drugs enhance risks of treatment failure and selects for resistant parasite genotypes. In turn, drug resistant parasites have a survival improvement over non-drug resistant parasites as drug resistant parasites have increased gametocyte carriage in primary and recrudescent infections [167]. Due to enhanced gametocyte carriage in patients with drug resistant infections as opposed to those infected with drug sensitive parasites, there is a correspondingly higher probability of gametocyte transmission, which explains the preferential spread of drug resistant parasites. Cures of patients with uncomplicated malaria are assured if drug concentrations of antimalarials are capable of a maximal biological effect that insures all malaria parasites are killed. For drugs that are slowly eliminated, drug exposure shown by the area under the curve (AUC) is a very useful PK tool to predict response to therapy capturing both drug duration and concentration of exposure [118, 168]. For antimalarials with half-lives greater than 24 hours, the plasma or blood concentration on day 7 correlates best with both the AUC and response to treatment [61, 170]. If the antimalarial drug used for treatment achieves greater than 1,000 fold reduction per asexual parasite replication cycle at these concentrations, one can reliably predict, given the *P. falciparum* life cycle, that a cure can be achieved [118, 169].

In severe malaria, the principal aim is to reduce the parasite biomass as quickly as possible. Achieving a complete cure is a secondary goal to be achieved after difficulties associated with severe malaria have been taken care of. Accordingly, the most relevant pharmacokinetic parameter that relates to patient outcome from a severe malaria infection is the duration from when treatment is started to the time point where the drug concentration in the blood exceeds the minimum parasiticidal concentrations (MPC). Given that the *in vivo* MPC is usually not well defined, the time required to achieve maximum drug concentration (T_{max}) correlates well to the

MPC and can be used instead [118]. This underlines the necessity of using an initial loading dose when administering quinine and this requirement also supports the use of water-soluble artesunate for intravenous administration as it is more rapidly absorbed rather than injection of the less soluble, not as well absorbed, oil-based artemether [171]. Sub-therapeutic concentrations of drug in a patient can result from a number of causes to include use of counterfeit drugs with insufficient active pharmaceutical ingredients, under dosing, inadequate absorption of drug, a large apparent volume of distribution or very rapid drug clearance. In addition to optimizing dosage regimens, patient compliance and drug quality require attention to ensure complete drug regimen administration.

Studies of artesunate and its principal metabolite, dihydroartemisinin (DHA), have shown that while artesunate is rapidly absorbed with a half-life of under one hour, oral artesunate is as effective given once a day or twice a day [78]. These findings suggest the biological effect of artemisinin drugs go well beyond their actual presence in the human body at therapeutic plasma concentrations. Artemisinin drugs have a broad stage specificity, which ensures that only two brief exposures in each asexual blood stage life cycle which, given a 48 hour duration, corresponds to daily administration are adequate to achieve the greatest antimalarial result. This finding is at odds with the traditional concepts that revolve around keeping antimalarial drug concentrations above parasiticidal levels during the entire dosing interval [160].

While pharmacokinetic parameters are generally discussed as mean or median values, extreme pharmacokinetic values are often more interesting as lower blood concentrations often result in treatment failure or provide selection pressure to induce emergence of resistant parasites. Higher extreme concentrations, by contrast, are more likely to result in toxicity [172]. PK sampling from patients who have treatment failures or adverse events can help explain issues with dosing. With increased inter-individual variability, the therapeutic range of a drug narrows and the fraction of patients with either sub-therapeutic drug levels or levels of drug that are toxic will increase. In many patients, poor oral bioavailability is known to be a significant driver of inter-individual variability in drug concentrations found in patient blood samples [61]. Inter-individual variability can be further increased by administration of other medications that interact with antimalarial compounds.

As therapeutic response to malaria infection can be altered by host factors, such as immunity acquired from past infections, therapeutic drug concentrations must be defined for non-immune populations which are primarily young children living in areas endemic for malaria (while travelers are also non-immune, the numbers of travelers in endemic areas is far smaller than the number of children). Most pharmacokinetic studies are not generally designed to describe adequately the drug concentration over time relationship to therapeutic response and drug safety. Consequently, most antimalarial drugs were dosed with treatment regimens devised from studies of non-pregnant adult patients, and these drug regimens are often designed to be not much above the bare minimum dose required to save money and minimize the risk of adverse events associated with higher dose drug treatment. The dosing regimens for amodiaquine, mefloquine, halofantrine, primaquine, the artemisinin derivatives, and lumefantrine were all increased after their initial deployment suggesting better up-front studies in infected individuals may provide data initially to more adequately define the proper dose regimen [25, 163].

4.2.3. Relationship between Dosing Regimens and Efficacy in Special Risk Groups

The pharmacokinetic processes that determine a concentration profile of drug over time such as absorption, distribution, metabolism, and excretion (ADME) can be quite different between non-pregnant adults and other important special groups, such as pregnant women, children, young infants, and patients co-infected with HIV/AIDS. There are varieties of reasons explaining why pharmacokinetic parameters would be altered in patients, who are malnourished; however, there are very few studies of this group of patients [1, 23]. Accordingly, dosage regimens for these special population groups from studies in adults who are non-pregnant may well be incorrect. These special groups are of great concern given their vulnerability to malaria infection because of diminished malaria immunity [163].

1) Young Children and Pregnant Patients

Drug treatment regimens in children have largely been derived from dosage regimens of milligram per kilogram body weight, a 'one dose fits all' approach, based on data derived from non-pregnant adults which fails to take into account the fact that drug disposition is very different in pregnant women, infants and children. Despite broad antimalarial treatment of children for many years, only recently have clinicians recognized that current recommended doses in mg/kg for both CQ and SP yield much lower plasma drug levels in younger children than in adults [173, 174]. In addition, lumefantrine concentrations achieved in the plasma of children under 5 are much lower than in adults or older children [175]. Decreased lumefantrine concentrations in the plasma of young children are known to be a risk factor for malaria recrudescence and earlier re-infections [61, 176].

In some cases, the relationship between age and drug disposition is complex. One example of this is found in the absorption and clearance of chlorproguanil, which is commonly administered in combination with dapsone, which is decreased in younger children than adults while clearance of the active metabolite of chlorproguanil, chlorcycloguanil, is increased in young children. In addition, the clearance and apparent volume of distribution parameters for dapsone have been shown to increase with body weight [177]. Piperaquine, which is commonly dosed with dihydroartemisinin for treatment of uncomplicated malaria, has been shown to have sub-therapeutic concentrations at the initial phase of terminal elimination in children, and sub-therapeutic piperaquine concentrations observed in the plasma of patients on day 7 have been shown to be a risk factor for treatment failure. In addition, there are some differences in quinine toxicity in young children infected with severe malaria who are more susceptible to quinine-induced cardiotoxicity than older children [178]. There is no published evidence to date that differences in exposure to artemisinin compounds are reduced in younger children, however, significant differences in inter-individual variability makes the use of small studies with limited statistical power problematic to accurately assess the role of age in artemisinin pharmacokinetics.

The physiological changes to a woman's body in pregnancy include decreases in drug concentrations and exposure (shown by reduced AUCs), which in turn results in diminished efficacy of antimalarial drugs. Pregnant women in areas with endemic malaria with high transmission are also at higher risk of adverse effects from malaria particularly, the risk of maternal anemia and delivering a baby with low birth weight [179]. Even in areas with lower transmission of malaria, pregnant women who are infected with malaria are at higher risk of severe malaria disease and maternal and fetal death [179]. Antimalarial drug concentrations have been shown to be significantly lower in pregnant women during the second and third trimesters for a number of orally administered drugs to include artemether, artesunate, lumefantrine, CQ, atovaquone, mefloquine, sulfadoxine, proguanil and cycloguanil after oral administration [180, 181].

The PK parameters for antimalarial drugs administered *via* intravascular or intramuscular routes, however, do not show any significant difference between pregnant women and non-pregnant women [182, 183]. Suboptimal dosing may explain poorer treatment responses for both pregnant women and young children. Despite these findings, there have been very few published studies of altered regimens for treatment in pregnant women. One study was conducted to examine differences between non-pregnant and pregnant women who are treated with quinine for uncomplicated and severe malaria. In pregnant and non-pregnant women with uncomplicated malaria treated with quinine, there were no differences in the pharmacokinetic parameters of quinine observed [184]. In patients with severe malaria, however, pregnant women were shown to have a smaller volume of distribution (Vd) and faster elimination of quinine was noted [185]. No data are published on the PK properties of piperaquine, clindamycin, or amodiaquine in pregnant women; however, all of these drugs are used to treat pregnant women with malaria.

2) Intermittent Preventive Treatment

This dearth of data is also of concern for pregnant women given intermittent preventive treatment (IPT) for malaria. Intermittent preventive treatment (IPT) is defined as administration of a curative dose of antimalarial drugs systematically at discrete, predefined time points in pregnancy to asymptomatic women who are pregnant and at risk of malaria infection due to their residence in endemic regions. This treatment strategy was initially focused on pregnant women in their second and third trimesters (IPTp). Later iterations of this program focused on children during infancy (IPTi), and the latest focus of IPT has been on children in the high intensity transmission areas of malaria. Of all the antimalarial drugs that might be used for IPT, SP is widely used. Of all of the studies published on IPT using SP, only one included a PK study element [186, 187]. The continued use and considerable research dollars being spent on implementation of SP for IPT is quite surprising given the consensus view that SP is contraindicated for prophylaxis given known problems with SP drug resistance. This gap in knowledge is concerning as IPT and other forms of prophylaxis for travelers are the only context where antimalarial drugs are administered as monotherapy.

The use of drugs such as SP, which are slowly eliminated, will result in a window of selection where decreased antimalarial drug levels selects for survival of drug resistant parasites while killing off drug sensitive parasites [73, 188]. If many recipients of IPT therapy obtain sub-therapeutic doses due to drug resistance and a lack of PK data on the proper curative dose, any benefits from SP IPT treatment may be short-lived, and future IPT treatments with SP and a related antifolate drug, chlorproguanil-dapsone, may be contraindicated. There is limited published PK data that supports this conclusion about sulfadoxine. The AUC of sulfadoxine in 30 pregnant women in their second trimester was shown in this study to be 40% lower when compared with the AUC observed in 10 of the same who were re-treated 2-3 months after giving birth [186]. There are no PK data published on the parameters associated with SP dosing of infants despite many published research articles on the use of SP for IPT in infants. Amodiaquine is another antimalarial drug that has been used for IPT despite the lack of published data on the pharmacokinetic properties of amodiaquine in either infants or pregnant women. There have been some attempts to model the impact of IPT therapy on drug resistance [189, 190]. These models have made assumptions, with no supporting data, that IPT treatment actually results in a curative dose in pregnant women or infants. The drug levels observed in patients treated for IPT programs cannot be derived from data obtained on malaria-infected children or pregnant women as acute malaria infection can alter drug disposition. This widespread use of amodiaquine and SP for IPT in pregnant women and children in the absence of data to support dosing poses risks for both the individuals who may not receive an adequate IPT dose and for the surrounding populations who may be affected by parasites who have been selected for resistance to both drugs.

3) HIV/AIDS Co-Infection

Recent evidence has shown that HIV infection and malaria co-infection have significant impacts on patients. As HIV infection and malaria infection are prevalent in tropical environments, the impact of each disease on the other must be considered. With regards to IPTp, studies have shown that failure to clear all parasites has been demonstrated in HIV-infected women [191], and this finding has led to a recommendation for monthly SP IPT for patients living in areas with an HIV seroprevalence over 10% as opposed to a two-dose SP regimen implemented in areas with HIV seroprevalence under 10% [187]. Patients infected with malaria are more likely than HIV negative-patients to develop severe malaria and to die from their malaria infection, and this is particularly true for patients residing in areas with low-intensity transmission of malaria [192]. Immune suppression associated with HIV co-infection has also been shown to enhance the risk of treatment failure with SP [193]. Clinically significant drug-drug interactions are more prevalent in patients who are being treated with HIV protease inhibitors, which have a known propensity to inhibit cytochrome P450 enzymes. In addition, treatment with non-nucleoside reverse transcriptase inhibitors can act to either induce or inhibit CYP enzymes, which further impacts on the clearance of antimalarial drugs. Both quinine and lumefantrine are all metabolized by CYP3A4, and inhibition of CYP3A4 by an HIV protease inhibitor or reverse transcriptase inhibitor can lead to increased risk of toxicity [194]. Simultaneous administration of antimalarial drugs such as artesunate or amodiaquine with anti-HIV drugs such as efavirenz in healthy volunteers has been shown to be associated with hepatotoxicity, which resulted in early discontinuation of this study and a clear warning on the potential problems of concomitant administration of antimalarial and antiretroviral drugs [195].

4.3. THE RELATIONSHIP BETWEEN DRUG EXPOSURE LEVEL AND TIME TO ANTIMALARIAL EFFICACY

Human and animal species studies have shown unambiguously that artemisinin derivatives are very potent drugs against *falciparum* and *vivax* malaria. These drugs initiate immediate decreases in parasitemia and, in most studies, clinical recovery of the patient is faster than with other antimalarials. A high rate of recrudescence (approximately 30-50% recrudescence for monotherapy for 3 days, 6-15% recrudescence for monotherapy for 5 days, and 2-6% for monotherapy for 7 days), however, is still a major disadvantage for artemisinin compounds used as monotherapy [71, 196]. Although the clinical significance of their rapid killing advantage, in terms of morbidity, has yet to be determined [197-199], at least two published trials have shown the potential of artemisinin compounds to reduce mortality. The two largest trials conducted for treatment of severe malaria in malaria endemic areas includes the South East Asian Quinine Artesunate Malaria (SEQAUAMAT) trial and the African Quinine Artesunate Malaria (AQUAMAT) trials. Both studies showed that treatment of adults and children infected with severe malaria with intravenous artesunate is superior to treatment with intravenous quinine. The mortality rate in patients treated with quinine was 22% in the SEQUAMAT trial and 10.9% in the AQUAMAT study. For AS-treated patients, the mortality rate in the SEQUAMAT trial was 15% and the mortality rate in the AQUAMAT trial was 8.5%. This amounts to a significant mortality reduction for artesunate of 35% *versus* quinine in the SEQUAMAT study and a 22.5% reduction in mortality in the AQUAMAT trial *versus* quinine. Patients with hyperparasitemia (>10% malaria-infected RBCs) have been shown to have a significantly greater treatment effect after therapy with AS than patients without hyperparasitemia. Treatment with intravenous AS has been better tolerated, easier, and safer to use than quinine [200, 201]. The benefit of intravenous treatment with AS over intramuscular artemether [202] for treatment of severe malaria was announced by the WHO in 2006, and intravenous AS has since been recommended as the initial treatment for severe *falciparum* malaria [1].

4.3.1. Influence of Drug Exposure Level and Time Studies Performed in Animal Species

Injectable AS is being developed for FDA approval for treatment of severe, complicated malaria by Walter Reed Army Institute of Research and Sigma Tau Pharmaceuticals. An assessment of the efficacy of AS and artelinic acid an experimental water-soluble artemisinin derivative, after daily IV injection for 3 days was conducted in rats infected with *P. berghei* and control rats without infection. The minimal effective suppressive dose to suppress parasitemia for AS in this model was 2.3 mg/kg, and the minimal suppressive dose required for artelinic acid to inhibit parasitemia was 2.5 mg/kg. The dose required to cut parasitemia by 50% (the 50% suppressive dose or SD_{50}) in animals treated with AS was 7.4 mg/kg while the dose required cutting parasitemia in half for artelinic acid 8.6 mg/kg (Table **13**). There seemed to be no significant difference between these two water-soluble compounds at suppressive dose levels [203].

Table 13: Definitive efficacy parameters of artelinic acid (ALA)/lysine salt at 96 µmoles/kg (40 mg/kg) and artesunate(AS)/$NaHCO_3$ at 96 µmoles/kg (36.7 mg/kg) given as daily intravenous treatment for three days in *P. berghei* infected rats (2.0 x 10^7 parasitized erythrocytes per adult rat) [203]

Pharmacodynamic (PD) Parameters	**ALA/lysine 95 µmoles/kg (40.6 mg/kg)**	**AS/$NaHCO_3$ 95 µmoles/kg (36.7 mg/kg)**
Initial PD parameters		
Number of rats	19	18
Parasitemia on day 6 (%)	5.5 ± 1.1	6.7 ± 2.1
Rat number of clearance	19/19	7/18
Mean time for parasitemia to clear completely (PCT, hr)	57.2 ± 10.6	52.8 ± 14.9
Time parasitemia cleared (days)	3.2 ± 1.2	2.7 ± 0.7
Recrudescence rate (%)	100	100
Time recrudescence (days)	6.5 ± 1.0	6.0 ± 0
Mortality	0/19	0/18
Secondary PD parameters (computer fitting)		
Lag time (hr)	3.36 ± 1.64	4.01 ± 2.5
E0 (%, drug effect on parasitemia at time 0)	6.2 ± 2.3	8.1 ± 2.7
E_{max} (%, maximum drug effect on parasitemia)	0.008 ± 0.01	0.339 ± 0.039**
EC_{50} (hr, time causes 50% of drug effect parasitemia)	10.85 ± 1.32	8.86 ± 2.87*
AUEC (%*hr, area under effect of parasitemia *vs* time curve)	313.3 ± 148.2	535.8 ± 252.4

Note. Values are means ± SD. Injection times are on day 6, 7, and 8 after infection day (day 0).
* $P = 0.0048$ (AS compared with ALA).
** $P = 0.0007$ (AS compared with ALA).

Concerning the parasite clearance times (PCT), artesunate dosed at equimolar doses of 96 µmoles/kg, (36.7 mg/kg) cleared parasitemia in 7 out of 18 rats (39% clearance rate). At this dose, the parasitemia clearance time (PCT) for AS was 52.8 hours and the clearance time lasted only 2.7 days with recrudescence observed in these same seven animals. In the seven rats who showed a clearance in parasitemia, the EC_{50} was 8.86 hours, and the area under the effect curve (AUEC) was 536 % of parasitemia x hr for this dose of AS/$NaHCO_3$. Using the same equimolar dose of 96 μmoles/kg (40.6 mg/kg), artelinic acid cleared parasitemia in all 19 rats treated with a 100% clearance rate. At this dose level, the PCT of artelinic acid was 57.2 hours with parasitemia clearance times lasting 3.2 days before recrudescence was observed. Computer fitting revealed that E_0, the drug effect achieved at initial administration, was 6.2 ± 2.3%, whereas E_{max}, the maximum drug effect achieved, was measured at 0.008 ± 0.01% of parasitemia. The EC_{50} was 10.9 hours, and the area under the effect curve (AUEC) was 313 % of parasitemia hr for this dose of artelinic acid (Table **13**) [203].

From this data, the authors of this study concluded that at an equimolar dose, artelinic acid (with 100% clearance) has increased efficacy over AS (with 39% clearance) in malaria-infected rats. The *in vitro* data, however, indicate that, AS has a 5-8 fold greater antimalarial activity than artelinic acid [204]. This leads to the question, why is there a discrepancy between the *in vitro* and *in vivo* data? A pharmacokinetic analysis may provide the answer to this question. Comparative pharmacokinetics and hydrolysis studies of intravenously administered artelinic acid and AS were conducted in *P. berghei* infected rats using 3 daily equimolar doses (96 μmoles/kg). The drug concentration of AS achieved after daily doses of 36.7 mg/kg on day 3 was one-third the concentration observed on day 1, and the mean C_{max} of AS on day 1 was 16,492 ng/ml and 1,377 ng/ml on day 3. Similar to its active metabolite, dihydroartemisinin (DHA), AS showed a maximum drug concentration in plasma of 10,842 on day 1 and 6,485 ng/ml on day 3, suggesting hepatic enzymes associated with drug metabolism had been auto-induced after AS administration [205-209].

Auto-induction of liver enzymes after dosing was similarly noted in 4 other artemisinins, artemisinin (QHS), DHA, artemether (AM) and arteether (AE) [205-209], but not for artelinic acid [210]. The pharmacokinetic parameters of artelinic acid were very similar on day 3 compared to day 1 with the same molar dose of compound administered compared to the AS dosed animals. The mean C_{max} of artelinic acid on day 1 was 48,453 ng/ml and 44,101ng /ml on day 3. AS is a pro-drug of DHA with a DHA/AS ratio of 5.26 as compared to artelinic acid, which shows a DHA/artelinic acid ratio of 0.01. The increase in artelinic acid's peak concentration can explain why artelinic acid has a much greater efficacy than AS *in vivo* (Fig. **6**). Other pharmacokinetic parameters revealed that the total $AUC_{1\text{-}3}$ on days 1-3 of artelinic acid (84.4 μg·h/ml) was 5-fold higher than that of AS (15.7 μg·h/ml of AS plus DHA). The elimination half-life of artelinic acid (7.1 hours) was longer than AS (0.36 hours) or DHA (0.72 hours) (Table **14**). The remarkable changes in PK parameters artelinic acid could be due to a limited conversion to DHA and enterohepatic circulation of this compound, which has been confirmed by pharmacokinetics and tissue distribution studies [210, 211]. The higher drug peak and AUC values of artelinic acid in rat blood compared to AS may explain its increased efficacy in malaria-infected rats.

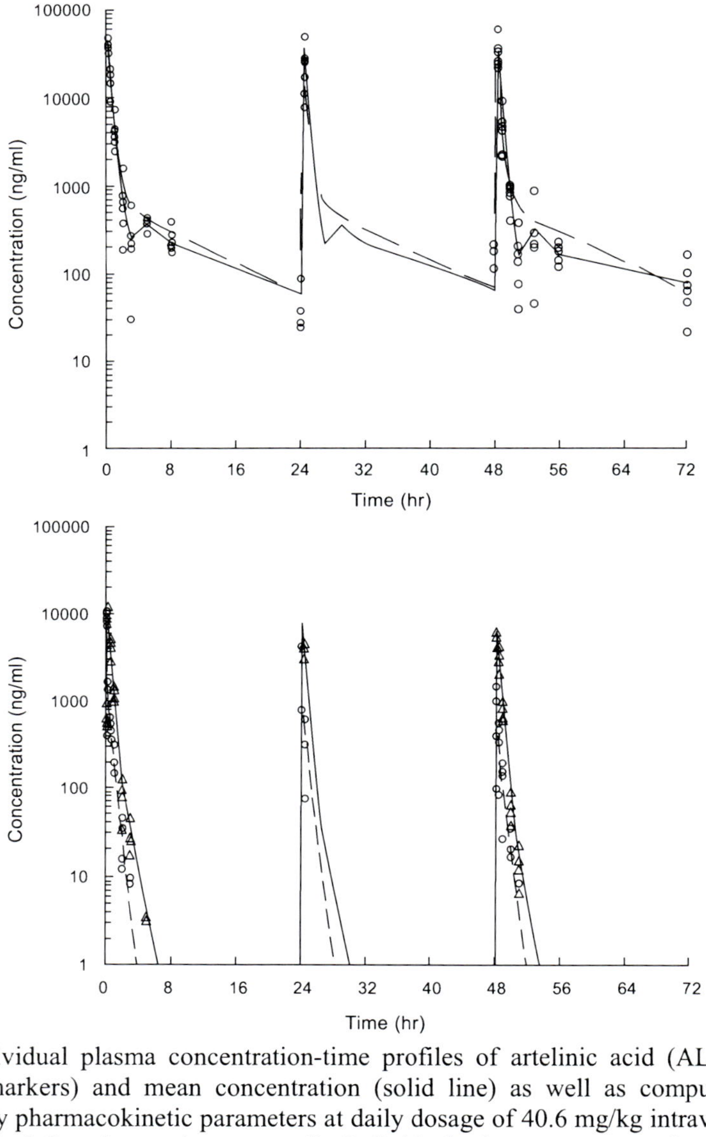

Figure 6: Individual plasma concentration-time profiles of artelinic acid (ALA) measured by LC/MS/MS (markers) and mean concentration (solid line) as well as computer fitted curves (dashed line) by pharmacokinetic parameters at daily dosage of 40.6 mg/kg intravenously for three days in malaria-infected rats (top, n = 6). Individual plasma concentration-time profiles of artesunate (AS) measured by HPLC-ECD (markers) and computer fitted curves for parent drug, AS (dashed line), and its active metabolite, DHA (solid line), by pharmacokinetic parameters at dosage of 36.7 mg/kg once daily intravenously for 3 days in *P. berghei* infected male rats.(bottom, n = 4) [210].

Table 14: Toxicokinetic parameters of artesunate (AS) and artelinic acid (ALA) at 96 μmoles/kg following multiple intravenous injections daily for three days in *P. berghei* infected rats by using a Culex automated blood sampler [210]

PK Parameters	AS (36.7 mg/kg, n = 4)		AL (40.6 mg/kg, n = 6)	
	Parent drug (AS)	Metabolite (DHA)	Parent drug (AL)	Metabolite (DHA)
Day 1				
C_{max} (ng/ml)	16492 ± 4205	10842 ± 1950	48453 ± 7177	124.2 ± 36.2
T_{max} (h)	0	0.19 ± 0.03	0	0.33 ± 0.18
$AUC_{inf.}$ (ng·h/ml)	1324 ± 242	4893 ± 779	25857 ± 2114	160.4 ± 86.2
$t_{1/2}$ distribution (h)	0.04 ± 0.01	0.20 ± 0.02	0.29 ± 0.06	-
$t_{1/2}$ elimination (h)	0.36 ± 0.03	0.72 ± 0.05	7.05 ± 2.01	-
Vss (liter/kg)	8.10 ± 1.70	-	4.57 ± 2.01	-
CL (ml/min/kg)	474.2 ± 89.8	-	25.93 ± 2.10	-
MRT (h)	0.62 ± 0.33	0.43 ± 0.04	2.89 ± 1.11	-
Day 3				
C_{max} (ng/ml)	1377 ± 898	6485 ± 1053	44101 ± 21452	116.6 ± 74.3
T_{max} (h)	0	0.18 ± 0.06	0	0.26 ± 0.12
$AUC_{inf.}$ (ng·h/ml)	490.6 ± 314.0	3327 ± 743	24650 ± 8663	204.2 ± 134
$t_{1/2}$ distribution (h)	0.12 ± 0.07	0.21 ± 0.02	0.30 ± 0.08	-
$t_{1/2}$ elimination (h)	0.46 ± 0.06	0.65 ± 0.06	6.06 ± 0.64	-
Vss (liter/kg)	76.87 ± 8.54	-	5.24 ± 3.50	-
CL (ml/min/kg)	2172 ± 1274	-	29.40 ± 8.24	-
MRT (h)	0.53 ± 0.01	0.60 ± 0.11	2.78 ± 1.34	-
Total $AUC_{1\text{-}3D}$ (ng·h/ml)	2717 ± 809	13051 ± 1926	84406 ± 19703	524 ± 277
Ratio of DHA/AS or AL	-	5.26 ± 2.22	-	0.01 ± 0.00

TK = toxicokinetics, DHA = dihydroartemisinin, MRT = Mean residence time; D = days.

Efficacy and pharmacokinetic experiments using two artemisinin derivatives, AE and AM, were performed in rats with two different intramuscular vehicles, sesame oil, and cremophore [65, 212]. AM and AE demonstrated similar efficacy against *P. berghei* in rodents when administered in a cremophore vehicle in place of the traditional sesame oil formulation for intramuscular treatment. There were significant differences in the 50% cure dose (CD_{50}) between the sesame oil and cremophore formulations required to treat *P. berghei*-infected mice. AM in sesame oil showed a CD_{50} value of 35.6 mg/kg (ranging from 7.6-63.6 mg/kg) while AE formulated in sesame oil showed a similar CD_{50} values of 34.1 mg/kg (ranging from 1.3-66.9 mg/kg) for treatment of malaria-infected mice. AE formulated with cremophore had a CD_{50} value of 14.2 mg/kg (ranging from 6.8-21.5 mg/kg) and AM showed a CD_{50} value of 21.0 mg/kg (ranging from 18.5-23.4

mg/kg) for treatment of *P. berghei* infected mice (Table **15**). The results demonstrated formulation of AE and AM in cremophore dosed at three daily multiple intramuscular injections was much more efficacious than the same drugs formulated in sesame oil dosed the same way [65].

Table 15: Antimalarial activity (50% cure dose, CD_{50})* and corresponding 95% confidence interval (95% CI) of arteether and artemether given intramuscularly dosed daily for 3 days against *P. berghei* in female mice (n = 8 for each dose level) [65]

Drug formulation	Arteether (CD_{50})		Artemether (CD_{50})	
	mg/kg	95%CI	mg/kg	95%CI
Sesame oil formulation	34.1	12.3-66.9	35.6	7.6-63.6
Cremophore formulation	14.2	6.8-21.5	21.0	18.5-23.4

* When the mice have survived and showed negative smears at 60 days, they were considered cured.

The mean plasma concentration-time profiles (n = 3) of AE formulated with sesame oil (AESO) and in a 1:2 cremophore/0.9% saline (AECM) after single intravenous and intramuscular doses is shown in Fig. **7** (bottom). AE formulated with sesame oil and cremophore showed a biphasic disposition pattern, which was fitted by a two-compartment open model after either intravenous or intramuscular injection. The concentration-time profiles of AE formulated with two different vehicles are shown in Fig. **7** after daily intramuscular injection for 7 days. The plasma trough concentrations were shown to increase up to the last dosing day in AESO treated rats, but not in AECM rats. Clearly, AESO administered rats demonstrated drug accumulation in the plasma (7.5 fold over 7 days of dosing). In the AECM rats, the AE level increased slightly (1.8-fold) on day 7 after multiple days of dosing over the level of AE observed on day 1.

Differences in PK parameters between AESO and AECM are summarized in Table **16** after multiple intramuscular doses of 25 mg/kg. Plasma peak concentration on day 1 showed the C_{max} of AECM (1,227 ng/ml) was 13-fold higher than AESO (92.2 ng/ml). The area under the curve (AUC) of AECM (4,165 ng·h/ml) was approximately 4-fold greater than AESO (1,135 ng·h/ml) on day 1. The total AUC of AECM (46,286 ng·h/ml) during the 7-day test period was approximately 2.7-fold higher than AESO (16,922 ng·h/ml). The elimination half-life observed was 7.0 hr for AECM and 17.7 hr for AESO on day 1. Based on AUC data, the bioavailability of AECM was 74.5% and the bioavailability of AESO was 20.3% after a single intramuscular injection. The data suggests that AECM, a less oily formulation, was more easily absorbed in muscle tissue with a higher C_{max} and AUC, which may explain its increased efficacy *versus* AESO [65].

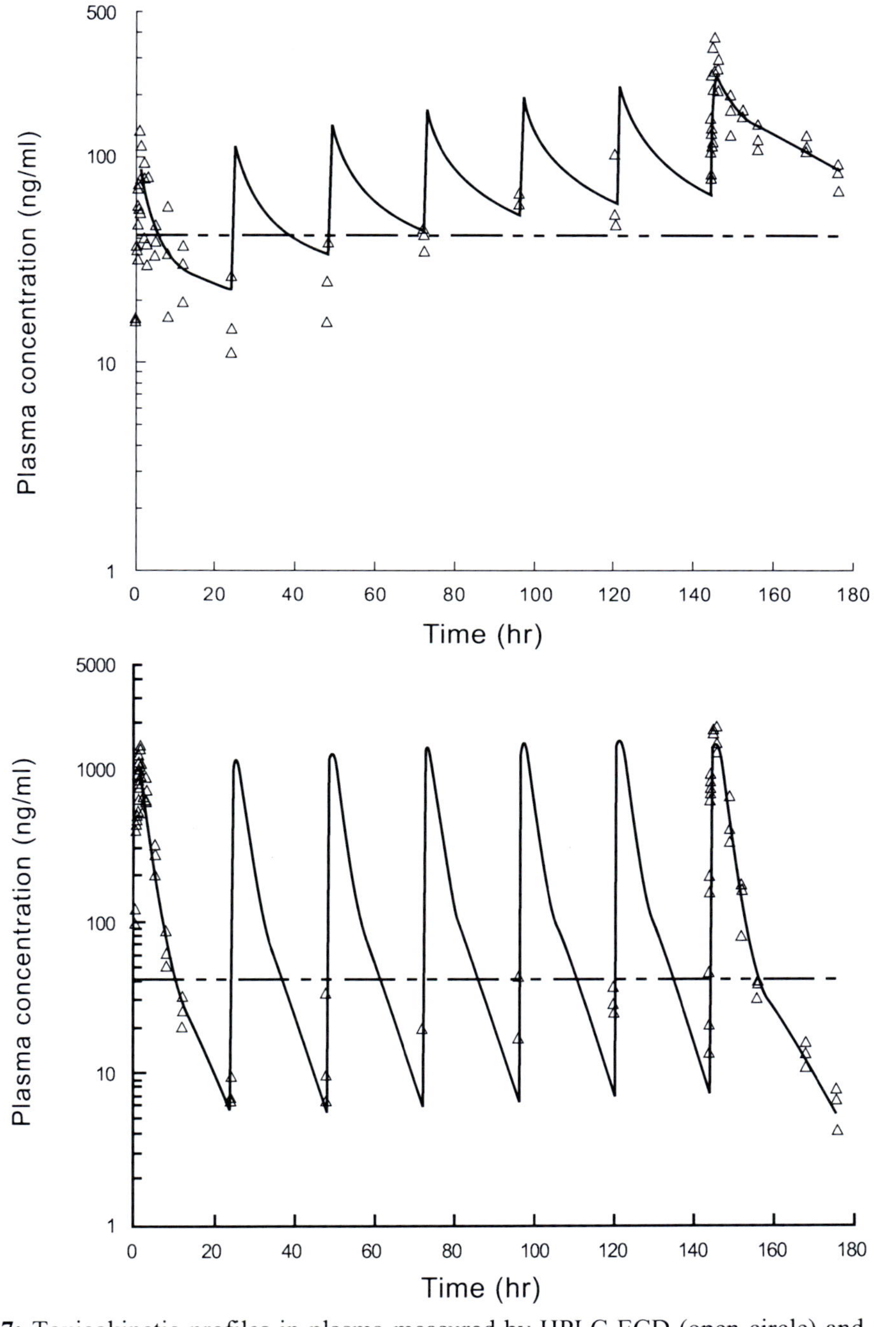

Figure 7: Toxicokinetic profiles in plasma measured by HPLC-ECD (open circle) and computer fitted curves (solid-line) of 25 mg/kg of arteether with sesame oil (AESO, top, n = 3) and arteether with cremophore (AECM, bottom, n = 3) following daily intramuscular injection for 7 days in male rats [250]. The minimal detected pathological effect level (MDPEL) was estimated at 41.32 ng/ml (dashed line).

Table 16: Pharmacokinetic parameters of arteether (AE) and dihydroartemisinin (DHA), a metabolite of AE, following single intravenous (25 mg/kg), and multiple intramuscular (25 mg/kg) administration with sesame oil and 1:2 cremophore (CRM)/0.9% saline daily for 7 days in male rats (n = 3-7) [65]

PK Parameters	Single IV CRM/Saline	Intramuscular Multiple)			
		Sesame oil (AESO)		1:2 Cremophore/Saline (AECM	
		Day 1	Day 7	Day 1	Day 7
Arteether					
C_{max} (ng/ml)	14482 ±1023	92.2 ± 19.9	311.9 ± 54.6	1227 ± 171	1826 ± 118
T_{max} (h)	0	1.42 ± 0.63	1.67 ± 0.58	1.33 ± 0.29	1.33 ± 0.58
$AUC_{inf.}$ (ng·h/ml)	5593 ± 591	1135 ± 277	8527 ± 1006	4165 ± 676	7312 ± 588
$AUC_{D1-8.}$ (ng·h/ml)			16922 ± 4038		46286 ± 2061
Vss (liter/kg)	0.98 ± 0.25	150.2 ± 33.7	54.1 ± 7.8	8.70 ± 1.21	5.06 ± 0.27
CL (ml/min/kg)	71.3 ± 9.11	73.7 ± 2.8	147.9 ± 6.19	76.3 ± 2.9	76.0 ± 1.9
$t_{1/2}$ distribution (h)	0.22 ± 0.04	0.71 ± 0.47	1.08 ± 0.49	1.00 ± 0.04	1.18 ± 0.14
$t_{1/2}$ elimination (h)	0.82 ± 0.05	17.66 ± 2.68	29.57 ± 2.07	6.96 ± 0.93	9.06 ± 1.69
MAT (h)	-	0.76 ± 0.40	0.87 ± 0.39	1.04 ± 0.03	1.07 ± 0.10
MRT (h)	0.74 ± 0.18	23.56 ± 3.42	41.51 ± 2.84	6.21 ± 0.66	5.83 ± 0.09
Bioavailability (%)	100	20.3 ± 5.0	152.4 ± 17.9	74.5 ± 12.1	130.7 ± 10.5
% of single daily dose in muscle		37.6 ± 8.2	91.4 ± 11.6	4.7 ± 1.8	17.3 ± 3.3
Dihydroartemisinin					
C_{max} (ng/ml)	815.8 ±164.2	16.02 ± 4.05	123.8 ± 28.9	171.1 ± 79.4	188.4 ± 91.0
T_{max} (h)	0	0.92 ± 0.14	0.86 ± 0.35	0.92 ± 0.14	1.33 ± 0.29
$AUC_{inf.}$ (ng·h/ml)	350.0 ± 97.1	117.1 ± 33.0	790.3 ± 221	607.7 ± 102	708.2 ± 29.2
$AUC_{D1-8.}$ (ng·h/ml)			3427 ± 759		5346 ± 831
$t_{1/2}$ elimination (h)	1.08 ± 0.16	9.17 ± 2.54	14.47 ± 2.17	4.71 ± 0.71	6.64 ± 1.25
Ratio of DHA/AE	0.06 ± 0.02	0.09 ± 0.03	0.08 ± 0.03	0.14 ± 0.03	0.11 ± 0.01

* On day 1 the amount of dose in the muscle was measured at 24 h after first dosing, and on day 7 the amount of dose was measured at 24h after last dosing. IV = intravenous, CRM/saline = 1:2 cremophore/0.9% saline.

This *in vivo* efficacy study showed that AM and AE formulated with cremophore were more efficacious than when both compounds were formulated with sesame oil. The most likely reason for the enhanced efficacy of AE in cremophore is due to the higher plasma concentration of AE produced by cremophore formulation (AECM). The plasma concentration measurement of AE in cremophore showed that the C_{max} of AECM was 13 fold higher and the AUC of AECM was 5-fold higher than that of AESO on day 1. The total AUC of AECM (46,286 ng·h/ml) throughout the 7-day period was 2.7-fold higher than AESO (16,922 ng·h/ml).

The elevated exposure of AE formulated in cremophore in rats significantly aided antimalarial efficacy, and antimalarial efficacy of AE in cremophore demonstrated a drug concentration dependency [164, 213-215], especially with the 13-fold higher peak concentration than AE formulated in sesame oil.

4.3.2. Influence of Drug Exposure Level and Time in Human Studies

In a clinical study of oral AM treatment of patients infected with *falciparum* malaria, Karbwang *et al.* reported results for four patients who failed treatment with an oral AM regimen used for malaria treatment. These patients were noted to have significantly decreased levels of DHA, a biologically active metabolite of artemisinin compounds, than other patients in the study [216]. These four patients were administrated the same amount of AM, however, they demonstrated a much lower DHA C_{max} (196 ng/ml at 6 hours and 54 ng/ml at 12 hours) than the DHA C_{max} (354 ng/ml at 6 hours and 158 ng/ml at 12 hours) in the 46 other subjects in the study. Also, a lower AUC (834 ng·h/ml) of DHA was shown in 4 patients but not the other 46 patients (3,684 ng·h/ml). The concentrations of the parent drug, AM, were similar in these four patients (1,044 ng·h/ml) compared to the drug concentrations of AM observed in the other 46 subjects (1,272 ng·h/ml). It is not known why those patients had such low DHA concentrations given the fact that they received the same AM regimen as the other subjects, however, low DHA concentrations observed in these patients may be the cause of treatment failure. An alternative explanation for this phenomenon may be the parasites themselves in these four patients may have been mature and thus required a higher concentration of AM and DHA than patients with similar parasitemia but less mature development.

More recently, Sharma reported results for two patients who died of cerebral malaria who had a correspondingly high degree of parasitemia (16% and 50%). The dose regimen of AM at 80 mg used to treat these two patients was injected intramuscularly twice on the first day and then daily for four days [217]. AM administered by intramuscular injection has been shown to result in very low plasma concentrations and low bioavailability [218] due to the prolonged injection site absorption [219]. This study showed that administration of a low dose AM regimen (total 480 mg) for *falciparum* malaria treatment may not elicit a high enough drug concentration in the blood to cure patients infected with *falciparum* malaria at high parasitemia levels (Fig. **8**).

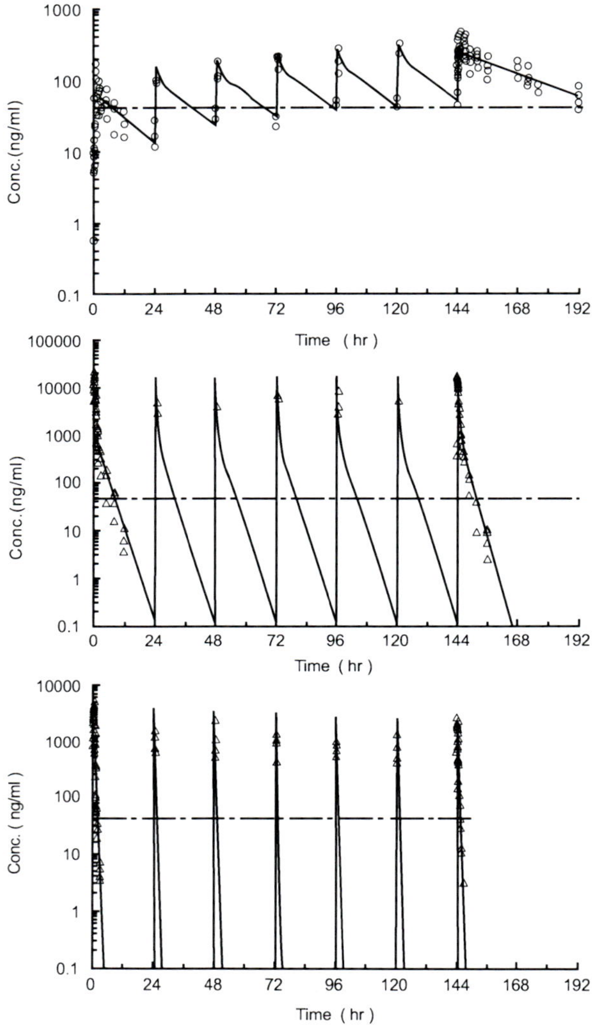

Figure 8: Pharmacokinetic profiles measured by HPLC-ECD (markers) and computer fitted curves (solid line) of 25 mg/kg of arteether with sesame oil (top, n = 4) [219]. Artelinic acid (middle) and artesunate (bottom) with 5% $NaHCO_3$/0.9% saline following daily intramuscular injection 25 mg/kg daily for 7 days in male rats. (n = 3) [65]. The minimal detected pathological effect level (MDPEL) from arteether measurement was estimated at 41.32 ng/ml (dashed line) in rats [12].

During a Phase 3 clinical trial of intramuscular AE (Artemotil), one patient was dosed by mistake intravenously with the intramuscular AE formulation on day 1 of treatment. The difference in concentration profiles *versus* time of AE and DHA for this patient (#151, high dose group) is shown in Fig. **9** (bottom). This patient received an initial dose of AE, which appeared to have been accidentally injected intravenously instead of intramuscularly. This injection resulted in a blood plasma drug profile with a very high C_{max} and a quick distribution phase. AE and DHA plasma concentrations in this patient decreased significantly after the first intravenous dose with an elimination $t_{1/2}$ of 1.1 hours over a 6-hour period. After a second IM injection of AE at hour 6, the elimination $t_{1/2}$ of AE was immediately extended to 9.35 hours when expressed as a daily half-life. The C_{max} (2,407 ng/ml) of this patient treated with AE was shown to be 22-fold higher than the average AE C_{max} value (110 ng/ml) observed in other patients in this study dosed only through intramuscular injection. The AE AUC value (12,259 ng·h/ml) was 2 times higher than the average AE AUC value (7,403 ng·h/ml) shown in other patients. Similar results showing increases in DHA levels were also reported for this patient dosed accidentally through intravenous injection. As expected, this patient was successfully cured with a parasitemia clearance time (PCT) of 36 hours and a fever clearance time (FCT) of 4 hours compared with other patients dosed intramuscularly with AE who showed a PCT of 64.4 hours and an FCT of 70.1 hours [220]. The 22-fold increase in the AE C_{max} achieved through intravenous injection *versus* intramuscular injection may also have contributed to the observed increase of drug efficacy. This clinical outcome suggests that intravenous injection of AE (like AS) plays an important role in rapid treatment of *falciparum* malaria due to the high peak concentrations (C_{max}) achieved, especially in cases of severe and complicated malaria.

Comparisons of the efficacy of oral *versus* IM administration of AM have been conducted in clinical trials with malaria-infected patients [171, 221]. A study was conducted in Vietnamese adults infected with severe *falciparum* malaria who were treated with IM AS *versus* oral AS *versus* oral AM. In this study, intramuscular AS was administered at a dose of 2.4 mg/kg followed by AS dosed orally at 1.2 mg/kg daily and AM dosed at 3.2 mg/kg intramuscularly followed by AM dosed orally at 1.6 mg/kg daily. Nineteen patients were in this study; nine of these patients received AS and 10 patients received AM. Intramuscular AS was shown to be rapidly absorbed, and plasma AS concentrations in these patients peaked between 523 and 3,221 ng/ml (median, 2,193 ng/ml) within 20 minutes of injection and subsequently declined with a median half-life of 30 minutes (ranging from 3 to 67 minutes). Peak plasma concentrations of DHA were shown to range between 488 and 2011 ng/ml (median concentration, 869 ng/ml), and these concentrations declined with at1/2 of 52 minutes (ranging from 26 to 69 minutes). Clearly, in these patients artesunate was rapidly hydrolyzed to the biologically active metabolite, DHA. The median fever clearance time (FCT) for these AS treated patients was shown to be 65 hours while the parasite clearance time (PCT) was shown to be 38 hours, and all patients survived.

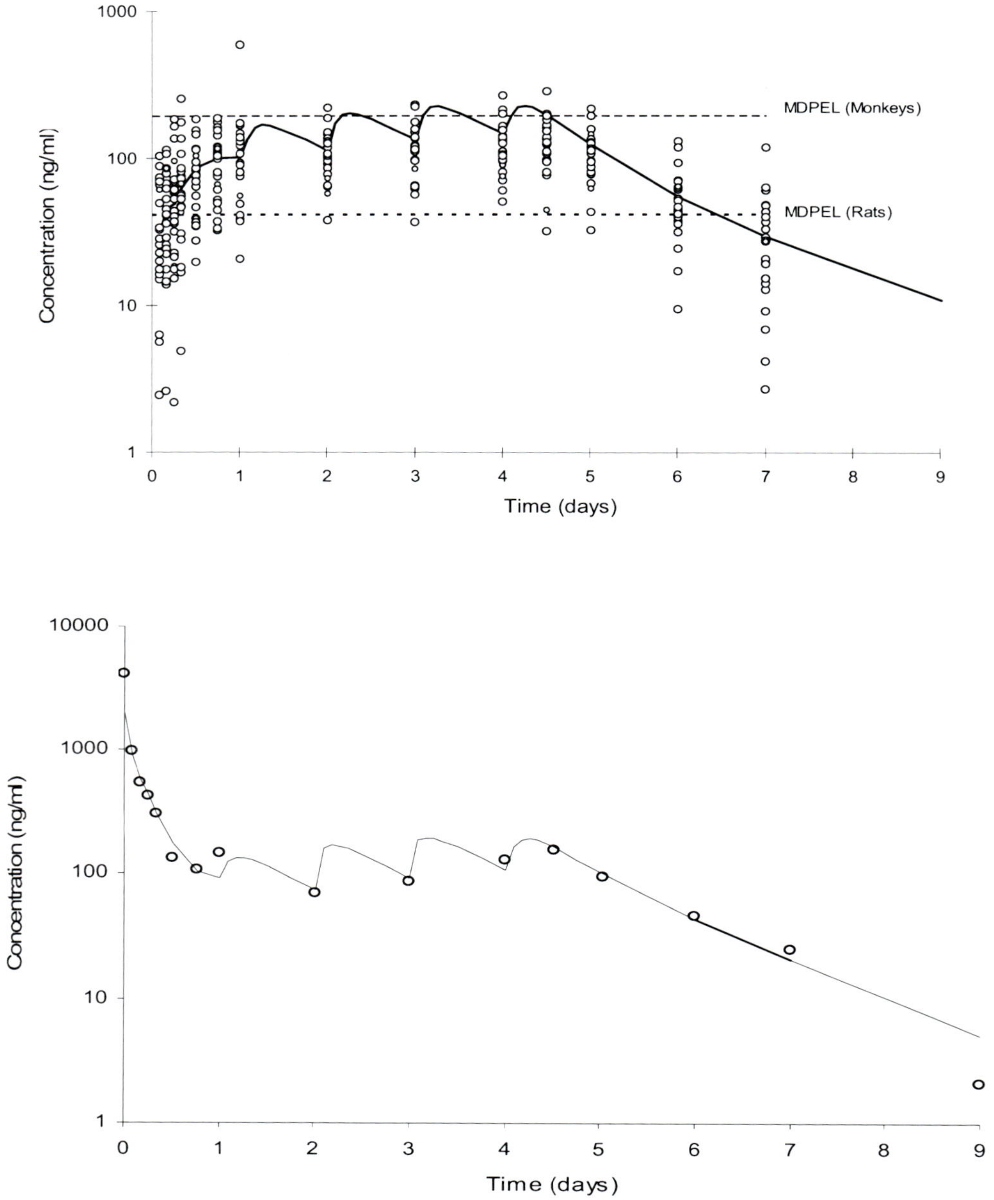

Figure 9: Pharmacokinetic profiles in plasma measured by HPLC-ECD (open circle) and computer fitted curves (solid-line) of 4.8 mg/kg at 0 hour and 1.6 mg/kg at 6, 24, 48, 72, and 96 hours of arteether (AE) with sesame oil in 42 patients. The summary of intramuscular administration in 42 patients is shown above (top chart), and in a single patient (bottom chart), whose drug was reported to have been erroneously injected into a blood vessel as an intravenous injection at the first dose [220].

In contrast, PK evaluation of patients treated in the previous study with AM demonstrated that the drug was absorbed slowly and erratically from the site of injection. The absorption profile for patients treated with AM appeared biphasic in nature. The maximum AM plasma concentrations observed in this study ranged from 20 ng/ml to 487 ng/ml (median concentration, 171 ng/ml), and these maximum concentrations were shown to occur at a median of 10 hours (range of 1.5 to 24 hours). In this group, there was relatively little conversion of AM to DHA. The median fever clearance time in the AM treated group was shown to be 56 hours while the median parasite clearance time was shown to be 48 hours. Two of ten AM treated patients died in this study (20% mortality rate). After IM injection for treatment of severe malaria, absorption of water-soluble AS is extensive and rapid, while absorption of AM, which is oil-based, is slow and erratic with low conversion to the more active metabolite, DHA. Based on this pharmacological study, the intramuscular injection of artesunate seems preferable to intramuscular injection of AM for initial antimalarial therapy, particularly in seriously ill patients. The findings that the peak plasma concentrations (2,193 ng/ml) of AS noted in this study were 13-fold higher than the peak plasma concentrations observed after AM injection (171 ng/ml) supports the hypothesis that a high peak plasma concentration makes a significant contribution to improving clinical antimalarial efficacy and reducing mortality [221].

Oral dosing of AS in this study resulted in a significantly larger drug plasma concentration than oral AM despite administration of a 29% lower molar dose. The average oral bioavailability of AM, when compared to oral AS (corrected for the molar dose), was 58%. The average relative bioavailability of AM, by contrast, was 31% the first day of dosing (95% CI, range of 17-100%), while on the second day the mean oral antimalarial bioavailability was shown to be 72% (95% CI, range from 44-118%, $P = 0.018$). The parasite clearance time and the time the drug levels remained above the *in vitro* IC_{90} were equal for AS and AM, despite significant differences in the AUC and C_{max}. The oral bioavailability of AM was shown to be lower in patients with acute malaria compared to the oral antimalarial bioavailability of AS, and the oral antimalarial efficacy of AM was much lower than the efficacy of oral AS. This difference in bioavailability may explain the increased antimalarial efficacy of oral AS over orally dosed AM at a similar molar dose [221].

All of the evidence in the literature has shown that artemisinin drugs with higher peak plasma concentrations (C_{max}) and increased AUC also demonstrate enhanced efficacy and utility as a treatment regimen. Given the life-threatening nature of *P. falciparum* malaria infections, these patients have a true medical emergency, and the best treatment should be started as soon as infection is suspected. The most appropriate antimalarial treatment equates to drug regimens with sufficient dosing to provide successful efficacy for definitive treatment of malaria-infected patients. It has been shown that 84% of malaria related deaths of African children occur within 24 hours of being admitted to a hospital [222]. Therefore, the first exposure concentrations of any artemisinin drugs administered are a critical clinical parameter.

4.4. Rapid Effects of Artemisinin Are Related to Peak Drug Concentrations

Pharmacokinetic and pharmacodynamic evaluations have shown that the effective rate of decrease in parasitemia in artemisinin-treated patients is significantly slower (2.8-8.9 hours) than the decline of artemisinin drugs present in the patient's plasma, reflecting a mean sum of the lag phase time, stage effect time, and even body elimination time with different compounds and dosage regimens. This suggests that the PD effects of artemisinin drugs are longer than the PK outcomes of artemisinin drugs. The PK elimination half-lives of artemisinin drugs have been shown to be in the range of 0.7-22.7 hours, while the times required to achieve a 50% reduction in the maximal parasite count (PC_{50}) were in the range of 8.48-19.68 hours suggesting an extended PD outcome [65]. In this evaluation, AS was shown to be superior both pharmacokinetically and pharmacodynamically to other artemisinins examined for malaria treatment. The PD analysis of AS showed that AS had the most rapid killing activity with a larger E_{max} (the maximum drug effect achieved) after oral administration. AS showed the highest peak concentration, the fastest and most reliable oral absorption rate, and the most limited drug exposure time than the other four artemisinins. Although AM and AE showed the longest half-lives and the highest exposure level (high AUC values), they had the worst efficacy (the longest lag time, the greatest AUEC, and the longest PC_{50}) likely due to their corresponding slow absorption rates and lowest peak concentrations (Table **17**). The poor treatment cure rates ranging from 48.0-86.8% for AM and AE dosed as monotherapies suggests that effective use of these two artemisinins should be as a combination therapy to enhance clinical outcomes (Table **3**).

Table 17: Pharmacokinetics/pharmacodynamic (PK/PD) parameters of AS (IV, 120 mg and oral 100 mg at 8h, then oral 750 mg mefloquine at 24h), AS (oral, 100 mg and then 50 mg b.i.d x 4), DHA (oral, 200 mg and then 100 mg x 4), QHS (oral, 500 mg and 250 b.i.d x 4 and then 500 mg on D6), AM (IM, 3.2 mg/kg and 1.6 mg x 4), and AE (IM, 4.8 mg/kg at 0 h and 1.6 mg/kg at 6 h and then day 2-5 daily) in human treatment with uncomplicated and severe/complicated malaria on day 1* [65]

PK/PD Parameters Administration Route	**AS Intravenous**	**AS Oral**	**DHA Oral**	**QHS Oral**	**AM Intramuscular**	**AE Intramuscular**
First loading dosage Maintaining dosage Total dose	120 mg Oral 100 mg at 8 hr 220 mg and mefloquine**	100 mg 50 mg b.i.d. x 4 500 mg	200 mg 100 mg x 4 600 mg	500 mg 250 x 2 x 5 3000 mg	3.2 mg/kg 1.6mg/kg x 4 9.6 mg/kg	4.8 mg/kg 1.6mg/kg x 5 12.8 mg/kg
PK parameters (Day 1)						
C_{max} (ng/ml)	2646 (DHA); 11343(AS)	1052 (DHA); 198 (AS)	437.5	588.0	74.9	110.1
T_{max} (hr)	0.13	0.75	1.4	2.4	6.0	8.2
Tlag (hr)			0.2	0.45		
$AUC_{0-24\,hr}$ (ng·h/ml)	2378 (DHA); 1146 (AS)	1334 (DHA); 210 (AS)	1329	2601	1230	4702
$t_{1/2}$ (absorption, hr)		0.36 (DHA)	0.67	1.21	1.88	3.2
$t_{1/2}$ (elimination, hr)	0.67 (DHA); 0.05 (AS)	0.70 (DHA)	0.85	2.3	7.83	22.7
MRT (hr)	0.90 (DHA)	1.95 (DHA)	2.71	7.41	13.94	42.9
PD parameters (Day 1)*						
Time of lag phase (hr)	1.92	2.81	4.03	5.76	7.26	8.89
AUIC (%·h/μl)	397.3	921.2	1167.9	1464.4	1613.4	2463.5
PC_{50} (hr)	3.18	8.48	10.05	13.95	15.63	19.68
E_{max} (%) or MPC	0.0011	0.0016	0.2132	0.0100	0.0030	0.5504
Curative rate (%)	100**	81.3	76.0	74.3	86.7	48.0

*The data was fitted with WinNonlin (V5.0) by author. **Oral 750 mg mefloquine at 24 hr after IV injection. PK = pharmacokinetics; PD = pharmacodynamics; MRT = Mean residence time; PC_{50} = Mean time for parasitemia to fall by half; AUIC = area under inhibitory curve; QHS = Artemisinin; DHA = Dihydroartemisinin; AM = Artemether; AE = Arteether; AS = Artesunate; MPC = minimum parasiticidal concentration; IM = intramuscular.

4.4.1. Effects of Artemisinin Drugs Against Cultured Parasites

An *in vitro* study of parasites in synchronous culture has shown that artemisinin treatment of parasites at concentrations ranging from 10^{-7}-10^{-5} M (30-3000 ng/ml) is rapidly effective against both ring and schizont stages of the parasite showing inhibition of 100% of parasites in these stages within a 6-hour period. The inhibitory effects of AM are slower and exposure up to 10 hours is needed to inhibit growth of 70% of ring stage parasites and 40-50% inhibition of schizont parasites. DHA was shown to be highly effective against all parasite stages and 100% parasite growth inhibition was achieved within 4 hours [215]. At concentrations ranging from 10^{-6}-10^{-5} M (280-2,800 ng/ml), artemisinin was shown to demonstrate a parasiticidal effect after 3 hours of exposure to drug, whereas treatment with artemisinin at 10^{-7} M (28 ng/ml) needed 24 hours of drug exposure for a parasiticidal effect [213, 223]. The results of this study show that treatment of *falciparum* parasites with a low concentration of artemisinin in turn requires a longer exposure time to achieve killing while treatment of *falciparum* parasites with a high concentration of artemisinin results in a decreased exposure time to achieve parasite death. Accordingly, this study supports the hypothesis that low dose treatments cannot be selected for artemisinin drugs in human treatments in malaria because; 1) the artemisinins have very short half-lives, and 2) the principle risk factor for fatal neurotoxicity after artemisinin treatment in animal models is longer exposure times [224].

In addition, when treating patients with complicated and severe *falciparum* malaria, where the ultimate survival of the patient is paramount, low effective doses of artemisinin drugs cannot be used without an undue delay in treatment time required to achieve clinical cures [214]. There is no evidence that rapid killing of malaria parasites with high sufficient doses of artemisinin drugs is harmful. In fact, all evidence points to the benefits of rapidly achieving therapeutic concentrations of artemisinin in the blood as quickly as is possible without running undue risks of drug toxicity [225]. Therefore, the plasma concentration of the artemisinin derivatives in humans against *P. falciparum* should at least be in the range of 10^{-6}-10^{-5} M (300-3000 ng/ml) or even higher for AS or DHA as they are more potent compounds. AE or AM should be administered in doses that will achieve higher plasma concentrations than AS or DHA as they are less potent. AL, being the lowest potency agent with regards to first drug exposure [204, 226], should be administered in the highest doses to achieve the highest plasma concentration.

4.4.2. Efficacy of Artemisinin Drugs in Animal Studies

Administration of artemisinin drugs reliably reduces initial malaria parasitemia by a factor of 10^4 every 48 hours. Therefore, modeling studies of asexual parasites have suggested six days of artemisinin treatment should be sufficient to kill parasites at burdens of up to 10^{12} parasites [24]. This model result does not track with the high rates of recrudescence observed (10-15%) in patients who have been treated with artemisinin monotherapy and this model result is difficult to reconcile with a higher potency agent, such as AS or DHA, or with the use of artemisinin drugs administered at higher concentrations. The poor efficacy of artemisinin monotherapies to achieve cures is not believed to be a consequence of drug resistance [227], but rather to the lower peak concentration of many artemisinins, which was demonstrated in the rat PK/PD evaluations described previously.

Table 18: The main pharmacokinetic parameters of artesunate (AS) and dihydroartemisinin (DHA), an active metabolite of AS, following oral, intrarectal (IR), intramuscular (IM) and intravenous (IV) administrations in malaria patients and volunteers*[65]

						Artesunate (AS)			Dihydroartemisinin (DHA)			Ratio of
Patients	**Where**	**Cases**	**Date**	**Route**	**Regimens**	**C_{max} ng/ml**	**AUC ng·h/ml**	**$t_{1/2}$ min**	**C_{max} ng/ml**	**AUC ng·h/ml**	**$t_{1/2}$ min**	**AUC_{DHA} /AUC_{AS}**
Children	Thailand	10	1998	IR	15.6 mg/kg	301	871	111.6	916	6145	40.2	7.06
Children	PNG	47	2004	IR	13 mg/kg	417	-	16.2	718	-	42.6	-
Children	Gabon	11	2002	IM	1.2 mg/kg	14 988	2000	11.5	2655	1585	32.0	0.79
Children	Gabon	10	2002	IV	2.4 mg/kg	29 683	3752	1.5	3012	3325	20.7	0.89
Children	Ghana	9	2001	IV	2.4 mg/kg				1593	1708	31.8	
Adults	Vietnam	13	1998a	Oral	100 mg/person	-	-	-	737	1289	39.3	-
Adults	Thailand	3	2000	Oral	2 mg/kg	198	210	-	1052	1334	-	6.35
Adults	Vietnam	5	1998b	Oral	100 mg/person	-	161	-	851	1161	40.1	7.21
Volunteer	Cambodia	15	2005	Oral	4 mg/kg	-	-	-	748	1673	78.0	-
Volunteer	Thailand	10	2004	Oral	4 mg/kg	-	-	-	519	657	44.4	-
Volunteer	Caucasia	6	2002	Oral	150 mg/person	112	154	-	546	825	-	5.36
Volunteer	Vietnam	8	2001	Oral	150 mg/person	-	-	-	1309	2532	53.0	-
Adults	Thailand	6	2001	Oral	100 mg/person	114	97	24.6	339	502	52.2	5.18
Volunteer	Malaysia	1	1997	Oral	200 mg/person	577	312	23.4	1141	1340	-	4.29
Adults	Vietnam	11	2002	IM	120 mg/person	887	999	41.0	1166	2475	64.0	2.48
Adults	Vietnam	9	2004	IM	2.4 mg/kg	2193	857	30.0	869	1497	52.7	1.75
Adults	Vietnam	13	1998a	IV	120 mg/person	11 343	1146	2.7	2646	2378	40.2	2.08
Adults	Vietnam	11	2002	IV	120 mg/person	16 149	1038	3.2	2760	2873	59.0	2.77
Adults	Thailand	2	2000	IV	2 mg/kg	-	1056	-	-	3999	-	3.79
Adults	Vietnam	12	1998b	IV	120 mg/person	13 688	877	2.2	2193	1846	36.7	2.10
Volunteer	Vietnam	10	2001	IV	120 mg/person	-	846	2.6	1508	1365	53.0	1.61
Adults	Thailand	17	2006	IV	2.4 mg/kg	130	49	13.2	605	418	20.4	8.53

*The drug measurements are by using HPLC-ECD or LC-MS/MS methods, and some drug evaluations by using bioassay are not selected in this summary.
PNG = Papua New Guinea.

The pharmacokinetic factors affecting artemisinin not only focus on the high peak plasma concentration achieved after dosing, but also involve tissue distribution of artemisinin drugs in red blood cells [228]. Recently, studies examining the tissue distribution of artemisinin drugs in rats and the protein binding of artemisinin drugs to human red blood cells were conducted at Walter Reed Army Institute of Research. Table **19** demonstrates the RBC/plasma ratios of five radiolabeled artemisinins in human whole blood at various levels [228, 229]. For equal volumes of plasma and red blood cells, the fraction of the five artemisinins found in the red blood cells of malaria-infected patients was reduced compared to the fraction found in the plasma of normal volunteer blood. The ratios are almost constant in human blood over an extensive concentration range. After correction for the 55:45 ratios of plasma and red blood cell volumes, the RBC/plasma ratios are 0.23 for ^{14}C-AE, 0.28 for ^{14}C-AM, 0.44 for ^{14}C-AL, 0.52 for ^{14}C-DHA, and 0.71 for ^{14}C-AS. The AS had the highest tissue distribution in normal human red blood cells while AE had the lowest tissue distribution in normal human red blood cells.

Table 19: The bound ratios* of human red blood cells (RBC) and plasma with ^{14}C-AE, ^{14}C-AM, ^{14}C-AL, ^{14}C-DQHS, and ^{14}C-AS in human whole blood from low to high concentration with incubated dialysis method at 37°C [65]

Concentration (MW)	**^{14}C-AE (312.4)**	**^{14}C-AM (298.4)**	**^{14}C-AL (418.5)**	**^{14}C-DHA (284.9)**	**^{14}C-AS (384.4**
0.125 nM	0.20 ± 0.01	0.28 ± 0.01	0.43 ± 0.01	0.52 ± 0.03	0.72 ± 0.05
0.25 nM	0.24 ± 0.03	0.27 ± 0.01	0.44 ± 0.02	0.53 ± 0.04	0.71 ± 0.03
0.5 nM	0.22 ± 0.02	0.28 ± 0.01	0.47 ± 0.02	0.52 ± 0.05	0.73 ± 0.05
1 nM	0.23 ± 0.02	0.27 ± 0.02	0.43 ± 0.03	0.51 ± 0.03	0.74 ± 0.04
2 nM	0.22 ± 0.01	0.26 ± 0.01	0.45 ± 0.02	0.50 ± 0.03	0.74 ± 0.06
4 nM	0.23 ± 0.01	0.29 ± 0.02	0.45 ± 0.01	0.51 ± 0.04	0.69 ± 0.06
8 nM	0.24 ± 0.03	0.27 ± 0.02	0.45 ± 0.02	0.53 ± 0.03	0.64 ± 0.04
16 nM	0.25 ± 0.03	0.29 ± 0.03	0.44 ± 0.02	0.51 ± 0.04	0.59 ± 0.08
Mean value	0.23 ± 0.02	0.28 ± 0.02	0.44 ± 0.02	0.52 ± 0.04	0.71 ± 0.08

*All values represent mean ± SD for n = 4 individual samples, AE = arteether, AM = artemether, AL = artelinic acid, DHA = dihydroartemisinin; MW = molecular weight.

These findings suggest that DHA and AS have significant advantages for entering human red blood cells (RBC/plasma ratio of 0.52 for DHA and 0.71 for AS) compared to AE and AM (RBC/plasma ratios of 0.23 for AE and 0.28 for AM). These data suggest that to reach the same distribution level in red blood cells, the drug peak concentrations for AE and AM should be two to three times higher than that of DHA and AS. In addition, the binding affinities for human plasma proteins are high for radiolabeled AE and AM. The half-maximal bound concentration value (BC_{50}) for AE is 1,945 ng/ml, and the BC_{50} for AM is 1,673 ng/ml. Conversely, the half-maximal bound concentration value (BC_{50}) for radiolabeled AS is 143 ng/ml, and the BC50 for DHA is 162 ng/ml. This data demonstrates the free drug concentrations of AS and DHA are much higher in human plasma compared to the free drug concentrations observed after administration of AE or AM.

Although DHA tablets and AM intramuscular formulations have a similar AUC compared to AS tablets (Table **17**), the speed at which they kill parasites is much slower than the speed at which AS tablets have been shown to achieve efficacy (Fig. **10**, bottom). Initial killing of parasites after administration of DHA tablets or injection of AM intramuscularly is poor because the pharmacokinetic outcome of drug administration is a peak plasma concentration that is not high enough to penetrate all red blood cells efficaciously. The uptake of DHA in infected erythrocytes has been shown to be 100-300 times higher than in uninfected erythrocytes, and the maximum uptake of the drug occurs after 1-2 hours [230]. In this case, as discussed previously, the plasma concentration of artemisinin derivatives in humans infected with *P. falciparum* should be much higher than the threshold range of 10^{-6}-10^{-5} M (300-3,000 ng/ml) for the first drug exposure in order to efficaciously cover all infected and uninfected RBC cells [214, 223]. In this animal study, compared to oral AS, the other four artemisinins administered as both oral and intramuscular formulations showed lower peak plasma concentration levels, and these artemisinin drugs could not inhibit parasite growth and efficaciously cover all RBCs in the initial several hours after first drug administration which in turn resulted in elongated half maximal parasite clearance (PC_{50}) times.

High peak plasma concentrations (C_{max}) are also more important than high overall drug exposures (AUC) to cure malaria because sufficient drug is needed to cover all RBCs, both infected and infected, in order to kill as many parasites as possible after the initial drug treatment. The AUC concentration observed during this period very often lacks the necessary high peak concentrations for maximal efficacy. For example, in clinical trials with AE, the observed AUCs are higher after administration of four other artemisinin drugs (Table **17**), and AE dosing results in lower C_{max} values that are also associated with poor efficacy. Therefore, high overall drug exposures (AUC) without high peak plasma levels do not result in coverage of all RBCs. This outcome could result in some infected RBCs left untreated. These untreated RBCs may be the reason for recrudescence after drug regimens of artemisinin monotherapy. One other example is native artemisinin (QHS) which has low efficacy against malaria [204, 226]. In clinical studies, oral doses of QHS 5-fold higher than AS have been given to patients, and despite the much higher doses given, QHS still showed poor efficacy which is likely due to its peak concentration which is only half the peak concentration achieved with AS. These data also support the hypothesis that any artemisinin drug with such poor antimalarial efficacy should not be used in malaria treatment.

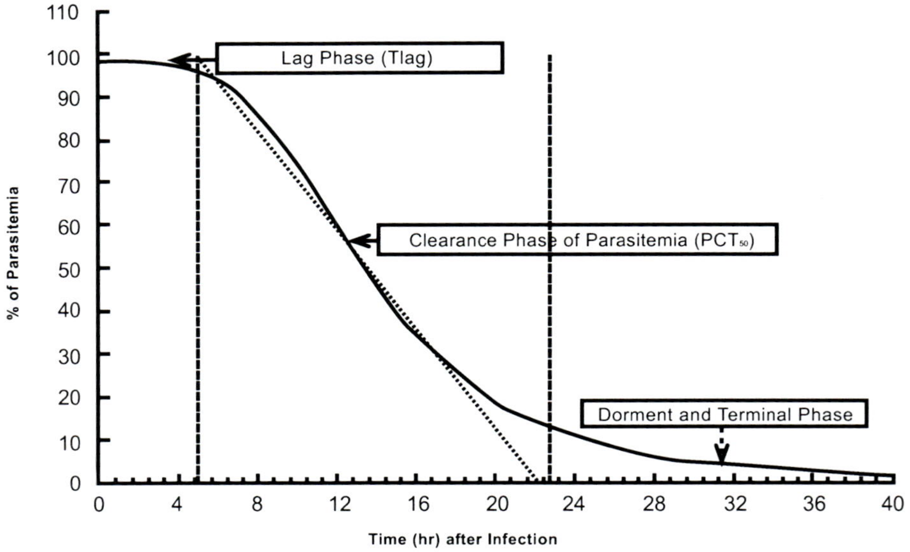

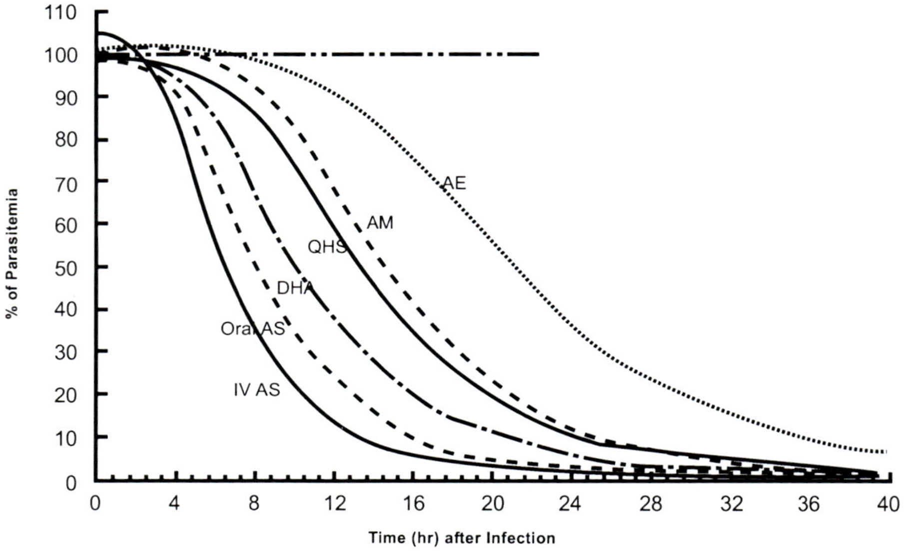

Figure 10: Standard parasite clearance curve in different stages (lag phase, clearance phase, dormant and terminal phase) and synchronicity of parasite development under antiparasitic drug received at 0 hour (top chart). The mean parasite clearance curves (bottom chart) from the shortest to longer time were AS (solid line) at single intravenous 120 mg, oral 100 mg at 8 hr then oral 750 mg mefloquine at 24 hr, oral AS (dashed line) at 100 mg first day and 50 mg b.i.d 2-5 days orally, oral DHA (dot & dashed line) at 200 mg first day and 100 mg 2-5 days orally, oral QHS (solid line) at 500 mg first day, 250 mg b.i.d 2-5 and 500 mg last day orally; intramuscular AM (dashed line) at 3.2 mg/kg first day and 1.6 mg/kg 2-5 days intramuscularly, and intramuscular AE (dot line) of 4.8 mg/kg at 0 hour and 1.6 mg/kg at 6 and then 2-5 days intramuscularly in malaria patients (bottom chart). The parasitemia at 0 hour was set as 100% of parasitemia [311].

In conclusion, the swift efficacy of artemisinins is primarily dependent on peak drug concentrations (C_{max}) after the first drug exposure and relative antimalarial drug potency. The relative antimalarial potency of the artemisinin drugs is demonstrated by the capability for killing malaria parasites at various stages, rapid oral drug absorption, high peak plasma concentrations, low plasma protein binding, drug distribution in targets (RBCs), and the actual membrane permeability of infected RBCs to artemisinin drugs. Other pharmacokinetic parameters such as drug exposure level (AUC) and drug exposure time tend to be less influential on drug efficacy.

4.4.3. Recrudescence of Patients Treated with Artemisinins Due to Reduction in Drug Levels

Decreases in plasma drug concentration after multiple oral drug doses have been shown in clinical trials of many artemisinin drugs (AS, QHS, DHA, AM) administered to both malaria-infected and uninfected patients. The C_{max} and AUC values of artemisinin drugs observed after multiple oral doses over time were substantially reduced by one-third to one-seventh on the last day of dosing compared to the first day of dosing. The decreases in drug exposure and drug levels noted during treatment were not believed to be disease-related, as the pharmacokinetic analysis of artemisinin on day 1 was similar to that reported in healthy subjects in other studies [205-209]. Similar time-dependent decreases after oral AM administration were also demonstrated experimentally in beagle dogs (Fig. **11,** bottom) [231]. One possible hypothesis to explain decreases in plasma concentration over time during treatment is a change in metabolism due to auto-induction of hepatic enzymes such as the CYP drug-metabolizing enzymes. This decrease in drug concentration observed over time was not observed after dosing patients intramuscularly with intramuscular administration of AE formulated in sesame oil [232]. The remarkable alteration of the pharmacokinetic shape of artemisinins administered as monotherapy through multiple doses may be a contributing factor to the reduced efficacy of artemisinin monotherapy regimens and, in turn, may be the explanation for parasite recrudescence often observed in patients treated with artemisinin monotherapy.

The therapeutic efficacy of all of the artemisinin drugs including derivatives administered as antimalarial monotherapy in varying dose regimens in 54 clinical trials is summarized in Table **3**. Treatments with 100% cure outcomes could not be achieved in 3-5 day monotherapy treatment regimens nor were they achieved

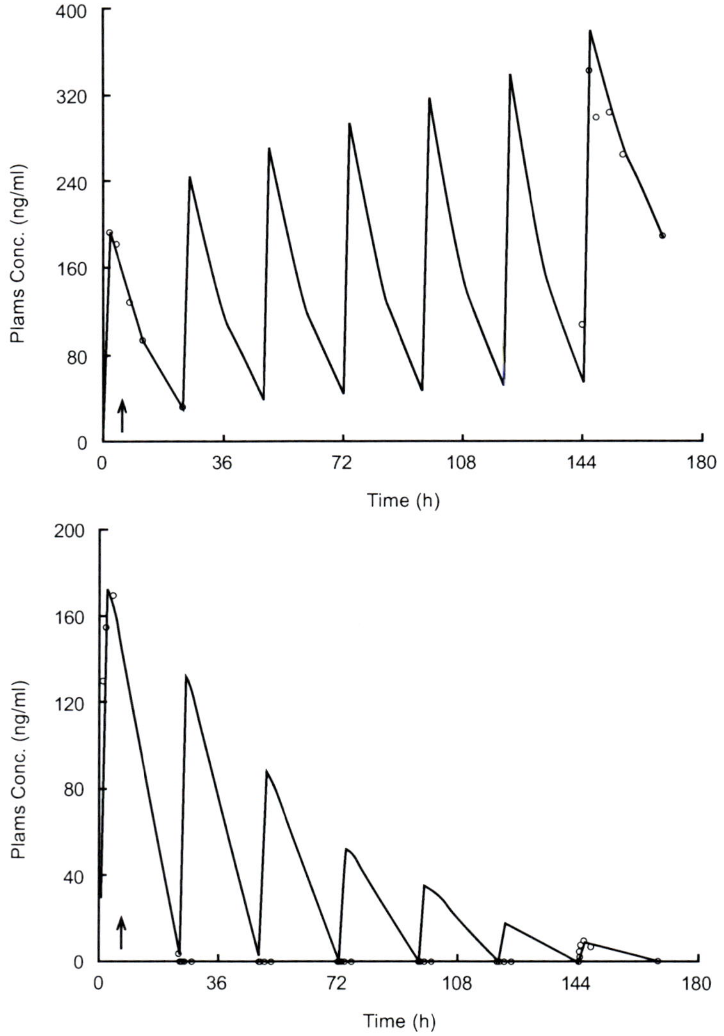

Figure 11: Pharmacokinetic profiles measured by HPLC-ECD (open circle) and computer fitted curves (solid line) of 20 mg/kg of artemether with sesame oil (top, showing drug accumulation) after intramuscular injection and 600 mg/kg of artemether in capsule (bottom, showing drug decline) following oral administration daily for 7 days in beagle dogs [231].

in high dose monotherapy regimens (4.8 mg/kg) [65, 233]. Table **3** shows the curative rates, fever clearance times (FCT), and parasite clearance times (PCT) for each regimen as these parameters are the most descriptive pharmacodynamic evaluation parameters known for comparing the antimalarial drug efficacy in man. This table of these three parameters illustrates the therapeutic potential of intravenous, intramuscular, and oral artemisinin agents in various regimens. One set of results, which is clear when looking at the data from Table **3**, is that arteether (AE) in sesame oil vehicle, is an inferior treatment when compared to oral and intravenous artesunate, oral dihydroartemisinin (DHA), intramuscular AE formulated with peanut oil, or intramuscular artemether (AM). These data all support the hypothesis that artemisinin drugs are best administered in combination therapy with long lasting, appropriately chosen, partner drugs [71, 196].

The outcomes data previously discussed helps explains the majority of *in vitro* and *in vivo* data observed following antimalarial treatment [234]. In particular, this data sheds light on why monotherapeutic treatment of <7 days duration with rapidly eliminated artemisinin drugs will likely not result in 100% cure rates, why infections with large biomass are more likely to recrudesce following antimalarial treatment (increased numbers of parasites require longer duration therapy). It also explains why recrudescence tends to occur two weeks after stopping treatment with short course antimalarials [234] and why recrudescence following treatment with slowly eliminated antimalarial drugs tends to occur later at periods of 28 days or later after treatment is initiated [78]. This data also explains why the mean time to recrudescence shortens as antimalarial drug resistance worsens. For many clinicians, prevention of recrudescence is not high priority when compared to achieving immediate patient cures, and it has been suggested that recrudescent infections should be re-treated with the same regimen that failed initially. This strategy may achieve success in achieving cures (particularly in cases of poor compliance), but it overlooks the real risk of selecting for drug resistant parasites which in turn become a public health threat to many instead of one. The utilization of combination therapy regimens is a far better tool to achieve radical cures in cases of recrudescence both in terms of patient outcomes and in terms of achieving worthwhile public health goals of decreasing the incidence of drug resistance of malaria parasite.

The parasite clearance time (PCT) is a measure of how well a drug therapy reduces parasitemia, and this assessment of initial drug treatment is commonly coupled with the fever clearance time (FCT) as a yardstick to gauge malaria drug treatment efficacy. Reviews of therapeutic efficacy from multiple clinical studies have shown that monotherapeutic use of AM (both oral and intramuscular administration), AS (oral and intravenous dosing), and DHA (oral administration) appear to have similar abilities to reduce PCT and FCT under various dose regimens (Table **3**). The finding that the therapeutic potential of AM and AS in oral formulation could be equal to DHA is surprising and may be explained by the high conversion rate of AM or AS to DHA in humans and development of high peak concentrations as described previously. Intramuscular AE injection appears to have lower efficacy than the other four drugs, even when administered at high doses. Intramuscular AE is inferior to AM intramuscular formulations (Table **3**), and this may be due to the much lower blood concentrations achieved after AE injection due to slow and prolong absorption [171, 221, 235].

The PCT does not always track with the total numbers of parasitized red blood cells, but better parameters are not available [236, 237]. As all of the artemisinin drugs are capable of rapidly reducing the parasite biomass, quick parasite clearance induced by artemisinin therapy provides a very simple pharmacodynamic measure that is useful for comparative efficacy assessments of antimalarial drugs. In the next section, we will discuss and compare the pharmacodynamic data derived from malaria treatment of patients in various clinical trials with the associated PK results.

4.5. THE INTERACTIONS OF PK AND PD AFFECT THE EFFICACY OF ANTIMALARIAL DRUGS

Theoretical research and speculation into the dynamics determining the evaluation of drug usage have focused on five main areas:

1) the widespread nature of single and multi-drug resistant parasites;
2) the variability in immunity ranging from semi-immune to non-immune subjects;
3) the relationship between parasitemia and malaria disease;
4) the large inter-individual pharmacodynamic variations; and
5) the dynamics of utilizing antimalarial drugs in special populations.

If the variables concerning an infection are known, then it is possible to define the PD properties for a drug required for a cure. Assessment of treatment responses in malaria are provided through clinical outcomes (speed of recovery, mortality, parasite clearance time, fever clearance time, *etc*.). The advantages of more precisely defining the pharmacodynamic properties of antimalarial drugs include coming up with better methods of assessing therapeutic response. A clear definition of PD properties required provides a means of designing drug-dosing regimens for antimalarial drugs (dose, duration, and frequency), predicting treatment failures, and reducing the emergence of drug resistance to antimalarials.

4.5.1. Inter-individual PK Variation Influences Drug Efficacy

There is significant inter-individual variation in plasma or blood drug concentrations observed in patients after administration of many antimalarial drugs at any given dose, and peak blood concentrations may differ by a factor of 10 or more. Several of the antimalarial drugs, such as mefloquine, atovaquone, halofantrine, and lumefantrine, share some similar characteristics of hydrophobicity and lipophilicity, and all of these drugs have been shown to have high variability in oral bioavailability [238, 239]. Absorption of antimalarial drugs administered orally is often poor in acutely ill patients who have not eaten. Co-administration of these drugs with fat may enhance absorption 10-fold or more [240].

Accordingly, some patients will have inadequate absorption of these oral drugs despite receipt of a full treatment dose. Inadequate blood concentrations will result, and malaria infections may recrudesce. The minimum parasiticidal concentration (MPC) of an antimalarial drug is defined as the minimum blood or plasma concentration which produces maximum inhibitory drug activity (*i.e.* IC_{99}), and blood drug levels of should therefore exceed the MPC concentration during four asexual reproduction cycles (>6 days) to achieve maximum cure rates [160]. For lumefantrine, for example, the plasma concentrations observed 7 days after starting treatment have been shown to be a very useful metric to predict a therapeutic outcome [241]. In the past, it was assumed that blood concentrations of artemisinin drug should be above the MPC throughout the period of treatment, which a general rule is found to be true for all previous antimalarial drugs. This general rule was overcome by the data showing that once-daily administration of artemisinin compounds with half-lives of <1 hour provides a similar outcome to artemisinin drugs dosed twice daily [78, 242].

Clearly, if the range of blood drug concentrations achieved in patients exceeds the drug concentrations associated with inhibition of 90% of parasite growth (IC_{90} values) for a drug resistant parasite (IC_{90R}), then it is not possible to select for drug resistance as resistant mutants are precluded from growing [243]. Provided a window of selection is possible, the odds of selecting a drug resistant parasite in a patient is largely dependent on the range of peak antimalarial drug concentrations observed. The closer the median drug concentration approaches the IC_{90R}, the lower the probability of mutation. Peak drug concentrations observed in a concentration time plot are, like all other pharmacokinetic parameters, dependent on the dose provided and the processes of drug absorption and distribution. Several antimalarials to include atovaquone, mefloquine, and lumefantrine are hydrophobic, lipophilic, and vary in their absorption as inter-individual bioavailability can vary up to 20-fold [61, 225]. Inter-individual variation in the volume of distribution is lower, generally in the range of 5-fold variability among individuals, however, when adding in the effects of variability of absorption overall outcomes show broad inter-individual variability in peak antimalarial blood concentrations.

The priority for treatment of severe and complicated malaria disease is intravenous administration of the most appropriate, safe dose of antimalarial drug capable of reducing parasite biomass and patient care conducted at the highest possible level. The range of supportive care required for patients with severe malaria can include care for complications to include convulsions, coma, fluid and electrolyte imbalance, metabolic acidosis, hypoglycemia, anemia, renal failure, bleeding disorders, and secondary infections. The most significant advance in decreasing mortality among patients with severe malaria has been the replacement of quinine injections with injections of intravenous artesunate [200], which may very well revolutionize the management of severe disease. Recrudescence rates are still relatively high, however, after administration of intravenous AS monotherapy [244]. Since recrudescence is not due to parasite resistance [245], one possible explanation of this parasitological failure may be a low peak concentration after administration of the first loading dose of intravenous AS.

Currently, the therapeutic dosages of injectable AS to treat severe and complicated malaria are in the range of 2-2.4 mg/kg. This dose was designed in accordance with prior experience of physicians with access to clinical trial data spanning twenty years. The principal concerns are associated with side effects caused by too much AS which include neurotoxicity and dose-dependent hemotoxicity, and the consequences of too little AS which include a poor antimalarial efficacy and diminished cure rates below 90% [196, 246]. This regimen will produce a highly variable C_{max} ranging from 735-18,909 ng/ml (Table **18**), however, and the lower range of peak concentrations achieved are at a lower concentration than needed for patients with hyperparasitemia. In theory, patients with severe malaria require a C_{max} ranging from 7,500-30,000 ng/ml peak concentration to efficaciously cover all infected RBCs. Infected RBCs absorb artemisinin compounds differently than uninfected cells, and an infected RBC can concentrate 100 to 300-fold more DHA than an uninfected, normal RBC during the first 1-2 hours after dosing. The large variability in pharmacokinetics and pharmacodynamics observed when using AS should also be considered. All of these factors translate into a dosing requirement for intravenous AS that is increased to a higher level (4-8 mg/kg) than the current level of 2.0-2.4 mg/kg. The question remains, however, is this intravenous dose safe for treatment of severe malaria?

Compared to oral AS, injectable artesunate is superior in both pharmacokinetic and pharmacodynamic terms to oral AS and the other four artemisinins in treating patients with severe malaria. Injectable AS shows the highest peak concentration (Table **18**), the fastest effective time, rapid elimination, and a very short exposure moment compared to oral AS (Table **20)** [247]. As discussed elsewhere, the drug exposure time of artemisinins is the principle factor responsible for induction of neurotoxicity in animal species. Therefore, the production of the active metabolite of artemisinin, DHA, the drug distribution in the CNS, and the drug exposure level play relatively less important roles than the drug exposure time. The water-soluble artemisinins, AS in particular, have very short half-lives and produce limited exposure times in animal species and in humans, suggesting that once-daily oral or intravenous administration of AS is relatively safe. In fact, these animal experiments demonstrated that no neurotoxicity (pathological or behavioral) has been shown in animals administered intravenous administration at any range of doses repeated up to the maximum tolerated dose tested (MTD). The MTD of AS tested in rats was 240 mg/kg administered through intravenous injection daily for 3 days, and no observable neurotoxicity effects were detected in these animals after treatment with injected AS at that dose [255, 256].

Table 20: Comparison of the main pharmacokinetic parameters of artemisinin derivatives (DHA, AM, AE, AS and AL) at 10 mg/kg in rats following single intravenous injection. Values are mean ± SD (n = 4) [247]

Parameters	**DHA**	**AM**	**AE**	**AS**	**AL**
MW =	**284.9**	**298.4**	**312.4**	**384.4**	**418.5**
Dose (mg/kg)	**10**	**10**	**10**	**10**	**10**
Dose (μM/kg)	**35.1**	**33.5**	**32.0**	**26.0**	**23.9**
IV Vehicles	**CMP**	**1:3 CMP/sal**	**1:3 CMP/sal**	**Saline pH 8**	**Saline pH 8**
C_{max} (ng/ml)	6683 ± 2405	6231 ± 1837	3724 ± 430	2106 ± 399	12706 ±1010
(μM)	23.5 ± 13.0	20.9 ± 6.2	11.9 ± 1.4	5.5 ± 1.0	30.4 ± 2.2
$AUC_{inf.}$ (ng·h/ml)	3184 ± 659	1857 ± 432	842 ± 154	738 ± 114	5481 ± 1754
(μM·h)	11.2 ± 2.3	6.2 ± 1.4	2.7 ± 0.5	1.9 ± 0.3	13.1 ± 3.8
Vss (liter/kg)	0.50 ± 0.19	0.67 ± 0.11	0.72 ± 0.09	0.87 ± 0.35	0.39 ± 0.12
CL (ml/min/kg)	55.4 ± 9.7	91.8 ± 21.0	200.0 ± 31.0	190.9 ± 30.3	32.1 ± 8.0
$t_{1/2}$ distribution (h)	0.22 ± 0.04	0.10 ± 0.01	0.10 ± 0.02	0.15 ± 0.02	0.19 ± 0.08
$t_{1/2}$ elimination (h)	0.95 ± 0.21	0.53 ± 0.14	0.45 ± 0.03	0.35 ± 0.08	1.35 ± 0.45

CMP = Cremophore EL, DHA = Dihydroartemisinin, AM = Artemether, AE = Arteether, AS = Artesunate, AL = Artelinic acid, MW = Molecular weight, IV = intravenous, sal = saline.
*pH adjusted to 8.5 with 1N $NaHCO_3$.

In another study, intravenous AS administration had no effect on behavioral neurotoxicity scores after administration at a dose of 120 mg/kg daily for 7 days (unpublished data derived at Walter Reed Army Institute of Research). IM injection of AS in rats at a dose of 420 mg/kg resulted in no observations of neuronal necrosis. In addition, administration of daily doses of AS orally to rats at a dose of 200 mg/kg for periods of 5-7 days showed neither neuronal changes nor any clinical signs of behavioral change [248]. Therefore, the 4-8 mg/kg dose administered intravenously should be safe concerning neurotoxicity [249, 250] and safe about hemotoxicity [203, 251]. One study in man used a high dose of oral AS, up to 6 mg/kg, and this AS regimen was well-tolerated [252]. In Phase 1 clinical trials conducted at WRAIR, doses of AS ranging from 2-8 mg/kg administered intravenously were exceedingly well tolerated following both single and multiple intravenous injections in volunteers with a new formulation [253, 254). In malaria patients, treatment with AS at higher doses is demonstrably safe and is unlikely to result in a sub-maximal antimalarial effect.

To further characterize dose responses *in vivo* for AS and design a more rational basis for dosing, Angus *et al.* [252], conducted a study of 47 random adults infected with uncomplicated *falciparum* malaria characterized by parasitemia >1% who were subsequently treated with one dose of AS ranging from 0-250 mg together with an oral mefloquine administered at a curative dose. The pharmacodynamic endpoint of this study was the parasite clearance time. The data from this study was fitted to a sigmoidal maximum inhibitory effect PD model (E_{max}) where dose was related to the PCT. The E_{max} derived from this model was estimated to be 28.6 hours, and the calculated 50% effective dose of oral AS was estimated to be 1.6 mg/kg body weight. These results suggest there is no reduction in the parasite clearance times through administration of a single oral dose of artesunate greater than 2 mg/kg, effectively reflecting the mean lower limit of a maximally effective dose [252]. The authors concluded that 2 mg/kg is a maximum effective dose in those selected patients. The authors also pointed out, however, that a dose of 2 mg/kg is the lowest capable of providing maximum effects in "average" patients. When taking into account the considerable and large PK/PD variances between individuals [246, 252, 257], a bigger dose is necessary to ensure that the population of patients receives a maximum effect. Therefore, it is reasonable to suggest increasing the loading dose of intravenous AS to a higher level (4-8 mg/kg) to achieve the goals of maximum treatment effect for all patients taking into account variables in PK and PD described previously. After the first drug exposure to reduce the parasitemia below 1%, follow-on maintenance doses could be significantly cut or switched sequentially to another slower acting and low dose non-artemisinin antimalarial agent in order to protect AS from recrudescence or induction of drug resistance [258, 259].

4.5.2. Pharmacodynamic Characteristics of Antimalarial Drugs

1) Effects of Antimalarial Drugs on Parasite Clearance

Falciparum malaria infections may exhibit rapid or slow declines in parasitemia following various treatment regimens because of parasite sequestration of a synchronous infection. The parasite clearance time or PCT is defined as the period from the initiation of antimalarial therapy to the point where parasites are no longer microscopically observed. Defining the PCT accurately is highly dependent on parasitemia observed at the time of patient admission and the frequency with which follow-on microscopy is conducted. PCTs will obviously be lower if the parasitemia at admission is low and may vary by 24 hours if microscopy is conducted only once per day. Accordingly, particularly in small clinical trials, parasitemia counts should be conducted every 12 hours and preferably every 4-6 hours with a consistent method. Given variability in microscopy associated with slide preparation and staining, length of assessment, and, most importantly, the experience of the microscopist, parasite clearance times should be defined by calculating more than one parameter [214]. One method of assessing parasite clearance time more accurately is to make multiple assessments. For example, in one study, investigators assessed parasitemia by defining the PC_{50} (time until the parasite count is reduced by 50%), PC_{90} (time until the parasite count is reduced by 90%), and the overall time until all parasites are cleared (PCT). Other investigators have used the PC_{95} and the PC_{99}. These measures are all misleading at low parasitemia levels due to the intrinsic variability associated with obtaining parasite counts disproportionally increases when parasite counts are close to the limits of detection. For comparisons of drug efficacy, it may be desirable to exclude patients whose parasite counts are under 10,000/ml [160].

The dihydrofolate reductase inhibitors (cycloguanil and pyrimethamine) and many of the quinolines such as quinidine, quinine, and mefloquine have been shown to have little effect on asexual malaria parasites in the first 24 hours of the 48-hour parasite life cycle [164, 260-262]. Due to this lack of activity of traditional antimalarial drugs, most circulating parasites will grow and mature, express adhesins on the surface of infected erythrocytes, and begin to clump and trigger formation of red blood cell rosettes in spite of the initiation of treatment. Accordingly, exposure of ring form parasites to traditional antimalarial drugs has no significant effect on preventing parasite sequestration [263]. Consequently, observations of a decline in parasitemia after initiation of treatment with traditional antimalarials are largely similar to what would have taken place if treatment had never been initiated. In contrast, artemisinin and its derivatives are capable of inhibiting the growth of young ring stage parasites *in vitro* and they are capable of triggering clearance of ring forms *in vivo* [164, 264, 265]. As a result, declines in parasitemia after artemisinin compounds are administered are more rapid than with drugs affecting only mature schizonts. Differences in stage activity may not be visible from the treatment record of an individual, however, these differences do become clear when patients with similar background immunity and parasitemia at admission are treated with drugs affecting different parts of the parasite life cycle, and the outcomes are directly compared [160].

Populations of patients with malaria have infections that vary in magnitude in terms of stage, parasitemia, and synchronicity, and therefore the time-parasitemia profile will vary. The clearance curve of parasite for a population shows an average of individual parasitemia *versus* time profiles normalized to a 100% baseline parasitemia. After treatment with mefloquine or quinine, the average parasitemia-time profile begins with a lag phase, where the population mean parasitemia is unchanged, followed by a decline in parasitemia. Parasite clearance curves in population after artemisinin therapy [266] shows a much shorter lag phase and thus a shorter PC_{50}, PC_{90}, and PCT, provided the infecting organisms are fully sensitive. These differences in the parasitemia *versus* time curve are too rapid to be explained through reductions in merogony, and this effect can only be explained by accelerated ring form clearance [267]. Enhanced sequestration through accelerated cytoadherence is not likely as a different explanation, as quick declines in parasitemia coincide with morphological changes in circulating parasites who also have reduced cytoadherence *in vitro* [160]. The drug action on stage specificity and the relative extent of drug effect can be determined from these clearance curves of population parasite [268].

Antimalarial drugs, in general, are most active on mature trophozoites, which correspond to the middle third of the life cycle [160, 164, 264, 265]. Assessment of stage specificity can be conducted *in vitro* using methods of parasite growth assessment conducted on synchronized parasites and visually through examination of inhibition of morphological development and multiplication. Stage specificity effects do vary between compounds and precise methodology varies. Available evidence suggests that dihydrofolate reductase inhibitors are most active during a narrow window of time in the second half of the parasite life cycle while mefloquine and quinine have a broader window of time during the same second half of the parasite life cycle. Chloroquine has a wide activity window; however, artemisinin analogues derivatives have the biggest time window of activity, with substantial effects on young, ring stage parasites. As parasite stages can be assumed to be randomly distributed in patient populations some of the patients will predominantly have mature schizonts present when drug treatment is provided. Accordingly, the effects of antimalarial drugs on schizont development can be determined by directly matching the fraction of patients whose parasitemia has an early rise within 6-12 hours after treatment is initiated. After treatment with oral artesunate, early increases in parasitemia are substantially reduced compared to the early increases in parasitemia observed after initiation of treatment with mefloquine or quinine. This data supports the hypothesis that artesunate affects mature schizont development later than other antimalarial drugs [160].

2) Influence of Antimalarial Pharmacodynamics on Drug Regimens

Although PD properties of antimalarial compounds *in vivo* are not entirely explained enough data has been published to make simple models to predict the duration of antimalarial treatment required to reduce the probability of treatment failure leading to parasite recrudescence. Mature schizonts and tiny rings have long been known to be drug-resistant stages of malaria blood infections [164]. The majority of antimalarial drugs in use are effective on sequestered parasites invisible to the microscopist. The aftermath of antimalarial drug treatment with most compounds is inhibited trophozoite development and a considerable decrease in the parasite multiplication rate. As susceptibility is stage dependent for many drugs, the matching the administration of a drug with the stage of a parasite (chronotherapy) may be of use to determine a therapeutic response, assuming exact matching of administration to stage is possible in a clinical setting [165].

Artemisinin compounds are peroxidic antimalarial drugs active against ring stage parasites. In early Chinese studies of artemisinin, drug treatment was initiated when the majority of parasites observed microscopically were at the tiny-ring stage of development [166]. Normally drugs are administered at intervals that correspond to drug half-life in patients with disease. If a drug were efficacious at levels above a therapeutic level, then biological half-life of this drug would correspond to drug half-life. If concentration-dependent killing is taking place and the effects *in vivo* continue after drug concentrations decrease below the therapeutic level, however, then a drug can reasonably be administered less often than one might predict from drug half-life parameters shown in a PK study [269]. The biological half-life data is independent of the antimalarial dose-response or concentration-effect relationships *in vivo*, so a holistic data analysis approach must consider any confounding pharmacodynamic effects not readily apparent from looking at one piece of data. *In vitro*, the relationship between the effects of antimalarial drugs and hypoxanthine uptake or on schizont maturation is displayed as a sigmoid curve [164].

These concentration effect relationships are likely not similar at different parasite development stages. Although therapeutic concentrations are believed to show activity of a drug at the top flat part of the sigmoidal concentration effect dose-response curve (*i.e.*, E_{max}), there is very little data to support this hypothesis for antimalarial drugs. These issues are relevant for other short-half-life antimalarial agents such as the artemisinin analogues. The published data shows despite the short half-life of artesunate (<1 hour) and the equally short half-life of its metabolite, DHA (<1 hour). Oral artesunate is as efficacious administered either once daily or twice daily [78, 268].This data supports a hypothesis that for artemisinin compounds, the biological pharmacodynamic effect extends beyond the actual presence of drug at therapeutic levels in the plasma. The broad activity of these drugs against a number of parasite life stages provides a biological effect where exposure of just a few hours in each asexual life cycle is adequate to achieve a significant antimalarial outcome. This data challenges the hypothesis that all antimalarial drugs must be present at therapeutic levels, which are above the minimal parasiticidal concentration throughout the interval between doses.

3) Effect of Drug Efficacy on the Parasite Reduction Ratio

The parasite reduction ratio (PRR) is defined by the reduction in parasitemia from the initiation of treatment to the parasitemia count observed 48 hours later [160]. The PRR represents the fractional reduction of parasitemia per asexual life cycle, which is a very simple useful tool to predict outcomes. Conventionally, parasitological recovery after a malaria infection is measured by peripheral blood parasite clearance assessed by microscopy. In patients who have infections with drug-resistant malaria, parasites remain in peripheral blood and their numbers may increase after antimalarial drug administration. Patients who are infected with less drug resistant parasites will vanish from the peripheral blood typically below detectable levels by microscopy but may recur later usually at the same time as symptoms recur. As antimalarial drug efficacy is assessed by how quickly signs and symptoms resolve, declines in parasitemia, and the fraction of patients who suffer recrudescence/new infection in a given period.

The number of new young parasites, which entering the circulation capable of invading red blood cells depends on a variety of factors. These factors include:

1) Stage of parasite development and the synchronicity of development,
2) The biomass of parasitemia that is sequestered,
3) The presence or absence of agglutinating antibodies directed against the merozoite,
4) The number of viable merozoites that are produced per schizont,
5) Drug levels achieved in the peripheral blood, the timing of administration of antimalarial drugs, and
6) The activity of the drug [214].

Antimalarial drugs vary in concentration-effect relationships, and they vary in their activity (Fig. **12**). Thus, the maximum drug effect (E_{max}) achieved for one particular drug will be varied *versus* another, and the minimum parasiticidal concentration (MPC) in the blood is required for maximal effect. Generally, drug concentrations of antimalarial drugs will have to be higher than the concentration required inhibiting parasite multiplication. In the presence of concentrations of antimalarial drug that are effective (*i.e.*, drug concentrations >minimum inhibitory concentration or MIC), parasitemia falls as a consequence of inhibited supply of new parasites, clearance of circulating ring stage parasites, and parasite sequestration.

Malarias that are non-sequestering such as *P. vivax*, *P. ovale*, and *P. malariae*, show a decrease in parasite burden after antimalarial treatment, and this can be assessed by looking at the parasitemia at baseline *versus* the parasitemia at 48 hours multiplied by blood volume. While the actual parasite burden for *P. falciparum* cannot be assessed in this manner (this is due to sequestration of parasites out of the peripheral blood circulation), this baseline-to-48-hour parasitemia ratio is useful information. The plasma reduction ratio (PRR) which is defined as the fractional reduction in malaria parasitemia demonstrated per asexual life cycle is analogous to the rate of killing. When comparing the substantial differences in PRR observed in patients treated with different between antimalarial drugs, actual differences in the intrinsic activity (shown by the E_{max} value) are illustrated [160].

The estimated PRR *in vivo* for artemisinin compounds is 10^3-10^5, while the PRR for 4-aminoquinolines such as chloroquine, and halofantrine range from 10^2-10^4. Quinine, mefloquine, pyrimethamine-sulfadoxine range from 10^1-10^3 while antimalarial antibiotics, show a PRR estimated to range from 5-10.

The highest PRR values observed are found in the artemisinin derivatives followed by the quinoline drugs (chloroquine, mefloquine, amodiaquine, piperaquine, quinine *etc.*) and the lowest PRR values observed *in vivo* are the antimalarial antibiotics such as doxycycline, tetracycline, sulfadoxine, and pyrimethamine. Patients treated with these drugs as monotherapy must have these drugs present at therapeutic concentrations for approximately 2 weeks or it is very likely the malaria infection will recrudesce, which is consistent with results of various clinical studies. There is a clear relationship between therapeutic drug levels observed in blood or plasma *in vivo* and the PRR, which reflects the parasite-killing rate, and the minimum parasiticidal concentration (MPC) equals the maximum PRR. Additionally, estimates of the PRR *in vivo* also allows for estimation of the length of time therapeutic concentrations of drugs are required (Fig. **12**). The PRR estimate makes the assumption that rate of parasite killing or reduction remains constant with succeeding lifecycles. The simple concept of a parasite reduction ratio does not explain all therapeutic responses observed for malaria treatment of infection.

One example of where the PRR estimate falls short is the combination of tetracycline with quinine as a single agent, which is consistently more efficacious than quinine monotherapy, even in locations where quinine-resistant parasites are present, but mean PRRs for quinine combined with tetracycline, however, are not significantly different if tetracycline is added in combination with quinine or not. For complete eradication of parasites, malaria drug concentrations must be at least at the MIC (minimum inhibitory concentration) and preferably at the MPC (minimum parasiticidal concentration) in the blood until all parasites are dead or the host immune defenses are capable of dealing with the residual parasites. Treatment with short-acting antimalarial agents for periods of less than 7 days in non-immune patients will not kill all of the parasites present in all patients, and significant rates of recrudescence in these patients treated with monotherapy should be expected (Fig. **12**). Treatment failure rates will be elevated in patients who present with a greater initial parasite burden as these patients have more parasites to remove.

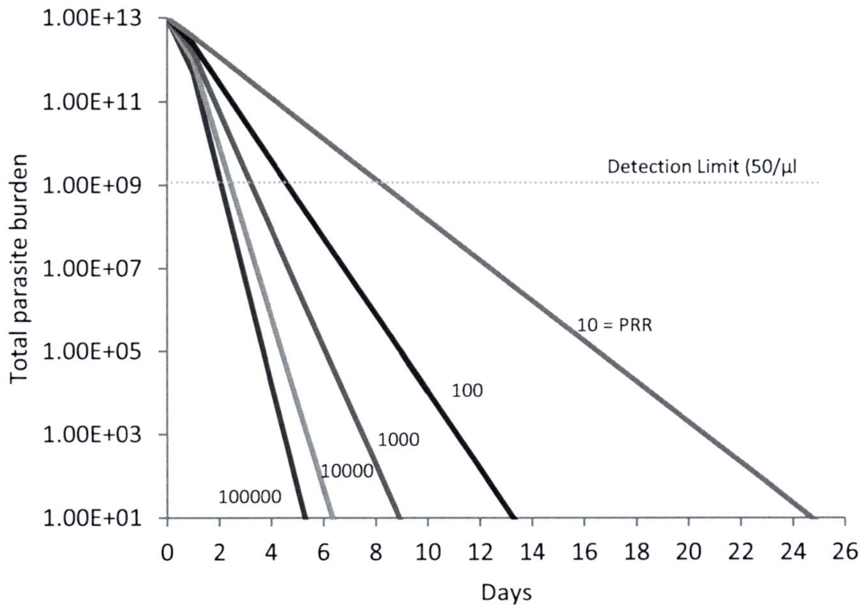

Figure 12: Parasite clearance shown following different antimalarial treatments. The initial parasite burden corresponds to a parasite count of approximately 100,000/ml, or 2% parasitemia, in an adult with *falciparum* malaria. The time taken to eradicate all parasites from the body is shown at different killing rates (PRRs), assuming constant fractional reduction and no contribution from induced immunity. It is evident that rapidly eliminated drugs with PRRs of 10^3 need to be given for 1 week [243, 438].

Calculations of parasite reduction after chloroquine treatment are more complex as chloroquine has a very long elimination half-life of 1 to 2 months; the drug profile for chloroquine reflects a multi-exponential decline post treatment. Concentrations of chloroquine in the blood rapidly fall after absorption, and chloroquine levels persist at sub therapeutic levels for weeks after treatment has ended at much lower concentrations compared to drug levels observed during treatment [225]. If chloroquine-killing rates are initially low due to drug resistance, then it is likely the malaria infection cannot be cured with this drug alone. Resistance to the antifolates has been shown to develop much more quickly than drug resistance to antimalarial drugs such as the quinolines [161]. Antifolate drug resistance arises from reductions in the affinity of the drug to bind to the dihydrofolate reductase enzyme (DHFR) of parasite. This loss of binding is usually associated with genetic mutations in the parasite DHFR gene at either one location (single base pair mutation) or at two locations (double base pair mutation).

Given only one or two base pair mutations are needed to provide drug resistance *in vivo*, high-grade drug resistance rapidly develop. After the introduction of the antifolate drug proguanil (chloroguanide) in peninsular Malaya, both *vivax* and *falciparum* malarias were shown to be very sensitive to proguanil, but over three years, the mean parasite reduction ratio after drug administration for treatment of uncomplicated *falciparum* malaria dropped from 500 in 1947 to 100 in 1948 to 25 in 1949. By mid-1949, the treatment failure rates had risen to 25% [160]. The parasite clearance time (PCT) and the parasite reduction ratio (PRR) are clearly related, although the PRR is far easier to assess and is a more precise measurement. The specificity and sensitivity of the PRR should be assessed for each drug tested in a clinical trial to understand its utility as a predictor of treatment failure due to antimalarial drug resistance.

4) Effects of Immunity on Therapeutic Response

Treatment responses to antimalarial drugs are always better in patients who are semi-immune. Even non-immune patients will develop a strain-specific immune response over time to a malaria infection, which will limit the extent of disease and aid in parasite eradication. Non-immune patients infected with parasites, which are drug resistant, may potentially need multiple rounds of antimalarial therapy before a final cure is achieved. In areas where malaria is endemic, semi-immune patients with a well-developed immune response benefit from the combined antimalarial activity of immunity together with antimalarial drugs. The combination of immune response with antimalarial therapy permits the use of briefer treatment doses, and patients often present good responses to therapy despite being infected with drug resistant parasites. Accordingly, response to treatment improves with age as immunity to malaria is acquired through multiple rounds of resolved infections. Accordingly, age is a relevant variable determining the response to therapy in endemic areas, and age must therefore be considered when conducting drug trials. Immunity is temporarily disrupted in women who are pregnant, and pregnant women are a tougher population to treat particularly given the more limited choices of appropriate drugs plus the added issues of insuring adequate dosing given altered PK parameters during pregnancy.

4.5.3. Prevention of Drug Resistance through Matching Antimalarial Pharmacodynamic Effects

Antimalarial drug combinations were implemented to decrease the development of parasite drug resistance. A similar strategy is utilized for treatment of tuberculosis, and in antiretroviral and cancer chemotherapy. This practice of combining drugs is most effective if the drugs in the antimalarial combination have well-matched pharmacokinetic properties and all of the drug partners have activity against circulating parasite strains. In a rodent model, the combination of mefloquine with sulfadoxine-pyrimethamine was shown to delay the onset of resistance to mefloquine in a drug sensitive strain of *P. berghei*, but this combination of three drugs was not efficacious against *falciparum* malaria in Thailand, where the combination was put into use in 1984 [162]. One reason for the efficacy failure was attributed to the mismatch in pharmacokinetic properties. Mefloquine has a much longer drug half-life than sulfadoxine or pyrimethamine, and *P. falciparum* parasites in Thailand were known to be resistant to sulfadoxine and pyrimethamine [269]. The pharmacodynamic properties of drugs used in an antimalarial combination are also important to prevent the emergence and spread of drug resistance.

If resistance potential is a function of the biomass of parasites (*i.e.*, more parasites increase the probability a resistant parasite will emerge), then the probability a drug resistant parasite will emerge from an initial infection will be substantially decreased if the biomass of parasites is also reduced. One example of this can be found with the combination of artesunate with mefloquine, which is commonly used for treatment of uncomplicated drug resistant malaria. This combination has been shown to provide high cure rates, even when used to treat patients infected with parasites with mefloquine-resistant [78, 161]. Administration of artesunate for 3 days substantially reduces the biomass of parasites. Thus, few parasites remain to be killed by mefloquine and the probability of a mefloquine-resistant parasite emerging from this primary infection is decreased. Therefore, the use of artesunate does not protect mefloquine from a new infection at a time when the levels of mefloquine are diminished to sub-therapeutic values. Mefloquine protects artesunate by killing off residual parasites exposed to artesunate, and therefore no selective pressure for development of artesunate is exerted, and similarly other combinations of a slowly eliminated partner and an artemisinin should be similarly protected.

4.5.4. Impact of Inter-individual Pharmacodynamic Variation on Antimalarial Drug Therapy

Antimalarial drugs are generally administered in doses that result in patient blood concentrations, which are well in excess of the minimum parasiticidal concentration, MPC. The maximum antimalarial effect observed differs when examining the varied responses between individuals. The results of studies conducted *in vivo* suggest there are considerably large variations in pharmacodynamics observed between patients within the same treatment group. Dose recommendations for many standard antimalarial drugs are quite variable; doses range from a 6-fold difference for chloroquine to an 8-fold difference for quinine. Observations of minor adverse effects after treatment have led to limits on dosing in cases of uncomplicated malaria, which unfortunately has also led to limiting antimalarial doses used for treatment of severe disease, where small adverse effects are not relevant, and the primary objective for treatment is to save human life.

Parasitemia decreases as circulating, drug-affected, ring form parasites are cleared, more mature stages are killed, and parasite multiplication is inhibited due to the loss of immature and mature parasites [160]. Thus, providing that drug concentrations remain above the maximum effect value, there is a constant fractional decline in biomass of parasites with each asexual cycle. This log-linear decline goes on until all parasites have been removed; the numbers of parasites have decreased low enough such that host defenses can contain the remainder, or until drug concentrations have fallen below the minimum parasiticidal concentration (MPC). Accordingly, the rate by which the parasite population declines or expands is dependent on the time profile of the blood concentration of the antimalarial drug, and the concentration effect relationship for the parasites that remain [160]. In symptomatic malaria there are typically between 10^8 and 10^{13} parasites in the body [214]. Although the parasite population may be exposed to elevated concentrations of antimalarial drug and up to 99.99% of all parasites can be killed in the first asexual cycle, significant numbers of viable malarial parasites will still be present in the body, and these residual parasites must all be killed in subsequent asexual cycles.

In general, antimalarial drug levels in the blood should exceed the MPC value (which corresponds to the IC_{99}, the concentration at which 99% of the parasite growth is inhibited) during four asexual-cycles over a 6-day period to achieve cures [160]. To treat patients with severe malaria, physicians have to face many critical and variable malarial conditions such as cerebral infection, hyperparasitemia, and renal failure. In addition, the parasitemia counts in patients with severe malaria could be in the range from 0.1-20% and some cases present with changes that are even more drastic. The overall individual parasitemia profile for *falciparum* malaria actually represents a complex interplay between parasite stage, drug treatment stage specificity, and the observable parasitemia, which reflects the number of circulating of ring and trophozoite parasites not the numbers of sequestered mature schizont parasites [160, 164]. A population of patients can provide an array of very different profiles of parasitemia. Accordingly, there is considerable inter-individual variability in profiles of parasite clearance. One can reasonably assume, however, that this distribution of different stages of parasites in a population is random in nature. Before even attempting to measure effects of antimalarial drugs *in vivo*, consideration must be given to the considerable inter-patient differences in pharmacodynamic variables [252].

The high parasitemia and drug-RBC binding factors, which influence the drug concentrations and the corresponding efficacy of AS, are effective when used to treat severe malaria [270, 271]. However, there is now convincing evidence in a milestone clinical trial called SEAQUAMAT that treatment of patients with severe malaria with intravenous AS will reduce the risk of death by approximately one-third *versus* treatment with standard quinine therapy [200, 253]. So far, this has been the largest trial ever performed with 1,461 patients with severe malaria enrolled, and this is the first clinical trial to demonstrate conclusively that intravenous AS treatment results in a mortality reduction over standard quinine therapy. Due to large variation in pharmacodynamic responses, large clinical trials are required to improve result accuracy. The World Health Organization now approves the use of injectable artesunate for treatment of severe malaria based on the SEAQUAMAT clinical trials [23, 200, 253]. To help make the case for the WHO and the international physician community to believe that injectable AS is the best therapy for severe malaria, we offer a number of arguments below on why injectable AS therapy is the best choice for treatment of severe malaria.

4.5.5. Intravenous AS is the Best Treatment Choice for Patients with Severe Malaria

The TropNetEurop network for Tropical Medicine and Travel Health recommends the use of intravenous AS for treatment of patients infected with severe malaria [272] on the basis of the large and successful SEAQUAMAT trial in Southeast Asia and the AQUAMAT trial in Africa [200, 202]. Patients infected with severe malaria in rural areas may be delirious or may experience vomiting making orally administration of antimalarial drugs impossible and lead to significant delays in definitive treatment without intravenous therapy. If intravenous treatment is not possible in a rural setting, the rectal route of administration is an excellent option as rural healthcare workers can identify patients presenting with moderate and severe malaria and provide rectal drug administration prior to the transfer of these patients to in-patient hospital facilities. The only alternative treatment for severe malaria is IV quinine, which is not as effective [200, 253], costs more, is harder to administer, and is not as well tolerated compared to injectable AS [273].

In addition, for pregnant patients in the second and third trimesters, injectable AS is a superior drug for treatment of uncomplicated malaria than parenteral quinine. Injectable AS treatment needs to be combined with a long-term antimalarial administered orally with a dose adjustment due to altered pharmacokinetics observed in pregnant women [181, 274, 275]. AS monotherapy is still needed for the initial treatment of severe malaria, and other antimalarial drugs are needed to insure a radical cure of disease. There is a distinct need for manufacturers who will supply injectable AS of good quality produced alone to be used in specific circumstances [276].

All cases of *falciparum* malaria can progress to severe malaria particularly when managed inappropriately. Delayed or missed diagnosis is a leading cause of disease progression from mild cases of malaria to severe disease. The most recent advance in decreasing mortality has been the use of intravenous AS instead of injection quinine [200, 253], which may very well revolutionize treatment of severe disease [254, 277]. Previous studies have shown that once-daily administration of artemisinin derivatives provides equivalent cure rates relative to more frequent administration [259, 278]. This suggests that exposure of the infecting parasite population to therapeutic concentrations of drug twice each life cycle is sufficient for maximum effect [160]. Walter Reed Army Institute of Research (WRAIR) and Sigma Tau Pharmaceuticals are in late stage development of a novel cGMP injection formulation of AS, which is currently in the process of achieving final US FDA approval. The WRAIR AS injectable drug candidate is currently available through the CDC under a treatment protocol for patients in the US who present with severe malaria [255, 277].

CHAPTER 5

PK/PD Evaluations of Antimalarial Drugs and Their Combinations

Abstract: Antimalarial drug treatment failures are often not fully investigated, and determining why a patient failed therapy requires not only examining the possibilities of infection with a drug resistant parasite, but also determining drug levels in these patients. Determining drug levels at the point of malaria treatment failure provides useful data even though this is not a routine element of routine patient care or even. Any clinical symptoms or signs at this time should be noted as well given the patient's illness which in and of itself may affect PK parameters, particularly the volume of distribution. Comparison of PK parameters at the time of late parasitological and clinical failure can be used to assess the impact of illness. In this chapter, the PK/PD parameters of artemisinin compounds will be reviewed. Although the body of literature describing the PK/PD of artemisinin agents is quite limited, the available literature on PK/PD evaluations of artemisinin drugs in man is reviewed in this chapter particularly artemisinin drugs administered in a similar manner as monotherapy. The PK/PD results for administration of artemisinin monotherapy may actually provide greater information than other studies of artemisinin dosage regimens. The PK/PD analysis of artesunate and other artemisinin drugs administered by intravenous, oral, and intramuscular regimens are discussed and derived from combined data with the same drug and dosage regimens. Detailed PK/PD evaluations have demonstrated that artesunate has superior PK/PD behavior among artemisinin derivatives. Among ACT combination drugs, the combination of dihydroartemisinin- piperaquine (DP) has demonstrated superior PK/PD qualities compared to all other ACTs recommended by WHO.

Keywords: ACTs, artemisinin derivatives, artesunate, cure, dihydroartemisinin-piperaquine, drug concentration, intramuscular, intravenous, oral, parasitemia, pharmacokinetics and pharmacodynamics (PK/PD), resistance, treatment failure.

Defining the most appropriate therapeutic drug levels *in vivo* requires analyzing associations between drug levels (PK inputs) and the risk of recurrent parasitemia, recrudescence and re-infection (PD inputs). For those antimalarial drugs where there is a known link between a particular parasite mutation and drug resistance, this analysis can be categorized by genotype. Associated PK data such as the levels of drug present at the time of treatment failure and clinical signs and symptoms shown at this time also must be recorded given the possibility that malaria disease itself may affect certain pharmacokinetic parameters, in particular, the volume of distribution. Comparison of PK parameters to a PD outcome such as treatment failure or drug resistance can be used to assess the impact of illness.

Qigui Li and Mark R. Hickman

In malaria disease, there are varieties of factors that contribute toward treatment *in vivo* that may be dissimilar between patients. Drug concentrations of antimalarials in the plasma are likely quite relevant, but some have suggested that as malaria is an intraerythrocytic parasite, drug concentrations within red cells may well be a better measurement. This view is likely too simple given most RBCs present in the blood are not infected, and assessing the drug concentrations inside red cells will be confounded by measuring the drug levels present in the much larger population of uninfected red blood cells. There are other important differences when comparing *in vivo* infections with antimalarial susceptibility testing performed *in vitro*. For *falciparum* malaria, asexual blood stage parasites multiply every 48 hours. Malaria infections have a tendency to be in synchrony from the beginning of an infection, and there are many differences in drug susceptibility for each stage throughout the parasite life cycle. The late trophozoite-schizont stage of the malaria life cycle is very sensitive to antimalarial drugs while ring stage, young parasites, and mature gametocytes are much less sensitive to most drugs [160].

Given circumstances where the concentrations of antimalarial drugs such as chloroquine and artemisinin can fluctuate widely, the parasite stage and synchronicity of the parasite population will become very relevant factors affecting therapeutic response. While short term treatments can be effective in patients who are semi-immune, non-immune patients require therapeutic antimalarial drug levels for at least 3-4 asexual blood stage parasite life cycles which translates into a treatment period over six to eight days, except if parasites are extremely drug sensitive. Unfortunately, studies relating antimalarial plasma drug concentrations achieved to clinical treatment failures have not been widely conducted.

In one study conducted on quinine treatment failures, recrudescent infections in children in Thailand occurred more frequently if serum drug concentrations declined below10 μg/ml in the second half of the treatment period [279]. In a similar study conducted in Tanzanian children infected with extremely resistant malaria parasites (*Res2* parasites) treated with chloroquine, parasitemia was shown to rise when the whole blood median chloroquine concentrations fell below 790 nmol/L [280]. The corresponding estimated median *in vivo* minimal inhibition concentration (MIC) for low grade resistant malaria infections was estimated to be 147 nmol/L. In Thailand where mefloquine resistance is rampant, parasitemia in resistant infections were shown to rise when the median mefloquine concentration in serum was 638 ng/ml [269]. In contrast, studies of mefloquine response in Malawi, where mefloquine treatment is more effective due to a lack of drug resistance, whole blood concentrations of mefloquine in children over 500 ng/mL were shown to be associated with cures [281]. These examples clearly refer to populations of patients infected with parasites at a particular stage who develop antimalarial drug resistance.

The MIC values derived from whole blood concentrations in a particular study conducted in a particular region with one patient population cannot be extrapolated to other geographic populations or locations. In patients infected with severe malaria, treatment is oriented toward halting the pathology of infection as quickly as possible. This goal is achieved best by turning off all the parasite's vital functions as rapidly as possible [214]. When treating other infectious diseases such as tick-borne fever, the death of invading spirochetes leads to a response called the Jarisch-Herxheimer reaction. This clinical reaction is caused by the rapid release of endotoxins and lipoproteins from dying organisms. In malaria, no such reaction is observed when killing the malaria parasite. Accordingly, there is no risk associated with rapid killing of the malaria parasite, and in patients with severe malaria, achieving therapeutic blood concentrations of antimalarial drugs quickly without toxicity is the most important goal. Where feasible, antimalarial drugs administered as a loading dose are best given through controlled IV infusion at a controlled rate although administration of artemether or quinine *via* intramuscular injection has been shown to be equally effective.

Stage specificity of antimalarial drugs is another consideration. Antimalarial drugs that act rapidly with broad stage specificity such as the artemisinin analogues would be preferable, in theory, when compared to drugs with a narrow spectrum of activity late in the parasite lifecycle such as pyrimethamine [214]. These theories should be tested in clinical studies. Finally, some of the practical realities associated with treatment of severe *falciparum* malaria in rural regions in the tropics must be considered. Intravenous treatment regimens that are complex may provide ideal levels of antimalarial drugs in the blood, but the bulk of severe malaria patients will never be treated in a hospital setting. The current approach for management of malaria infection is oriented to assessment at a primary health clinic where oral antimalarials are administered, and patients who progress to severe disease are then referred to higher echelons of care. Given the delays in treatment associated with patient referral that may be life threatening, easy, robust methods of drug administration suitable for administration to severe malaria patients in rural regions who cannot take oral medication must be developed. Accordingly, the safety, efficacy, and pharmacokinetics of a variety of drug administration methods such as intramuscular injections, nasogastric instillation, and suppository administration should be evaluated prospectively. Treatment recommendations on the best method of drug administration should be made only when this information is available.

5.1. PK/PD EVALUATION OF MONOTHERAPY WITH ARTEMISININ AND ITS DERIVATIVES

5.1.1.PK/PD Evaluation of Artemisinins in Malaria Patients

In general, pharmacokinetic (PK) studies show an absorption phase of artemisinin drugs following oral or intramuscular administration. The time-concentration curve of these drugs shows peak concentration at 1-3 hours followed by a sharp decline in the subsequent elimination phase. No absorption phase, however, is observed after intravenous injection of artesunate (AS). After multiple administrations, the drug concentrations of artemisinins (artemisinin, AS, artemether, and dihydroartemisinin) have been shown to decline daily because of an auto-induced metabolic response [205-209]. Patients dosed orally with DHA and AS have shown short mean residence times (MRT) in a range of 0.9-2.7 hours while QHS has been shown to have a longer mean residence time of 7.4 hours at sites of injection in human patients. Arteether (AE) and artemether (AM) have been shown to have very long MRTs ranging from 13.9-42.9 hours because of prolonged periods of drug absorption and drug accumulation at sites of injection. Table **17** shows PK analysis data of five different artemisinin drugs (QHS, DHA, AM, AE, and AS) used for treatment of malaria in man [65].

Pharmacodynamic (PD) profiles are similar to PK profiles but they differ by measuring efficacy parameters of parasitemia over time instead of measuring drug concentrations over time. When reviewing a parasitemia-time curve in human patients treated with antimalarial drugs, an initial lag phase is noted which is characterized by a sharp rise in parasitemia followed by a sharp decrease in parasitemia. This sharp decrease in parasitemia characterizes entry into the clearance phase, which is then followed by a slow decrease of parasitemia to a very low level, which represents the terminal, and dormant phases of infection. Observations on malaria parasitemia over time are conducted by microscopy, which has limitations with regard to quantitative assessment, which, in turn, may affect accurate assessment of the final phases of the parasitemia- time relationship during infection (Fig. **10**, top). Artemisinin drugs have been shown to affect these parasitemia-time profiles in a number of ways. First, artemisinin drugs appear to inhibit the continuation of asexual parasite replication at a later parasite stage than either mefloquine or quinine. This activity inhibits the occasional significant increases in parasitemia often observed following initiation of treatment in the lag phase described previously. Second, artemisinin drugs trigger a decline in parasitemia that is accelerated when compared to other antimalarial drugs. This rapid decline can only be explained by the rapid clearance of ring-stage parasite-infected erythrocytes in the clearance phase [267, 282]. After a rapid decline from the clearance phase into the final terminal stage, the surviving unaffected parasites are present in low numbers in a dormant state [230], which is characteristic of parasite recrudescence observed in the terminal and dormant phases. Studies of different artemisinin drugs administered at different doses present variable parasitemia-time profiles (Fig. **10**, bottom).

Although the body of literature of the pharmacokinetics and pharmacodynamics (PK/PD) of artemisinin agents is limited in nature, PK/PD evaluations have been published for artemisinin drugs administered in a similar manner as monotherapy for treatment of human malaria. The PK/PD results for administration of artemisinin monotherapy may actually provide greater information than other studies of artemisinin dosage regimens [283]. To provide more data on this subject, a PK/PD analysis of intravenous AS and oral artemisinin (QHS) was conducted using the same subjects in one study. The PK/PD evaluations of four other artemisinin drugs with oral and intramuscular regimens (oral AS, oral DHA, IM AE, and IM AM), are derived from combined data from two separate publications where the studies were conducted with the same drug and dosage regimens [182, 220, 284-288].

1) Intravenous AS

To investigate the PK/PD properties of AS and DHA, its active metabolite, for treatment of *Plasmodium vivax* infections, 12 male Vietnamese adults with confirmed *vivax* malaria were treated with IV AS(120 mg) or an alternative formulation administered 8 hours later. The PK/PD profiles observed in treatment of malaria infections in man have been assessed after IV administration of AS at doses of 120 mg/person administered on the first day of treatment at hour 0 followed by oral treatment with AS administered at 100 mg 8 hours later (Fig. **13**, IV AS). The mean peak level (C_{max}) of AS was shown to be 11,343 ng/ml, and this concentration rapidly declined giving an elimination half-life of 0.05 hours. The C_{max} of DHA, a metabolite of AS, was shown to be 2,646 ng/ml, and this concentration rapidly declined giving an elimination half-life which was calculated to be 0.67 hours (Table **17**). In this trial, the mean AUC of DHA observed in patients treated with AS was estimated to be 2,378ng•h/ml, which is two times higher than the AUC of AS, the parent compound, which was shown to have an AUC of 1,146 ng•h/ml [283].

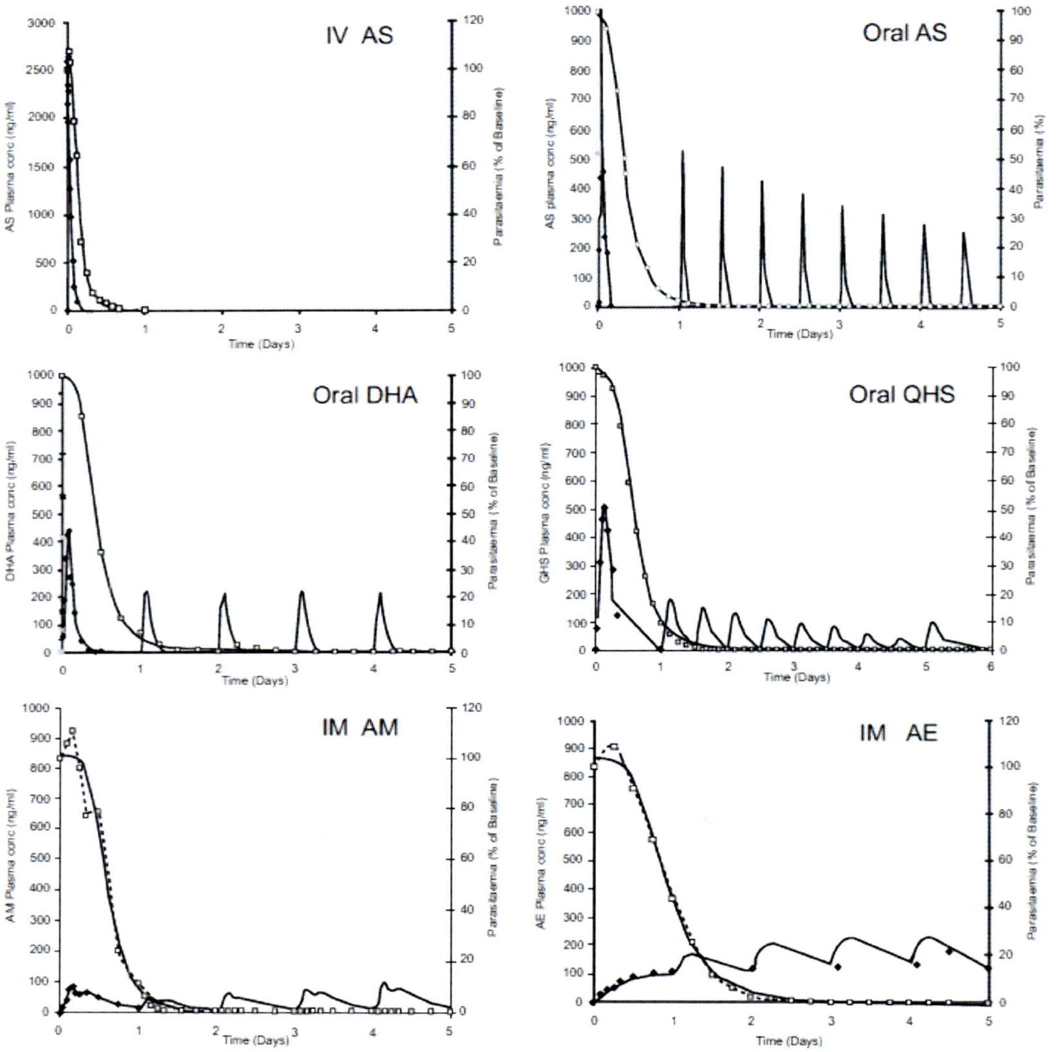

Figure 13: Pharmacokinetic/pharmacodynamic profiles in plasma derived from patients in human malaria trials following administration of intravenous and oral artesunate (AS, with DHA measurement), oral dihydroartemisinin (DHA), oral artemisinin (QHS), intramuscular artemether (AM) and arteether (AE) with various regimens measured by HPLC-ECD or LC-MS (solid markers) [311].

When dosed with the same regimen, the length of the lag phase in the parasitemia curve of patients treated with intravenous AS was shown to be 1.92 hours, which was quite short compared to the lag times of oral AS and four other artemisinin drugs (Fig. **10**, bottom). This is consistent with the rapid half-maximal parasite clearance time (PC_{50}) of 3.18 hours and the lowest area under the inhibitory curve of 397.3% observed after AS injection of (Table **17**). After computer fitting, an E_{max} of 0.00111% parasitemia was predicted because of day one IV AS treatment of *falciparum*-infected patients. In this evaluation, the E_{max} was the most useful pharmacodynamic parameter to assess the maximum antimalarial activity of artemisinin derivatives, which were shown to have steep relationships between concentration and effect. The very sharp relationship between concentration and effect observed may be related to the period of time drug blood concentrations exceeded the minimum inhibition concentration (MIC), as opposed to the C_{max} or AUC [267]. The E_{max} of 0.0011% observed after administration of AS at a dose of 100 mg per patient, reflected the lowest residual parasitemia observed when compared to the other four-artemisinin derivatives in this data set (Table **17**).

2) Oral AS

The PK properties of oral AS were studied in six patients with uncomplicated *falciparum* malaria who received artesunate dosed at 100 mg for 5 days in a randomized crossover study design [209]. A larger PD trial, which assessed the efficacy and safety of AS, was conducted in patients both during treatment of their infection with *falciparum* malaria and after infection. Forty adults with confirmed *falciparum* malaria were randomly treated with oral AS dosed at 100mg on the first day and 50 mg administered twice per day for a five-day period. The PK/PD profiles of individuals treated for malaria with oral AS at doses of 100 mg/person on the first day followed by treatment with 50 mg administered two times daily for two to six days have been assessed through clinical study (Fig. **13, Oral AS**).

In the first PK study of six patients treated with oral AS at 100 mg/person for 5 days, the mean peak plasma concentration of dihydroartemisinin, the principal AS metabolite, shown to be 1,052ng/ml, which decreased with an elimination half-life, estimated to be 0.75 hours (Table **17**). In addition, the concentration of AS observed waned daily throughout the 5-day dosing period [209]. The mean AUC of DHA in this study was predicted to be 1,334ng·h/ml, 6.4 fold higher than the AUC of AS, which had an AUC of 210 ng·h/ml [182]. In the second PD study of 40 adults treated with oral AS at 100 mg/person for 5 days the duration of the parasitemia lag phase was 2.81 hours, which was the shortest lag time observed compared to the other four drugs tested (Fig. **10**, bottom). It is possible the efficacy or oral AS yielded quick parasite killing with an absorption period of

0.36 hours and a C_{max} of 1,052 ng/ml [284]. Similarly, very rapid parasite clearance by oral AS in this study translated to a mean time of 8.48 hours to reduce parasitemia by half (PC_{50}), which was the lowest PC_{50} observed in this study, and also produced the lowest area under the inhibitory curve (AUIC) of 921.2%·h/µl (Table **17**).

Computer modeling of the E_{max} showed a value of 0.0016% parasitemia for orally administered AS treatment of infected patients on day 1 (Table **17**). The E_{max} calculation was shown to be the principal pharmacodynamic parameter to determine the maximum effective antimalarial response of artemisinin compounds. From the data presented here for oral AS administered at a dose of 100 mg per patient, the calculated E_{max} of oral AS, which reflects a parasitemia of 0.0016%, was the lowest observed compared to the calculated E_{max} of the other four artemisinin derivatives (Fig. **13, Oral AS**).

3) Oral Dihydroartemisinin (DHA)

PK and PD analysis of dihydroartemisinin was conducted in individuals infected with uncomplicated *falciparum* malaria who were treated with 600 mg total of dihydroartemisinin at administered over a 5-day duration. All of the patients assessed in this study were actually in the hospital as inpatients to assess DHA safety and efficacy over a period of 28 days. By day 3 of treatment, most patients had undetectable parasitemia by microscopy and no patients showed any significant adverse effects. The PK/PD profiles of patients with malaria treated with oral DHA at a dose of 200 mg/person on day1 followed by treatment with 100 mg per day from days 2-5 are shown in Fig. **13** (Oral DHA). After oral administration of 200 mg of DHA, the mean peak plasma concentration of DHA observed was 437 ng/ml, and this concentration subsequently declined with a half-life estimated to be 0.85 hours. The mean AUC of DHA in this study was calculated to be 1,329 ng·h/ml. The duration of the parasitemia lag phase for patients in this study was 4.03 hours. The lag time observed for DHA was longer than AS (2.81 hours) and shorter than for AM (7.26 hours), AE (8.89 hours) and QHS (5.76 hours) (Table **17,** Fig. **10**, bottom). The data suggests that the efficacy of DHA might not be as effective as oral AS treatment, but the lag time observed was shorter than the AM, AE, and QHS treatments. The rapid parasite elimination observed after DHA administration resulted in a mean half maximal parasite clearance time of 10.05 hours (PC_{50}) and an AUIC of 1,168 %•h/µl.

Computer modeling of oral DHA administered to human patients on the first day yielded an estimated E_{max} of 0.2132% parasitemia. Based on the data, administration of 200 mg of DHA per patient yielded a result showing more parasites were still present in these patients compared to the other artemisinins assessed (Table **17**). The absorption half-life of DHA tablets was shown to be 0.67 hours, which was 50% slower than the absorption half-life shown for AS (0.36 hours) in this trial which suggests the slow pace of parasite reduction may be due to slow absorption of DHA. In addition, the AUCs of the AS and DHA treatments were the same, however, the C_{max} observed after AS administration was twice as high as the C_{max} observed after DHA treatment, suggesting elevated peak drug levels (C_{max}) of AS may be another reason for the differences in E_{max} observed [284, 285]. Compared with the AS study, the bioavailability of DHA was much lower (< 50%). If calculated based on an equal dose level, the C_{max} observed after AS treatment is 4 times higher than the C_{max} observed for DHA and the AUC_{DHA} estimated after AS treatment is two times higher than the C_{max} and AUC_{DHA} observed after dosing with DHA. In a study conducted at WRAIR in beagle dogs, we observed that the bioavailability of the DHA tablet Cotexin was only 24.4% [246]. Patients treated with DHA tablets in clinical studies showed a recrudescence rate of 24% with rebound parasitemia of 3% on day 3 [285]. In this comparison study, the 3% rebound parasitemia was only found in patients undergoing oral DHA treatment (Fig. **13, Oral DHA**).

4) Intramuscular Artemether (AM)

Artemether (AM) is strongly plasma protein bound (76%) and distributes rapidly throughout the body into red blood cells and the brain. In contrast to AS, the biotransformation of AM into DHA is slow. PK and PD profiles from patients with malaria treated with intramuscular AM formulated in sesame oil dosed at 3.2 mg/kg on day 1 and then 1.6 mg/kg daily from days 2-5 can be seen in Fig. **13** (IM AM). The mean peak plasma concentration observed in these patients was 74.9 ng/ml, and the concentration subsequently decreased showing a calculated half-life of 7.83 hours (Table **17**), suggesting that this formulation had a C_{max} that was the lowest compared to the other four artemisinin derivatives in this study. The mean AUC of AM was estimated to be 1,230 ng·h/ml [286]. At a similar dose, the duration of the parasitemia lag phase was 7.26 hours, the second longest parasitemia lag time observed compared to the three artemisinin drugs tested with the exception of AE, suggesting the injected intramuscular AM formulation was absorbed slowly from muscle injection sites [219]. Initial parasitemia counts observed after AM dosing increased to 110% by 4 hours (parasitemia was counted as 100% at time zero when the first dose was administered). The prolonged absorption may explain the observed parasitemia lag time of 7.26 hours with no decrease of parasites, observed after intramuscular AM injection at hour 4.

Parasite clearance was shown to be slow with a mean PC_{50} time of 15.63 hours, the most elongated PC_{50} period *versus* the other three drugs (Table **17**). Intramuscular AM injection produced the highest AUIC of 1,613 %·h/μl, which suggests that this intramuscular artemisinin drug, was not as efficacious in reducing malaria parasitemia [287].

Although the injection of intramuscular AM did not yield a rapid decline in parasitemia in study patients, the long exposure time observed in patients treated with intramuscular AM (7.83 hours elimination half-life) was associated with significant reductions in malaria parasitemia. Computer modeling of PD parameters in this study estimated an E_{max} of 0.0030% parasitemia. The parasitemia observed was two times higher than the parasitemia observed after administration of oral AS in the first day, but much less than the parasitemia noted after administration of oral DHA, AE and QHS (Table **17**).

5) Intramuscular Arteether (AE)

PK data were derived from a study of Artemotil (ß-arteether) administered to 56 patients in Thailand infected with severe *P. falciparum*. Artemotil was administered intramuscularly at 3.2 mg/kg on day 0 followed by administration of 1.6 mg/kg/day for another 4 days. In a second arm, AE was administered at a dose of 4.8 mg/kg on day 0 at 0 hours, 1.6 mg/kg at 6 hours, and 1.6 mg/kg/day over the next four days. The PK and PD profiles in patients with malaria given AE administered intramuscularly formulated in sesame oil at a dose of 4.8 mg/kg at 0 hour and 1.6 mg/kg at 6 hours on day 1 followed by daily dosing of 1.6 mg from days 2-5 are shown in Fig. **13** (IM-AE). The mean peak plasma concentration was observed to be 110.1 ng/ml, and the concentration of drug then waned with a clearance half-life estimated to be 22.7 hours (Table **17**), suggesting this sesame oil formulation has a lower peak drug concentration compared to QHS, AS, and DHA. The mean AUC of injected intramuscular AE was estimated to be 4,702 ng·h/ml [220].

At a similar dose, the observed parasitemia lag time was 8.89 hours, which was the longest lag time seen in this study when compared with the other four drugs tested suggesting that the injection of the AE formulation intramuscularly resulted in extended absorption from muscle injection sites [219]. Initial parasitemia counts observed after injection did not decline as a consequence of the low C_{max} of AE, but the parasitemia counts did increase to 108% by 6 hours (the initial parasitemia was established at 100% when the patients was initially treated. The increased parasitemia count may explain the extended lag time of 8.89 hours with no parasite killing observed after AE injection at 6 hours. Similarly, a very slow clearance of parasites was observed with a mean PC_{50} of 19.68 hours, the longest PC_{50} observed *versus* the other four drugs (Table **17**). Intramuscular AE formulation injection yielded the highest AUIC of 2,464 %•h/μl suggesting that this intramuscular artemisinin drug was not as efficacious in reducing parasitemia [287]. Intramuscular AE injection was not able to kill parasites rapidly, nor was it capable of reducing parasitemia as well compared to the other four drugs. Computer modeling estimated that the E_{max} was 0.550% parasitemia in this trial. Even with two doses of Artemotil on the first day (4.8 mg/kg at 0 hours and 1.6 mg/kg at 6 hours), the observed parasitemia was still very high *versus* the other drugs tested in this study (Table **17**).

6) Oral Artemisinin (QHS)

The PK profile of the antimalarial artemisinin exhibited an unusual time dependency during a study of oral artemisinin administered at 500 mg/day over a 7-day period to 10 healthy, male Vietnamese adults. The AUC of artemisinin observed decreased over time to 34% (median) by day 4 and decreased further by day 7 to only 24% of values obtained after the first day of administration. In seven subjects restudied after a two- week washout period, the AUCs of artemisinin had almost normalized, demonstrating the reversibility of this time-dependent drug disposition. The results suggest artemisinin exhibits an auto-inductive effect on drug metabolism of an unusual magnitude [206]. The PK/PD evaluations of patients with malaria treated with artemisinin (QHS) administered orally at a dose of 500 mg/person on day 1 followed by 250 mg twice daily for four days followed by administration of another dose of 500 mg on the sixth day is shown in Fig. **13** (Oral QHS).

After administration of 500 mg of artemisinin orally, the average peak concentration of QHS in plasma observed was shown to be 588 ng/ml, and the concentration of drug declined with an elimination half-life estimated to be 2.4 hours. The mean AUC of QHS was estimated to be 2,601 ng•h/ml, which was the highest AUC observed likely due to the high oral dose taken. At an oral dose of 500 mg, the lag time in the parasitemia curve was shown to be 5.76 hours, which was longer than the lag time observed after administration of oral AS (2.81 hours) and DHA (4.03 hours) but was shorter than the lag times observed in AE and AM trials (Fig. **10**, bottom). The data suggests QHS capsules were not as efficacious as oral AS and DHA even given the higher doses given [206, 207, 284]. The patients administered oral QHS showed a half-maximal parasite clearance time (PC_{50}) of 13.95 hours and an AUIC of 1,464 %·h/μl. (Table **17**). The absorption of QHS capsules showed an absorption half-life of 1.21 hours which was slower than the absorptions of DHA and AS, which suggests the slow pace of parasitemia reduction observed after oral QHS dosing may have resulted due to extended absorption of this drug. Compared with studies of oral DHA and AS, oral QHS has a poor bioavailability of 30% [290, 291] and poor antimalarial potency [204, 226, 288].

To review the PK/PD evaluations discussed, five artemisinin drugs were evaluated, and the summary of the findings of the data derived for each drug/regimen tested are as follows:

1) Intravenous or oral artesunate are the most rapid malaria killing drugs when compared to the other four artemisinins. Intravenous AS administration provides the highest peak drug concentrations accompanied by limited exposure times, and, orally administered AS provides increased peak drug concentrations with shorter durations of exposure. The high peak drug levels are a key element in the ability of these two drugs to eliminate parasites rapidly (Fig. **10,** bottom) and the short exposure time is essential to avoid artemisinin-associated neurotoxicity [224] and it is an important element in preventing drug resistance [289].

2) While DHA is comparable in potency to AS *in vitro* [204, 226, 288], this drug does not have a rapid PD effect like AS, even with oral doses twice that of AS. The PK/PD explanations for this difference include a lower bioavailability than AS [80, 81], extended absorption and a long efficacy lag time. The most important reason for this difference is likely due to lower peak concentrations observed in patients compared to peak concentrations achieved clinically in patients given oral AS.

3) Intramuscular AE or AM administration yields a lower efficacy and slower parasite killing. When formulated in sesame oil, intramuscular AE and AM have low, extended absorption from sites of muscle injection [219]. Initial parasitemia counts after drug administration have been shown not to decline likely as a consequence of low, delayed peak concentrations of AE and AM (75-110 ng/ml). The low peak concentrations of AE and AM may explain why the parasitemia lag time is extended (7.2-8.9 hours) with no parasite killing observed after injection. Slow clearance rates of parasites were observed with mean PC_{50} times of 15.63-19.68 hours, which may explain AE trial failures [220]. While the drug exposure times for AE and AM are

higher than QHS, AS, and DHA, these extended exposure times did not enhance efficacy. Instead, this enhanced exposure time increases the risk of neurotoxicity, and these formulations are likely not good choices for administration into man for treatment of severe malaria.

4) Artemisinin does not demonstrate favorable PK/PD parameters compared to other artemisinin drugs due to poor efficacy. The high dose of QHS administered (500 mg/person) resulted in a high plasma concentration (AUC of 2,601 ng·h/ml) and a high peak concentration (C_{max} of 588 ng/ml). However, the time-dependent drug disposition due to auto-induction of drug metabolism coupled with [204, 226, 288] low bioavailability [291] are all factors that likely translate into poor clinical efficacy. The PK data suggests that some of the artemisinin derivatives with lower antimalarial efficacy cannot produce rapid antiparasitic effects even at elevated doses.

5.1.2. Intravenous Artesunate is the Treatment of Choice for Severe Malaria

The artemisinin derivatives are highly effective compared to other traditional malaria drugs, and the combinations of artemisinin derivatives and traditional antimalarial drugs routinely provides efficacy above 90%, which, a few decades ago, would have been unheard of. Drug resistance to artemisinin compounds associated with delayed parasite clearance times has occurred *in vivo* only in certain geographic areas in Asia. Short durations of monotherapy treatment with artemisinins over 3-5 days have been shown to lead to recrudescence. The data that emerged from clinical studies of all artemisinin drugs on market administered as monotherapy is the length of monotherapy ultimately determines whether recrudescence occurs or does not occur. A comparison chart showing the utility of various artemisinins administered as monotherapy over a 3-5 day treatment period derived from a variety of clinical studies is shown in Table **17**. The pharmacodynamic parameters of fever clearance time, parasite clearance time, and the recrudescence rates commonly used measures of efficacy comparisons of antimalarial drugs in humans. Examination of these parameters derived from various clinical studies suggests that treatment with IM arteether formulated in sesame oil (Artemotil) is less efficacious [292]. Arteether is less efficacious than intramuscular artemether (AM), oral and IV artesunate (AS), oral dihydroartemisinin (DHA) or when compared to intramuscular administration of a/ß -arteether in a peanut oil formulation [293]. Data derived from clinical studies of artemisinin drug monotherapy in man have been shown to be highly variable [65].

Artemisinin monotherapy use was strongly discouraged after 2001 as a means of preventing development of artemisinin drug resistance. For severe malaria, monotherapy with intravenous AS is still the treatment of choice for children and adults in Asia and some regions of Africa [23]. Comparisons of intramuscular AM to quinine to treat severe malaria (quinine has been first-line treatment for severe *falciparum* malaria for almost 400 years) demonstrated less toxicity associated with intramuscular AM administration *versus* quinine but no clear mortality advantage [202]. Two of the largest severe malaria clinical trials showed IV AS treatment of children and adults was superior to treatment with IV quinine. The mortality rate for patients treated with quinine was 22% in the SEAQUAMAT study and 10.9% in the AQUAMAT study, while AS treatment showed a mortality rate of 15% in the SEAQUAMAT study and 8.5% in the AQUAMAT study. Patients with hyperparasitemia (>10% of RBC) showed a much better treatment response to AS than patients without hyperparasitemia. Intravenous AS was Intravenous AS was shown to be well tolerated, safer, and much simpler to dose than quinine [200, 201]. The life-saving benefits of AS treatment *versus* quinine or intramuscular artemether [202, 294] treatment for severe malaria led to the WHO advocating AS be used in place of these drugs in 2006 [1, 23].

The SEAQUAMAT and AQUAMAT trials were the largest trials conducted in severe malaria patients and these studies were first to demonstrate intravenous AS is a better treatment with a clear benefit in reducing mortality compared to the previous standard therapy with quinine. After the SEAQUAMAT trials, IVAS was also suggested as the treatment of choice for severe malaria patients by The European Network on Imported Infections Disease Surveillance (TropNetEurop) [272], and WHO [1]. The most significant changes in malaria mortality have been due to the implementation of artemisinin compounds for treatment of severe malaria [254]. Accordingly, AS monotherapy still has a use for this particular indication [23, 295, 296]. There are currently no intravenous AS products available, however, that are GMP produced and FDA approved to use in the US. Walter Reed Army Institute of Research (WRAIR) and Sigma Tau Pharmaceuticals are developing a novel cGMP AS injection product, which is currently under development to achieve US FDA approval [297].

5.1.3. The Impact of PK/PD Evaluations on Assessment of Artemisinin Efficacy Studies

The high recrudescence rates associated with artemisinin monotherapy (30-50% after 3 days of treatment, 6-15% after 5 days of treatment, and 2-6% after 7 days of treatment) is a major disadvantage for all artemisinin compounds including injectable AS [14, 71, 196]. It is still unclear, however, how high the dosage or the blood concentration of artemisinins should be for efficacious chemotherapy of severe malaria. In order to estimate the most efficacious blood concentration, three aspects should be considered.

Aspect 1: Effects of High Parasitemia on Drug Concentration

Some reports have shown that the uptake of DHA in infected erythrocytes *in vitro* is between 100-300 times higher than the uptake of DHA in uninfected erythrocytes [230, 298, 299]. This may be due to the induction of nonselective actin conductance in RBC membranes after infection with *P. falciparum* that alters the membrane permeability [300]. Other mechanisms to explain the increase in artemisinin concentrations in malaria-infected erythrocytes have also been investigated by many scientists. For normal erythrocytes, studies have shown that DHA is absorbed by red blood cell membranes that have been isolated *in vitro* but not by red blood cells that are intact. The difference between uptake of DHA in isolated membranes but not by red blood cells that are still intact is consistent with the fact that the proteins that bind DHA, alpha- and beta-spectrin, protein 4.1 and protein 4.2, glyceraldehyde-3-phosphate dehydrogenase, and actin, are membrane proteins facing the cytoplasmic side of the red cell membrane [301]. Thus, binding of DHA to membranes may require its exposure to the membrane's inner surface. These observations may explain why radiolabeled artemisinin and DHA are taken up by infected red blood cells but not by intact red blood cells [302]. The outer erythrocytic membrane of parasite- infected red blood cells has alterations in the distribution of phospholipids between the outer and inner membrane sheaths [303] and may contain clefts, pores [304-306], and parasite-produced proteins [307, 308]. These studies have shown that when *P. falciparum*-infected erythrocytes are treated with radiolabeled DHA and AE, the radioactive drugs are bound to six *P. falciparum* malarial proteins. The binding of artemisinin drugs to parasite proteins occurs at physiological concentrations, and no proteins have been bound by radiolabeled artemisinin drugs when they were incubated with uninfected erythrocytes [309].

Accordingly, the level of malaria parasitemia affects artemisinin drug concentration. The patients with 1.0% of erythrocytes infected with malaria show an AS+DHA combined C_{max} of 1,250 ng/ml [182, 284]. The amount of drug entering infected RBCs can easily reach the minimal concentration to inhibit 99% of malaria parasites with efficacious equilibrium of drug between infected and uninfected erythrocytes. In 5%-20% of patients, the uptake of DHA in infected RBCs can be significantly increased. The free plasma drug concentration can be decreased, suggesting that the drug concentration (1,250 ng/ml) of AS+DHA observed in malaria patients after treatment with oral AS may not be not sufficient to distribute the drug to every erythrocyte (infected and uninfected) in each patient (from 1-20% infected RBCs). Therefore, it is clear that the peak drug level of AS+DHA at 1,250 ng/ml in plasma is far from enough to cure patients with severe malaria associated with hyperparasitemia.

AS+DHA concentrations were measured at WRAIR *in vitro* where AS and DHA were co-cultured with two *P. falciparum* strains (W2 and D6) at varying parasitemia (0.2, 0.5, 1.0, 2.0, and 5.0%) in 5.0 x 107 RBC/ml utilizing a 3H-hypoxanthine based growth- inhibition assay [310]. The drugs were determined when the drug concentration reaches equilibrium between the plasma and infected and uninfected erythrocytes in patients with hyperparasitemia. The results showed that responses to AS and DHA were more consistently altered by parasite burden against resistant and susceptible *P. falciparum* strains. For the drug susceptible strain D6, increasing the parasitemia from 1.0 to 5.0% resulted in a 7.6 and 7.0 fold increase in the IC90 of AS and DHA, respectively. For the W2 chloroquine-resistant strain, increasing the parasitemia from 1.0 to 5.0% resulted in 6.3 and 4.6 fold increase in the IC_{90} of AS and DHA, respectively (Table **21**). Based on this data, we assume an average IC_{90} increase of 6-fold *in vivo* when parasitemia is increased from 1.0 to 5.0% [310]. The minimum plasma peak concentration of AS+DHA required for patients to exterminate parasites at a 5% parasitemia level would be at least 7,500 ng/ml while a minimum plasma peak concentration of 30,000 ng/ml would be required to kill parasites at a 20% parasitemia level. This calculation was based on the drug concentration observed at equilibrium after oral administration of AS where a plasma peak concentration of 1,250 ng/ml (AS plus DHA) was required to reach IC_{99} levels and kill parasites at a 1.0% parasitemia. With this estimation, for patients with severe malaria, the concentration of AS plus DHA (11,343 + 2,646 ng/ml) achieved following injection of AS at a dose of would not be satisfactory to achieve an efficacious drug level inside of every erythrocyte, infected and uninfected, in patients with hyperparasitemia [283].

Table 21: Drug concentrations (ng/ml) and molecules per single red blood cell (molecules/RBC) needed to inhibit 50% and 99% of parasites (IC_{50} and IC_{99}) in culture with 0.8% (Part A) and 1-5% (Part B) parasitemia and 5.0 x 10^7/ml RBC (1% of whole blood) to dihydroartemisinin (DHA) and artesunate (AS) against chloroquine-resistant clones of *P. falciparum* from Indochina (W2) and mefloquine-resistant clone of *P. falciparum* from Sierra Leone (D6). Two clinical trials (Part C) of AS after oral and intravenous administrations were compared to the *in vitro* results [65]

Part A. Efficacy of AS and DHA against *P. falciparum* clones (n = 3) with 0.8 parasitemia [1]						
Parasite Strain	Test Compound	IC_{50} ng/ml	IC_{99} ng/ml		IC_{50} Molecules/RBC*	IC_{99} Molecules/RBC*
W-2	AS	0.26 ± 0.04	7.22 ± 3.36		0.11 x 10^5	0.31 x 10^6
	DHA	0.36 ± 0.13	17.16 ± 6.17		0.15 x 10^5	0.73 x 10^6
D-6	AS	0.32 ± 0.12	9.69 ± 2.74		0.14 x 10^5	0.49 x 10^6
	DHA	0.24 ± 0.08	9.30 ± 0.85		0.10 x 10^5	0.39 x 10^6
Part B. IC_{90} of AS and DHA against *P. falciparum* clones at different starting parasitemia						
		Starting Parasitemia (%)				
Parasite Strain	Test Compound	0.2	0.5	1.0	2.0	5.0
W-2	AS	0.3	0.2	0.5	1.3	3.8
	DHA	0.2	0.2	0.4	0.8	2.8
D-6	AS	0.3	0.3	0.7	1.6	4.4
	DHA	0.1	0.2	0.5	1.0	2.3
Part C. Clinical trials after oral or intravenous AS on day 1 (n = 12-13)						
Drug (dose)		AS C_{max} ng/ml	DHA C_{max} ng/ml	Drug molecules/RBC*		
				AS	DHA	AS + DHA
Oral AS (100 mg)		198	1052	0.06 x 10^6	0.44 x 10^6	0.51 x 10^6
IV AS (120 mg)		11343	2646	3.56 x 10^6	1.12 x 10^6	4.671 x 10^6

*Drug molecules were calculated in according to Avogadro's number (mole = 6.024 x 10^{23} molecules) of drug/mole divided by RBC counts in culture. Values are mean or mean ± SD; W-2: Indochina clone, resistant to chloroquine, sensitive to mefloquine. D-6: Sierra Leone clone, sensitive to chloroquine, resistant to mefloquine. IC_{50} = 50% inhibitory concentration; IC_{99} = 99% inhibitory concentration. IV = intravenous.

Aspect 2: Effects of Protein and RBC Binding on Drug Concentrations

Pharmacokinetic factors affecting drug efficacy are not simply limited to plasma peak concentrations. Other PK factors include drug tissue distribution, RBC drug distribution, and binding of artemisinin drugs to plasma proteins [228]. At WRAIR, we have conducted studies of artemisinin distribution in rat tissues and protein binding to human blood. Table **19** shows the RBC/plasma ratios of five radiolabeled artemisinins in human whole blood at various concentrations [228, 229]. For equal volumes of normal volunteer RBCs and plasma, the fraction of the five artemisinins found in RBCs is lower than the fraction found in plasma. The ratios of drug found in RBCs *versus* plasma are almost constant in human blood over a broad range of drug concentrations. After correction for the normal ratios of 55:45 between plasma and RBCs found in normal blood, the RBC/plasma ratios of drug observed are 0.23 for ^{14}C-arteether (^{14}C-AE). The next lowest ratio is 0.28 for ^{14}C-artemether (^{14}C-AM), 0.44 for ^{14}C-artelinic acid (^{14}C-AL), 0.52 for ^{14}C-dihydroartemisinin (^{14}C-DHA), and 0.71 for ^{14}C-artesunate (^{14}C-AS), showing that AS has the lowest capability of binding plasma proteins and AE has the highest capacity of binding plasma proteins. In unpublished studies conducted at WRAIR, comparisons of the 50% bound concentration (BC_{50}) of ^{14}C-AM, ^{14}C-AE, ^{14}C-AL, ^{14}C-AS and ^{14}C-DHA at various concentrations in human plasma samples were performed by the micro-dialysis equilibrium method at 37°C for 6 hours. The BC_{50} calculations for ^{14}C-AE showed a concentration of 1,945 ng/ml, 1,673 ng/ml for ^{14}C-AM, 482ng/ml for ^{14}C-DHA, and 143 ng/ml for ^{14}C-AS (Fig. **14**) in human undiluted plasma. DHA and AS have significant advantages in their capacity to enter human red blood cell (RBC/plasma ratio of 0.52 for DHA and an RBC/plasma ratio for AS of 0.71) compared to AE and AM (RBC/plasma ratio of 0.23 for AE and an RBC/plasma ratio for AM of 0.28, Table **19**). Accordingly, to penetrate the same RBC targets the drug peak concentrations for AE and AM would need to be two to three times higher than that of DHA and AS. In addition, the binding affinities to plasma are high for radiolabeled AE (BC_{50} of 1945 ng/ml) and AM (BC_{50} of 1673 ng/ml). Conversely, the binding affinity to plasma is low for radiolabeled AS (BC_{50} value of 143 ng/ml) and DHA (BC_{50} of 162 ng/ml), supporting the hypothesis that the free drug concentrations of AS and DHA can be much higher in human plasma than the free drug concentrations of AE and AM.

Aspect 3: Effects of High PK/PD Variability on Drug Concentrations

1) Human PK Variability

Fortunately, intravenous AS is capable of providing high peak drug concentrations in patients with rapid exposure times. In a recent clinical trial, the

C_{max} of AS was shown to range from 605 to 18,909 ng/ml (total AS plus DHA levels) at a dose of 120 mg/person or 2.4 mg/kg to treat malaria infections including severe malaria (Table **18**). The variability of AS drug concentrations, however, has been shown to be 25-fold higher in a number of different trials [63, 182, 311]. In clinical trials with oral AS formulations, the C_{max} was demonstrated to range from 453 to 1,718ng/ml (total AS plus DHA levels) as a consequence of dosing AS administered orally at 100 mg/person or 2-4 mg/kg in patients with uncomplicated malaria [311, 312]. The variability observed in C_{max} in this oral AS trial and others is approximately 4-fold. In addition, in each trial, large inter-individual variability has also been detected among patients. It is obvious that such low AS and DHA peak drug concentrations presented in some patients may be the cause of treatment failure [216].

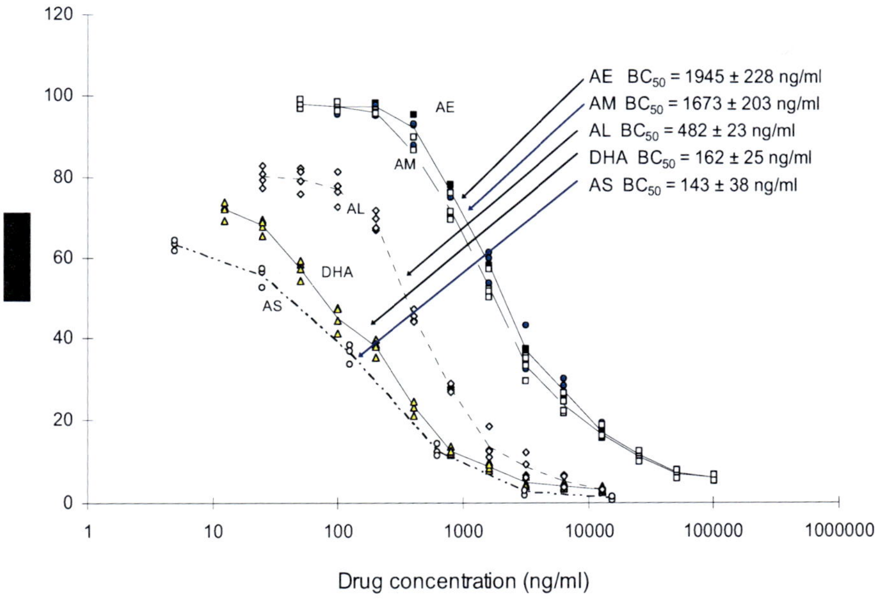

Figure 14: Comparison of 50% bound concentration (BC_{50}) of ^{14}C-artemether (AM), ^{14}C-arteether (AE), ^{14}C-artelinic acid (AL), ^{14}C-artesunate (AS) and ^{14}C-dihydroartemisinin (DHA) at varied concentration in human plasma samples by microdialysis equilibrium method at 37 °C for 6 hours (n = 4) [65].

2) Human PD Variability

Physicians face highly variable and serious conditions such as cerebral infection, hyperparasitemia, and renal failure in severe malaria patients. In addition, the parasitemia counts of severe malaria patients can range from 0.1-20% and some cases present with changes that are even more drastic. In an individual, a number of factors have a role in determining the drug PK/PD profile. Parasite development stage and the synchronicity of the overall population of parasites and the rate by which sequestered mature schizont stage parasites multiply determines the initial time profile of parasitemia immediately after an antimalarial drug is administered [160]. If a patient is admitted during a period when the majority of parasites are undergoing schizogony, then the parasitemia will increase after administration of antimalarial drugs as schizonts rupture red blood cells and merozoites are released which will invade other RBCs to start the blood stage life cycle over again with new ring stage parasites. While blood stage parasites can be observed microscopically and counted, the development stage of sequestered parasites are not observed and not counted.

When an antimalarial without effect on ring stage parasites was administered, the observed parasitemia counts will flatten and decrease later because of parasite sequestration [160, 164]. Overall, an individual patient's parasitemia profile can be a mix of varying parasite life cycle stages. When looking at entire patient populations, therefore, an array of varying profiles in parasitemia are observed. Consequently, there is large inter-individual variability in parasite clearance. One can assume, however, that parasite stage distribution is random in a group of patients given there is no biological reason to explain why one patient would possess one stage of development but not another upon hospital admission. When assessing the effects of an antimalarial drug *in vivo*, a number of inter-patient pharmacodynamic variables that must be considered [252].

Aspect 4: Recrudescence Associated with Artemisinin Drug Concentration Reduction

A variety of studies have shown declines in artemisinin drug concentration (QHS, AS, AM, and DHA) observed over time in the blood plasma of patients administered repeated dose of oral artemisinin compounds in both patients with malaria and healthy controls. The C_{max} and AUC values observed were significantly reduced by 15-33% on the last dosing day *versus* the first dosing day. The decline in exposure to drug observed is not related to disease given the same decrease is observed in healthy subjects [205-209]. Similar time-dependent decline of oral AM drug concentrations over time was also found in beagle dogs (Fig. **11** bottom) [231]. One hypothesis, which has been mentioned previously, to explain decreases in plasma drug concentration profile over time throughout therapy shows elevated liver metabolism due to auto-induction of cytochrome

P450 liver enzyme that metabolize drugs. The drug decrease, however, was not noted in patients after administration of intramuscular AE formulated in sesame oil [232].

The alteration of the pharmacokinetic shape of artemisinin drugs used as monotherapy may in turn result in a decrease in efficacy following administration of multiple doses over time and finally result in recrudescence. The therapeutic potentials of all artemisinin and its derivatives used in monotherapy in various dose regimens for treatment of malaria in 54 clinical trials have been summarized in Table **3**. Successful (or 100% cure) were not noted in the 3-5 day treatment regimens nor the high dose (4.8 mg/kg) monotherapy treatment regimens [65, 233].

5.2. PK/PD CHARACTERISTICS OF IV ARTESUNATE USED IN SEVERE MALARIA THERAPY

The drug C_{max} or peak drug concentration has been shown to be a more important parameter than drug exposure time (AUC) for efficacy when treating patients with severe malaria. Intravenous AS provides the highest peak drug levels in malaria-infected patients and provides the quickest efficacy available of any drug to kill parasites. Accordingly, injected artesunate has both a superior PK and PD profile when compared to other artemisinin derivatives tested in various regimens (Table **17**). There is now compelling data showing intravenous AS will reduce deaths in patients infected with severe malaria by approximately one-third[19, 34, 313, 314]. The extraordinarily high antimalarial activity of intravenous AS in the blood of infected patients in the first few hours after first administration of this drug is critical from a therapeutic standpoint, for patients with severe malaria whose mortality rates can reach between 15% and 20%, despite antimalarial treatment and supportive treatment. Intravenous AS is a safer drug than injectable quinine that is also easier to administer for patients with severe malaria [315].

Oral AS treatment of patients has been shown to have the best pharmacokinetic and pharmacodynamic profile for treatment of uncomplicated malaria when compared to data derived from studies of the other four artemisinins (Table **17**). Severe malaria kills upward of one million people every year, and the malaria death rate for children under the age of five approaches 1% [316]. A small fraction of children may be afflicted with neurological deficits after infection with severe malaria. Severe malaria is often accompanied by metabolic abnormalities or organ failure. Cerebral malaria with coma is a form of severe malaria resulting in a mortality rate of 20% [316, 317]. Some of the cerebral malaria survivors demonstrate neurological problems that persist after their infection is cured. In malaria endemic regions, children under five are at high risk for death by severe malaria while in areas that are not highly endemic for malaria, both adults (particularly travelers) and children are vulnerable to severe malaria [318]. There are three treatments for severe malaria, intravenous artesunate (AS), injected artemether (AM), and injectable quinine or injectable quinidine that are recommended for therapy of severe malaria.

5.2.1. Limitation of Quinine for Treatment of Severe Malaria

Intravenous quinine is the most broadly used drug for severe *falciparum* malaria treatment. For 400 years, quinine has served as the treatment of choice for severe malaria. While quinine is efficacious for malaria treatment, this drug does have significant limitations. Case-fatality rates for severe malaria patients treated with quinine often exceed 20% even with prompt drug administration [202]. To avoid adverse effects, controlled IV infusion is the best route for administration of quinine, which may not be feasible in rural areas, so quinine is also administered *via* intramuscular injection. Some studies have demonstrated that rectal administration of quinine is well tolerated and efficacious with none of the problems associated with IM injection and none of the complexity associated with slow, constant IV administration [319, 320].

Adverse effects associated with quinine administration known as cinchonism are quite common. Cinchonism frequently occurs at after administration of quinine at recommended dose levels, and this complex of symptoms, which is usually reversible, consists of dizziness, vomiting, tinnitus, and deafness, which has an impact on treatment adherence. Hypoglycemia can be observed which can be a significant adverse effect. Some patients demonstrate allergies to quinine, and these allergies manifest as skin rashes and edema even after administration of small doses. Toxic quinine drug concentrations can occur after fast IV injection, which can lead to coma, cardiotoxicity, death, and blindness, and cardiac monitoring is recommended during intravenous treatment [202].

Quinine is also administered *via* intramuscular injection as an alternative to intravenous dosing. In order to cut down on the time required to reach the most appropriate concentration of quinine in the blood, injection of a quinine-loading dose administered at 20 mg/kg is suggested [321]. A Cochrane Review demonstrated a decrease in the parasite clearance time and fever clearance time in patients treated with a quinine-loading dose *versus* to patients treated without a loading dose [319]. As per the WHO policy on antimalarial drugs used to treat severe malaria [316, 322], quinine is still the recommended treatment for children if intravenous AS is not available In the USA, quinidine gluconate, a quinine diastereoisomer, is the only IV treatment available for severe malaria.

Quinidine is associated with cardiac arrhythmias, which can lead to sudden cardiac death, and, due to a short elimination life, quinidine must be given two to three times daily. Quinidine should be administered in an ICU setting where continuous cardiac electrographic and blood pressure monitoring can be conducted due to the risk of cardiotoxicity with monitoring [323]. Rapid administration of quinidine can frequently lead to cardiovascular adverse events, and adverse cardiac events may also occur with an increased risk with existing conditions of hypokalemia, bradycardia, and hypomagnesaemia or if a patient has been administered another drug, which could extend the QTc interval such as macrolide antibiotics, chloroquine, or mefloquine [324].

5.2.2. Artemether Shown Not To Be Superior to Quinine

While not common, drug resistance to quinine has been observed more frequently in the literature [325]. This leads to the question of whether artemisinin compounds are better than quinine to treat severe malaria. Based on other work presented previously, intravenous AS has been shown to be superior to quinine. Intramuscular AM (AM cannot be administered by IV injection) has been compared in a number of studies to intravenous quinine in over 3,000 patients in Africa and Asia [235]. Large randomized trials comparing IM AM to IV quinine were conducted in Gambian children [197] and Vietnamese adults [198]. A meta-analysis of individual treatment data derived from 1,919 patients in eleven clinical studies of injected AM *versus* quinine treatment [202] showed no difference in efficacy in the two treatments with death serving study end-point.

A group of adults, however, showed decreased death after treatment with AM. AM has been shown to provide variable drug uptake, and AM therefore requires a longer period to reach peak plasma levels compared to AS [326]. While AM provided enhanced survival to a subgroup noted in one trial, and AM is safer and easier to administer than quinine, overall these trials did not show AM to be superior to [202]. This data did not demonstrate a compelling reason to change drug treatment policies from quinine to AM. Compared to AS, AM shows slow, erratic absorption from sites of injection, and AM is not metabolized as well to DHA, unlike AS. Given these drawbacks, surprisingly, intramuscular AM still managed to provide equivalent efficacy to quinine in these studies. As AM showed no survival advantage *versus* quinine, subsequent trials discussed in this next section involved comparing the efficacy of AS *versus* quinine to treat severe malaria.

5.2.3. Use of Artesunate for Treatment of Severe Malaria in the SEAQUAMAT and AQUAMAT Clinical Trials

Artesunate has a better PK profile than AM, it can be dosed either IV or IM while AM can only be dosed intramuscularly, and AS rapidly achieves peak plasma levels when dosed either IV or IM [65]. AS was therefore considered to have greater potential to treat severe malaria than AM, given the results showing AM was as efficacious as quinine for severe malaria treatment. Initial trial results in small studies comparing the two drugs in adults showed AS demonstrated evidence of a survival benefit compared to quinine [327]. With this encouraging initial data, the Southeast Asian Quinine Artesunate Malaria Trial (SEAQUAMAT) trial was initiated between 2003 and 2005.

1) Southeast Asian Quinine Artesunate Malaria Trial (SEAQUAMAT)

The SEQUAMAT trial was a large, multicenter, randomized, trial performed at trial sites in Bangladesh, India, Bangladesh, Indonesia, and Myanmar. This comparative efficacy study was conducted in 1,461 patients (to include 202 children) in Asia, with 730 patients enrolled in the AS treatment group and 731 in the quinine treatment group. The severity of disease was shown to be similar between these groups, and the patients had similar baseline characteristics. The observed mortality in the quinine arm was 22%, as compared to mortality rate of 15% in the AS arm, a reduction in mortality risk of 34.7% [200].Large variability in mortality rates were observed between the studies conducted in different countries. For example, at the Bangladesh site, a mortality rate of 28% was observed compared to a mortality rate of 9% in Indonesia. The survival benefit provided by AS compared to quinine was consistently shown in all of the sites. The majority of the survival benefit provided by AS was noted early after hospital admission, and rates of mortality after this period were similar.

Efficacy was similar in adults compared to children, however, the population of children in this study was much smaller than the adult population, and the mortality difference was not statistically significant [328]. AS treatment resulted in minor adverse events, and hypoglycemia was much more frequently noted in patients treated with quinine. Only one type 1 hypersensitivity reaction was noted after AS administration in 3000 patients. Quinine, however, is locally toxic at sites of injection and it often causes damage to the sciatic nerve. Quinine cannot be administered by bolus IV injection, it must be dosed three times per day, and its administration is well known to result in serious hypoglycemia. A systematic meta- analysis of five randomized comparative efficacy trials comparing IV AS and IM AS to IV quinine showed AS to be superior with large decreases in the relative death risk (relative risk, 0.62), decreased hypoglycemia incidence, and faster parasite clearance times *versus* quinine. Neurological after effects in patients treated with AS were very rare. Because of this study, intravenous AS has been recommended to be first-line treatment by WHO to treat severe malaria areas of low malaria transmission and to treat pregnant women in their later trimesters [1, 23].

The SEAQUAMAT trial showed severe malaria treatment with intravenous AS provides a survival benefit *versus* quinine. This trial was definitive to the point where other trials of its kind are unlikely to be conducted given the ethical risk of providing quinine, an inferior treatment, to patients with severe disease at risk of death. The next question to be answered was this data applicable to Asian children or to children and adults in Africa, where the majority of severe *falciparum* malaria is found. Unfortunately, while intravenous AS has been used for 30 years in Asia, no GMP-prepared formulation of intravenous AS is available. Affordable, GMP-produced intravenous AS should be innovated and manufactured to provide drug that is openly available in malaria endemic areas as soon as possible [329]. Severe malaria is a leading cause of death in children in Africa and the most frequent cause for hospital admission in sub-Saharan Africa. Quinine has been first-line treatment for severe malaria in Africa for many years, and given the promising data derived from the SEQUAMAT trials in Asia, a follow-on trial was conducted to assess artesunate treatment for children and adults in Africa with severe disease. The African Quinine Artesunate Malaria Trial was conducted to ask the next question not answered in the SEAQUAMAT trial regarding the potential survival advantage provided by intravenous AS *versus* intravenous quinine.

2) African Quinine Artesunate Malaria Trial (AQUAMAT)

The AQUAMAT trial was conducted at 11 centers in nine African countries. 5,425 children less than 15 years of age were randomly enrolled in this study; 2,712 were in the artesunate treatment group and 2,713 were in the quinine treatment group. The principle study endpoint was in-hospital mortality, analyzed by intention to treat. Total 230 patients (8.5%) in the artesunate arm died compared to 297 patients (10.9%) enrolled in the quinine arm. No differences in the frequency of neurological after effects were noted, however, coma was observed to occur in 65 of 1,832 patients (3.5%) treated with artesunate *versus* 91 patients out of 1,768 (5.1%) treated with quinine. Artesunate was shown to be safe, and no serious adverse effects were noted associated with drug treatment.

Artesunate was shown to reduce substantially the death of children in Africa with severe disease compared to quinine with fewer side effects. By contrast, quinine has long been associated with potentially serious hypoglycemia and in this study, 22 children died prior to administration of quinine *versus* six who passed away prior to administration of artesunate. This observation may be due to the challenges of dosing quinine, particularly in rural areas. Based on this study and on other studies of artesunate therapy, the treatment guidance to treat severe malaria in patients from areas of low malaria transmission should be conducted by dosing AS at 2.4 mg/kg bodyweight administered either IV or IM at hospital admission. Subsequent treatment should be conducted by dosing AS at 2.4 mg/kg 12 hours later and at 24 hours post admission followed by dosing every day until parasitemia is reduced.

Treatment of patients in high transmission areas involves the use of the following drugs only based on the published data for efficacy: 1) AS administered intravenously or intramuscularly at 2.4 mg/kg bodyweight at hospital admission followed by treatment at 12 hours, 24 hours, and daily. 2) Artemether dosed at 3.2 mg/kg bodyweight IM after hospital admission followed by treatment at 1.6 mg/kg bodyweight daily thereafter. 3) Quinine dosed at 20 mg salt/kg bodyweight administered intravenously or through divided intramuscular injection at hospital admission and then administration at10 mg/kg bodyweight every 8 hours thereafter at an infusion rate of no more than 5 mg salt/kg bodyweight per hour. Any delay of a severe malaria patient increases the risk of mortality. The advantages of easy and safe administration of artesunate are significant advantages compared to quinine. While artesunate is more expensive to purchase than quinine, quinine is demonstratively more expensive to dose given the requirement for slow intravenous dosing three times a day. The preponderance of data derived from analysis of many clinical trials supports the hypothesis that IV artesunate treatment is the treatment of choice for children and adults with severe *falciparum* malaria worldwide [201].

Changes in drug policy as suggested will potentially save thousands of children's lives every year. For example, if 4 million children in Africa are infected with severe malaria yearly, and all of them were treated with intravenous artesunate then 100,000 lives could potentially be spared every year given the results of this trial [201]. The data from the AQUAMAT and SEQUAMAT studies also confirmed the choice we made at Walter Reed Army Institute of Research (WRAIR) in 2002 to develop a GMP formulated injectable artesunate over other possible replacements for quinidine [65, 255, 330].

One of the most significant issues encountered at WRAIR early in the development program was the lack of a commercial partner. Given the low incidence of severe malaria in the US, there was little interest by many pharmaceutical companies to co- develop injectable AS. Fortunately, a few new companies that have emerged specialize in small orphan drug markets like injectable AS. As the time approached to file a New Drug Application for injectable AS, WRAIR researchers met with representatives of the Sigma-Tau Pharmaceuticals Inc. who specialize in producing drugs for rare diseases. A partnership between Sigma Tau and WRAIR was created in 2009 to bring IV artesunate made under GMP to market as quickly as possible [330].

5.2.4. The Advantages of Artesunate Compared to Artemether and Quinine

The water solubility of artesunate enhances absorption, and AS has distinct advantage over other artemisinin derivatives such as intramuscular AM and intravenous quinine as AS can be dosed rectally, orally, and injected either IV or IM to treat severe malaria. The other advantage is the rapid hydrolysis of AS to dihydroartemisinin, which is a very potent schizonticidal compound. As discussed previously, intravenous administration of artesunate provides higher peak plasma concentrations more quickly than injectable intramuscular AM. This pharmacokinetic advantage clearly provides a clinical benefit for severe malaria treatment [65]. One question regarding AS administration in any form is the potential effects on fetuses in early pregnancy particularly in the first trimester. Animal data testing of the effects of AS on fetuses early in pregnancy have shown administration of artemisinin compounds is associated with fetal re-sorption and fetal abnormalities.

While animal data has provided a warning of what might take place if AS were administered to pregnant human patients, no increase in rates of stillbirth or abortion were shown in a study conducted on the Thai-Myanmar border of 461 pregnant women treated with AS. While possible embryolethality after AS injection in patients in their first trimester is concerning in patients with uncomplicated malaria, pregnant patients with severe disease may not have the luxury of avoiding AS given the adverse outcomes from severe malaria. Severe malaria in pregnant women is commonly linked to significant adverse outcomes and the highest priority when treating pregnant women with severe malaria is rapid administration of effective treatment. Given the increase in quinine resistance and the known enhanced survival of severe malaria patients with intravenous AS, pregnant women will likely be treated with IV AS as opposed to being treated with quinine. The rates of fetal death were similar in the IV AS treated group and the IV quinine treated group in the SEAQUAMAT and AQUAMAT trials, however, the numbers of patients in this study were small and outcomes from surviving pregnancies were not assessed.

The risk of fetal death is highest in a narrow window of pregnancy in the first trimester from artesunate exposure, and this risk must be balanced against the known risk of death by severe disease for both fetus and mother. For this reason, artesunate is the treatment of choice for all women who are pregnant in Asia who are afflicted with severe disease, as quinine resistance is a significant concern in this region. In Africa, pregnant patients in their first trimester have a different set of risks as quinine is still effective, the potential for artesunate-induced embryolethality is the same, and the advantage of treatment with artesunate is not as clear [328]. Intramuscular AM and intravenous AS have been shown to be effective treatments for severe malaria. As AM did not show superiority against quinine administered either intramuscularly or intravenously [171, 197, 198, 326], intramuscular AS injection merits consideration for treatment of severe malaria, as IM AS will likely be efficacious and useful in rural, resource limited areas [171]. Intramuscular quinine administration has become commonly used in many countries, and this is the treatment of choice in Tanzania for severe disease. IM quinine decreases the risk of dosing problems associated with cardiotoxicity, however, the risk of developing hypoglycemia is not changed.

Given the drawbacks for using IM quinine in terms of adverse events, intramuscular AS has potential to replace IM quinine in these rural areas that do not have the resources for intravenous injection. IM artesunate has been assessed in clinical trials to treat patients with both severe and uncomplicated malaria [270, 271, 331]. Results of a number of studies on patient outcomes of children in Africa with severe malaria admitted to a hospital disease have shown there are a variety of factors that can influence patient outcomes. Two of the most important factors include speed of diagnosis and time required to administer effective therapy swiftly as the majority of deaths from severe malaria in children in Africa occur within the first 12 hours after hospital admission. This data reinforces the hypothesis that intramuscular AS administration is a valid alternative to treatment with IM quinine.

Many African children die of malaria prior to hospital admission. One potential route of administration for AS discussed previously to treat patients infected with severe disease in rural areas is *via* rectal dosing. Rectal AS is not likely to replace intravenously administered quinine or AS in hospitals, but this product may play a prominent role in rural Africa where the majority of deaths from malaria take place. While intravenous AS is demonstrably the best treatment for severe malaria, this treatment is impractical for patients who develop severe disease in resource constrained rural areas. For these patients, AS suppositories provide an efficacious treatment that can be provided in rural areas to prevent further increases in parasitemia and buy time to reach inpatient care in a hospital. The WHO has been involved as a sponsor to develop GMP formulated AS suppositories, which are well absorbed and have been shown to be efficacious for treatment of moderately severe malaria [329].

Rectal AS deployed in homes or villages in rural regions of Asia and Africa may be important tools to reduce mortality from severe disease. A trial in Uganda, which compared rectal AM dosing *versus* IV quinine, did show a trend of more rapid clearance of parasites, but this trend was not statistically significant [332]. Rectal AS may well provide a mortality benefit given its more rapid absorption and rapid biotransformation into DHA [329]. A multicenter trial of rectal AS administered in rural areas to patients who were not able to travel to a hospital within 6 hours has shown increased survival for these patients [333]. The use of suppository treatment for malaria in rural Africa can potentially save many lives, and this novel route of administration warrants additional clinical trials. One potential issue to be addressed is the potential consequence of widespread use of artemisinin rectal suppositories concerning induction of drug resistance.

Recent systematic reviews have been conducted to compare artemisinin rectal suppositories with IV quinine to treat severe malaria [333, 334]. The results of all of the meta-analysis showed that both AS and artemisinin rectal suppositories demonstrate a better parasite killing compared to intravenous quinine in the first 24 hours of treatment. The treatment dose of the rectal suppositories made a clear difference in the parasitological outcome as treatment with a series of low dose. This data is consistent with other studies of artemisinin derivatives used to treat severe malaria. Treatment with a water soluble, highly efficacious product like artesunate provides rapid peak drug levels [329, 335] that are most likely to kill rapidly parasites in severe malaria patients, and exposure of drug sustained over time through multiple lower doses does not provide a clinical benefit [336].

The SEAQUAMAT trial comparing intravenous quinine to intravenous AS showed a 35% lower mortality in the AS treatment arm *versus* the quinine treatment arm, which supports the hypothesis that rapid initial parasite clearance provides a clinical benefit and reduced mortality in cases of severe malaria [200]. Unfortunately, the analysis of the pooled data discussed did not have adequate power to utilize death as a study endpoint. The rate of parasite killing shown by rectal artemisinin suppositories is superior compared to intravenous quinine, and the rates of parasite clearance shown between different rectal artemisinin dosing procedures are excellent indicators of efficacy differences, which translate into differences in clinical outcomes. Future studies designed with mortality as a study endpoint for efficacy comparisons among rectal suppository products will likely need a patient population size so large that the study will likely not be conducted. The use of parasite clearance provides a surrogate marker, which was used in this meta-analysis, and this metric is likely the best obtainable evidence to conduct efficacy comparison studies for rectal artemisinin drugs [337].

Based on the body of evidence from many clinical trials conducted using intravenous, intramuscular and rectal administration of AS, quinine, and AM, AS is clearly the superior product to treat severe malaria in adults and likely the best treatment for children in regions of high transmission [200, 253, 338, 339].

5.3. PK/PD CHARACTERISTICS OF ARTEMISININ AND ITS DERIVATIVES FORMULATED AS ACTS

5.3.1. The PK Advantage of Artemisinin Drugs Acting as an ACT Partner Drug

Given the number of studies conducted utilizing oral AS, a complete PK/PD, data set is available for review. In a number of previously mentioned studies, PK/PD evaluations have shown oral AS is pharmacokinetically and pharmacodynamically superior to artemisinin, arteether, artemether, and DHA for treatment of uncomplicated malaria. The absolute bioavailability observed after a single dose of oral AS in uncomplicated adult malaria is approximately 60% [182]. The peak drug concentration (C_{max}) of DHA observed after oral AS dosing was shown to range from 339 and 1,309 ng/ml in many clinical trials (Table **18**). This PK data and the abundance of clinical trial data using AS explains why the WHO Expert Consultative group recommended AS as an artemisinin partner drug for 3 different combinations (AS-MQ, AS-AQ, and AS-SP). The other two drug combinations recommended by the WHO include fixed dose artemether-lumefantrine (Coartem) and DHA-piperaquine [342-349].

AS-mefloquine has been widely used since 1994 for first-line treatment of uncomplicated malaria in Southeast Asia particularly, Thailand and Cambodia, and in many parts of the world outside Southeast Asia, this combination is still effective. Recently, DHA-piperaquine as a fixed-ratio drug combination was developed to treat uncomplicated malaria in China [350]. DHA-piperaquine has been widely used in Southeast Asia in controlled clinical trials. In March 2004, Oxford University, Chongqing Holley Holding, and Sigma Tau S.P.A. joined forces with Medicines for Malaria Venture (MMV) to develop this promising antimalarial drug to international standards. Clinical trials of DHA-piperaquine conducted over the last 5 years have shown this combination is efficacious, safe, and well tolerated [351]. DHA-piperaquine is likely to replace AS-mefloquine for treatment of uncomplicated malaria in Southeast Asia.

Artemether-lumefantrine was the first fixed dose combination ACT drug, and this combination is used most widely around the world as AL represents 70% of all ACTs used today for treatment [2]. In the PK/PD evaluation discussed previously, intramuscular AM administration did not show large gains in efficacy, pointing to pharmacokinetic disadvantages when intramuscular AM is given to humans. Given this data, how could AM constitute a successful oral therapy combined with lumefantrine to treat uncomplicated malaria. Pharmacokinetic studies have shown that oral administration of AM, which has a pharmacokinetic advantage over administration of IM artemether in man [340].

The plasma concentrations of artemether (AM)in 15 adults infected with *falciparum* malaria was measured after intramuscular or oral administration. The C_{max} or peak AM concentrations in blood plasma surprisingly were shown to be higher in patients after oral AM administration (median DHA C_{max} of 541.8 ng/ml)which is 16 times higher than the median drug concentrations observed after intramuscular administration of AM (DHA level of 34.4 ng/ml). The ratio of the AUC observed over the first 24 hours (AUC_{0-24}) following oral administration of AM was 3.3 fold higher than the AUC_{0-24} observed after intramuscular administration, which is likely due to the slow and incomplete absorption of intramuscular AM in patients [340]. Other studies have shown administration of oral AM provided a C_{max} ranging from 406-818 ng/ml, which translates to a drug level 5.5 to 11.2 fold higher than the C_{max} observed in patients dosed with intramuscular AM [246, 341].

5.3.2. Artemisinin Drugs Demonstrate a Significant PD Advantage When Administered as an Orally Dosed ACT

Artemether combined with lumefantrine (Coartem) is a well-tolerated oral antimalarial combination drug that has been shown to be effective even against multidrug resistant *falciparum* malaria. The artemether component is absorbed rapidly and biotransformed to dihydroartemisinin and both are eliminated with terminal half-lives of around 1 hour. These are very active antimalarials, which give a rapid reduction in parasite biomass and consequent rapid resolution of symptoms. The lumefantrine component is absorbed variably in malaria-infected patients, and is eliminated more slowly (half-life of 3 to 6 days). Absorption is very dependent on co-administration of this combination with fat. Artemether clears most of the parasite biomass, and the lumefantrine drug that remains at the end of the 3- to 5-day treatment course is responsible for eliminating the residual 100 to 10,000 parasites. Its correlate, the plasma concentration on day 7, has been shown to be an important determinant of therapeutic response [17, 355-359].

Another ACT treatment, AS-mefloquine, has been widely used in Southeast Asian countries such as Thailand and Cambodia since 1994, and AS-MQ is still highly effective for treatment of drug resistant *falciparum* malaria. Under the WHO system of efficacy assessment, more than 95% of patients will remain free of malaria 28 days after such treatment [138]. The failure rate of the AS-mefloquine combination, however, has been reported to be up to 13% in Thailand and Cambodia [346], and the neuropsychiatric side-effects of mefloquine as well as its relative expense are problematic [347]. Other studies of mefloquine in combination with DHA have been conducted to investigate the efficacy of this combination and the PK/PD interactions between the two drugs. These aspects of DHA combined with mefloquine were studied in a three-way crossover design study of 10 healthy Thai males [354].

The subjects were randomized to receive one of three different drug treatments on three separate occasions to include the first regimen, a single dose of 300 mg of orally administered DHA. The second regimen included a single dose of 750 mg of orally administered mefloquine, and the third regimen included a single dose of 300 mg of orally administered DHA co-administered with a single dose of 750 mg of orally administered mefloquine. All of the treatment regimens were well tolerated, and oral DHA was rapidly absorbed and metabolized within 8-10 hours. Mefloquine absorption and disposition are much slower by comparison. The pharmacokinetics of DHA and mefloquine when co-administered were similar, however, the rate of mefloquine absorption was shown to be much quicker when mefloquine was co-administered with DHA than by itself. The combination of DHA and mefloquine together has also been shown to yield drug synergy as shown in an *ex vivo* blood study of schizonticidal activity.

The maximum pharmacodynamic activity observed, E_{max}, for DHA combined with mefloquine increased by 2- to 20-fold, while the E_{max} for DHA as monotherapy increased by 4-fold, and the E_{max} for piperaquine as monotherapy increased by 2-fold. The AUEC of mefloquine observed during the first 24 hours ($AUEC_{0\text{-}24h}$) increased by roughly 50 fold in patients co-administered mefloquine and DHA [354]. Recently, DHA- piperaquine (DP) was developed in China and Africa as a fixed ACT [350]. This combination therapy has been shown to be safe, efficacious, and well tolerated over the last 5 years, and DP administered orally every day for 3 days has been shown to have a 99.4% effective at achieving cures [360-363]. DP is registered in several Southeast Asian and Africa countries and has been adopted as a national treatment policy in Vietnam, and it is likely DP will replace mefloquine as the treatment of choice in this region due to the rising incidence of treatment failure with AS-MQ [147, 364].

Measurement of PD outcomes from these ACT comparative efficacy studies often involves the utilization of parasite counts and parasite clearance times. Parasite count and clearance time (PCT) are not always the best method of assessing total parasite burden in *falciparum* malaria due to parasite sequestration in the periphery, however, better pharmacodynamic parameters are not currently available. All of the artemisinin compounds had been shown to yield a very swift reduction of parasitemia, which begins right after administration [352, 353]. Fortunately, rapid parasite clearance induced by artemisinin drug treatment provides a simple pharmacodynamic metric that is useful for drug comparisons (Figs. **10** and **13**). Parasitological cure is the best end measure of efficacy for patients infected with malaria, and this metric is even easier to measure as an endpoint. The available parasitemia reduction data for the artemisinins is shown in Fig. **10** along with the associated PK profile noted during treatment of uncomplicated malaria. While none of the artemisinin agents showed 100% curative effects in a 5-day monotherapy regimen, artemisinin drugs demonstrate a well-established clinical benefit of rapid parasite killing which leads us to the best use of these drugs: oral ACTs for uncomplicated malaria and intravenous AS sequential therapy for severe and complicated malaria.

5.4. PK/PD EVALUATION OF QUINOLINE AND ANTIFOLATE DRUGS AS PARTNERS IN ACTS

The traditional antimalarial drugs, the quinolines (chloroquine, quinine, piperaquine, mefloquine, and primaquine) and the antifolates (sulfadoxine, pyrimethamine), have been utilized as long-acting ACT partner drugs (Table **22**). When these slowly eliminated antimalarials are given in combination with artemisinin drugs, the duration of artemisinin treatment can be reduced to 3 days. As ACTs are administered over a 3-day period, killing all parasites present requires the antimalarial activity of the partner drug persisting at parasiticidal concentrations. Thus, the partner compounds must be eliminated slowly. A slowly eliminated partner drug also protects the artemisinin component from development of drug resistance, and the partner drug has some partial protection by the artemisinin partner drug. Mutual protection from drug resistance aids efforts to control malaria and this is very helpful in areas that have low-to-moderate endemic infection rates. To reduce parasitemia by 90%, artemisinin treatment is required over a 3 day period to provide coverage through 3-4 a sexual parasite growth cycles. By killing 90% of the malaria parasites with the artemisinin partner, only 10% of infecting parasites are still present to be killed by the long-lived partner drug in the ACT, which in turn reduces the likelihood of drug resistance developing.

5.4.1. Quinine and its Derivatives

Quinine is the first drug used for malaria treatment, and quinine was originally derived from bark stripped from the *Cinchona calisaya* tree. Four antimalarial compounds have actually been derived from cinchona tree bark to include quinine, cinchonin, quinidine, and cinchonidine. Quinine was finally successfully synthesized in 1944, and no cinchona trees are required for its production. Other analogues of quinine that have been developed include halofantrine, lumefantrine, and mefloquine. Quinine does not prevent parasite sequestration nor is it active against *P. falciparum* parasites in the circulating ring stage of development. Quinine is capable of killing the gametocytes of *vivax*, *malariae*, and *ovale* parasites but cannot kill mature *falciparum* gametocytes. The mechanism of action of quinine differs from other quinolines such as the 4-aminoquinolines; however, it is not precisely known how they vary. Arylaminoalcohols have been shown to interfere with digestion of heme rather than interfering with the elimination of toxic byproducts of heme digestion. Increasing the copy number of the pfmdr1 gene (Plasmodium falciparum multi-drug resistance) which codes for a transport protein has been shown to be a principal means of parasite resistance to the arylaminoalcohol class of drugs [365].

Table 22: Drug classes of current antimalarial drugs according to chemical structure [65]

	Generic Drug Classes	**Drug Example**
1	Arylaminoalcohols:	Quinine, quinidine (cinchona alkaloids), mefloquine, halofantrine, lumefantrine,
2	4-aminoquinolines	Chloroquine, amodiaquine (bisquinoline piperaquine)
3	8-aminoquinolines	Primaquine, tafenoquine (WR238605), 4-methyl primaquine diphosphate. (WR181023)
4	Folate synthesis inhibitors (Antifolates)	Type 1 - competitive inhibitors of dihydropteroate synthase - sulphones (dapsone), sulphonamides (sulphadoxine) Type 2 - inhibit dihydrofolate reductase - biguanides like proguanil and chlorproguanil; diaminopyrimidine like pyrimethamine; cycloguanil, trimethoprim
5	Peroxides (Sesquiterpene lactones)	Artemisinin (Qinghaosu) derivatives - dihydroartemisinin artemether, arteether, artesunate, artelinic acid
6	Antimicrobials:	Tetracycline, doxycycline, clindamycin, azithromycin, fluoroquinolones, chloramphenicol
7	Naphthoquinones (Respiratory chain inhibitors)	Atovaquone
8	Iron chelating agents	Desferrioxamine
9	Drug combinations	▪ Sulphadoxine-pyrimethamine ('Fansidar') ▪ pyrimethamine + sulphadoxine + mefloquine ('Fansimef') ▪ atovaquone + proguanil ('Malarone')

Quinine

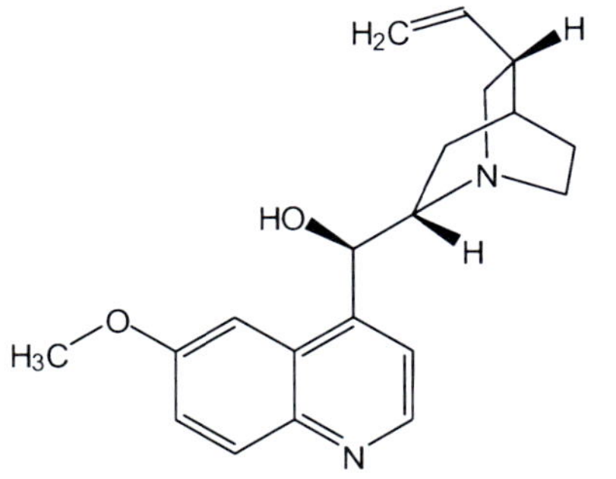

Quinine is a stereoisomer of quinidine, and it acts rapidly on mature trophozoite parasites. Quinine cannot prevent parasite sequestration nor is it active against *falciparum* parasites in the circulating ring stage of development.

PK/PD Properties of Quinine

Oral quinine is formulated as a sulfate or bisulfate, and it is rapidly absorbed from the gastrointestinal tract providing peak plasma drug levels 1-3 hours after dosing. Quinine is absorbed after injection intramuscularly into severe malaria patients. Quinine is 70% bound to plasma proteins in healthy subjects, and the percentage of plasma protein binding increases to 90% in malaria patients. Quinine is distributed throughout the body including the CSF (2-7% of plasma drug levels), breast milk (30% of plasma drug levels), and the placenta. Small amounts of quinine have been shown to accumulate in the bile and saliva. Quinine is metabolized by CYP3A4 in the liver, and the metabolites of quinine are cleared primarily through the kidneys. The initial metabolite produced by CYP3A4, 3-hydroxyquinine, has been shown to contribute 10% of the antimalarial activity of quinine, however, the concentration of this metabolite and its activity may increase in patients who have renal failure. Quinine excretion is enhanced in acidic urine. The mean half-life of quinine is approximately 11 hours in healthy humans, 16 hours in patients with uncomplicated malaria, and 18 hours in patients with severe malaria [23].

Quinine, as has been discussed previously, is primarily used to treat severe *falciparum* malaria although quinine's supremacy as first-line treatment for severe malaria has decreased since the introduction of intravenous artesunate, particularly in Southeast Asia. Until the 1980s, intravenous quinine was given in regimens that had evolved from empirical observations of efficacy and toxicity, but these regimens were not derived with the benefit of pharmacokinetic guidance. Because of the increasing incidence of chloroquine resistance in Africa during the 1980s, the use of quinine increased, and doctors tended to follow the guidelines developed for use of quinine in Thailand. This necessitated the use of infusion devices, which were generally available only in African hospitals. The "Thai regimens" were derived to yield quinine drug levels in plasma above 10 mg/L as quickly as possible. This target concentration was chosen because some local strains of the parasite had minimum inhibitory concentrations approaching 10 mg/L *in vitro*. African strains are generally sensitive to quinine compared to parasites found in Southeast Asia, which suggests a lower target concentration would be effective. Moreover, in Africa, severe malaria mainly occurs in young children, whereas the Thai regimens were developed for adults with severe malaria [366, 367].

PK simulations have suggested that the standard regimen developed in Thailand would result in unbound quinine concentrations that exceed the upper end of the therapeutic range after each dose, and these concentrations are several-fold above the MIC_{99} at the trough concentration. Alternative regimens were therefore designed that would: 1) rapidly achieve, and maintain, unbound drug concentrations within the therapeutic range; 2) allow dosage regimens that did not depend on the use of infusion devices to be employed; and 3) reduce the number of daily maintenance doses from 3 to 2. Administration of quinine at 12-hourly instead of 8-hourly intervals has reduced the workload of healthcare personnel in overburdened healthcare centers. Based on the therapeutic range and pharmacokinetic data obtained following intramuscular administration of quinine, similar dosage recommendations have been made for use of the drug in rural settings where facilities for intravenous administration are unavailable [368].

Mefloquine

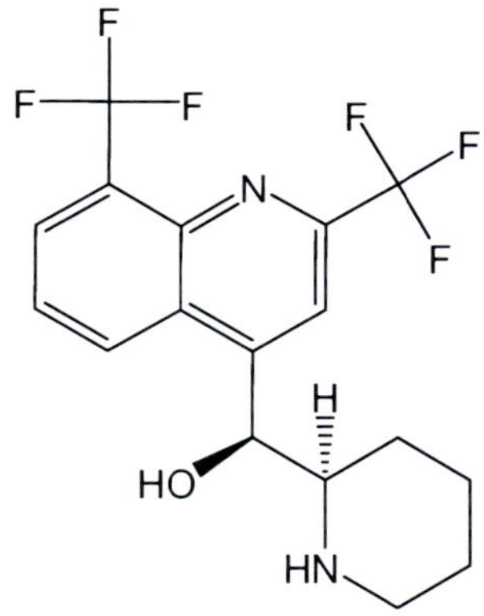

Mefloquine (MQ) is a 4-methanolquinoline and is structurally similar to quinine. MQ was developed by the U.S. Army Medical Research and Development Command, Hoffman-La Roche, and WHO. By screening over a quarter million compounds *in vivo* at Walter Reed Army Institute of Research (WRAIR), mefloquine (MQ), a 4-quinoline methanol was identified. Mefloquine is readily dissolved in alcohol but it is not as soluble in water, and as mefloquine is light sensitive, it must be protected from light. MQ is structurally related to quinine, and it is used to treat uncomplicated malaria. Mefloquine efficacy against *falciparum* malaria was demonstrated in a number of clinical trials, and it was shown to be highly useful for prophylaxis and treatment of US soldiers in clinical trials conducted in South America and Southeast Asia. After introduction of mefloquine in 1985, evidence of drug resistance to MQ was quickly noted in Southeast Asia [23].

PK/PD Properties of Mefloquine

In general, MQ is slowly absorbed, and the C_{max} is achieved within 8 to 24 hours. As mefloquine has significant inter-individual differences in bioavailability, this extended absorption is a potential site for drug interactions. Combination of mefloquine with artesunate yields drug synergy and absorption of mefloquine is enhanced. Food intake has been shown to increase the bioavailability of mefloquine, similar to other antimalarials, and diarrhea has been shown to reduce the bioavailability of mefloquine. Mefloquine plasma protein binding is another possible site for drug interactions as mefloquine is 90% plasma protein bound. The C_{max} of mefloquine is increased in patients infected with malaria and the half-life is shorter, however, the AUC is similar in healthy patients and malaria infected patients, which suggests during acute disease the Vd is decreased with no change in mefloquine binding to plasma proteins. The large variability in results observed in various studies is another confounder when trying to compare the efficacy of various MQ combinations. As MQ is combined primarily with artemisinin derivatives, which have short half-lives, potential interactions between MQ and an artemisinin compound can be addressed by simply adjusting dose timing. MQ has been combined with antibiotics such as tetracycline, and it has been combined with sulfadoxine-pyrimethamine (Fansi-Mef) [232].

MQ is effective against multidrug resistant *P. falciparum*, and its half-life of approximately 20 days demonstrates treatment is suitable in a single dose regimen. The combination of MQ and SP treatment was previously used to counter mefloquine drug resistance. The problem with this combination, which was pointed out before it was introduced, is that due to the differences in half-lives (SP has a half-live of no more than 10 days), no protection was provided for MQ in an environment that is admirably suited to the selection of resistant organisms. Moreover, even before the development of this combination therapy, there seemed to be little reason to be optimistic that this combination would be successful because *falciparum* parasites in Asia were already highly resistant to pyrimethamine and sulfadoxine prior to development of MQ. While this combination did lead to an improved treatment response, utilization of this combination has also resulted in an increased incidence of adverse effects and enhanced drug resistance. Therefore, it is important to recognize that knowledge of the pharmacokinetic profile of a compound is essential to predict the clinical utility of the drug alone or in combination [368].

Halofantrine

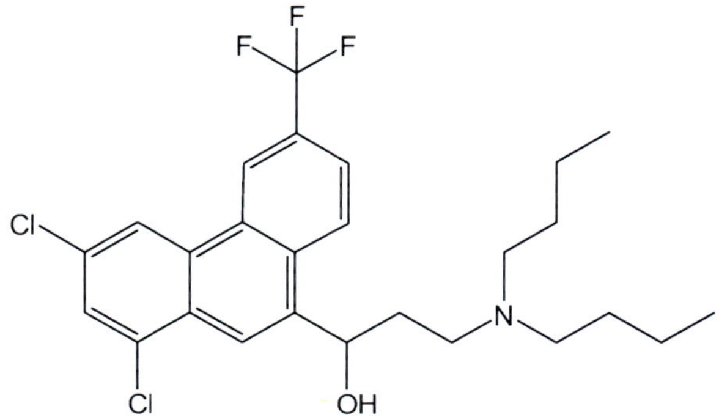

Halofantrine was also developed at Walter Reed Army Institute of Research (WRAIR). Halofantrine is a phenanthrene methanol structurally similar to quinine. Halofantrine is an effective antimalarial drug, which provides rapid parasiticidal activity against the trophozoite stages of *P. falciparum*. Halofantrine is not widely used due to cardiotoxic side effects with potentially fatal cardiac arrhythmias. Halofantrine use results in QT interval prolongation measured by electrocardiogram (ECG) preclude the use of this drug to treat patients with known prolongations in the QT interval. Adverse events may occur through drug interactions of halofantrine with other compounds, which may also affect the QT interval or enhance the concentration of halofantrine.

PK/PD Properties of Halofantrine

The pharmacokinetics of halofantrine has been previously studied, and few studies have been conducted since then due to the known cardiotoxicity risk associated with halofantrine's use. Halofantrine's absorption is quite variable, and drug absorption is enhanced when halofantrine is administered with a fatty meal. When halofantrine first came on market, the dosing recommendation was to do administer the drug along with a fatty meal to enhance absorption. With increased drug resistance against halofantrine in Thailand, higher doses than the recommended dosing were needed which led to cardiotoxicity in patients with underlying cardiac problems. When adverse cardiac effects were noted, dosing of halofantrine beyond the recommended dose was discouraged, and the recommendation to administer this drug with a fatty meal was rescinded in favor of administration without food. Halofantrine is rarely used today as dosing cannot be conducted with prior ECG screening to detect any underlying cardiac problems. Clearly, halofantrine has a poor therapeutic index, and halofantrine is vulnerable to development of adverse effects in combination with other drugs.

The elimination of halofantrine is exceedingly variable, with average half-life ($t_{1/2}$) values that range from 10 to over 100 hours; however, the majority of this data was obtained from orally administered halofantrine. An intravenous formulation of halofantrine was assessed for antimalarial efficacy in *falciparum*-infected patients. In a two-compartment PK model, average half-life of halofantrine was shown to be 14.4 hours in patients infected with malaria and 7.5 hours during the convalescent period. The Vd was shown to be less than 0.5 L/kg. Halofantrine's highly variable bioavailability, cardiotoxicity risks at increased dose, poor therapeutic response in regions of Southeast Asia, and the poor therapeutic index to avoid cardiotoxicity are the most relevant factors when considering the potential for drug interactions. Given its limited use, there is very little published data regarding halofantrine's propensity to cause drug interactions [232].

Circulating halofantrine concentrations following administration of a standard dosage are very unpredictable, and this may result in an unacceptable incidence of cardiovascular toxicity, principally, concentration-dependent prolongation of the QT interval. Similar QT effects are seen with quinine and quinidine, which is the only drug approved to treat severe malaria in the USA. Similar to halofantrine, these effects appear to relate to the circulating plasma concentrations of the parent drug. Given that it may be necessary to increase the dose of halofantrine in areas with halofantrine-resistant strains of *P. falciparum*, it would seem prudent to keep observe treated patients closely for cardiotoxicity. Interestingly, patients treated with halofantrine after mefloquine failure showed a longer QT prolongation. This observation is important because halofantrine was shown to be highly effective for recrudescent mefloquine-resistant malaria infections [368].

Lumefantrine

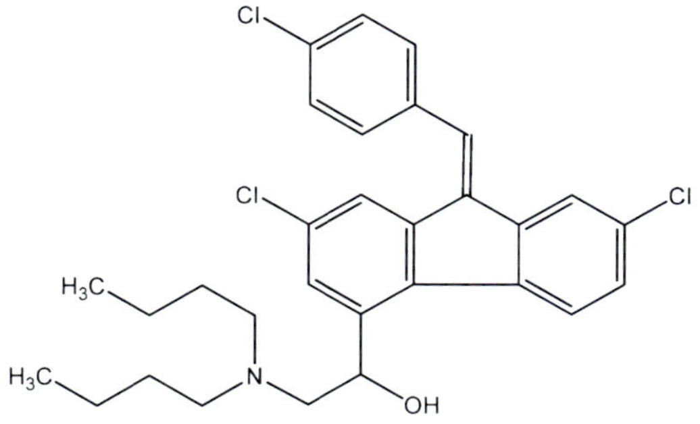

Lumefantrine is structurally similar to quinine, halofantrine, and mefloquine, and its mechanism of action is similar against the malaria parasite. Lumefantrine was developed by the Academy of Military Medical Sciences in Beijing and by Novartis Pharmaceuticals as a fixed dose combination called Coartem. Lumefantrine is only available co-formulated with artemether as an orally administered ACT. Artemether-lumefantrine has been to shown to be very efficacious against both drug sensitive and multidrug resistant *falciparum* parasites [65].

PK/PD Studies of Lumefantrine

Lumefantrine's oral bioavailability is highly variable and dependent on administration with fatty foods [23]. Absorption of lumefantrine has been shown to increase by 108% after consuming a meal, and absorption has been shown to be diminished in patients infected with malaria compared to recovering patients. Peak drug levels in plasma of lumefantrine occur 10 hours after dosing, and the half-life is approximately 3 days. Lumefantrine pharmacokinetics data is sparse in the published literature as most preclinical studies of this drug were conducted in China, and very little of this data was ever published. Based on published studies, drug absorption is slow with significant variability in bioavailability. Lumefantrine is 99% bound to plasma proteins. *In vitro*, lumefantrine was metabolized in the liver principally by CYP3A4 to desbutyl-lumefantrine, and it is ultimately excreted *via* the bile and feces. The reported half-life is also quite variable ranging from 33 hours to 6 days. In healthy volunteers, administration of lumefantrine with artemether had no effect on CYP3A4 activity. Some inhibition of CYP2D6 has been described in other studies; however, the clinical significance of this is unclear. Possible drug interactions involve the highly lipophilic nature of lumefantrine, which affects drug absorption and plasma protein binding [232].

Lumefantrine is chemically related to halofantrine; however, it does not share halofantrine's adverse cardiac effects. The four-dose regimen of artemether-lumefantrine has been shown to be more efficacious than chloroquine in geographic regions with high chloroquine resistance, but this combination was shown to be less effective when compared against other drugs. A number of clinical studies have shown that the six-dose artemether-lumefantrine treatment is as efficacious as other artemisinin based combination therapies and antimalarial combinations. A meta-analysis of 32 comparative efficacy trials demonstrated artemether-lumefantrine is highly efficacious. The reduction in gametocyte carriage observed after treatment with artemether-lumefantrine is believed to be due to the direct gametocidal effect of artemether, and the reduction in gametocyte carriage may be the result of the death of asexual stages of the parasite, which were prevented from developing to the gametocyte stage. No serious cardiotoxicity or neurotoxicity to artemether-lumefantrine has been reported, and this finding is particularly important when considering the treatment regimen recommended is six-doses administered for 3 days [369].

Artemether-lumefantrine meets the WHO efficacy criteria which is >95% efficacy for malaria treatment of adults and children in malaria-endemic regions. Drug resistance to artemether-lumefantrine *in vivo* has not been observed in Africa, however, resistance to this drug combination has been observed in Southeast Asia [370].

5.4.2. 4-Aminoquinoline Compounds

The 4-aminoquinoline group of antimalarials has been shown to complex with ferriprotoporphyrine IX (FPPIX), a toxic breakdown product of hemoglobin, which prevents its polymerization into hemazoin, which is not toxic to the parasite. FPPIX is produced in large amounts by malaria parasites digesting hemoglobin, and the detoxification of this waste product is essential for parasite survival [371]. Drug resistance against compounds of the 4-aminoquinoline class has been associated with a K76T mutation in the chloroquine resistance transporter gene (*pfcrt*) which is located in the digestive vacuole membrane, which removes 4-aminoquinolines from the digestive vacuole where they are effective in inhibiting hemazoin formation by the parasite.

Chloroquine

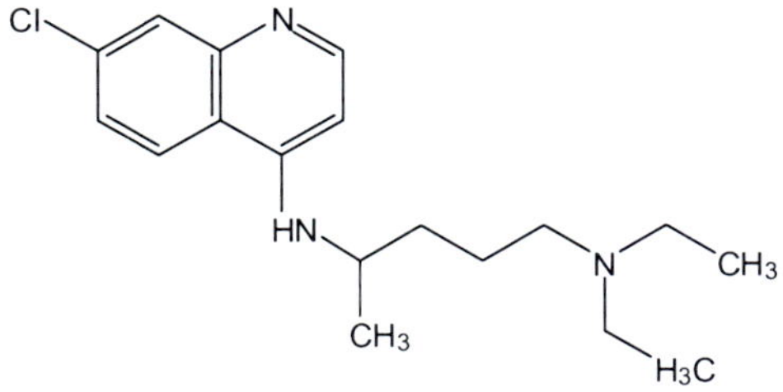

Chloroquine has been the mainstay of malarial chemotherapy for over 40 years. Many drugs were created as malaria prophylaxis drugs by the US Army to protect soldiers from malaria during the 1940s and 1950s to include chloroquine, primaquine, amodiaquine, proguanil, and sulphadoxine-pyrimethamine, which were all innovated and clinically developed during this era. Chloroquine was the first 4-aminoquinoline and it was widely used for treatment and prophylaxis in the 1950s and 1960s. Worldwide resistance has made chloroquine useless for treatment and prophylaxis against *falciparum* malaria in many malaria endemic areas; however, chloroquine is still efficacious against blood stage *vivax*, *malariae*, and *ovale* infections. Like other drugs in this class, chloroquine cannot kill the dormant hypnozoite form of *vivax* malaria.

Chloroquine's mechanism of action involves interfering with the detoxification of heme in the parasite, and CQ resistance is related to mutations in parasite drug transporters to include pfcrt and pfmdr1, which diminish the CQ drug concentration at the drug site of action in the parasite food vacuole. Ten to twelve years after chloroquine was introduced, resistance to chloroquine appeared against *P. falciparum* in two initial resistance foci developed at the same time in Colombia and in Southeast Asia on the border of Cambodia and Thailand. From these initial locations, CQ drug resistance spread throughout Southeast Asia and South America. Chloroquine drug resistance was observed in Africa by the late 1970s, and it has spread throughout the continent [2, 23].

PK/PD Studies of Chloroquine

Chloroquine is absorbed quickly and completely from the GI tract after oral administration, although peak plasma concentrations of chloroquine have been shown to vary considerably in both healthy subjects and malaria-infected patients. The volume of distribution (Vd) of chloroquine is very high from 100-1000 L/kg, and the given limited distribution into the central compartment, transient levels of chloroquine that are cardiotoxic can occur after IV dosing without slow administration. Chloroquine plasma protein binding ranges from 50-60% and this drug is metabolized by the liver to an inactive metabolite, desethyl-chloroquine, and subsequently metabolized to 7-chloro-4-aminoquinoline, bisdesethyl-chloroquine, and other metabolites. The metabolism of chloroquine is likely mediated through CYP enzymes in the liver, but in humans, the mechanism of metabolism is unclear. Chloroquine is 50% cleared by the kidneys, and chloroquine clearance follows multi-compartment kinetics. This may explain the significant inter-individual variability in half-lives observed which may range from 8 to 58 days. The half-life of chloroquine is not clinically significant for malaria treatment, but it is widely believed to contribute to emergence of chloroquine drug resistance. Administration of chloroquine intramuscularly or subcutaneously results in rapid absorption, which in turn may lead to transient toxic concentrations so parenteral administration is no longer recommended.

Chloroquine shows similar pharmacokinetic properties when administered to both children and adults with little change shown due to disease severity. There are data *in vitro* which suggest chloroquine inhibits CYP2D6. *In vivo* this inhibitory effect on CYP2D6 activity is weak, however, and other trials have shown chloroquine may be a CYP3A inhibitor or a substrate. No *in vivo* inhibitory effects on CYP2C19, CYP1A2, CYP3A4, or CYP2E1 have been shown. Chloroquine has used in combination with a variety of drugs, and no significant drug interactions have been shown [232].

Amodiaquine

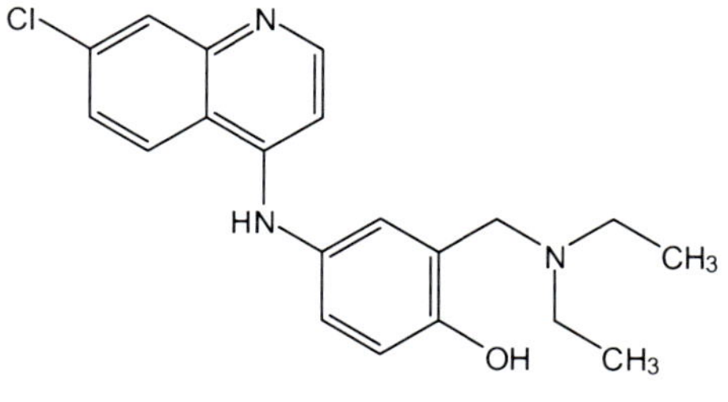

Amodiaquine is a 4-aminoquinolinewitha Mannich base component whose mechanism of antimalarial activity is the same as chloroquine. Amodiaquine was innovated and developed as an alternative to chloroquine given its efficacy against *falciparum* parasites resistant to chloroquine. Amodiaquine was commonly used for malaria chemoprophylaxis in travelers between 1948 and 1990; however, it is no longer used due to adverse effects on bone marrow and liver. Amodiaquine is not marketed in the US, but is widely available in Africa. Amodiaquine was combined with artesunate by DNDi in 2007 to create an orally administered fixed-dose combination to treat uncomplicated *falciparum* malaria

PK/PD Studies of Amodiaquine

Amodiaquine is rapidly absorbed through the GI tract and metabolized by the liver to create an active metabolite, desethylamodiaquine, which provides most of amodiaquine's antimalarial effect. Amodiaquine is similar to chloroquine pharmacokinetically with a lower volume of distribution ranging from 17-34 L/kg and a half-life of 1-3 weeks [23]. The half-life of desethylamodiaquine is not well characterized, and desethylamodiaquine and amodiaquine have been detected in the urine of patient's months after their treatment. Comparisons of amodiaquine to other drugs been conducted in 40 separate trials. In 24 studies, patients with symptomatic malaria were enrolled in trials comparing the efficacy of amodiaquine (n = 1,071) to chloroquine (n = 1,097). Amodiaquine was shown to be much more efficacious chloroquine, with an odds ratios and 99% confidence interval of 4.29 (3.30-5.58) by day 7 and 6.00 (3.97-9.06) by day 14. The parasite clearance time for amodiaquine is much shorter than chloroquine, and the fever clearance time of amodiaquine was shown to be slightly shorter. Studies comparing amodiaquine to sulfadoxine-pyrimethamine have been conducted, and the two drugs did not show significant efficacy differences on day 7, however, the odds ratio favored SP on day 14 and on day 28. Amodiaquine is more toxic than chloroquine, which initially limited the use of this drug. There are no data implicating amodiaquine in drug interactions [232].

Piperaquine

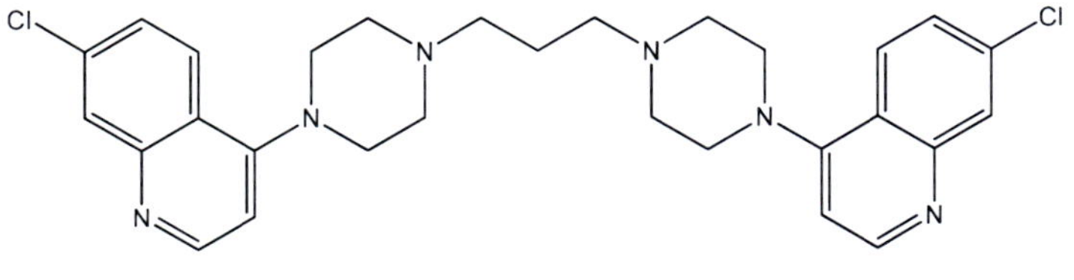

Piperaquine was innovated in the 1950s at Rhone Poulenc, France, [372], but this compound was set aside as no pharmaceutical company was interested in development (a common problem for malaria drug developers to this day). Piperaquine was resurrected by the Shanghai Research Institute of Pharmaceutical Industry in 1966. Piperaquine is an orally active bisquinoline, which was developed for antimalarial use in China in 1973. Piperaquine has been used extensively in Asia for both malaria treatment and prophylaxis over the last 20 years. A number of Chinese studies have shown that piperaquine is as effective as chloroquine for treatment of *falciparum* and *vivax* malaria, but no PK characterization was conducted. In the 1980s, strains of *falciparum* malaria resistant to piperaquine emerged, but despite this, piperaquine was piperaquine was chosen in China to be a partner drug with an artemisinin derivative of the first piperaquine ACT was China-Vietnam 4 (CV4). CV4 consisted of DHA, piperaquine, primaquine, and trimethoprim.

The follow-on piperaquine ACT drug was called CV8 which contained the same drugs but in larger doses. Subsequent piperaquine combinations include Artecom (containing no primaquine) and Artekin (DHA combined with piperaquine) have been produced. Recent studies in Indochina have shown that piperaquine-DHA combinations have excellent clinical efficacy with28-day rates of cure >95% and these studies have also shown DHA-piperaquine is not associated with cardiotoxicity. The PK properties of piperaquine have been characterized, and piperaquine is shown to be highly lipophilic with a long half-life and a high volume of distribution. Clearance of piperaquine is much more extensive in children compared to adults. Comparable efficacy, tolerability, low cost, and favorable pharmacokinetic profile of piperaquine have all been reasons why piperaquine has been promoted as an ACT partner drug [373].

PK/PD Studies of Piperaquine

The first pharmacokinetic and efficacy studies of piperaquine to treat malaria were conducted in Cambodia enrolling adults and children infected with uncomplicated *falciparum* and *vivax* malaria who were administered Artekin 2 tablets containing 40 mg of DHA and 320 mg of piperaquine or Artekin 2 granules dissolved in water. Four drug doses were at 0, 6, 24, and 32 hours providing an average total piperaquine total dose of 32-35 mg/kg. A two-compartment open model with first-order absorption fitted the data best using a population pharmacokinetic approach. Absorption of piperaquine was slow as the mean absorption period was shown to be 9.1 hours in adults and 9.3 hours in children. The mean half-life was 543 hours in adults and 324 hours in children, and the mean volume of distribution was shown to be large as adults have a Vd of 574 L/kg and children have a Vd of 614 L/kg. The clearance/bioavailability (CL/F) was shown to be two times higher in children (1.85 L/h/kg) *versus* adults (0.9 L/h/kg).The plasma protein binding of piperaquine is estimated to be approximately 97%, however, this has not been measured directly [373].

The bioavailability of piperaquine was assessed in a stud of healthy Caucasian subjects administered 500 mg of piperaquine phosphate(289 mg of piperaquine base) in patients who were either fasting or given a standard high-fat breakfast. Significant increases in C_{max} and AUC were noted in patients who were dosed after a high-fat meal suggesting that the piperaquine absorption may be enhanced by co- administration with fat. Administration of atovaquone and mefloquine with a fatty meal has also been shown to enhance the AUC.

Pyronaridine

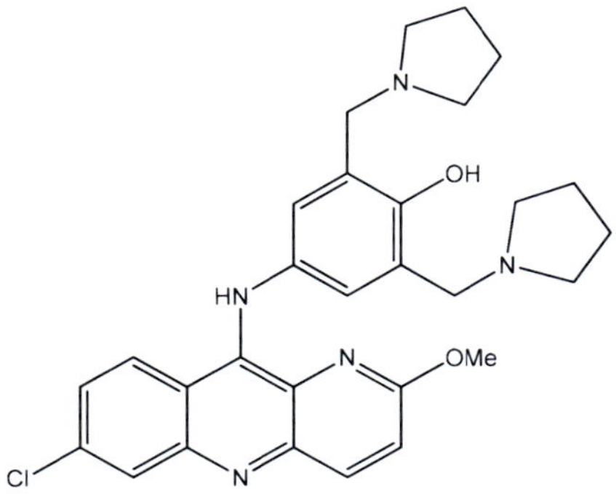

Pyronaridine has been used in China for over 20 years. While pyronaridine was shown to be 100 percent effective in Cameroon, the efficacy of pyronaridine in Thailand was shown to be 63 to 88 percent. Medicines for Malaria Venture (MMV) has collaborated with Shin Poong Pharmaceutical to develop a fixed dose combination of artesunate and pyronaridine called Pyramax®.

PK/PD Studies of Pyronaridine

Pyronaridine is a bis-Mannich amodiaquine analogue, with an acridine nucleus. Pyronaridine has been used for malaria treatment in China as monotherapy and combined with other drugs. The PK parameters of pyronaridine have not been thoroughly investigated. In healthy subjects, pyronaridine was administered as a single dose intramuscularly, which was rapidly absorbed with a C_{max} of 525 µg/L, a T_{max} of 0.66 hours, and an elimination half-life of roughly 64 hours. Pyronaridine has been used as an alternative first-line drug in chloroquine-resistant area. Shin Poong Pharmaceuticals recommends liver function testing during administration, does not have guidance on a safe interval between drug treatments, and does not recommend the use of pyronaridine for malaria prophylaxis, which suggests a liver toxicity liability for repeated use.

5.4.3. 8-Aminoquinoline Compounds

Primaquine is the only 8-aminoquinoline antimalarial in use today. 8-aminoquinoline drugs have activity against the dormant hypnozoite liver-stage parasites of the relapsing parasite, *Plasmodium vivax*. 8-aminoquinolines are the only antimalarial compounds capable of providing a radical cure for *vivax* malaria.

Primaquine

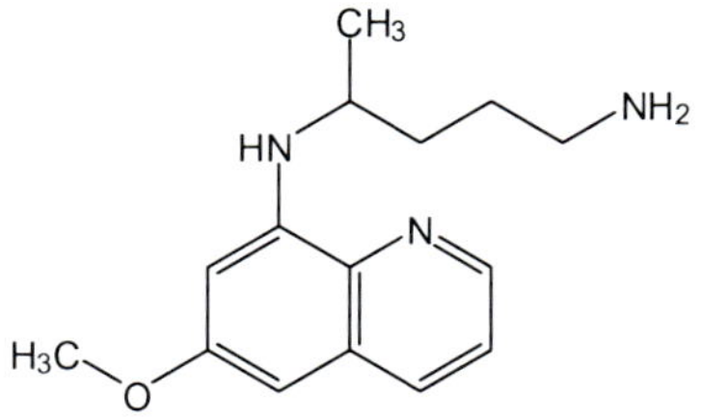

Primaquine is an 8-aminoquinoline originally developed by the US Army and other development partners, which came on market in 1952. Primaquine is capable of killing liver stage parasites of all *Plasmodium* species. Primaquine is used to treat dormant liver stage infections from both *vivax* and *ovale* parasites. Blood stage parasite killing requires combination of primaquine with a blood stage antimalarial compound as primaquine has very limited blood stage activity. Primaquine also has activity against *P. falciparum* gametocytes, which makes it a valuable tool for malaria eradication. Primaquine's mode of action is not known, but recent reports support the hypothesis that primaquine is a prodrug generating a wide variety of reactive metabolites with anti-hypnozoite activity. Primaquine is not routinely used to prevent malaria in travelers, and this drug is only used when no other alternatives are appropriate. It is not licensed for this use in the U.S. or the UK.

PK/PD Studies of Primaquine

Primaquine is formulated as a diphosphate salt, and it is easily absorbed from the gastrointestinal tract and widely distributed into many tissues of the body. Peak drug levels in plasma occur approximately 1-2 hours after dosing and primaquine is subsequently eliminated by the liver with a half-life of 3-6 hours [23]. The principle metabolite of primaquine is carboxy-primaquine, which demonstrates plasma accumulation with repeated administration. The metabolism of primaquine is primarily through liver CYP enzymes, and recent data has supported the hypothesis that CYP2D6 metabolism is required for primaquine activation. Malaria infection has been shown to decrease primaquine clearance. Primaquine induction of extravascular hemolysis is a known toxicity risk for individuals with deficiencies in glucose phosphate dehydrogenase (G6PD), however, G6PD deficiency does not change the PK parameters of primaquine. Given the many pathways of metabolism for primaquine, predicting sites of drug interaction for primaquine is difficult. Drug interactions with other antimalarials may not be an issue as primaquine is rarely used with other drugs beside chloroquine for radical cure of relapsing malaria [232].

Tafenoquine

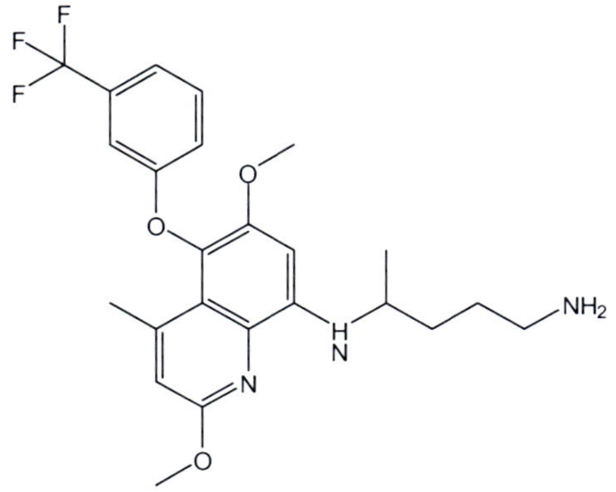

Tafenoquine, a synthetic analog of primaquine, was innovated at Walter Reed Army Institute of Research (WRAIR) as WR-238605, and this drug is currently being tested in clinical trials for treatment of relapsing *vivax* malaria by Glaxo Smith Kline. Tafenoquine is efficacious against both liver and blood stages of malaria. Tafenoquine may have considerable value for prophylaxis indications for travelers because of its long half-life of 14 days *versus* primaquine, which has a half-life of 6 hours. Given its properties, tafenoquine may be capable of serving as an agent for Single Encounter Radical Cure and Prophylaxis (SERCAP) malaria treatment. Similar to primaquine, tafenoquine can trigger acute hemolytic anemia in G6PD deficient patients.

PK/PD Studies of Tafenoquine

Tafenoquine is slowly absorbed and T_{max} is not reached until 12 hours after administration. The half-life of tafenoquine as mentioned previously is roughly 14 days. While the bioavailability of tafenoquine has not been precisely determined, the volume of distribution is estimated to be very large. Recent data has also demonstrated that CYP2D6 is required for activation of tafenoquine, similar to primaquine. This supports the hypothesis that 8-aminoquinoline drugs in general are prodrugs requiring metabolic activation for efficacy.

5.4.4. Antifolate Compounds

Antifolates were shown to be effective against malaria as early as the 1930s, and sulfonamide drugs with better pharmacokinetic profiles were developed in the 1940s and 50s. Antifolates were not commonly used for antimalarial treatment given the availability of highly efficacious quinoline analogues such as chloroquine. Sulfadoxine- pyrimethamine came on market in 1971 for second-line malaria treatment, and drug resistance developed soon thereafter. Resistance to antifolate drugs which have a specific enzyme target emerged more quickly than resistance to chloroquine, which has no specific parasitic target [366].

Antifolate drugs are usually used as a partner drug for combination therapy. These combination drugs include different combinations of DHFR inhibitors (chlorproguanil, proguanil, pyrimethamine, and trimethoprim) and sulfa drugs (sulfalene, dapsone, sulfadoxine, sulfamethoxazole, and others). Current antifolate combinations in use for infectious disease treatment include sulfadoxine-pyrimethamine (SP), sulfamethoxazole-trimethoprim, and sulfalene-pyrimethamine. Proguanil has been used the combination with chloroquine for malaria prophylaxis in areas with moderate chloroquine resistance; however, proguanil provides minimal added benefit in this combination particularly with prolonged exposure. The latest antifolate combination to be introduced is dapsone and chlorproguanil, also known as LapDap [374].

Antifolates target two enzymes involved in the synthesis of folic acid, dihydrooperterate synthase, and dihydrofolate reductase (DHFR). Sulfonamides such as sulfadoxine or sulphone inhibit 4-aminobenzoic acid or act as false substrates for dihydropteroate synthase. DHPS inhibitors are weak antimalarials, but these drugs have synergy with inhibitors of dihydrofolate reductase. Many malaria parasites have accumulated point mutations, which have resulted in drug resistance against inhibitors of dihydropteroate synthase. Pyrimethamine and the metabolite of proguanil, cycloguanil, inhibit dihydrofolate reductase. *In vivo*, the open-chain proguanide proguanil is transformed into cycloguanil, and cycloguanil actually acts as an efficacious metabolite. The principal determinant of antifolate treatment success is the presence or absence of mutations in the parasite DHFR enzyme. Stepwise accumulation of mutations in DHFR in many field isolates of *P. falciparum* has resulted in drug resistance. The most relevant DHFR mutation is a triple mutation, which renders the parasite insensitive to both proguanil and pyrimethamine but still sensitive to chlorcycloguanil, which has weak activity against the malaria DHFR enzyme. Unfortunately, the activity of chlorcycloguanil is weak and not useful clinically [374].

Sulfa Drugs: Sulfadoxine, Sulfalene, Sulfamethoxazole

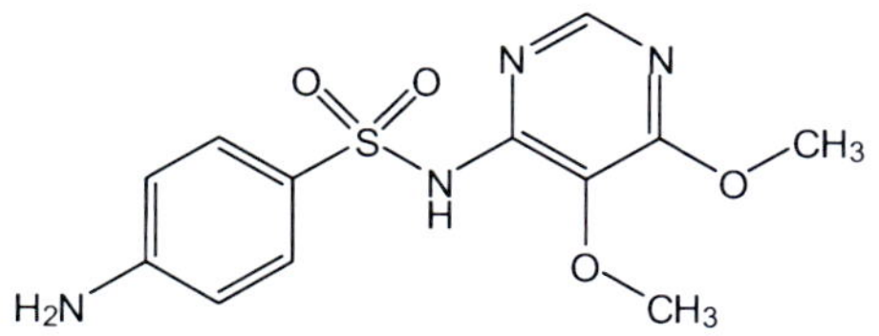

Sulfonamides act as competitive antagonists to p-aminobenzoic acid and act as a competitive inhibitor of dihydropteroate synthase, which utilizes p-aminobenzoic acid to synthesize folic acid.

PK/PD Studies of Sulfonamides

The sulfonamides act as DHPS inhibitors, and while they are not specifically antimalarial agents, they are widely used as part of drug combinations to treat malaria. The sulfonamides in use as antimalarial drugs include sulfadoxine, sulfamethoxazole, and sulfalene. These drugs are primarily dosed in fixed combinations. Sulfalene and sulfadoxine are dosed in combination with pyrimethamine, and sulfamethoxazole is combined with trimethoprim. These drugs are quickly absorbed with T_{max} ranging from 2-6 hours after dosing. The majority of sulfonamides are cleared metabolically through acetylation and glucuronidation. While the metabolites of dapsone have antimalarial activity, the metabolites of sulfadoxine have no antimalarial activity. The CYP enzymes have no role in metabolizing most sulfonamides. The most significant PK differences observed among members of the sulfonamide family are the rate of elimination. Sulfalene and sulfadoxine are cleared slowly, while the half-life of sulfamethoxazole is much shorter. Sulfadoxine is highly plasma protein bound and similar to other drugs in this class, sulfadoxine will compete for binding sites on plasma proteins, which may lead to issues with drug interactions. In the blood, only a small fraction, less than 10%, of sulfadoxine is metabolized through acetylation or glucuronidation. Sulfadoxine is excreted largely in its acetylated form *via* the urine, and a small fraction is excreted *via* the stool [232].

Pyrimethamine

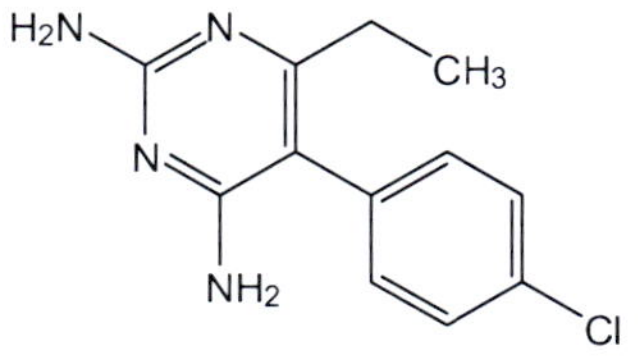

Pyrimethamine is a diaminopyrimidine, which is commonly used as an antimalarial drug combination combined with a sulfa drug, typically sulfadoxine or dapsone. Pyrimethamine inhibits the plasmodial dihydrofolate reductase, which indirectly blocks nucleic acid synthesis of the malaria parasite. Pyrimethamine is a slow-acting schizonticidal drug, which has been shown experimentally to inhibit liver stage forms of malaria, and it has been shown to inhibit development of sporozoites in the mosquito vector. Pyrimethamine is efficacious toward all four species of *Plasmodium,* and it is commonly used to treat isosporiasis and toxoplasmosis, and for *Pneumocystis carinii* prophylaxis. Pyrimethamine cannot be used for antimalarial treatment as monotherapy due to drug resistance, and it is only administered a synergistic combination with other antifolate drugs such as the sulfonamides for malaria treatment or combined with dapsone for prophylaxis.

PK/PD Studies of Pyrimethamine

Pyrimethamine is a dihydrofolate reductase inhibitor which is readily absorbed is readily absorbed from the gastrointestinal tract, and peak drug levels in plasma have been shown to occur 2-6 hours after oral administration. It is primarily concentrated in the lungs, kidneys, spleen, and liver and approximately 80-90%of pyrimethamine is plasma protein bound. Pyrimethamine is metabolized by the liver, and it is slowly cleared through the renal system. The half-life of pyrimethamine is approximately 4 days. Pyrimethamine has been shown to cross the placenta and the blood-brain barrier and has been detected in breast milk. Absorption of intramuscular pyrimethamine is poor, and this route of administration is not reliable for administration [23]. Absorption of pyrimethamine is slow after oral administration with a T_{max} ranging from 2-12 hours, and pyrimethamine is 90% plasma protein bound. The half-life of pyrimethamine ranges from 50-106 hours, and it is mainly metabolized in the liver with some excretion of unmetabolized drug through the kidneys.

Pyrimethamine is widely combined with dapsone and the sulfonamides for both malaria prophylaxis and treatment. In all of these drug combinations, drug interactions have not been shown to be clinically significant. Pyrimethamine-sulfadoxine is considered a useful substitute for chloroquine; however, sporadic resistance to pyrimethamine-sulfadoxine is commonly encountered particularly in Asia. In Africa, this combination generally remains effective, it is well tolerated, cheap, and, as a fixed dose combination, it is easy to administer. The disposition of pyrimethamine-sulfadoxine has been described in healthy individuals, in patients receiving the drug as malaria prophylaxis, and in patients with uncomplicated malaria.

The disposition of pyrimethamine after intramuscular administration is probably absorption rate-limited in children with mild malaria. This finding may be clinically relevant, but the single most important point concerning the disposition of pyrimethamine-sulfadoxine is its very slow rate of elimination. This fact is associated with the major disadvantage of the drug, namely the selection of resistant parasites. *P. falciparum* develops resistance to pyrimethamine by genetically determined variation in the target enzyme. Thus, a single mutational amino acid substitution reduces susceptibility to the drug 10 to 100-fold. A further mutation causes a higher level of resistance. In Kenya, one study showed that although parasites in patients treated with pyrimethamine-sulfadoxine were uniformly cleared, re-infections that occurred during the long period of elimination were primarily due to pyrimethamine-resistant parasites. When pyrimethamine-sulfadoxine was used as a substitute for chloroquine in Indochina, it remained useful only for a very short period. It appears that this rapid reduction in efficacy was a consequence of the pharmacokinetic and pharmacodynamic properties of the drug [367].

Malarone^{TM} (Atovaquone/proguanil)

In 1998, a novel combination drug consisting of two partners, atovaquone and proguanil, was first released by Glaxo Smith Kline in Australia under the trade name Malarone^{TM}. Atovaquone came on market in 1992, and it has been used with some success for treatment of *Pneumocystis carinii*. Proguanil was developed in 1945, and it is a biguanide derivative, which is converted metabolically to a metabolite called cycloguanil pamoate, which has antimalarial activity. Drug combination studies conducted at Walter Reed Army Institute of Research showed the combination of atovaquone and proguanil had unexpected synergy against malaria when dosed in combination. The drug synergy provided by combining atovaquone with proguanil provides more effective prophylactic and antimalarial efficacy than either drug alone.

Atovaquone

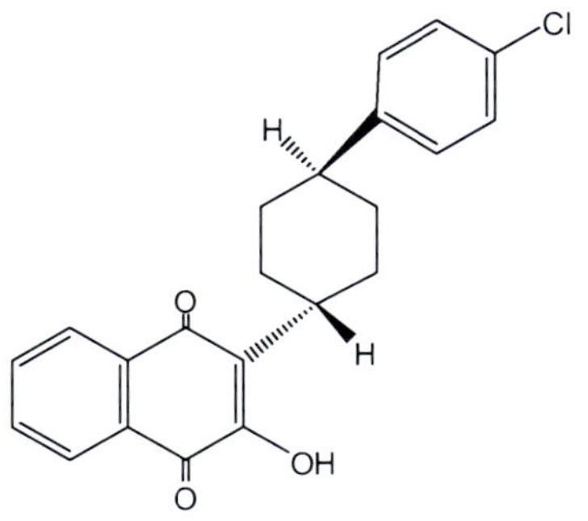

Atovaquone is a hydroxynaphthoquinone that has active against all *Plasmodium* species. Atovaquone inhibits parasite liver stage development and oocyst development in the mosquito. Atovaquone is only administered in combination with proguanil for the synergistic treatment and prophylaxis of malaria. Atovaquone interferes with cytochrome electron transport and consequently kills the *Plasmodium* parasite through interference with cellular respiration.

PK/PD Studies of Atovaquone

Atovaquone is not well absorbed from the gastrointestinal tract, but drug bioavailability after oral administration is enhanced by administration of atovaquone with fatty foods. Bioavailability is decreased in HIV patients. Atovaquone is 99% plasma protein bound, and it has a plasma half-life from 66-70 hours as a consequence of enterohepatic recycling. Atovaquone is excreted in the feces as unchanged drug. Plasma concentrations of atovaquone are sharply decreased in late pregnancy [23]. Atovaquone's pharmacokinetic properties are characterized by its poor oral bioavailability of roughly 23%, which increases from 3- to 6-times if atovaquone is administered with fatty foods [232].

In HIV patients, the AUC and C_{max} observed after atovaquone is administered have been shown to be higher when multiple doses are administered daily as opposed to dosing with the standard single daily dose. Dose-limited absorption of atovaquone has not been noted, however, in a population pharmacokinetic study conducted with a number of patient treatment groups infected with malaria. No significant interracial PK differences of atovaquone have been observed. In theory, the poor and variable bioavailability combined with high percentage of atovaquone bound to plasma proteins of atovaquone are possible drug interaction sites.

Proguanil

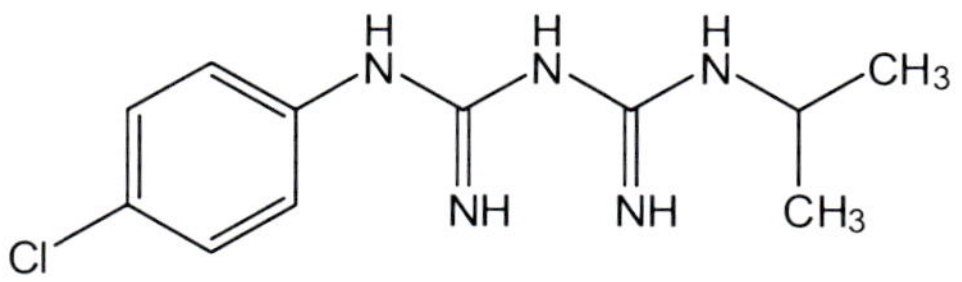

Proguanil is a biguanide drug metabolized in the liver by CYP2C19 to cycloguanil, a metabolite with antimalarial activity. Approximately 20% of Asians and 3% of Caucasian and African populations are poor CYP2C19 metabolizers, and these individuals have decreased metabolism of proguanil and corresponding decreased levels of cycloguanil. Cycloguanil actively inhibits the plasmodial dihydrofolate reductase enzyme, while proguanil, the prodrug, has modest antimalarial activity whose mechanism is not known. Proguanil may be active against liver stage parasites, and it is known to be a slow blood schizonticidal drug. Proguanil has also has been shown to have sporonticidal activity which makes the gametocytes of *Plasmodium* uninfective to mosquitoes. Proguanil is administered as a hydrochloride salt with atovaquone. Proguanil is never administered as monotherapy due to rapid emergence of drug resistance. Cycloguanil has been administered in the past *via* intramuscular injection of the embonate or pamoate salt, but administration in this era is solely by oral means.

PK/PD Studies of Proguanil

Proguanil is well absorbed in the gastrointestinal tract, and peak drug concentrations in plasma have been observed at approximately 4 hours after dosing. Peak plasma concentrations are diminished in the third trimester of pregnancy, which underlines the need for PK studies of antimalarial drugs in pregnant women. Roughly 75% of proguanil is plasma protein bound, and metabolism of proguanil to cycloguanil in the liver provides peak cycloguanil concentrations in plasma one hour after the peak drug level in plasma is reached for proguanil. The half-lives for cycloguanil and proguanil are roughly 20 hours. Proguanil is eliminated by 50% through the kidneys, and 60% of drug eliminated through the renal system is not metabolized while 30% is cycloguanil. The other 50% of proguanil is eliminated in the feces. Low levels of proguanil have been shown in breast milk. The clearance of cycloguanil is a function of the amount of proguanil absorbed and metabolized, and the metabolism of proguanil to cycloguanil through the action of CYP2C19 is reduced in women who are pregnant and in women taking oral contraceptives [23].

Proguanil and chlorproguanil act as DHFR inhibitors, and the successful use of proguanil for malaria treatment is dependent on whether drug resistance mutations in the DHFR gene of blood stage *falciparum* parasites. Proguanil has also been used for malaria prophylaxis in combination with chloroquine in vivax endemic regions such as Afghanistan. Proguanil is very well absorbed, and the C_{max} is reached 2-5 hours after administration. While proguanil acts as a prodrug of cycloguanil, the parent compounds itself has synergistic activity with atovaquone. Cycloguanil, however, does not show drug synergy with atovaquone. As proguanil is metabolized by CYP2C19 to cycloguanil, this is a drug interaction site. The half-life of proguanil is 12 to 20 hours in both healthy volunteers and in malaria infected patients, but the half-life is longer in poor metabolizers while the half-life of cycloguanil is roughly 12 hours [232].

Proguanil and chlorproguanil are prodrugs for cycloguanil and chlorcycloguanil, respectively. While chlorproguanil is commonly combined with dapsone to treat malaria, proguanil is recommended in the UK for chemoprophylaxis, and it is usually given in combination with chloroquine. Unfortunately, breakthrough infections can develop in individuals receiving proguanil and chloroquine prophylaxis. While these infections may result from resistance, it has been speculated that they may be due to a reduced ability of individuals to metabolize proguanil to cycloguanil. Strong evidence exists *in vitro* and *in vivo* to suggest that the cyclisation of proguanil to cycloguanil is mediated *via* the cytochrome P450 isozyme CYP2C19. Patients who are poor metabolizers show a reduced ability to cyclize proguanil, and these patients have a lower circulating plasma cycloguanil concentration [367].

5.4.5. Antibacterial Drugs

Clindamycin

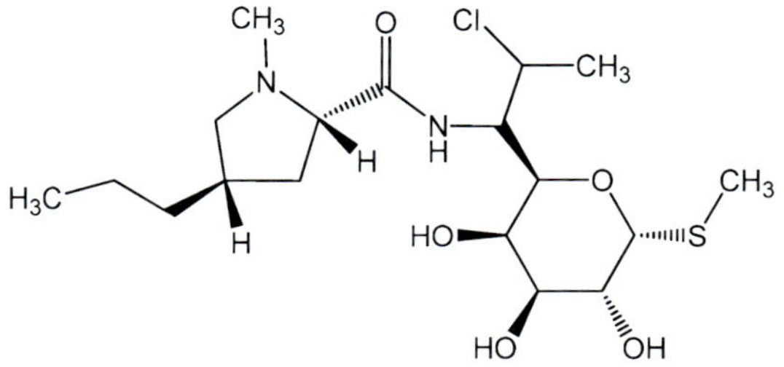

Clindamycin is an antibiotic that has weak antimalarial activity. Clindamycin should never be used as antimalarial monotherapy and must be administered combined with a schizonticidal drug in blood stage like quinine or one of the artemisinins, particularly when patients with no or little immunity to malaria are being treated. Clindamycin is on market by itself and combined with a variety of other drugs under different trade names.

PK/PD Studies of Clindamycin

Approximately 90% of clindamycin is well absorbed through the gastrointestinal tract after oral administration. Concomitant consumption of food does not stop absorption; however, absorption may be delayed. Peak plasma concentrations can be achieved in children one hour after administration while adults require 3 hours to reach C_{max} after oral administration. Clindamycin is well distributed in the body has been observed in breast milk and has been noted to cross the placenta; however, it does not appear in CSF fluid. Clindamycin is 90% plasma protein bound, and it does accumulate in white blood cells and in the bile. The half-life of clindamycin is 2-3 hours, but the half-life may be longer in individuals with kidney disease or in neonates. Clindamycin is metabolized to active N-methyl and sulfoxide metabolites, and it is metabolized to inactive forms. Approximately 10% of clindamycin is excreted through the urine as either as an active metabolite or as active drug and approximately 4%of clindamycin is excreted in the feces. The remaining drug is excreted as metabolites that are inactive metabolites. Excretion of clindamycin is slow, and this process may take place over a period of days [23].

Tetracycline

The tetracyclines are antibiotics derived originally from *Streptomyces*, but today, tetracyclines are produced synthetically. Tetracycline can be administered intravenously as a hydrochloride or orally as a phosphate. Both of the salt forms of clindamycin are soluble in water, but the IV hydrochloride form is not very stable and lasts just a few hours. In areas where the efficacy of quinine is weakened, tetracyclines are often dosed with quinine to improve efficacy. Tetracyclines can also be administered with shorter quinine treatments to decrease the side effects associated with quinine. Tetracyclines inhibit the binding of aminoacyl-tRNA during the synthesis of proteins, and these drugs are broadly used in treatment of a variety of diseases beyond malaria to include infections from bacteria, rickettsia, chlamydia, mycoplasma, brucella, tularemia, cholera, and plague. Doxycycline is a synthetic form of tetracycline with a better half-life, making it more advantageous for dosing compared to tetracycline drugs.

PK/PD Studies of Tetracycline

Approximately 60-80% of tetracycline is absorbed through the gastrointestinal tract after oral dosing, absorption is impaired by metal ions as tetracycline drugs form insoluble, stable complexes with these ions, and absorption is impaired by concomitant consumption of milk or food. Formulation of tetracycline drugs with phosphate is one method to enhance absorption. Peak plasma levels of tetracycline occur 1-3 hours after administration, and tetracycline is 20-65% plasma protein bound. Tetracycline drugs are widely distributed in the body; however, doxycycline is less well distributed due to its lipophilic nature. High concentrations of tetracycline drugs can be found in breast milk at 60% of the plasma concentration, tetracycline easily cross the placenta, and these drugs are retained in the teeth and in areas of new bone formation. The half-life of tetracycline is approximately 8 hours, and 40-70% of the drug is excreted *via* glomerular filtration in the kidneys. The remaining drug is excreted through the feces and in bile. Enterohepatic recycling has been shown to slow down complete elimination.

Doxycycline

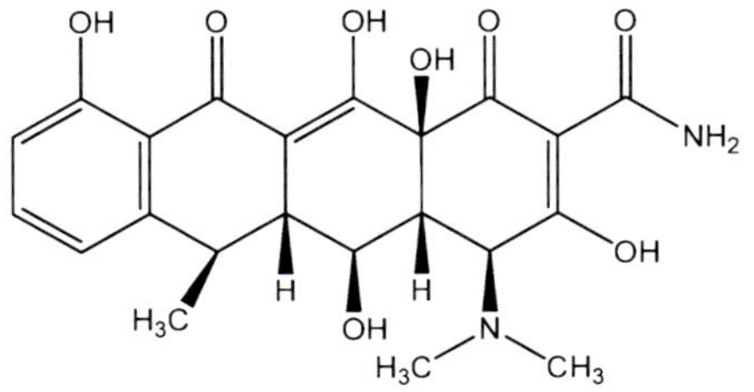

Doxycycline is a tetracycline analogue used in place of tetracycline. It has advantages over tetracycline due to better absorption, longer half-life, and its improved safety profile in patients with kidney disease. It is not very water soluble, but it is quite soluble in lipids. Doxycycline may be administered either orally or intravenously.

PK/PD Studies of Doxycycline

Doxycycline is readily absorbed through the gastrointestinal tract, and unlike tetracycline, absorption of doxycycline is not significantly changed by concomitant food consumption. Peak plasma levels occur 2 hours after ingestion. Some 80-95% of doxycycline is protein-bound, and the half-life is 10-24 hours (78). Doxycycline is broadly distributed in body fluids and tissues. 40% of doxycycline has been shown to be excreted through the kidneys and this percentage will rise if the urine is more alkaline. Doxycycline may accumulate in the body in patients with kidney disease, however, the majority of doxycycline that is administered ends up being excreted in the feces.

5.5. PK/PD COMPARISON OF CURRENTLY USED ACTS RECOMMENDED BY THE WHO

5.5.1. Currently Used ACTs Recommended by the WHO

WHO has recommended treatment of *falciparum* malaria with combination drugs to avoid induction of drug resistance. Artemisinin derivatives in ACTs rapidly decrease the parasite biomass, while the presence of a second antimalarial with a dissimilar mode of action reduces the probability of the emergence of resistant strains. WHO encourages the development of fixed-dose combination (FDC) versions of ACTs, *versus* co-blistered tablets that can be misused to facilitate administration of artemisinin as monotherapy. Two ACT combinations, artesunate-SP (AS-SP) and artesunate-amodiaquine (AS-AQ), have been used in areas where parasites are still susceptible to SP and amodiaquine. In other areas where these partner drugs are not effective, artemisinin combinations such as artemether-lumefantrine (AL) or artesunate-mefloquine (AS-MQ) are used. More recently, dihydroartemisinin-piperaquine (DP) has been developed as a new ACT showing efficacy and safety in clinical trials, and DP has become the treatment of choice for uncomplicated malaria in Asia. Artemisinins will soon be on market combined with other partner drugs to create fixed dose ACTs containing atovaquone-proguanil, pyronaridine, and chlorproguanil-dapsone [23].

Artemether-Lumefantrine (AL)

Artemether-lumefantrine (AL) is fixed dose combination approved in several European countries and is the only ACT approved for use in the United States to treat malaria. AL is recommended as first line treatment in a number of African countries, as well as in some Asian and South American countries. Currently, lumefantrine has been shown to be active against drug resistant *falciparum* malaria, however, cross-resistance of lumefantrine with halofantrine and mefloquine has been noted. AL is dispensed as tablets containing 80 mg artemether and 480 mg of lumefantrine. When AL is administered as a 4-dose treatment, the plasma levels of lumefantrine in the third and fourth treatment cycles (4-8 days) were shown to be insufficient to kill all parasites. A 6-dose treatment was created to enhance the AUC and the cure rate, and this regimen has been shown to be both efficacious and well tolerated. When compared to artesunate-mefloquine, the 6 dose AL regimen has been shown to be equally efficacious and much better tolerated. AL has been shown to have an excellent adverse effects profile and provides a very cost-effective option for treatment as costs are now down to less than US $1 per adult. While AL has been shown to be safe for pregnant women in the last two trimesters, plasma levels of artemether, its active metabolite dihydroartemisinin, and lumefantrine have been shown to be decreased in late pregnancy, which suggests a longer treatment regimen, may be warranted [375].

Artesunate-amodiaquine (AS-AQ)

AS-AQ is a fixed dose combination manufactured by Sanofi-Aventis, ("Coarsucam")as the treatment of choice for uncomplicated malaria in some African countries, although there is considerable resistance to amodiaquine in East Africa but not West Africa. Amodiaquine, similar to chloroquine, is a 4-aminoquinoline, and it is efficacious for treatment of chloroquine-resistant *falciparum* parasites. Amodiaquine drug resistance has increased in parts of East and Southern Africa. Amodiaquine is well tolerated, and the most significant adverse effects of liver toxicity and agranulocytosis are associated with prophylactic use and these adverse effects are rarely noted when amodiaquine is used short-term for treatment. AS-AQ is administered as 4 mg/kg of body weight of artesunate and 10 mg base/kg body weight of amodiaquine daily for a 3 day period. AS-AQ has been shown to be efficacious in areas where the 28-day rates of cure for amodiaquine monotherapy exceed 80%.

Artesunate-mefloquine (AS-MQ)

AS-MQ is a fixed dose combination created through a partnership between Farmaguinhos and Drugs for Neglected Diseases Initiative (DNDi), with tech transfer to Cipla, but this combination has obtained neither stringent regulatory approval nor WHO pre-qualification. It was used as the treatment of choice for uncomplicated *falciparum* malaria in Cambodia until Dec 2010, after which the country will switch to dihydroartemisinin-piperaquine, and it has been used for first line treatment in Thailand, Laos, Bolivia, Peru, and Venezuela. The tolerability and safety data for AS-MQ at 25 mg/kg were deemed insufficient to support the use of MQ combinations for children in Africa [23].

A number of mefloquine drug formulations have been innovated with varying levels of oral bioavailability. Long-term use of mefloquine as monotherapy to treat malaria has led to emergence of drug resistant *falciparum* malaria occurring through increase in copy number of the multi-drug resistance (MDR) gene, *pfmdr1*. It has been suggested that administration of mefloquine at 15 mg/kg led to this resistance and higher doses at the 25 mg/kg level, combined with an artemisinin analogue may be less vulnerable to drug resistance. The mefloquine dose should be either split with 15 mg/kg dosed first followed by 10 mg/kg dosed second or administered at 8.3 mg/kg daily for 3 days to achieve enhanced bioavailability and decreased adverse effects from vomiting, the most common adverse effect.

Neuropsychiatric adverse effects are common if a patient was treated with mefloquine within a two-month window, therefore, mefloquine is not recommended to treat recrudescent infections. Vomiting is more common in young children, and repeat administration after vomiting can still result in low blood levels and elevated risk of treatment failure. A drug combination of mefloquine with artesunate provides enhanced parasite killing and diminished adverse effects if the dose of mefloquine is reduced over a 3-day treatment period. A fixed combination of AS-MQ was developed as a tablet containing 200 mg of artesunate and 400 mg of mefloquine. A number of studies have shown this new fixed dose combination is well tolerated compared to the standard treatment of mefloquine at 25 mg/kg. The AS-MQ combination has been tested and used in Southeast Asia and South America, and additional data on safety, tolerability, and efficacy may be needed to inform use in Africa [374].

Artesunate-sulfadoxine-pyrimethamine (AS-SP)

AS-SP is only available co-blistered, and no FDC version is available nor is an FDC in development. AS-SP is not approved for use in either Europe or the US. SP resistance is widespread across sub-Saharan Africa and much of the rest of the world.

Sulfadoxine and pyrimethamine have drug synergy against parasites that are sensitive to anti-folate treatment. Adverse effects of sulfonamide or pyrimethamine treatment are not common. SP is commonly combined with artesunate in separate tablets; 50 mg of artesunate in one tablet and other tablets administered contain 500 mg of sulfadoxine and 25 mg of pyrimethamine. No company or NGO has shown interest in a fixed dose combination likely due to the increase in SP failures due to drug resistance. The total treatment provided equates to 4 mg/kg body weight of artesunate administered once per day over a 3-day period and a single dose of sulfadoxine-pyrimethamine (SP) at a dose of 1.25/25 mg base/kg body weight at hospital admission. This dose of SP dose was created for use in adults, however, in children under 5, weight-adjusted doses for this combination result in blood drug concentrations for both artesunate and SP half of what has been observed in adults. This example points out the need for testing antimalarial drugs in vulnerable populations such as pregnant women and young children who are frequently under-dosed as a consequence of pharmacokinetic differences compared to women who are not pregnant or healthy adults. This combination of artesunate-sulfadoxine-pyrimethamine was assessed for efficacy in children and adults infected with *falciparum* malaria and this ACT is efficacious in regions where the 28-day rates of cure with SP alone exceed 80%. AS-SP is in use n of the Middle East, South America, and South Asia where SP drug sensitive parasites are present. As SP, sulfalene-pyrimethamine, and sulfamethoxazole-trimethoprim are broadly used by themselves SP drug resistance will likely become even more widespread [374].

Dihydroartemisinin-piperaquine (DP)

DP was submitted for approval in July 2009 to the European Medicines Agency (EMA). It is noteworthy that the second edition of WHO's Guidelines for the Treatment of Malaria [23] was expanded to include DP as a treatment option for the "first-line treatment of uncomplicated *P. falciparum* malaria worldwide". This addition was categorized as a "Strong Recommendation" and was included due to "High Quality Evidence".

Piperaquine is a bisquinoline compound similar to other 4-aminoquinolines such as chloroquine. Piperaquine was used as monotherapy in China in the 1970s and after over 200 metric tons were used in China, including use of piperaquine for mass treatment, drug resistant to *falciparum* parasites emerged in the late 1980s. Piperaquine monotherapy was not conducted outside China, which did limit the geographic spread of earlier drug resistant parasites. Piperaquine has a volume of distribution greater than 500 L/kg and an elimination half-life of 2-3 weeks. The more accurate half-life is likely similar to chloroquine, which has a half-life of 1-2 months. The oral bioavailability of piperaquine is enhanced by concomitant administration with fatty foods.

The DP fixed dose combination is created in a tablet form with 40 mg of DHA and 320 mg of piperaquine, and this treatment is on market in a number of countries in Asia and Africa. A number of studies have shown this fixed dose combination DP treatment is safe and well tolerated. Commonly observed side effects include gastrointestinal upset, however, this is generally mild in nature. The principle source of DP's efficacy is the long piperaquine half-life. DP is very simple to dose, and this combination is efficacious against multi-drug resistant parasites. DP's safety and efficacy against multi-drug resistant *falciparum* malaria makes the DP combination on the best available [374].

5.5.2. Efficacy of ACTs for Treatment of Uncomplicated *falciparum* and *vivax* Malaria

There is a significant body of published data to support the hypothesis that ACTs are the best treatments available for uncomplicated malaria even for treatment of drug resistant parasites.

ACTs with rapid treatment responses are well tolerated in patients and they provide excellent rates of cure with treatment courses for only three days. ACTs also provide reductions in gametocyte carriage, and decrease drug resistance by providing protection for combination partner drugs.

DHA-piperaquine is now available as an inexpensive, efficacious, fixed-dose artemisinin combination therapy for uncomplicated *falciparum* or blood-stage *vivax* malaria. Fourteen studies on DP malaria treatment were conducted from

2002 to 2006 [376, 377]. There were 2,636 patients in 22 treatment groups administered DP to treat drug-resistant uncomplicated *falciparum* malaria. Eleven of these studies were performed in Southeast Asia (Laos, Thailand, Myanmar, and Cambodia), one study was conducted in Rwanda, and one study was conducted in China. The efficacy in these studies of DP for treatment of multidrug-resistant *falciparum* malaria was outstanding with overall 28- day cure rates of 97-98%. In these comparative studies, the efficacy of DP was comparable to artesunate-mefloquine (AS-MQ) and in Rwanda; the efficacy of DP was superior to amodiaquine-sulfadoxine-pyrimethamine and artesunate - amodiaquine. Notably, DP was shown to be highly efficacious against multidrug-resistant *falciparum* malaria in Asia. DP has a number of advantages over AS-MQ, which has been the standard first-line ACT treatment in Asia [158].

From 2007 to 2010, other studies have been published reporting similar results, and the PCR corrected cure rate observed with DP was equal to other comparator ACTs such as AS-MQ, AL and AS-AQ. The PCR uncorrected cure rate was consistently in favor of DP, suggesting a lower incidence of new infections during the follow up period (day 42 and/or 63). This lower incidence of new infections after DP treatment is likely due to the extended half-life of piperaquine which provides a post treatment prophylactic effect that is superior to other ACT combination partners with shorter half-lives such a amodiaquine, SP, or mefloquine (D'Alessandro U *et al.*, 2010). Recently, more trials that are clinical have been reported studying in the comparative efficacy of DP *versus* other ACTs. In Uganda, an area of very high malaria transmission, 421 children ranging in age from 6 months to 10 years infected with uncomplicated *falciparum* malaria were enrolled in a comparative study-testing efficacy of AL *versus* DP. Treatment of malaria with artemether-lumefantrine (AL) or DP was conducted following a standard 3-day dosing regimen. The risk of recrudescent *falciparum* malaria was lower for patients treated with DP than those treated with AL after 28 days to 42 days of follow-up. Patients in the DP arm also showed a lower risk for infection with non- *falciparum* malaria, showed diminished gametocyte carriage, and also demonstrated increased mean hemoglobin compared to the patients treated with AL. Both drugs were well tolerated, and serious adverse events were uncommon and unrelated to study drugs [378-380].

In the Cambodia-Thailand border area, artemisinin-piperaquine (AP), DP, and AL were compared to treat patients infected with uncomplicated malaria. The mean parasite clearance time was quite similar for all three treatment arms and no significant differences were noted (66.7 hours for AP, 65.6 hours for DP, and 65.3

hours for AL. The fever clearance times were also similar (31.6 hours for AP, 34.6 hours for DP and 36.9 hours for AL). Over a 28-day follow-up period, the cure rates achieved were 95.1% for AP, 98.2% for DP, and 82.4% for AL and the recrudescence rates were 4.9% for AP, 1.8% for DP and 17.6% for AL. The data from this study clearly showed that the 28-day cure rate in the AP and DP groups were clearly superior to the AL group [381].

In China, patients aged 1 to 60 with uncomplicated *P. falciparum* infection and parasites were enrolled in a comparative efficacy study of DP *versus* AL. Both AL and DP combinations showed a high cure rate and acceptable tolerability for treatment of patients with uncomplicated *falciparum* malaria in Hainan [382]. In five African countries, the non-inferiority of DP *versus* AL for treatment of children aged 6-59 months old with uncomplicated *P. falciparum* malaria was tested. DP was shown to be as efficacious as AL for treating uncomplicated malaria in African children from different endemicity settings, and demonstrated a comparable safety profile. The occurrence of new infections within the 42-day follow up period was significantly lower in the DP group, indicating a longer post-treatment prophylactic effect [383].

A comparative efficacy study was conducted in Vietnam to compare two fixed-dose ACT formulations, artesunate-amodiaquine (AS-AQ), and artemisinin-piperaquine (ARP) for treatment of *falciparum* malaria. The primary efficacy endpoint was the PCR-corrected parasitological cure rate at day 42. Secondary endpoints in this study included safety, the parasite clearance time and the fever clearance time. Of the 128 patients enrolled, 63 received ARP and 65 were given AS-AQ. The PCR-corrected parasitological cure rate at day 42 for both formulations by day 42 was 98%. The median parasite clearance time (PCT) of 48 hours was much slower in the ARP group compared with a 36 hour PCT for the AS-AQ group ($P < 0.001$) and the median fever clearance time of 12 hours was also shorter in the AS-AQ group *versus* 24 hours in the ARP group. The two ACTs were equally well tolerated and no serious adverse events were noted [384].

4,116 African children less than 5 years of age with uncomplicated *falciparum* malaria were treated with four ACTs: 1,226 with AL, 1,002 with AS-AQ, 413 with chlorproguanil-dapsone-artesunate (CDA) and 1,475 with DP. There were 10 investigational sites in 7 African countries (Burkina Faso, Nigeria, Gabon, Zambia, Uganda, Rwanda and Mozambique). The PCR- corrected cure rate on day 63 showed no differences between DP, AL, and AS-AQ, while these three ACTs were statistically superior in comparison with CDA. The PCR-uncorrected cure rate at day 63 indicated that DP was statistically superior to AL, AS-AQ, and CDA [386].

In southern Papua, Indonesia, where patients are routinely infected for infections with both *falciparum* and *vivax,* a number of studies were conducted to compare treatment regimens. A randomized trial to compare the safety and efficacy of DP with AS-AQ was conducted in 334 patients. Of the 334 patients in the patient population, 185 patients were infected with *P. falciparum*, 80 patients were infected with *P. vivax*, and 69 patients were infected with both species. The overall parasitological failure rate at day 42 was 45% for the AS-AQ treatment group and 13% for the DP treatment group ($P<0.001$). The rate of recrudescence for both *P. falciparum* and recurrence of *P. vivax* infection were much higher in patients administered AS-AQ compared to patients treated with DP ($P < 001$). AS-AQ treated patients were 2.95-fold more likely to have clinical anemia *versus* the DP treated patients, and the AS-AQ patients were 14.5-fold more likely to demonstrate carriage of *P. vivax* gametocytes. The prolonged post treatment prophylactic effect of piperaquine aided in reducing the time to *P. falciparum* re-infection, cut the rate of *P. vivax* recurrence, and diminished the risk of *P. vivax* gametocyte carriage and anemia [389].

5.5.3. Delayed Clearance of *P. falciparum* Infections after ACT Treatment

Recently, artemisinin-resistant *falciparum* malaria has developed on the border between Thailand and Cambodia. The development of artemisinin resistance is likely a consequence of patient treatment with artemisinin monotherapy likely with substandard, counterfeit, or adulterated drugs for over 30 years. This artemisinin resistance phenomenon is characterized clinically by much slower parasite clearance rates after artemisinin treatment [37].

One hypothesis to explain this phenomenon is delayed parasite clearance derived from a stage-specific decrease in artemisinin sensitivity of circulating young asexual ring stage parasites. Another hypothesis to explain this phenomenon is dormancy of ring stage parasites *in vivo*, which would render them resistant to artemisinin treatment. A related hypothesis is that reduced sensitivity to treatment with artemisinins renders the ACT partner drug vulnerable to development of resistance. This very ominous development accompanied with the development of resistance over time in Asia to all of the partner drugs used for ACTs suggests that all of the current ACT regimens would be predicted to fail in Southeast Asia. This phenomenon will lead to malaria recurrence after treatment of malaria episodes, and decreased efficacy of artemisinin-based treatment of severe malaria. A clinical trial of 151 subjects infected with uncomplicated *falciparum* malaria was conducted using AS-MQ. Patients were followed over a 42 day period or until recurrent parasitemia was observed. The PCR-corrected treatment failure rate at 28 days was 13.1%, and the treatment failure rate at 42 days after treatment was 18.8%. These treatment failures were associated with longer parasite clearance times, increased *pfmdr1* copy number, increased initial parasitemia, and elevated mefloquine IC_{50} values These data demonstrate the combined effects of artesunate resistance and mefloquine resistance in southern Cambodia [395-397].

A retrospective analysis of 31 different comparative efficacy studies conducted from 1997-2007 involving 1,327 patients treated with AS-MQ was conducted by the Thai National Malaria Control Program, and some surprising geographic changes in parasitemia were noted. The prevalence of patients with parasitemia on day 2 was higher in the eastern part of Thailand compared to the western part of Thailand. In addition, the prevalence of day 2 parasitemia increased over time. The presence of parasitemia on days 2 and day 3 were specific, but not sensitive, predictors of treatment failure [398]. An open-label, multicenter, non-inferiority trial was conducted that included 1, 271 patients ranging in age from 3 to 60 years of age from Asia (81.3%) or Africa (18.7%) infected with *falciparum* malaria. Patients were randomized for treatment with a fixed-dose combination of pyronaridine-artesunate or AS-MQ. Pyronaridine-artesunate was shown to be non-inferior to AS-MQ for the primary endpoint which was adequate clinical and parasitological response in the per-protocol population on day 28, corrected for re-infection using PCR. In Cambodia, where 211 patients were enrolled, the median parasite clearance time was extended for both treatments from 64 hours in Cambodia to PCT times ranging from 16.0 to 38.9 hours in the other countries ($P<0.001$). The 42-day recrudescence rate in Cambodia 42 was higher with pyronaridine-artesunate than with AS-MQ, but the rates were similar for the other countries combined. While fixed-dose pyronaridine-artesunate was shown to be efficacious in this study for treatment of uncomplicated *falciparum* malaria, the extended parasite clearance times observed in Cambodia suggest *in vivo* resistance to artemisinin [399].

5.5.4. Reducing Transmission of Parasites from Malaria Patients by Treatment with ACTs

Slower parasite clearance was also associated with increased gametocyte carriage, thereby increasing the risk of transmission of drug-resistant parasites. Given that it would be highly desirable for candidate drugs to have activity against both hepatic and sexual forms of the malaria parasite, it is surprising that few clinical trials, to date, have examined whether gametocyte carriage can be reduced following drug treatment. The only drugs found to be effective at reducing gametocyte carriage include artemisinin [400], ACTs [401, 402], methylene blue [403], and primaquine [402, 404].

In some studies, the gametocytes were cleared faster in the AS-MQ group, and new gametocytes tended to appear more frequently in patients treated with DP, whereas in other studies gametocyte carriage for *P. falciparum* was either similar to the comparator drug or significantly lower. In Kenya, gametocyte carriage was assessed with the quantitative nucleic sequence-based amplification technique (QT-NASBA), a more sensitive method than microscopy, in patients treated with either DP or AL. Gametocyte clearance was significantly better in the AL treatment group, and the development of gametocytes was significantly higher and longer at days 3, 7 and 14 in the DP group, though after 28 days no difference could be observed between treatment arms. Similarly, in the multicenter trial in Africa mentioned previously, patients treated with DP had a significantly higher rate of person-gametocyte-weeks compared with those who received AL. Such an effect has been attributed to the low dose of dihydroartemisinin in the combination treatment, though it is unclear whether this translates into higher infectiousness to biting anophelines and hence increased transmission potential [405].

In a clinical trial conducted in the Republic of the Congo, 298 children aged 6-59 months were randomized to receive AS -SP, AS-AQ, or AL. There was no significant difference between groups concerning fever and parasite clearance time, improvement of anemia and gametocyte carriage at day 28. The results showed that the proportion of cases with gametocytes present increased during the first two days of treatment, but overall decreased during the four weeks of follow-up, from 23% to 3% in the AS-AQ group, from 26% to 5% in the AS-SP group and from 8% to 1% in the AL group (Fig. **15**) [406-408]. In one clinical trial examining gametocyte carriage, a non-ACT combination, amodiaquine-SP, was compared to an ACT combination, AS-SP or AL. In a second trial examining gametocyte carriage, an ACT, AS-SP, was compared to an ACT in combination with a single dose of primaquine, AS-SP +PQ. The mean circulation time of gametocytes was shown to be 4.6-6.5 days. After non-ACT treatment, patients were estimated to carry gametocytes for an average of 55 days. ACT treatment reduced the duration of gametocyte carriage fourfold to 13.4 days. Addition of PQ to ACT resulted in a further fourfold reduction of the duration of gametocyte carriage. These findings confirm previous estimates of the circulation time of gametocytes, but indicate a much longer duration of low-density gametocyte carriage after apparently successful clearance of asexual parasites. ACT treatment shortened the period of gametocyte carriage considerably, and ACTs showed the most pronounced effect on mature gametocytes when combined with PQ [402]. Eurartesim®, is the only DP combination formulation that meets international good manufacturing practice standards.

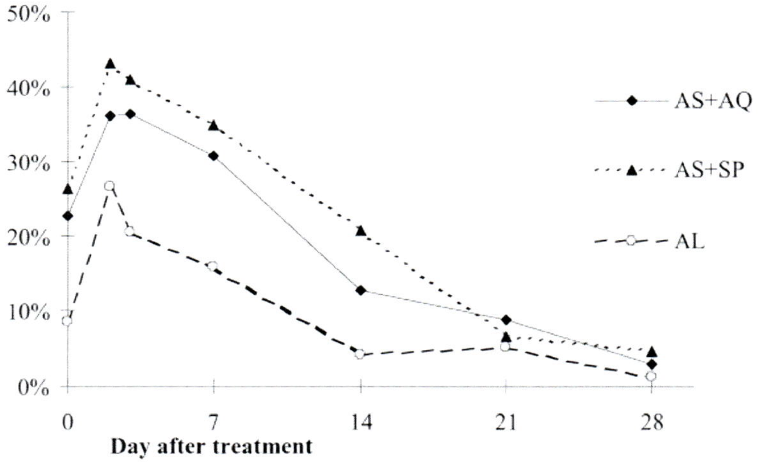

Figure 15: Gametocytemia inhibition following 3 different artemisinin-based combination therapies (Artesunate + Amodiaquine; Artesunate + Sulfadoxine-pyrimethamine; and Artemether-lumefantrine) treatment groups during follow-up [406].

5.5.5. Economic Considerations for Use of ACTs

Global mortality from infection with *falciparum* malaria has always been enormous, and mortality has increased in recent decades because of drug resistant malaria parasites. To protect the few remaining drugs available for malaria treatment, combination therapy is now considered to be the best option to prevent the further rapid loss of antimalarial drugs. Artemisinin combination therapy is clearly an appealing choice, as these drug combinations work quickly, are safe and well tolerated, and demonstrate activity against gametocytes that may decrease transmission of malaria by killing gametocytes. Several ACTs are on market that differs either in the choice of artemisinin analogue or in the partner drug. Researchers have noted that DP (approximately US $1. 00 per adult treatment) is far cheaper than AS-MQ (approximately $3. 85) due to the cost of mefloquine. Should all countries switch to DP? Most countries in Africa are switching to AL (approximately $1.47) from existing regimens.

Until recently, this was the only co-formulated ACT on market. Co- formulation prevents inappropriate use of drugs that occurs when drug regimens consist of different pills administered together (Table **23**) [388]. As of today, most commercially available formulations of DP are available either by gift (typically government-to-government donations) or through private sector sellers who command a significant premium in private pharmacy sales. Thus, a comparative cost and cost effectiveness basis for this product based on international open tender procurement for use in the public sector has yet to be established. Sigma-Tau has announced they will register the Eurartesim DP combination for use in the Affordable Medicine Facility-Malaria (AMF-M), as well as for public sector tenders financed, for example, by the Global Fund. Participation in the AMF-M will result in price negotiations designed to ensure affordability for customers in the non-premium private sector, as well as price comparability for public sector procurement of ACTs.

Table 23: Costs of artemisinin-based combination therapies compared with chloroquine [388]

Drugs	Total Dose for Full Adult (60 kg) Course (60kg)	Minimum Cost Per Full Adult Course (US$)	Additional Pur hase Cost Per Course (US$)	Additional Global Purchase Cost Per Year* (US$)
Artemether-lumefantrine	120/720mg	1.474	1.405	98-549 million
Artesunate-amodiaquine	600/1836mg	0.918	0.849	60-332 million
Artesunate-mefloquine	600/1500mg	3.85	3.781	0.26-1.5 billion
AS-sulfadoxine/pyrimethamine	600/2000/100mg	1.38	1.311	92-513 million
Dihydroartemisinin-piperaquine†	135/1080mg	1.00	0.931	65-364 million
Chloroquine	1500mg	0.07		

*Assumes: a) there are 70-435 million *P. vivax* infections per year, b) all of these infections are treated, c) adherence to World Health Organization dose recommendations and d) the average total dose administered is 2/3rds of a full adult dose. †As DHP is not yet manufactured according to International Good Manufacturing Practice standards, the cost in this table is conservatively set at one US dollar per treatment course based on a predicted public sector price of "less than one US dollar in adults and less than 0.5 US dollars in children"

Sigma-Tau has committed to making DP accessible and affordable for public sector use, with a target price of USD $1.00/treatment. This should place the product in line with currently available ACTs [386]. A systematic economic evaluation of existing ACT products was conducted examining the cost effectiveness and efficacy of ACTs used to treat children, adults, and pregnant women in endemic areas. Total 24 studies were evaluated investigating the cost-effectiveness of malaria treatments for uncomplicated malaria, severe malaria, or pre-referral treatment, combined with adequate diagnosis, and prevention of malaria by intermittent preventive treatment. In areas with both *P. falciparum* and *P. vivax* transmission, AL and DP, are at present the most cost-effective efficacious treatment options [411, 412].

CHAPTER 6

Use of PK/PD Assessments for Selecting the Best ACTs

Abstract: Most of the antimalarial drugs and their combination formulations in current use came on market before the modern use of PK and PD principles for dosage design to maximize drug efficacy. Antimalarial dose regimens have been empirical in nature based on clinical studies with drug half-life, PK inter-individual variation, drug exposure level and time variables have been derived from experimental data or referred to by data from public trials. PK studies involve investigating the relationship between drug absorption, distribution, metabolism, and excretion, while PD studies investigate relationships between the drug target and the drug itself, the mechanism by which the drug works, and the clinical effect the drug provides. Both kinds of studies are involved when assessing drug interactions. Many drugs are metabolized into a similar metabolism pathway or shared an identical target that provides an opportunity to match the proper partner drugs for an antimalarial combination. The ideal PK properties of antimalarial drugs have long been deliberated. From a perspective of preventing drug resistance, drug combination partners should have a similar PK profile. The implications of a PD mismatch on ACTs are not clear at present, particularly in regions with high malaria transmission. Current recommended ACTs have repeatedly shown in a variety of clinical studies that the PD match between ACT partner drugs is good, the combinations are efficacious, well-tolerated, and provide protection against new infections. As discussed in other chapters, PK/PD mismatched ACTs have a known risk of encouraging drug resistance to partner drugs where drug resistance has yet to emerge, and drug combinations that are mismatched will not aid in the important public health job of limiting the spread of resistance.

Keywords: Chemoprophylaxis, chemotherapy, clinical trials, combination, combination partner, dosage design, dosage regimen, metabolism matching, PD matching, PD mismatch, PK matching, PK mismatch, PK/PD mismatch.

Antimalarial drugs and their combination formulations in current use came on market before the advent of utilizing PK/PD principles in clinical trials to aid in dosage design to maximize drug efficacy. Antimalarial dose regimens have been empirically derived based on clinical studies. Many factors that might influence efficacy of antimalarials for both chemotherapy and chemoprophylaxis indications include convenience of the prescribed antimalarial regimen (daily or weekly) for both indications. While the aim of antimalarial drug therapy for severe *falciparum* malaria is saving a patient from death, in uncomplicated malaria, the goal of therapy it is to decrease the biomass of parasites to undetectable levels or to a low level where host defenses can eliminate the remaining parasites. Current treatment regimens of combination therapies (CTs) or artemisinin-based combination therapies (ACTs) must generally cover four asexual life cycles to eliminate blood-stage malaria parasites. For slowly eliminated drugs, blood drug levels must go beyond the minimum inhibitory concentration and if possible exceed the minimum parasiticidal concentration to kill all infecting parasites. Similar to other infections of HIV and tuberculosis, patients infected with malaria undergoing therapy with CTs or ACTs may not always respond satisfactorily to treatment. It is easy to understand why malaria infections might fail to respond to antimalarial treatment or prophylaxis-assuming drugs were dosed on schedule unless the parasites were intrinsically resistant to the drugs given.

The most significant problem with antimalarials today is the growing incidence of drug resistance to *P. falciparum*. Drug resistance implies that there is a shift to the right in the relationship between drug concentration and efficacy. Although treatment failures in malaria are generally a consequence of poor patient drug compliance, insufficient dosing, pharmacokinetic (PK) and pharmacodynamic (PD) factors, some malaria infections will recrudesce, and none of these factors may adequately explain why a recrudescence occurred. How parasites persist and survive in the presence of apparently adequate antimalarial treatment is an unanswered question. Unless the patient was observed during the administration of antimalarial treatment and for a minimum of 1 hour after drug administration, inadequate compliance or vomiting must be evaluated as a reason for treatment failure.

In general, patients do not like to take drugs after disease symptoms have subsided. Thus, patient compliance with 3-day treatment regimens of ACTs is usually quite good, and compliance with 7 day regimens of artemisinin analogue monotherapy has been shown to be poor. Patients who demonstrate poor compliance will have low and ineffective blood concentration of antimalarials and suboptimal drug exposure of parasites to drug concentrations high enough to kill the remaining parasites [234]. A number of limitations are well known to contribute to decreased ACT efficacy, and these limitations include a significant reservoir of parasites existing in semi-immune persons as an asymptomatic infection, elevated malaria transmission rates, inappropriate drug use, inadequate laboratory testing, poor drug control policies, and inadequate systems of public health, particularly in Asia and in Africa. Accordingly, understanding how PK, PD, and PK/PD variables of antimalarial drugs relate to efficacy enhances selection of the best drug combination(s) for treatment, and helps insure the most appropriate use of these drugs.

6.1. REVIEW OF CURRENTLY USED ACTS TESTED IN COMPARATIVE TRIALS

Effective treatment of malaria plays a crucial role in reducing morbidity and mortality as an effective malaria vaccine is not likely to be developed over the next ten years. Malaria parasite resistance to an array of antimalarial drugs from different classes has been noted all over the world, accordingly, monotherapeutic malaria treatment and some older antimalarial drug combination treatments are now ineffective. New antimalarial treatments are quickly needed to replace ACTs that are now the best antimalarial regimens possible today which may fail in the near future due to drug resistance. ACTs have been shown to enhance the efficacy of treatment cut down the length of treatment, and they have been shown to diminish the emergence of drug resistant parasites. Despite these advances, better treatments are required, and this leads us to the associated requirement to insure comparative efficacy assessments are well- designed and easily interpreted.

Antimalarial cure rates should be greater than 90% [1, 23]. The companion idea that malaria drug policies must be altered if the rates of malaria cure drop below 90% is still under consideration, but the current goal of cure rates >90% is a considerable advance from past years when lower cure rates were considered to be acceptable. Combination drug therapy involves combining the additive or synergistic potential of two or more drugs to provide better treatment. The total effect of ACTs is to diminish the probability of disease recrudescence, cut down on selective drug pressures within patients, and preclude parasite transmission. If the cure rate of any ACT is below 90%, the recommendation for the use of that combination for treatment should be changed, and a better ACT should be selected based on data from a comparative efficacy study demonstrating clinical superiority.

There are a number of published clinical studies comparing ACT efficacy for malaria treatment. One challenge in understanding the data from these studies revolves around the different endpoints utilized to evaluate comparative efficacy studies. In low-transmission areas, the traditional treatment goal is to kill all infecting parasites from a patient to insure no disease is transmitted, while in high malaria transmission regions is the goal is a clinical cure which may not necessarily kill all of the infecting parasites. The WHO has changed its endpoints in an effort to standardize study endpoints in a manner that encompasses both parasitological and clinical outcomes [2]. Comparative efficacy studies in Asia or Africa typically discuss patient outcomes at day 14 or day 28 day as a primary endpoint, which is too short to examine all aspects of malaria treatment particularly the parasitological outcome. Additional data on parasitological outcomes at later time points using PCR is an important public health goal. The ongoing presence of blood stage parasites post treatment can lead to anemia, recrudescent infections, and severe malaria. Studies over longitudinal time, where the clinical and parasitological endpoints for patients are followed for an extended period where each patient is provided the same drug treatment after each malaria infection, may provide the best comparison of malaria treatment efficacy in areas with high-malaria transmission. Currently ACTs are formulated based on various well-conducted and randomized comparative trials, and the efficacy comparison data is summarized below:

1) Non-ACT Combinations are not Recommended for Malaria Treatment

Non-artemisinin combination treatments such as amodiaquine combined with sulfadoxine- pyrimethamine, or sulfadoxine-pyrimethamine combined with chloroquine are no longer recommended. The existing levels of drug resistance to these combinations used without an artemisinin partner have decreased their efficacy. The combination of chloroquine and sulfadoxine-pyrimethamine has no data showing a benefit over SP alone, and, therefore, this drug combination treatment should not be used. Amodiaquine combined with sulfadoxine-pyrimethamine is a better combination than amodiaquine monotherapy or SP alone, but the efficacy of the amodiaquine-sulfadoxine-pyrimethamine combination is generally lower than the efficacy of ACT treatment, and this combination is not the best antimalarial drug choice either [23].

2) The Six Dose Dosing Regimen of Artemether-Lumefantrine (AL) is Superior to a Four Dose Regimen

The data derived from one clinical trial conducted in Thailand from 1996-1997 (238 adults and children) has shown a much higher cure rate at day 28 using a 6 dose artemether- lumefantrine (AL) regimen administered over 3 days *versus* a 4-dose AL regimen also given over 3 days. The new oral fixed dose combination of AL has been shown to be a well-tolerated and effective treatment for multi-drug resistant *falciparum* malaria, although four-dose cure rates have been lower than the cure rates observed with artesunate-mefloquine (AS-MQ). A comparative efficacy study of the six dose and four dose AL regimens was conducted to definitively answer this question. Two six-dose AL regimens with a total adult dose of 480 mg of artemether and 2,880 mg of lumefantrine were assessed against a four dose AL regimen of 320 mg of artemether and 1,920 mg of lumefantrine in 359 patients infected with multi-drug resistant uncomplicated *falciparum* malaria. The fever and parasite clearance times were no different in the three treatment groups, and there were no differences in adverse events reported. The two 6 dose AL treatments yielded PCR adjusted cure rates at day 28 of 96.9% and 99.12%, which was much better than the four dose regimen which had a cure rate of 83.3% (P <0.001). These 6-dose AL treatments clearly provide a clinical benefit when compared to four-dose regimens of AL [357, 414].

3) A Six-Dose Regimen of AL is Not Superior to Treatment with AS-MQ

In another set of clinical trials (537 participants), the efficacy of a 6 dose AL regimen was compared to treatment with AS-MQ. For the six-dose regimen, two studies compared the antimalarial efficacy of AL to treatment with AS-MQ with an endpoint of day 28 parasitemia, and no differences in fever or parasite clearance times were detected. There were 11 failures to clear all infecting parasites in the AL treatment arm and none with AS-MQ [344]. The data from this study suggests that AS-MQ therapy is more effective than AL treatment [386, 391].

4) The Six-Dose Regimen of AL Is Similar to the Efficacy Achieved with AS-AQ Treatment

A randomized, open label, clinical trial, was conducted in Nigerian children 6 months to 10 years of age infected with uncomplicated *falciparum* malaria. The 132 patients in this trial were split into two groups of 66 and received artesunate (4 mg/kg daily) combined with amodiaquine (10 mg/kg daily) or AL at different doses based on body weight range. AL was dosed daily with one tablet for children ranging in weight from 5-14 kg, two tablets for children ranging in weight from 15-24 kg, and three tablets for children ranging in weight from 25-34 kg. Both of the malaria treatment compared in this study was administered over a 3-day period, and clinical follow-up occurred until day 28. Day 28 cure rates were 93% for AS-AQ and 95% for AL (OR = 0.71, 95% CI = 0.12- 3.99, rho = 0.66). The PCR adjusted cure rates by day 28 per protocol of the two patient treatment groups were 98.4% for AS-AQ and 100% for AL. Both combination treatments were well tolerated and the efficacy comparison demonstrated that AS-AQ was non-inferior to AL, and both treatments were shown to be both efficacious and safe [386, 415]. Another clinical trial was conducted in Burundi to compare children treated with AS-AQ *versus* AL with a 14-day follow-up period [416].

Total 149 children were treated with AS-AQ, and 142 or 95.3% demonstrated both parasitological and clinical cures while 5 patients or 3.3% presented with parasitological failure late in the treatment period, one patient or 0.7% was a late treatment failure and one patient or 0.7% was an early treatment failure. 141

children were treated with AL, and 140 children or 99.3% demonstrated both parasitological and clinical and one patient or 0.7% was a late parasitological failure. The adverse effects of drug treatment were similar in both treatment arms. Both ACTs resulted in diminished carriage of gametocytes but did not achieve full gametocyte clearance in all of the patients treated. The Burundi Ministry of Public Health subsequently decided AS-AQ would be their best choice for first line treatment of uncomplicated *falciparum* malaria [416].

5) Efficacy of DP is Superior to AS-AQ for Treatment of Uncomplicated Malaria

A comparative efficacy study was conducted to compare treatment with dihydroartemisinin-piperaquine (DP) to treatment with AS-AQ. This trial compared the efficacy of DP *versus* AS-AQ in 334 patients infected with *P. falciparum*, *P. vivax* or both species of *Plasmodium* with a 42-day follow-up period. Of the 334 patients, 185 had *P. falciparum* infections, 80 patients presented with *P. vivax* infections, and 69 patients were co-infected with both *falciparum* and *vivax* malaria. At day 42, parasitological failure rates were 45% (95% CI ranging from 36%-53%) for AS-AQ, and 13% (95% CI ranging from 7.2%-19%) for DP. The recrudescence rates for *falciparum* infections and for *vivax* recurrence were significantly greater in patients treated with AS-AQ than in patients treated with DP. AS-AQ treated patients were 2.95-fold more likely to have anemia and 14.5-fold more likely to carry *P. vivax* gametocytes. DP was shown to both superior and better tolerated than AS-AQ for treatment of uncomplicated multi-drug resistant *P. falciparum* and *P. vivax* infections. The extended post-treatment therapeutic effect of piperaquine was shown to delay *falciparum* re-infection, diminish recurrence of *vivax* infection, and decrease anemia and gametocyte carriage [389, 417].

6) The Efficacy of DP is Superior to a Six Dose Regimen of AL

Uganda implemented artemether-lumefantrine (AL) as the drug of choice to treat uncomplicated *falciparum* malaria. AL treatment does have a number of drawbacks, however, which include a dosing requirement twice per day, concomitant administration with fatty food, and an elevated probability of re-infection after treatment in regions with high malaria transmission. DP is dosed once a day, and it demonstrates a prolonged post-treatment prophylaxis effect due to the long half-life of piperaquine. AL was compared with DP in Kanungu, Uganda, which is a region with moderate transmission of malaria. Patients ranging in age from 6 months to 10 years infected with uncomplicated *falciparum* malaria were divided into two treatment arms and followed for 42 days. Genotyping was employed in this study to distinguish a recrudescent infection with *falciparum* from a new infection. DP treated patients had a deceased risk of recurrent parasitemia (33.2% *vs.* 12.2%; risk difference = 20.9%, 95% CI 13.0-28.8%) but there was no statistically significant difference treatment failure risk due to recrudescence (5.8% *vs.* 2.0%; risk difference = 3.8%, 95% CI -0.2-7.8%). Patients who were treated with DP showed a decreased risk of gametocytemia after treatment (4.2% *vs.* 10.6%, p = 0.01) [379]. Similar studies were performed by other scientists in different regents, and these studies showed DP regimens were more efficacious than AL regimens to uncomplicated *P. falciparum* malaria [350, 378, 418].

7) The Efficacy of DP is Similar to AS-MQ

Multi-drug resistant *falciparum* malaria is a significant health burden in many parts of the world to include the Amazon region of Peru. A randomized open label clinical trial was carried out comparing AS-MQ with DP. Total 522 patients with uncomplicated *falciparum* malaria were recruited into this trial and followed for a period of 63 days post-treatment. The PCR-adjusted response, estimated by the Kaplan Meier survival and per protocol analyses, was very high for AS-MQ and DP (99.6% for AS-MQ and 98.4% for DP). All incidents of recrudescence noted were late parasitological failures. Gametocytes were cleared more quickly in the AS-MQ group (28 days for AS-MQ *versus* 35 days with DP), and new gametocytes appeared more commonly in patients treated with DP (day 7: 8 (3.6%) *vs.* 2 (0.9%), RR: 3.84, 95% CI [0.82-17.87]). The adverse events noted for patients in this study were more frequent in adults and children in the AS-MQ group. DP was shown to be equally effective as AS-MQ in treating uncomplicated *falciparum* malaria, and this combination was shown to be better tolerated and cheaper than AS-MQ [410]. Two other clinical trials that generated similar data to this study have also been conducted [351, 364].

8) Other Clinical Trials

A meta-analysis of 16 drug trials clinical malaria drug trials was conducted to compare the outcomes of patients treated with 3 days of any artemisinin after patients were treated with SP, CQ, AQ, or MQ monotherapy. The conclusion drawn in this study from all of the clinical trial data examined is adding 3 days of artemisinin treatment to a standard monotherapy treatment significantly reduced parasitological failure observed on day 14 and day 28. Gametocyte carriage was diminished in the patients treated with artemisinin.

6.2. EFFECTS OF METABOLISM MATCHING ON THE EFFICACY OF ACTS

6.2.1. The Effects of Metabolism Matching on the Efficacy of Non-ACTs

PK studies involve investigating PK and PD parameters of drug-drug interactions, which primarily take place during the phases of drug absorption, and distribution, that is dependent on plasma protein binding of drugs, metabolism, and excretion. Most drugs are given orally, and subsequently, drug absorption occurs in the mucosa of the intestine mucosa, mainly in the duodenum. Drug bioavailability is dependent on expression of a P-glycoprotein found in the intestinal absorption cells, or enterocyte, which is capable of actively pumping drugs back into the lumen of the intestine, and on cytochrome P450 (CYP450) enzymes also found in enterocytes, which metabolize drugs before they reach systemic circulation. Inhibition or induction of the P-glycoprotein and enterocyte CYP450 enzymes can alter drug bioavailability. After absorption, drugs bind to transport proteins in the plasma such as albumin. The percentage of drug bound to a plasma protein plays a significant role in drug distribution, and a number of drugs alter plasma protein binding of other drugs. When any drug passes through the liver, it is further metabolized to more soluble metabolites, which may be active or inactive.

Drug metabolism has an enormous impact on the efficacy of any drug. Drug metabolism is dependent on several phases, Phase I, Phase II, and Phase III metabolism. Phase I metabolism consists of processes of hydrolysis, oxidation, and reduction carried out by CYP450 enzymes. Phase II metabolism consists of conjugation and this phase is carried out by enzymes to include uridine diphosphoglucuronosyl transferase, glutathione S-transferase, and N-acetyl transferase. These enzymes are critical to the processes of drug detoxification and excretion. Phase III metabolism is carried out by drug transporters in the cell plasma membrane mediating both efflux and influx, such as the multidrug resistance protein, MRP, the P-glycoprotein, and the organic anion transport proteins, OATP1 and OATP2. These enzymes are located in the liver and in the GI tract, kidneys, and other organs, and they are significant players in the physiological processes of drug pharmacokinetics and pharmacodynamics (PK/PD).

In the liver, OATP1 and OATP2 insure drugs are taken up to be metabolized. MRP2 and P-glycoprotein are also found in hepatocytes, and these enzymes pay a role in pumping drugs out to the biliary canals. These enzymes can influence the processes of absorption, distribution, metabolism, and elimination, and they can also influence drug concentrations inside target cells, and ultimately, have an impact on drug treatment efficacy. Acute malaria infection can alter metabolism and distribution of some drugs, but it does not influence drug absorption through increased binding of drugs to proteins in plasma. Inhibition of metabolism of hepatocytes such as the CYP3A4 enzymes during infections with acute malaria has been shown to lead to diminished quinine clearance [232].

Atovaquone and Proguanil

One example of drug interactions of malaria drugs is found in the combination of atovaquone and proguanil. Atovaquone-proguanil is used for prophylaxis and treatment for *falciparum* malaria. The activity of atovaquone against *Plasmodium* is known to occur *via* inhibition of electron transport in mitochondria. Atovaquone is 99% bound to plasma proteins, and it has a highly variable half-life that can range as high as 70 hours. Atovaquone metabolism is marked by enterohepatic circulation, and atovaquone is metabolized to some extent by the liver resulting in most of the dosed drug being excreted without metabolism in the feces. There is *in vitro* evidence of CYP3A4 inhibition by atovaquone, and studies of atovaquone used to treat patients with infections caused by *Toxoplasma gondii* have shown decreases in the area of the curve of atovaquone (AUC) by 50% when atovaquone was combined with rifampicin but by 34% when atovaquone was combined with rifabutin. Administration of rifampicin and atovaquone at the same time is not suggested, and the clinical impact of a modest decrease in the concentration of atovaquone when combined with rifabutin is not clear.

In addition, while there are no efficacy studies on the effects of rifabutin and atovaquone when using atovaquone-proguanil for malaria treatment or prophylaxis, there are a number of studies on co-administration of these two drugs for treatment of opportunistic infections. The combination of atovaquone and rifabutin has been shown in mice to have synergy for prophylaxis of *Pneumocystis carinii* pneumonia and *T. gondii* infections. Given proguanil is metabolized by CYP2C19 to cycloguanil, concomitant administration of proguanil with rifampicin could affect antimalarial activity, as rifampicin is known to induce CYP2C19. Data on proguanil-rifampicin interactions are not available, and additional studies will be needed to understand the impact of rifabutin and rifampicin co-administration on proguanil efficacy and pharmacokinetics.

Doxycycline and Clindamycin

Doxycycline is a tetracycline derivative, which is commonly combined with quinine for treatment of malaria, and its mechanism of action involves disrupting mRNA and transfer RNA. 80-95% of doxycycline is plasma-protein bound, and this drug is known to be metabolized by the liver in a poorly understand manner. Inducers of CYP enzymes such as rifampicin, and likely rifabutin, have been shown to accelerate the metabolism of doxycycline and influence plasma exposure as the AUC of doxycycline and the half-life of doxycycline are decreased by 40% when co-administered with rifampicin. The question of altered drug efficacy through CYP induction is not clear concerning doxycycline.

Clindamycin is a lincosamide antibiotic that functions by inhibiting protein synthesis in the ribosome. Clindamycin is used for malaria treatment as a doxycycline alternative in women who are pregnant. Ninety percent of clindamycin is plasma protein bound, and it is metabolized by CYP3A enzymes to create an array of metabolites, both active and inactive, excreted in the feces. Clindamycin is known to inhibit CYP3A *in vitro* and concomitant administration with rifampicin could influence the metabolism of clindamycin and shorten its half-life as rifampicin induces CYP3A4. These drugs should be co-administered with caution [413].

6.2.2. Metabolism Matching of WHO Recommended ACTs

Oral administration of mefloquine has been shown to have no effect on the absorption, distribution, metabolism, and excretion (ADME) of AS and DHA, which does support the hypothesis that combinations of mefloquine with AS or DHA will be effective. AM has been found to significantly elevate the C_{max} and diminish the Vd of lumefantrine in healthy Zambian volunteers when AM is co-administered with lumefantrine. Drug interactions mediated by CYP enzymes was anticipated in patients administered both AM and mefloquine given AM is a substrate for CYP3A4 and mefloquine is known to be an inhibitor of CYP3A4. In healthy volunteers, however, no risk of drug-drug interaction was noted when AM was co-administered with mefloquine. The absorption of mefloquine was altered in patients infected with *falciparum* malaria who were co-administered mefloquine and AM. A lower C_{max}, AUC, and delayed T_{max} were observed in patients infected with *falciparum* malaria who are treated with mefloquine, however, these findings were not found to be clinically important. Quinine is also metabolized by CYP3A4 similar to AM and lumefantrine. A study conducted in

42 healthy subjects examined both PK and electrocardiographic interactions because of therapy with AM-lumefantrine and IV quinine. AM was not shown to have any influence on the metabolism of quinine or lumefantrine, and the drugs used in this study were noted to be well tolerated and safe [419].

The effects of ketoconazole were assessed in 16 subjects to determine the impact of ketoconazole, a known CYP3A4 inhibitor, on the PK parameters of lumefantrine, AM, and DHA. This trial was conducted in two-periods where patients were given a single dose of AL, in combination with ketoconazole or alone. The average exposure (C_{max} and AUC) to lumefantrine, DHA, and AM amplified twofold when ketoconazole was co-administered with AL. No increase in adverse events was noted in this study, and therefore the drug-drug interaction was not deemed significant. Adjustment of AL dosing does not appear to be required when ketoconazole or other CYP3A4 inhibitors are co-administered. There is an increased incidence of co-administration of anti-tubercular and anti-retroviral drugs with potent CYP modulating activity with antimalarials given the common presence of these ailments in patients in various parts of the world. In addition, there are a number of studies on the potential for clinical pharmacokinetic interactions of artemisinins and their partner drugs. ACTs have been used to treat malaria for more than a decade, and no clinically significant interactions have been reported. Given the wide therapeutic margins, short half-lives and the preferred uptake of artemisinins by parasitized RBCs, this issue of drug interactions may not be of clinical concern.

Given the known significant differences in bioavailability of long acting partner drugs like lumefantrine, differences in bioavailability may also mask clinically relevant drug-drug interactions. Often, the clinical significance of a drug-drug interaction is not noticed due to the fact the efficacy of an antimalarial combination therapy is the consequence of the antimalarial activities of rapidly acting and rapidly metabolized artemisinin drugs and long acting, slowly metabolized partner drugs. Despite the lack of available data on ACT drug interactions from clinical studies to date, *in vitro* and *in vivo* drug interaction studies of new artemisinins with combination partners and other drugs that are co-administered should be conducted to examine potential problems. The short residence time of artemisinins is an advantage in avoiding clinically relevant interactions through appropriately timing the administration of other drugs.

The advantages of combination therapy must be balanced with the enhanced risk of drug interactions. The pharmacokinetics of ACTs is complex. All of the artemisinin derivatives are metabolized by CYP3A4 to DHA, an active antimalarial metabolite. Artemisinins have also been shown to induce the activity of CYP2C19 and, in turn, induce their metabolism. This auto-induction phenomenon has been discussed previously, and this factor alone can play a significant role in modulating the efficacy of artemisinin therapy over time. The influence of CYP enzymes on the metabolism of partner drugs used in combination with artemisinin compounds also merits discussion given these compounds are slowly metabolized with long half-lives. Accordingly, the most significant drug interactions will be discussed here for the commonly prescribed artemisinin combination therapies.

Artesunate-Amodiaquine (AS-AQ)

Amodiaquine is quickly absorbed and metabolized to desethylamodiaquine, an active antimalarial metabolite, by CYP2C8. Administration of artesunate and amodiaquine co-administered with other drugs could result in altered drug exposure leading to either drug toxicity or insufficient treatment for malaria. Amodiaquine and DEAQ have been shown *in vitro* to have moderate inhibitory activity against the P-glycoprotein. In addition, metabolism of two drugs metabolized by CYPs such as losartan and debrisoquine has been inhibited *in vivo* after amodiaquine administration to healthy subjects. Debrisoquine is metabolized by CYP2D6 and losartan is metabolized by CYP2C9.

Amodiaquine drug exposure has been altered by other drugs. After administration of a three day malaria drug treatment regimen of amodiaquine combined with artesunate to two healthy subjects by itself and co-administered with the antiretroviral drug, efavirenz, the exposure of amodiaquine in patients treated with amodiaquine and artesunate increased by 115% and the exposure of amodiaquine increased by 302% when co-administered with efavirenz. The AUC of DEAQ decreased by 24% when combined with artesunate and by 9% when combined with efavirenz. Both volunteers showed prolonged hepatotoxicity that was delayed and asymptomatic several weeks after the study were completed. The hepatotoxicity observed in this study is a concern as this data suggests liver function testing may be required when administering amodiaquine to HIV-positive patients who are being treated with efavirenz. In addition, inhibition of the metabolism of amodiaquine *in vitro* has been shown by efavirenz and by another HIV drug, the protease inhibitors tipranavir, lopinavir, and saquinavir at concentrations that are relevant clinically. Inhibition of CYP isoenzymes and possible inhibition of the P-glycoprotein suggests further study of drug-drug interactions is necessary for antimalarial drug combinations containing amodiaquine. The dose of amodiaquine administered may require adjustment given changes in plasma concentrations when amodiaquine is co-administered with other drugs [420].

Artesunate-Mefloquine (AS-MQ)

In patients with *falciparum* malaria, co-administration of artemisinin with mefloquine has been shown to significantly increase the AUC and decrease the clearance of artemisinin. In contrast, oral co-administration of mefloquine and dihydroartemisinin (DHA) to healthy volunteers has been shown to have no effect either partner drug, except for a slight increase in the absorption rate of mefloquine. The absorption of mefloquine was affected by AM when these two drugs were administered together in patients infected with *falciparum* malaria. A lower C_{max}, AUC, and delayed T_{max} were observed in patients infected with *falciparum* malaria who are treated with mefloquine, however, these findings were not found to be clinically relevant. Mefloquine is metabolized by hepatocytes in the liver by CYP3A4. Given CYP3A4 is involved in the metabolism of 50% of drugs available today, interactions of other drugs with this enzyme result in frequent drug-drug interactions. Co-administration of 500 mg of mefloquine with 600 mg of rifampin, which is known to induce CYP3A4, to healthy Thai volunteers, was shown to lead to the decreases in the AUC of mefloquine by 68%, decreases in C_{max} by 19% and decreases in the half-life. In addition, a 281% increase in oral clearance (CL/F) of mefloquine was observed; however, the T_{max} of mefloquine was not altered. Given this data, monitoring mefloquine efficacy in patients who have been also co-administered rifampin is necessary to ensure complete malaria treatment.

Artesunate-Sulfadoxine/Pyrimethamine (AS-SP)

Several case reports have been published that suggest that drug-drug interactions might occur either when pyrimethamine is co-administered with cotrimoxazole drugs (trimethoprim and sulfamethoxazole) or lorazepam. Two women prescribed pyrimethamine as prophylaxis for malaria presented with megaloblastic anemia after co-administration of cotrimoxazole to treat a urinary tract infection or for malarial prophylaxis. The mechanism of this anemia was hypothesized to involve additive effects of two dihydrofolate reductase inhibitors. In two of five women who were co-administered pyrimethamine with lorazepam, increases in bilirubin and hepatic transaminases were observed. No hepatotoxicity was observed in these two women administered these drugs by themselves. The underlying hepatotoxicity mechanism is not yet clear and merits further investigation [420].

Artemether-Lumefantrine (AL)

Artemether has been reported to significantly increase the C_{max} and reduce the Vd of lumefantrine in healthy Zambian volunteers after co-administration of both drugs. Given mefloquine is a CYP3A4 inhibitor and both artemether and lumefantrine are CYP3A4 substrates. In healthy volunteers, however, this combination was tested and no risks associated with pharmacokinetic drug-drug interactions were observed. Co-administration of a single dose of AL to healthy volunteers with ketoconazole has been shown to result in modest increases in AUC for artemether (by 131.6%), dihydroartemisinin (by 51.3%), and lumefantrine (by 60.9%). These changes in the AUC were not believed to be clinically relevant. Quinidine is a potent inhibitor of CYP2D6, however, this enzyme does not appear to mediate metabolism of other antimalarial drugs. Quinine, similar to AM and lumefantrine, is metabolized primarily by CYP3A4. A study conducted in 42 healthy subjects examined drug-drug interactions after administration of oral AM-lumefantrine and IV quinine using electrocardiographic and pharmacokinetic endpoints. AM was shown not to have an influence on the pharmacokinetics of either quinine or lumefantrine, and no adverse events were noted [419].

Dose adjustment of AL when used to treat patients infected with malaria might not be required when AL is co-administered with a potent CYP3A4 inhibitor such as ketoconazole. When AL was co-administered with mefloquine to healthy volunteers, a 42% decrease in the AUC of lumefantrine was observed. The decrease in AUC of lumefantrine was not believed to have an impact on efficacy outcomes due to the well-known differences in oral bioavailability of lumefantrine due to dependence on administration with fatty foods and the wide therapeutic index of this combination. Clearly, patients receiving oral AL or the combination of AL with mefloquine should be encouraged to take their medication with foods high in fat. *In vitro*, lumefantrine has been shown to inhibit significantly CYP2D6 at therapeutic drug concentrations. Co-administration of known substrates of CYP2D6 or inhibitors of CYP3A4 may result in significant drug-drug interactions. Pharmacokinetic studies evaluating interactions between AL and co-administered antiretroviral drugs are needed due to the known ability of antiretroviral drugs to module the activity of CYP enzymes [420].

Dihydroartemisinin-Piperaquine (DP)

A single dose of DP consisting of 120 mg of dihydroartemisinin and 960 mg of piperaquine was administered to a healthy male subject after consuming a fatty meal to increase drug absorption. Piperaquine drug concentrations obtained from this subject provided an estimate of 33 days for the elimination half-life, which suggests that the published half-life data of 23 days is likely an underestimate of the true half-life of piperaquine. Another study reported metabolism of piperaquine into five metabolites (Ml-M5), and two metabolites, MI, a carboxylic metabolite, and M2, a mono-N-oxidated metabolite, were noted to be the two principle products. Ml might be created through either monoamine oxidase or CYP activity, and this metabolite showed a half-life of roughly 53 days. Two other metabolites, a di-N-oxidated metabolite and a urinary monohydroxylated metabolite were obtained. The clinical relevance of these piperaquine metabolites on piperaquine efficacy for malaria treatment is unknown and merits study.[420].

The effects of a co-administered fatty meal on piperaquine oral bioavailability were studied in a random crossover study composed of eight healthy Caucasian volunteers dosed with 500 mg of piperaquine while fasting and after a fatty meal. Piperaquine administration with a fatty meal was shown to be associated with a significant rise of 213% increase in the C_{max} and a 98% escalation in the AUC_{inf}. Piperaquine oral bioavailability after a fatty meal increased by 121% compared to administration of piperaquine without a fatty meal.

In conclusion, the pharmacology of quickly metabolized artemisinin analogues with short half-lives is complex in nature, and this complexity is further increased by the metabolism of slowly metabolized partner drugs with long elimination half-lives. Drug metabolism is heavily dependent on CYP isoenzymes, which increases the probability of clinically significant drug interactions. Changes in the plasma drug concentration of both the parent drug and the metabolite(s) of the parent drugs, when co-administered with other drugs, particularly anti-retroviral and anti-tubercular drugs, may have an impact on treatment outcomes leading to drug toxicity or reduced efficacy.

6.3. EFFECTS OF PK MATCHING ON MALARIA DRUG RESISTANCE TO ACTs

6.3.1. Simply Matching Half-Lives May Not Be Sufficient to Avoid Malaria Drug Resistance

The ideal PK properties of antimalarial drugs are continually debated, however, from a perspective of prevention of drug resistance, combination partners of malaria drug should ideally have comparable pharmacokinetic properties or a PK profile match. Parasite mutations that result in a drug resistance phenotype occur at a predictable rate of 10^6 per parasite generation. A parasite would have to develop mutations at two different genes to survive treatment with a combination of two drugs. Given the probability of developing two mutations simultaneously is only 10^{12} (10^6 x 10^6), the odds of this occurring are very small [25].

Rapid drug elimination provides a means to ensure residual drug concentrations are not present to provide a filter to select for drug resistant parasites, but such rapidly eliminated drugs used as monotherapy must be administered for 7 days, which creates problems with patient compliance given patient compliance with 7-day drug treatment regimens is notoriously poor. Treatment with artemisinin monotherapy for seven days has been associated with treatment failure rates of 10% [71, 196]. For a combination drug treatment to be efficacious over a three-day treatment period, the half-life of one of the partner drugs must be longer than 24 hours. For an ACT, the artemisinin derivative component is eliminated very rapidly leaving the non-artemisinin partner with the burden of providing coverage throughout the rest of the treatment period. The combination of mefloquine with artesunate, for example, includes artesunate, which has a half-life of 1 hour, with mefloquine whose half-life 21 days. The fraction of residual parasites that is actually exposed to mefloquine by itself after exposure of two asexual cycles to artemisinin, is very small, which helps ensure mefloquine is capable of inhibiting parasite growth of the small numbers of parasites. In addition, these remaining parasites are actually exposed to elevated concentrations of mefloquine, and in cases of moderate resistance, these drug levels are generally sufficient to kill off the remaining parasites. In this example of a mismatched PK profile, artesunate is well covered by the mefloquine partner drug, but mefloquine is vulnerable to development of parasite mutations given the slowly eliminated "tail" of mefloquine drug concentrations over time.

In the northwestern region of Thailand near the border which is a region of low malaria transmission, where resistance to mefloquine is present, use of the combination AS-MQ treatment was shown to be very efficacious, and incidence of drug resistance and the numbers of malaria cases was shown to decline [361, 421]. This approach would be expected to be inhibit *de novo* emergence of drug resistant parasites in regions of high malaria transmission, where infections with elevated parasite biomass is a significant source of the development of *de novo* resistant parasites.

The principle barriers to use of ACT drugs to prevent the development of drug resistance will involve incomplete drug coverage, monotherapy, or inadequate treatment. Unfortunately, drug counterfeiting is quite common in malarious regions of the world, antimalarial drugs of dubious quality are readily available for purchase on the open market without a physician's prescription, and full compliance with antimalarial treatment is often incomplete. Regardless of the epidemiological setting, patients with high parasitemia infections must receive a full and complete drug treatment regimen to help decrease the probability of emergent drug resistant parasites.

Rational choices of the most appropriate partner drugs for antimalarial treatment requires defining and matching selective windows, the time interval during which antimalarial drugs persist at low levels sufficient to suppress growth but too low to prevent parasite replication [422]. In the past, PK matching was required by the US FDA for licensure of new drug combinations for treatment of infectious disease, however, simply matching drug half-lives is not sufficient as the drug half-life does not adequately represent the time above the minimum inhibitory concentration [422]. For example, the half-life of chloroquine ranges from 1-2 months, and therefore, simply based on the half-life, chloroquine should be protected against emergence of drug resistant parasites. Chloroquine is naturally stored in the human liver in high concentrations, however, and while initial concentrations of drug are high, the concentration of chloroquine in the liver will drop quickly over time and the remaining drug will slowly leach out for months. In this example, chloroquine has an excellent half-life but the time above the minimum inhibitory concentration, while not defined, is likely relatively short.

Artemisinins have been commonly combined with quinoline drugs such as, amodiaquine, mefloquine, and lumefantrine pharmacokinetically; the artemether-lumefantrine combination is better matched than other combinations in terms of half-life as the half-life of lumefantrine ranges from 3-6 days while the half-life of artemether is 1-3 hours. Artesunate-amodiaquine also has a PK mismatch as the half-life of its main metabolite, desethyl amodiaquine, ranges from 9-18 days, and half-life of artesunate is less than 2 hours. The time above MIC for both lumefantrine and amodiaquine has not been established, and this data would help inform the risk of emergent drug resistance for each combination [77, 423, 424]. Antibiotics have been combined with artemisinin drugs, and the half-lives of antibiotics, which range from 2 to 4 hours are much more similar to artemisinin compounds. Cure rates of 87% have been observed in patients treated with combinations of artemisinin drugs and antibiotics [425].

There are significant concerns that drug combinations with mismatched PK profiles will facilitate selection of parasites with drug resistance to slowly eliminated partner drugs, which may undermine the benefits of ACTs. Accordingly, drug combinations should have partner drugs exhibiting an adequate time above MIC to kill infecting parasites but not long enough to exhibit a selective window sufficiently long enough to select for resistant parasites. Given the lack of data on time above MIC, similarity in drug half-life is the only metric readily available to make an initial selection of combination partners. Drug partners with short half-lives are best to avoid issues with emergence of resistance because of exposure of reinvading parasites to sub-therapeutic drug concentrations. In recent years, the phenomenon of artemisinin 'resistance' has been identified in Southeast Asia [2]. This phenomenon, which is characterized by extended parasite clearance times, has been linked at the genomic level to mutations in the PF3D7_1343700 kelch propeller domain (K13-propeller region) [6]. This phenomenon underlines the need for partner drugs that are not also vulnerable to mutation to create new ACTs capable of treating drug resistant malaria in Southeast Asia. PK/PD data that quantitates the minimum *in vivo* concentrations of drug that are inhibitory or parasiticidal and helps define the duration of the drug selective windows will be necessary data required to design rational antimalarial drug combinations capable of preventing selection of drug resistance after initial infections are cleared.

6.3.2. Potential Effects of Mismatched Pharmacokinetics on Drug Resistance

The emergence of multidrug resistance malaria parasites has triggered the requirement for combination antimalarial treatments. This requirement for new, effective combination treatments has resulted in the combined use of antimalarial drugs that have worked in the past as monotherapies. When combinations are used, mismatched pharmacokinetics can play a role in facilitating the development of drug resistance. Use of drugs with mismatches in their PK profiles has the potential to permit evolution of sequential drug resistance to a combination treatment given the exposure of the longer half-life partner which persists as a vulnerable monotherapeutic agent (Fig. **16**). The results of mismatched pharmacokinetics can almost completely undermine the benefits of combination therapy.

One example of drug resistance to ACTs that has been shown to emerge is resistance to the combination of artemether-lumefantrine. Artemether-lumefantrine (brand name CoArtem) was one of the first fixed dose ACTs to be deployed, and data on drug resistance does suggest problems with drug resistance to lumefantrine that will cause a loss of efficacy over time [426]. In this study, parasites possessing the 86N mutation in the *pfmdr1* gene were killed by artemether-lumefantrine; however, increased tolerance to residual drug levels was shown to allow these mutant parasites to re-infect more rapidly after initial treatment, compared with parasites possessing the 86Y form of the *pfmdr1* gene. The 86N mutation in *pfmdr1* clearly provides increased tolerance to the artemether-lumefantrine combination to rather than clinical resistance, and parasites with this mutation will spread due to their ability to infect successfully people soon after drug treatment (Fig. **16**).

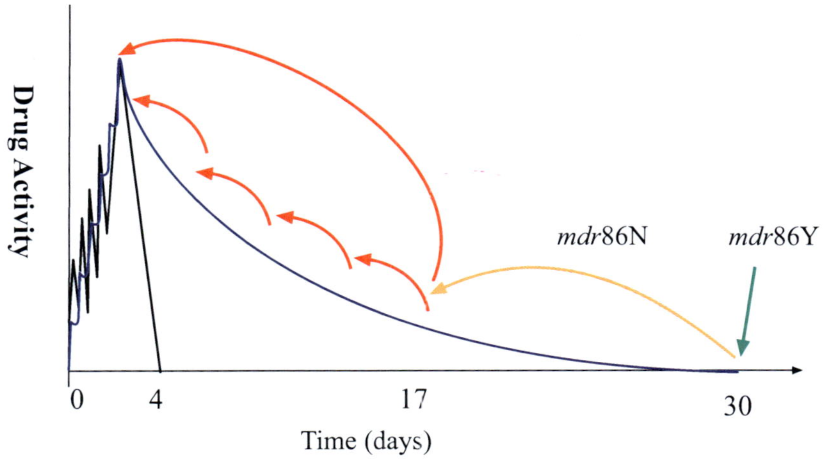

Figure 16: The graph represents the likely evolution of resistance to AL (artemether-lumefantrine), showing the drug levels in the serum of a patient starting a 3-day Coartem therapy regimen, an artemisinin-based combination therapy (ACT) comprised of lumefantrine *(blue)* and artemether *(black)*. The drugs have decayed to non-therapeutic levels when they cross the *X*-axis (defined as the concentration at which the drug, if present as a monotherapy, would be unable to prevent infection by drug-sensitive parasites). The *pfmdr1*86N mutation *(orange arrow)* increased parasite tolerance to lumefantrine allowing the parasite to infect a person 17 days post-treatment, compared with 30 days post-treatment for the *pfmdr1*86Y mutation. Two scenarios are given for subsequent mutational steps. Scenario 1 is a single large increase in drug tolerance *(red arrow),* in which the presence of artemether in the ACT is powerless to stop the spread of this mutation. The increased tolerance of lumefantrine allows it to infect a person 4 days post-treatment and to spread through the parasite population, displacing the 86N form, which can infect no earlier than 17 days post-treatment. Scenario 2 is a subsequent increase in tolerance, which occurs as a series of small increments *(black arrows);* the presence of artemether in the ACT will slow this process when it reaches day 4, and Coartem may remain clinically effective for a longer period [427].

These findings raise a new question: can ACT use accelerate development of drug resistance to artemisinin derivatives? Other data suggests the presence of the 86N mutation in the *pfmdr1* gene confers diminished sensitivity to artemisinin *in vitro* [426]. Although artemisinin or an artemisinin analogue may not select for the *pfmdr1* 86N mutation due to the intrinsic short artemisinin half-life drugs, lumefantrine, which has a longer biological half-life, is likely the main selective force on emergence of this mutation, which results in loss of sensitivity to both compounds. The results of this study underlines the idea that understanding the mechanism at the molecular level for ACT drug resistance is fundamental for maintaining the efficacy of antimalarial drugs in a combination. Since combination therapy is the best strategy for long-term malaria treatment, the conclusions that must be drawn from recent studies on artemisinin and partner drug resistance is that ACTs are not a panacea and these drug combinations may have a time-limited life span for therapeutic use. In order to maximize the useful lifetime of a therapeutic antimalarial combination, a number of measures must be taken. The first measure that needs to be considered is development of ACTs whose half-lives and time above MIC are better matched likely through use of partner drugs with half-lives shorter than lumefantrine. The second measure that should be considered is development of formal mechanisms for monitoring drug resistance to provide early indications of resistance, which will provide time to develop address regional drug resistance problems and a means to obtain the maximum benefit from ACTs [427].

Drug elimination rates of many combinations are mismatched [74]. The elimination half-life of artemisinins ranges from 0.5-2.6 hours, but the elimination half-life of pyrimethamine has been shown to range from 80-100 hours. The elimination half-life for sulfadoxine ranges from 80-100 hours, and the elimination half-life of mefloquine have been shown to range from 336- 432 hours. Accordingly, there is an extended period when sulfadoxine is "unprotected" by synergy with pyrimethamine, and there is an extended period, when mefloquine is unprotected with artesunate [152]. This sort of mismatched pharmacokinetics occurs with other combinations such as MQ+SP, AS-SP, AS-MQ, AS-AQ, DP and the combination of atovaquone-proguanil used in Asia and Africa [74, 428]. Artemisinin derivatives are protected from rapid emergence of drug resistance as these drugs circulate with a much more long-lived partner, but the partner drug is not protected by artemisinins [429].

6.3.3. PK Mismatching Has Not Yet Led to Widespread Emergence of Significant Resistance against ACTs

Other infectious diseases are commonly treated with combination therapy. One test of the PK mismatch hypothesis as a mechanism of drug resistance was conducted with *Mycobacterium tuberculosis*. Drug resistant tuberculosis is a significant issue similar to multidrug resistant malaria. One of the mechanisms that have been suggested to explain development of drug resistance is a pharmacokinetic mismatch. The hypothesis that was tested in this study was the pharmacokinetic mismatch between isoniazid and rifampin. Isoniazid has drug half-life of 6 hours, and rifampin has a half-life of 3 hours. Exposure of subpopulations of tuberculosis organisms that are resistant to both rifampin and isoniazid-resistant will result in a population of resistant microbes that grows over time.

To test this hypothesis, investigators examined the bactericidal and sterilizing effects of studies conducted with hollow-fiber-systems in experiments lasting of up to 42 days to mimic the pharmacokinetic effects of rifampin and isoniazid given to patients. Rifampin was initially administered, and then isoniazid at time intervals of 0, 6, 12, and 24 hours. Statistical analysis of the data showed that the mismatched regimens consistently killed more effectively at 12 and 24 hours than matched regimens when considering both sterilizing and bactericidal effects ($P < 0.05$). This data suggests that sequential administration or schedule ordering of combination drugs could lead to improvements in microbial killing. The authors concluded that subpopulations of bacteria that were resistant to rifampin and isoniazid were not increased due to a PK mismatch, and instead the authors concluded that a scheduled sequential administration of-tuberculosis drugs might be the best paradigm for treatment of tuberculosis. This *in vitro* study does lead to some interesting thoughts on patient treatment, which should be tested further in clinical studies [430].

Concerning antimalarial combination treatment, questions about the impact of PK mismatched therapy demand similar analysis. The fate of partner drugs in an ACT left unprotected by the elimination of an artemisinin partner drug due to a pharmacokinetic mismatch implies a selective pressure that could lead to development of parasite drug resistance and a corresponding rise in ACT treatment failures. The implications of a "pharmacokinetic mismatch" [73] are not well studied particularly in high malaria transmission regions in Africa. The best method of conducting malaria treatment to avoid providing selective pressure and discouraging emergence of drug resistant parasites is use of a partner drug with a half-life as brief as possible that provides clearance of parasite in a three-day period of treatment. This outcome is very challenging to accomplish with the drugs at hand. As discussed by Hastings and Watkins [73], drug combinations with a PK mismatch do not have a significant impact to limit the emergence of drug resistant parasites and use of mismatched drug combinations potentially may jeopardize the efficacy of component drugs where resistance has not been observed, such as the artemisinins. Therefore, drug combination ideally should have similar half-lives, which maintains dual pressure on existing and new parasites [74].

The *in vitro* susceptibility of parasites to mefloquine was followed in patients treated with the combination of AS-MQ to examine the efficacy of this drug combination in the face of drug resistance pressures. Although the combination of mefloquine and artesunate (AS-MQ) constitutes a PK mismatch, *falciparum* malaria parasites were shown to remain susceptible *in vitro* to mefloquine throughout the 5-year period of study period, and susceptibility to mefloquine has been to increase significantly. In contrast, mefloquine monotherapy was shown to result in a 40% efficacy decrease in drug susceptibility *in vivo* in the 5 years prior to this study [104]. Rates of cure with AS-MQ have been shown to be almost 100%, and AS appears to provide a protective benefit on mefloquine when both drugs are administered in a combination regimen. This protection is believed to be due to the elevated artesunate efficacy against mefloquine resistant parasites, which results in massive decreases in the parasite biomass, which, in turn, reduces the probability of selecting mefloquine-resistant parasites, and further reduces parasite transmission by reducing gametocyte carriage rates [68, 154]. All of these factors reduce the selection and differential transmission advantages of parasites with resistance to mefloquine [62]. In this study, extensive monitoring did not show evidence of a decrease in efficacy and potency of the artesunate-mefloquine combination despite the substantial PK mismatch in their half-lives [3-5, 431].

DP is an ACT with a very large PK mismatches piperaquine characterized by the longest mean terminal elimination half-life when compared to other long-lived partners (Table **24**). Given the disparity in the half-lives of DHA (rapidly eliminated in a few hours) *versus* the half-life of piperaquine (4 weeks), one would expect that DP use would result in rapid development of piperaquine resistance and a rise in treatment failures. Surprisingly, the cumulative risk of any parasitological failure, however, was greater for the AL, AS-MQ and AS-SP combinations than for DP, which may reflects the prophylactic half of long biological half-life of piperaquine. A number of trials have shown that DP is similar or superior to AL, AS-MQ, AS-AQ, and AS-SP for malaria treatment in adults and children despite a considerable mismatch in the DHA and piperaquine component drugs in Asia and Africa [389].

Another important finding that does affect the pharmacological mismatch hypothesis as applied to antimalarial drugs is clinical data that shows that mismatched combinations have regularly been associated with enhanced parasite killing compared to combinations that are better matched. From a PK perspective, artemether-lumefantrine is the best matched ACT given the short half-life of lumefantrine, which ranges from 3-6 days (Table **24**). It appears to be less efficacious, however, compared to AS-MQ in regions with multidrug-resistant parasites [76]. In one clinical trial (537 participants), the efficacy of a six-dose regimen of AL was compared to AS-MQ. No differences in day 28 parasitemia were noted, and no differences in fever or parasite clearance times were detected. There were, however, 11 parasitological failures in patients treated with AL and none with AS-MQ [344]. The results of this clinical trial suggest that AS- MQ therapy is more effective than AL therapy [386, 391]. The clinical trial data to date does not seem to support any significant impact of PK mismatch on the development of clinically relevant drug resistance and treatment failure.

Table 24: Plasma half-lives of drugs used in artemisinin-based combination therapies [388, 390-393, 405]

Antimalarials	Half-Life of Artemisinin Derivative	Half-Life of Partner Drug Per Full Adult Course (US$)	Regions Currently in Use Purchase Cost Per Course (US$)
Artemether-lumefantrine	~3 hr	4-5 days	Africa, EM, SE Asia, WP and SA
Artesunate-mefloquine	<1 hr	14-21 days	Africa, SE Asia, WP and SA
Artesunate-amodiaquine*	<1 hr	9-18 days‡	Africa and EM
Dihydroartemisinin-piperaquine	45 min	~5 weeks	SE Asia
Artesunate-pyronaridine	<1 hr	16 days	NA
Chloroquine[1]	NA	1-2 months	Africa, EM, SE Asia, WP and SA
Sulphadoxine-pyrimethamine	NA	~4 days (S) or ~8 days (P)	Africa, EM (IPT in Africa, EM and WP)

*This refers to the $t_{1/2}$ of the active metabolite monodesethylamodiaquine; the $t_{1/2}$ of amodiaquine is ~3hr.
[1]These former first-line antimalarials are included as a reference. EM, eastern Mediterranean; IPT, intermittent preventive treatment; NA, not applicable; P, pyrimethamine; S, sulphadoxine; SA, South America; SE Asia, Southeast Asia; $t_{1/2}$, half-life; WP, Western Pacific.

The rejection of the pharmacokinetic mismatch hypothesis to explain long-lived drug resistance may not be applicable, however, to all malaria areas. In regions of high transmission of malaria, use of artemisinin derivatives may not have an effect on malaria incidence. Immune individuals can harbor circulating sexual and asexual and remain symptom-free without treatment. Therefore, there is a large reservoir of gametocytes, which may be vulnerable to development of resistance because of periodic treatment with slowly eliminated partner drugs [154]. Optimal treatment plans should consider malaria transmission intensity as patients in these regions have a higher probability of acquiring new infections in the post-treatment drug clearance phase.

Treatment plans should be optimized to consider the impact of malaria transmission intensity as increases in the probability of acquiring a new infection during the post-treatment drug clearance phase translates into a trade-off between

ACT partner drugs with shorter half-lives *versus* partner drugs with longer half-lives. Exposure to new malaria infections every day may lead to use of drugs with longer half-lives as total parasite elimination may not be as important as period of post-treatment prophylaxis and this clinical benefit may be worth the increased risk of selecting for drug resistance by longer-lived drugs. In regions where transmission is low and the probability of acquiring a new infection is low, complete parasite eradication is more important, and PK mismatches between shorter lived and longer-lived drugs may not be important [417].

6.4. EFFECTS OF PD MATCHING ON THE EFFICACY AND SAFETY OF ACTS

ACTs are the malaria treatment of choice in many areas. The most common combinations consist of an artemisinin paired with a quinoline or antifolate drug. Drug combinations with other antimalarials have been tested, but they are not widely used. Combining artemisinins with quinolines has provided mixed outcomes. The different mechanisms of action should provide good drug synergy, however, the PK half-life differences observed between artemisinin drugs with short half-lives and longer-lived quinolines raise concerns over long-term problems with emergence and spread of drug resistance.

The advantages of ACTs are related to the unique properties of the artemisinin component, which include rapid reduction of the parasite biomass, swift resolution of clinical symptoms, and efficacy against drug-resistant *falciparum* malaria, decreases in gametocyte carriage and parasite transmission and limited artemisinin resistance in certain regions of Southeast Asia. Few reports of adverse events have been published regarding the ACTs; however, pre-clinical toxicology data on artemisinin compounds are limited. Combining the artemisinin component with a longer-lived partner drug provides a three-day malaria treatment rather than the seven-day period required for artemisinin monotherapy. Efficacy of ACTs is higher than the efficacy observed with artemisinin monotherapy, and the probability of drug resistance developing to both artemisinin and the partner drug is reduced. A number of studies have shown that the combination of artesunate with mefloquine has reduced drug resistance to mefloquine in low malaria transmission areas in Southeast Asia [68, 154, 361, 431]. The effects of AS-MQ or other ACTs on drug resistance in high malaria transmission areas is not yet studied. Current recommended ACTs have repeatedly shown in a variety of clinical studies that pharmacodynamically partner drugs of ACTs are well matched, efficacious, and provide protection against new infections.

6.4.1. PD Matching Between Different ACT Partners with Different Modes of Action

Artemisinins have a number of pluses over other antimalarial drugs. They act rapidly with efficacy against young ring stage parasites and more mature trophozoite and schizont parasite, and they are capable of rapidly reducing parasite burden [35]. There are some disadvantages to artemisinins as well. The artemisinin compounds are effective for a limited period as they have short half-lives. Consequently, monotherapy treatment of malaria with artemisinins for periods of less than 7 days is not effective due to recrudescence [2]. Artemisinins are paired with longer-lived partners to provide shorter, 3 day treatment periods with consistent efficacy >90%.

The best way forward to improve therapeutic efficacy and prevent drug resistance to ACTs involves using partner drugs that are novel antimalarials with different mechanisms of action from the standard list of quinoline compounds. The antimalarial activity of artemisinins is dependent upon the integrity of its peroxide bridge. Although the exact mechanism by which artemisinin compounds act has not been identified, it is believed that breaking the endoperoxide bridge of the artemisinin compounds leads to free radical damage to parasite organelles and also leads to alkylation of parasite proteins. Release of free radicals is catalyzed by intra-parasitic iron or heme, which may partly explain the selectivity of artemisinin compounds for the malaria parasite. Although the endoperoxide bridge of artemisinin and its analogues is essential for antimalarial efficacy, the intrinsic activity of the artemisinins is too great to be simply explained by nonspecific oxidative damage.

Quinolines and related compounds are believed to act by chemical inhibition of heme polymerization, a critical detoxifying pathway for the malaria parasite, [61]. Two factors are most important when choosing drug combination partners to enhance antimalarial efficacy and contain the development of parasite drug resistance: the partner drugs must have different mechanisms of action that are synergistic, and they should be matched both pharmacokinetically and pharmacodynamically. Mature schizonts and tiny rings are the most drug-resistant stages of the blood infection of *Plasmodium*. Most of the available quinoline antimalarial drugs are active predominantly on sequestered parasites that are not visible to the microscopist. The consequences of this are inhibition of trophozoite development and a considerable reduction in the parasite multiplication rate.

Artemisinin and its derivatives are peroxidic antimalarial agents, which are particularly active against ring stage parasites. The drugs of quinoline and antifolate are long acting agents killing mature parasites, while the artemisinins act quickly to kill immature parasites. This is an example of a complementary PD match between partner drugs. The combination of these two classes of drugs provides low risks of drug resistance and recrudescence, and shorter periods of treatment with increased patient compliance [14].

6.4.2. Drug Synergism and Antagonism Interactions and the Effects on PD Matching

Piperaquine was widely used as monotherapy in the 1980s until drug resistance emerged. Piperaquine is now back as a long-acting partner drug combined with DHA as an ACT. Piperaquine is highly active *in vitro,* and *in vivo* drug interaction studies have shown that dihydroartemisinin shows no antagonism when combined with piperaquine, chloroquine, and amodiaquine [99]. As a novel combination approach, retinol has been shown to be a good candidate partner with artemisinin derivatives as there is evidence of drug synergy when artemisinin is combined with retinol against *Plasmodium* [100]. There are several reports of drug synergism between artemisinins and quinine or mefloquine and this could be a result of the different but related actions of the two drugs on heme in the digestive vacuole of the *Plasmodium* parasite. Mefloquine is being increasingly combined with artemisinins in the clinic, especially in Southeast Asia where drug resistance is particularly prevalent.

Various synergistic and antagonistic interactions of artemisinins among quinolines (*e.g.*, chloroquine, quinine, mefloquine, amodiaquine) and related agents (*e.g.*, halofantrine, pyronaridine) have been reported and the picture that emerges is quite confusing. One example of such confusion lies in the reports of strain-specific antagonism between the artemisinins and chloroquine that have been reported in the literature [99] (Table **7a** & **b**). Another observation, which is somewhat consistent, is antagonism between chloroquine and mefloquine, and the related phenomenon of reciprocal susceptibility to the two agents where some strains selected for increased resistance to chloroquine have been shown to become increasingly susceptible to mefloquine [432]. Mefloquine can inhibit the uptake of chloroquine, and this fact may provide some basis for effects of drug antagonism that have been reported.

Famin and Ginsburg [433] have shown that the ability of chloroquine to cause accumulation of undigested hemoglobin in *Plasmodium* is antagonized by mefloquine. Host erythrocyte hemoglobin is normally degraded by *Plasmodium* parasites in an acidic parasite organelle, the digestive vacuole [88]. The heme component represents a toxic waste-disposal problem for the parasite, which is solved by biomineralization of heme into an insoluble complex, hemozoin. Interference with this process by chloroquine, and possibly other drugs, is believed to lead to membrane damage and death [432]. Famin and Ginsburg hypothesized that mefloquine inhibits endocytosis of the erythrocyte cytosol by the parasite, which in turn leads to reduced concentrations of free heme which chloroquine binds in the digestive vacuole [433].

Synergistic interactions have been extensively reported between combinations of antifolates, generally between an inhibitor of dihydropteroate synthase (DHPS) and an inhibitor of dihydrofolate reductase (DHFR) [88]. This synergism is so strong and so consistent that these agents are seldom used other than in combination. In spite of the long history of antifolate synergism, there is still a debate as to the mechanism of antifolate drug synergy in *Plasmodium*.

Proguanil has been shown to have strong synergism with atovaquone, and this synergism phenomenon has subsequently confirmed by others in almost all strains tested. A fixed-dose atovaquone-proguanil combination is now marketed (Malarone™) for both malaria prophylaxis and treatment indications. Interestingly, although proguanil is extensively metabolized to cycloguanil *in vivo* and the latter compound is a much more potent antimalarial than proguanil, there is no consistent pattern of synergism between atovaquone and cycloguanil (Table **7a**). Moreover, patients carrying cycloguanil-resistant strains with mutations in the DHFR gene can often still be cured with atovaquone-proguanil [434]. This suggests that the synergism of proguanil with atovaquone is limited to proguanil that has not been metabolized. Srivastava and Vaidya [435] have proposed a mechanism of atovaquone-proguanil synergism in which proguanil enhances the collapse of electrical potential across the inner mitochondrial membrane of *Plasmodium* parasites caused by atovaquone [88].

Azithromycin has been shown to be efficacious against malaria infections and when combined with faster-acting artemisinins has proven effective for treatment of *falciparum* malaria in Phase 2 clinical trials. *In vitro* studies have shown that azithromycin combined with artemisinin analogues or quinine demonstrates additive to synergistic interactions, has antimalarial activity on its own, and is not cross resistant to traditional antimalarials [102]. Using a continuous *in vitro* culture system, the sensitivity of *P. falciparum* to artemether and lumefantrine, alone and in combination, was investigated utilizing a chloroquine-resistant strain (LS-21) from India and a multi-drug resistant strain (T-996) from Thailand. Both strains showed similar 50% inhibitory concentration (IC_{50}) levels when challenged with either artemether or lumefantrine alone. When the combination of artemether-lumefantrine was tested in combination at lumefantrine ratios between 100:1 and 1:100, significant synergism was seen against both strains, especially at the IC_{90} and IC_{99} levels.

Recent experience with the simultaneous therapeutic treatment of patients infected with mefloquine-resistant *P. falciparum* using mefloquine and artemether or artesunate has shown that the earlier laboratory-based observation of synergism between mefloquine and artemisinin derivatives actually does translate into clinical reality. Such synergism has also been confirmed in a P. *falciparum in vitro* model simulating the interaction of artemisinin and mefloquine *in vivo* [103]. Preliminary pharmacokinetic information suggests that the intended oral dose regimen of artemether ($t_{½}$ of 1-2 hours) combined with lumefantrine ($t_{½}$ of 60 hours) over a 3 or 5 day period provides a brief increase in the artemether and dihydroartemisinin concentrations, while lumefantrine produced concentration increases until day 4 and a relatively slow reduction until day 7.

The additive and synergistic effects of artesunate when combined with other drugs have been tested *in vivo* in mefloquine and chloroquine sensitive and drug resistant strains of *P. falciparum*. The data derived from these combination studies have shown that artesunate and mefloquine show synergy against strains of *falciparum* malaria that are sensitive and resistant to mefloquine and a synergistic inhibitory effect against strains of *falciparum* malaria that are sensitive and resistant to chloroquine [104]. Today, it is generally accepted that additive and synergistic effects are shown *in vivo* when AS is combined with mefloquine which increase the clinical utility of both drugs, and these synergistic effects are a valuable attribute that delays the emergence of drug resistance [105]. Recently, an additive antimalarial effect was shown when doxycycline was combined with DHA in a murine malaria treatment model, and an additive antimalarial effect was noted for the combination of pyronaridine and artesunate [92, 107]. These additive and synergistic effects have helped support the recommendations made by the WHO to make ACTs the treatment of choice for uncomplicated multi-drug resistant *falciparum* malaria [23] (Table **7b**).

The synergistic effects observed *in vitro* with a new artemisinin drug, artemisone, when it is combined with lumefantrine or mefloquine are similar to synergy observed for artesunate-mefloquine, and these effects have been reproduced *in vivo*. Artesunate and artemisone have shown a similar pattern of synergistic drug interactions with standard antimalarials [106]. Another new drug, tafenoquine (TQ), a novel 3-phenoxy- substituted 8-aminoquinoline, has been shown to possess causal prophylactic, blood schizonticidal and gametocytocidal activity against rodent malaria parasites. Against the asexual, intra-erythrocytic stages of the drug-sensitive *P. berghei* N strain, it is approximately nine times as active as primaquine (PQ). TQ is from four to 100 times as active as PQ against strains of *P. berghei* or *P. yoelii* that are resistant to currently used antimalarials. In combination with chloroquine (CQ), tafenoquine and PQ have been shown to display a synergistic or 'resistance-reversing' action against CQ-resistant *P. yoelii* NS parasites. No such effects are seen when tafenoquine is combined with mefloquine against mefloquine-resistant strains or when TQ is combined with artemisinin against an artemisinin-resistant strain, and TQ has been shown to be antagonistic to halofantrine when the combination was tested against a halofantrine-resistant parasite [112].

ACTs have been used for treatment of uncomplicated malaria from more than a decade; however, clinically significant synergistic or antagonistic interactions have not been widely reported. Artemisinin compounds demonstrate wide therapeutic margins, short half-lives and the selective uptake of artemisinins by parasitized RBCs may decrease the probability of clinically relevant interactions. Large variability in the bioavailability of partner drugs like lumefantrine may overshadow the implications of synergistic or antagonistic interactions. Clinical significance of a drug interaction is not necessarily clinically observed, as the efficacy of a drug combination is the sum of the individual activities of both long acting and rapid drugs. Despite the lack of widespread clinical findings of artemisinin drug interactions, *in vitro* and *in vivo* drug interaction studies are still relevant and should be conducted for new artemisinin-based combinations particularly with novel antimalarial partner drugs and other co-administered drugs. The short half-lives of the artemisinins is an advantage in avoiding clinically relevant interactions, as concomitantly administered drugs can be administered after the artemisinin drug has cleared.

The first-generation artemisinins such as artesunate, artemether, and dihydroartemisinin have limitations including high recrudescence rates when used as monotherapy, short half-lives, and poor oral bioavailability. Second and third-generation artemisinins being developed are less expensive and have improved properties. To date, no clinically relevant drug interactions have been reported with first generation artemisinin combinations, and further investigation of drug interactions with second and third generation artemisinin drugs should be conducted. These compounds exhibit variable PD profiles, and investigation of the PK/PD relationships between artemisinin drugs with partner and concomitantly administered drugs will assist in supporting rational dosage regimen for treatment of malaria and understanding how to be better match future ACTs in terms of their PK and PD properties.

6.4.3. The Role of the Rates of ACT-Driven Parasite Killing on PD Matching

New antimalarial drugs with new mechanisms of action are needed to replace drugs lost to drug resistance and to address malaria eradication-specific objectives [436]. ACTs are under pressure due to evolving resistance to artemisinin drugs and long-term issues of drug resistance against legacy partner drugs, particularly the quinolines [437, 438]. The most pressing current need is for drugs with potency against ring stage parasites that act as quickly as the artemisinins to provide efficacious treatment of malaria with a low probability of selecting for drug resistance. Antimalarial drugs are measured by their *in vivo* properties to clear parasites, achieve cures, and avoid recrudescent infections. Killing rates against the malaria parasite can be estimated *in vivo* by calculating the parasite reduction ratio (PRR), which is defined as the ratio between the parasitemia observed when treatment begins and the parasitemia observed 48 hours later, which corresponds to one asexual life cycle of malaria [160].

The reduction in circulating infected red blood cells typically follows a log-linear curve, and the PRR can be used as a predictive therapeutic index. PRR values vary widely, and fast-killing drugs, such as the artemisinins, achieve up to a 99.99% decrease in parasitemia during a single life cycle, resulting in an *in vivo* apparent PRR of 10^3 ranging from 10^3-10^4. Slower acting drugs such as clindamycin, however, demonstrate a PRR of only 10 [266]. Beyond the parasite reduction ratio itself, the efficacy of antimalarial drugs is also dependent on the whether growth is inhibited or is parasites actually killed. Cytotoxic drugs, which actively kill parasites, are highly efficacious while cytostatic drugs, like atovaquone [439], are less efficacious and might not completely kill circulating parasites. The use of cytostatic drugs may lead to failures in treatment and selection for resistance.

Drug treatment may also directly affect metabolic pathways measured in an *in vitro* assay, without altering the viability of the parasite, which may lead to PRR measurement errors. These different situations demonstrate that metabolic activity and parasite viability are two different parameters, which are not necessarily linked, and relying on metabolism to measure viability could lead to measurement artifact and error. Moreover, assays based on metabolism do not permit directly measurement of how quickly antimalarial compounds are capable of killing, which is a crucial parameter to assess antimalarial potency and clinical efficacy. One way of estimating speed of killing more precisely is using *in vitro* methods to assess the viability of *falciparum* malaria insides the erythrocyte directly over time after drug treatment, which helps avoid some of the limitations of metabolism-based methods. *In vitro* PRR and PCT values can be estimated from these assays. In addition, the lag phase, which is the time necessary for a drug to reach the maximum kill effect, can be measured with precision [440].

1) Killing Rate of Classical Antimalarial Drugs Commonly Used as Combination Partners

One very interesting study compared the *in vitro* kill rates of standard antimalarial drugs such as the quinoline drugs, piperaquine, mefloquine, chloroquine, the amino-alcohols, pyronaridine and lumefantrine the dihydrofolate reductase inhibitor, pyrimethamine, artemisinin, and atovaquone with parasite clearance times. For all the drugs tested, the number of living parasites observed after 120 hours of drug exposure *in vitro* fell below 0.0001% of the original parasite population, suggesting that this period is an appropriate period to assess fully antimalarial activity. Two drugs showed a lengthy lag phase: pyrimethamine and atovaquone. Atovaquone demonstrated a lag phase of 48 hours and pyrimethamine showed a lag phase of 24 hours, and these drugs also were shown to be the slowest acting of those tested. Atovaquone showed a log value of parasite reduction ratio (PRR) of 2.9 and a parasite clearance time (PCT), where 99.9% of the parasites were killed, of 90 hours while pyrimethamine showed a log PRR of 3.5 and a PCT of 52 hours.

Artemisinin, on the other hand, was shown to kill much more quickly with a log PRR higher than 8 and parasite viability reduced below 0.1% in less than 24 hours. The rank of order of parasite clearance time is as follows: artemisinin is followed by pyronaridine (PRR of 4.8), lumefantrine (PRR of 4.8), piperaquine (PRR of 4.6), chloroquine (PRR of 4.5), mefloquine (PRR value of 3.7), pyrimethamine (PRR of 3.5) and atovaquone (PRR 2.9). No correlation could be made between the PRR or PCT values and the *in vitro* IC_{50} determination, which suggests there is no linkage between antimalarial potency and killing rate. Accordingly, how quickly a compound kills cannot be assessed through traditional metabolic methods of measuring parasite growth through incorporation of tritiated hypoxanthine. Experiments have shown that parasite clearance times for antimalarial drugs vary widely with 99.9% parasites cleared in times ranging from less than 24 to 90 hours. The parasite clearance time of antimalarial drugs appears to be a function of the lag phase, which is specific to the compound and PRR, and their speed of action is independent from potency [440].

2) Determination of the Optimal Drug Dose to Achieve the Maximum Malaria Kill Rate

Relatively large differences in parasite kill rates were shown in the different compounds tested in the study discussed previously. Considering that, all of these drugs were tested at concentrations of 10 times their respective IC_{50}s, these results may reflect under-dosing and, consequently, these results may underestimate kill rates for some of the antimalarial drugs tested. Atovaquone exposure at concentrations equivalent to the IC_{50}s have been shown to achieve a plateau level with constant parasitemia suggesting the killing rate at this concentration was equaled by the growth rate. Increasing the concentration of atovaquone to three times the IC_{50} was shown to decrease the parasitemia at which a growth plateau level is attained. This result suggests that atovaquone concentrations of 3 times the IC_{50} result in an overall kill effect as expansion of the residual parasites only partly compensates for the degree of killing, and the final growth plateau was reached at a parasitemia two logs below the starting parasitemia. Atovaquone drug exposure at concentrations 10 times the IC_{50} resulted in complete clearance of all parasites with a log (PRR) of 2.9 and a 99.9% PCT of 90 hours. An additional increase of 10 times the concentration of atovaquone did not increase the rate of killing seen, which suggests that the maximum kill rate for this drug is observed at drug concentrations 10 times the IC_{50}.

Pyrimethamine testing demonstrated a similar outcome and exposure of parasites *in vitro* to pyrimethamine at concentrations equivalent to the IC_{50} did not clear all parasites in the culture within 120 hours. The killing rate observed was increased over the rate observed when parasites were exposed to atovaquone at a concentration equivalent to the IC_{50} and, in fact, was similar to the atovaquone rate of killing where parasites were exposed to this drug at concentrations of 3 times the IC_{50}. This last concentration (3 times the IC_{50}) appears to be high enough, however, to reach the maximal kill rate of pyrimethamine, and the log PRR and 99.9% PCT values at this concentration were similar to those observed after pyrimethamine dosing at concentrations sufficient to achieve plasma concentrations 10 times and 100 times the IC_{50}. The artemisinin concentrations of the drug equivalent to the IC_{50} were not shown sufficiently to clear parasites within 120 hours. Kill rates similar to those observed at drug concentrations of 10 times the IC_{50} were observed in parasites exposed to artemisinin *in vitro* at concentrations as low as 3 times the IC_{50}, and the kill rates of artemisinin were not shown significantly altered when parasites were exposed to drug levels equivalent to 100 times the IC_{50}.

This data shows that the highest kill rate of all antimalarial compounds tested is reached at concentrations equal to 10 times the IC_{50}. This was found to be the case for compounds that kill slowly, as well as those that kill quickly, as illustrated by the results observed after administration of artemisinin, pyrimethamine, and atovaquone. This finding has been shown to be accurate for other antimalarial compounds, including lumefantrine and chloroquine, which were shown to achieve maximum killing rates at drug concentrations below 10 times the IC_{50}. Interestingly, concerning chloroquine, the maximal kill rate was seen at drug levels equivalent to the IC_{50}. For both pyrimethamine and atovaquone, altering the concentration of compound did not change the duration of the lag phase, which suggests the lag phase observed after treatment with these two drugs is not dependent on exposure of parasites to high drug levels but rather on the intrinsic mechanisms of compound action. In summary, this study suggests that drug concentrations of 10 times the IC_{50} are optimal doses to investigate the speed of action of antimalarial drugs at the maximum kill rate and these data demonstrate variability in the ability of antimalarial compounds to kill *falciparum* parasites [440].

3) Rate of Killing Observed in Antimalarials Correlates with the Compound Mode-of-Action

All things being equal, it is likely that the killing rates of antimalarial compounds are a function of the drug mechanism of action, and kill rate profiles represent a specific killing mechanism. To prove this possibility, the killing rate profiles (PRR and 99.9% PCT) of two different groups of compounds possessing an identical pharmacophore and target the same biological pathway were evaluated. The first set of compounds included artemisinin and two analogues, artemether and artesunate, and all of these compounds contain an endoperoxide bond responsible for antimalarial activity [441]. The second set of compounds was included drugs affecting mitochondrial function of the malaria parasite, and this set includes atovaquone, triazolopyrimidine, and pyridone. Parasites treated *in vitro* with atovaquone, triazolopyrimidine, pyridone, and artemisinin were tested for periods up to 120 hours. Given the known rapid killing action of artemisinin compounds, the response to artemether and artesunate was measured at 0 and 24 hours only. The number of living parasites observed after drug exposure was decreased by more than 4 log units for all compounds, except for pyridone, which demonstrated a delayed reduction in parasitemia when compared with triazolopyrimidine and atovaquone. This was believed due to a delay in the lag phase of pyridone to 72 hours, which is 24 hours beyond the lag phase of 48 hours observed with atovaquone exposure, as the log (PRR) values for all of these anti-mitochondrial compounds are virtually identical. The 99.9% PCTs observed for atovaquone, triazolopyrimidine, and pyridone were shown to be quite similar ranging from 90 to 108 hours.

This approach also showed atovaquone to be a slow acting compound, halofantrine was shown to be a fast acting drug, and the azithromycin was shown to be a slow acting drug. Interestingly, myxothiazol, which is an electron transport inhibitor with a similar mode of action to atovaquone, was shown to induce a similar reduction in parasitemia as atovaquone, which supports the hypothesis that parasite kill rates correlate with the antimalarial mechanism of action. These data also suggest parasite viability testing at one time point of 72 hours will reliably identify fast killing compounds among a set of possible drug candidates [440]. Further studies of this nature on a large set of antimalarials proposed for use as partner drugs in combination with artemisinins are needed to understand the results derived from current treatment and future combinations. PD matching research will also be helpful in defining the lead quality attributes of any artemisinin compounds for future replacement.

6.5. ROLE OF PK/PD MATCHING IN CHOOSING DOSAGE 3-DAY REGIMENS FOR ACTS

As recently discussed by Hastings and Watkins [73], mismatched drug combinations do not significantly affect the spread of resistance, and PK/PD mismatched ACTs have a known risk of jeopardizing the efficacy of partner drugs where resistance has not yet been widely observed, such as the artemisinins. Accordingly, the ideal drug combination would consist of drugs with similar half-lives in order to keep a constant dual pressure on current and reinvading parasites. From this perspective, drugs with short half-lives should be preferable in order to reduce the exposure of re-invading parasites to suboptimal drug levels, which may induce the selection for tolerance and eventually the development of resistance [74]. Once the artemisinin component has been eliminated, the partner drug is therefore left unprotected once the artemisinin has been eliminated from the body, and selective pressures on that partner drug will lead to development of resistance. The implications of this "pharmacokinetic mismatch" are not fully understood at present, particularly in areas of high transmission in Africa, and trade-offs between prevention of resistance and protection of patients from recrudescence and development of new infections may be considered [73]. The safest approach from a perspective of preventing development of drug resistance is to use a drug partner that has a residual half-life as short as possible, while still enabling parasite clearance with a 3-day treatment. This ideal PK matched combination may be difficult to develop given the limited range of antimalarial drugs available.

If the minimum parasiticidal concentration (MPC) is defined as the minimum blood or plasma concentration which produces maximum inhibitory activity of drug (*i.e.* the IC_{99}), then, in general, blood levels of an antimalarial drug should exceed MPC values during at least four asexual-cycles for maximum cure rates (>6 days) [6]. If the reduction in parasite biomass (parasite reduction ratio) is 1,000-fold per cycle then the MPC must be maintained for more than four cycles to ensure high cure rates. For both halofantrine and lumefantrine, the plasma concentrations 7 days after starting treatment have been shown to be a useful predictor of therapeutic outcome [241]. In the past, it was generally assumed that antimalarial blood concentrations should remain within the therapeutic range throughout the dosing interval. This has been challenged by observations that once-daily administration of artemisinin derivatives, which have elimination half-lives of <1 hour, are not associated with inferior immediate responses compared with more frequent administration [242]. In experimental animals, on the other hand, the timing of chloroquine administration to coincide with the greatest period of susceptibility in the parasite life cycle has been associated with improved parasitological clearance [165].

Artemisinin and its derivatives (artesunate, artemether, artemotil, and dihydroartemisinin) produce rapid clearance of parasitemia and rapid resolution of symptoms. They reduce parasite numbers by a factor of approximately 10,000 in each asexual cycle, which is 10 fold higher than other current antimalarials, which reduce parasite numbers in a range of 100 to 1,000-fold per cycle. Rapid elimination ensures that the residual concentrations of artemisinin do not provide a selective filter for resistant parasites, but the use of artemisinin drugs as monotherapy requires dosing for 7 days, and adherence to 7-day regimens is poor. Seven-day regimens of artemisinin derivatives have been shown to be associated with approximately failure rates of 10%. In addition, when artemisinin drugs are given in combination with rapidly eliminated compounds (tetracyclines, clindamycin), a 7-day course of treatment with an artemisinin compound is required; but when given in combination with slowly eliminated antimalarials, shorter courses of treatment (3 days) are effective. In order to be highly effective in a 3-day regimen, the terminal elimination half-lives of at least one drug component need to exceed 24 hours. Clear evidence for the superiority of ACTs over artemisinin monotherapy has been documented in a variety of clinical studies [7].

In 3-day ACT regimens, the artemisinin component is present in the body during only two asexual parasite life cycles (each lasting 2 days, except for *P. malariae* infections). This exposure to 3 days of artemisinin treatment reduces the number of parasites in the body by a factor of approximately one hundred million ($10^4 \times 10^4 = 10^8$). Complete clearance of parasites, however, is dependent on the partner medicine being effective and persisting at parasiticidal concentrations until all the infecting parasites have been killed. Thus, the partner compounds need to be eliminated relatively slowly. When artemisinin drugs are combined with slowly eliminated partner drugs, the artemisinin component is "protected" from resistance by the partner medicine provided it is efficacious and the partner medicine is partly protected by the artemisinin derivative for a limited period. ACT therapy over a period of 1-2 days is not recommended as these regimens have been shown to be less efficacious, and such a regimen provides even less artemisinin protection for the slowly eliminated antimalarial partner [2, 23].

The 3-day ACT regimen combination still provides protection against the emergence of resistance to the partner drug, but once resistance has developed, the residual concentrations of unprotected partner drug do provide a selective filter enhancing the spread of resistance to the partner compound [7]. Thus to be highly effective in a 3-day regimen, the terminal elimination half-life of at least one drug component must exceed 24 hours (longer for less active drugs) such that concentrations in the fourth drug-exposed asexual cycle (7 to 8 days after starting treatment) are still sufficient to suppress multiplication of the most resistant prevalent parasites encountered. Provided there is not high-level resistance to the partner drug, ACTs provide complete protection for the artemisinin derivatives from selection of a *de novo* resistant mutant if adherence is good, but this does leave the partner's slowly eliminated "tail" unprotected by the artemisinin derivative. Furthermore, these residual parasites are exposed to relatively high levels of partner drug and, even if susceptibility was reduced, these levels are usually sufficient to eradicate the infection. The long elimination phase "tail" of the partner drug does provide a selective filter for resistant parasites acquired from elsewhere, and thereby contributes to the spread of resistance once it has developed. Although the greatest use of antimalarials is in high-transmission areas, historically, resistance has emerged and spread most rapidly in low-transmission settings. This illustrates the important role of host immunity in delaying the emergence and spread of resistance [375].

Combinations of artemisinin derivatives given for 3 days with a slowly eliminated drug such as mefloquine (artemisinin combination treatment) provide complete protection for the artemisinin derivatives from selection of a *de novo* resistant mutant if adherence is maintained (*i.e.*, no parasite is exposed to artemisinin during one asexual cycle without mefloquine being present). This does leave the slowly eliminated "tail" of mefloquine unprotected by the artemisinin derivative as discussed in the previous paragraph. The residual number of parasites exposed to mefloquine alone, following two asexual cycles, is a tiny fraction of those present at the peak of the acute symptomatic infection. On the northwestern border of Thailand, an area of low transmission where mefloquine resistance has already had developed, systematic deployment of the artesunate-mefloquine combination therapy was shown to be dramatically effective, both in stopping resistance and in reducing the incidence of malaria [361, 421]. This strategy would be expected to be effective at preventing the *de novo* emergence of resistance at higher levels of transmission, where high-biomass infections still constitute the major source of *de novo* resistance.

6.6. IMPACT OF PK/PD MATCHING ON THE DRUG EFFICACY AND RESISTANCE OF ACTS

Drug combinations that were originally developed for Asia are now in use in Africa where higher rates of transmission are present. Future combination regimens must consider the drug mechanism of action, epidemiology of the parasite, pharmacokinetics, and pharmacodynamics, in order to maintain efficacy over time in the face of the constant threat of emergence of resistance.

6.6.1. Consideration of PK/PD matching to deter resistance to ACTs

Mefloquine was combined with sulfadoxine-pyrimethamine (SP) in Southeast Asia to provide enhanced efficacy in a region with emerging resistance to mefloquine, which had been widely used as monotherapy. This failure was predictable given the PK data showing that the half-life of mefloquine is approximately twice that of pyrimethamine and sulfadoxine that would leave mefloquine unprotected circulating mefloquine-resistant parasites encountered during its long elimination phase. By contrast, when artesunate was combined with mefloquine and used in the same region, significant reductions in mortality from malaria were observed in areas with multidrug resistant parasites, and this combination has been shown to deter and even reverse mefloquine resistance. If SP could be predicted to have failed based on a PK mismatch, why did the combination of artesunate-mefloquine succeed given the even more mismatched half-lives of artesunate (2-3 hours) and mefloquine (20 days). Mathematical modelling has suggested that given the presence of low-grade selection for drug resistance and spread of higher-level resistance is a function of the parasite's ability to survive exposure to drugs at treatment concentrations, and survival of the parasite is insensitive to drug kinetics after treatment [422].

Resistance to mefloquine may or may not follow this model, however, and artesunate has been shown to far more effective at killing malaria parasites quickly and efficiently which may explain the success of AS-MQ in Southeast Asia. The efficacy of AS-MQ has been under pressure in limited areas on the Cambodian border, and trials are in progress to understand if this is a consequence of artesunate resistance, characterized by delays in parasite clearance, decreasing efficacy of mefloquine, or other factors. Given the successful use of ACTs in Asia, these combination therapies are widely used for first-line malaria treatment in Africa, where drug resistance to SP and chloroquine resistance is rampant. There are excellent reasons to be concerned about the long-term prospect of ACTs deterring resistance in Africa given the higher rates of malaria re-infection and given that elevated consumption of antimalarial drugs will result in a larger fraction of the population with drug at sub-therapeutic concentrations after treatment in their blood. These circumstances will translate into a need for drugs whose post-treatment kinetics support inhibiting the development of resistance.

Matching PK/PD profiles to deter drug resistance is made more complex by other factors to include the period of protection and the length of the selective window of a drug in need of protection given by a partner drug, which may be altered by mechanism of action, killing rates, and other intrinsic components of a drug's antimalarial activity. For the majority of drugs, it is not clear whether killing of parasites depends on achieving drug concentrations above the minimum inhibitory concentration (MIC) or is killing dependent on the duration that that drug concentrations are sustained above the MIC, or is parasite killing dependent on the total drug exposure or AUC. As shown in Fig. **17**, even after complete antimalarial cures at initial infections with artemisinins eliminated, the partner drugs cleared more slowly for new drug resistant parasites when drug concentrations fall in an area below the minimum concentration required to kill a drug resistant parasite but are above the concentration required to deter infection with a drug sensitive parasite. This period called the selective window has been accurately characterized for lumefantrine and pyrimethamine. Pyrimethamine selects resistant parasites for 52 days while lumefantrine selects parasites for 30 days [422].

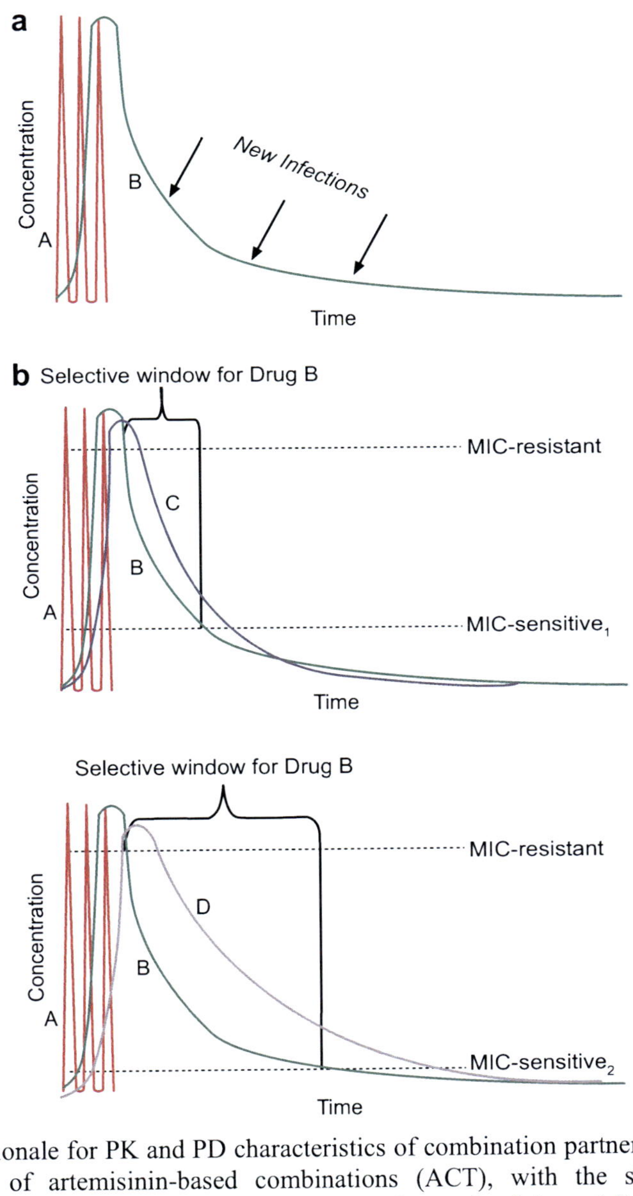

Figure 17: Rationale for PK and PD characteristics of combination partner drugs is defined. (a) A typical profile of artemisinin-based combinations (ACT), with the short-acting artemisinin derivative (Drug A, red line), eliminated quickly after each of three daily doses. Drug B (green line) should help prevent emergence of resistance to Drug A by killing parasites that evolve resistance to Drug A. Although the short-acting Drug A may reduce the probability of *de novo* resistance to Drug B emerging from the original infection, it does not prevent selection of resistant parasites that may be present in new infections occurring while selective concentrations of Drug B

persist after Drug A is eliminated. (b) MIC of Drug B for parasites that are resistant (MIC resistant) or sensitive (MIC-sensitive1) to Drug B. At concentrations of Drug B above MIC-resistant, Drug B kills both resistant and sensitive parasites. At concentrations below MIC-sensitive1, Drug B kills neither sensitive nor resistant parasites. The time during which the concentration of Drug B is between the MIC-resistant and the MIC-sensitive1 concentrations represents the time during which Drug B kills sensitive parasites but not resistant parasites and is referred to as the selective window for Drug B. This is the time when a partner drug (Drug C) is needed to prevent selection of parasites resistant to Drug B. (c) If the MIC for parasites sensitive to Drug B is lower (MIC-sensitive2), this would result in a longer selective window for Drug B, requiring a partner drug with a longer duration of action (Drug D) to protect Drug B. MICs and selective window times are undefined for most antimalarial drugs [73, 422].

The ACTs in current use include AS-SP, AS-AQ, AS-MQ, AL, and DP, which is currently the most popular ACT on market. For all of these combinations, the ACT partner drug has half-life that is much longer than the artemisinin component. All of these classic antimalarials are compromised by drug resistance in many regions of the world. While partner drugs may protect against new development of drug resistance to artemisinins by killing residual parasites surviving artemisinin treatment, and artemisinins prevent selection of partner drug resistant parasites in the original infection, long-acting partner drugs are unprotected during the post-treatment period and new drug resistant parasites may be encountered (Fig. **17**). Mathematical modeling suggests the probability of a drug resistant parasite being exposed to selective drug concentrations is entirely dependent on the fraction of patients with residual drug remaining from previous treatment not on the odds of encountering a new malaria infection in the drug clearance phase after treatment has been completed. If this model is accurate, the intensity of transmission may have no effect on selection for drug resistance [73].

Reviewing the PK/PD profiles of partner drugs in a combination is necessary as ACTs are constantly under review by policy makers to choose the best combination for use in African countries. While decreased use of drugs in Asia may resulted in temporary reversal of mefloquine resistance in that region because of implementing an AS-MQ combination, however, recent published reports show declining efficacy of the artesunate-mefloquine combination, which suggests that earlier concerns about drug combinations with large mismatches in half-life profiles may have been justified. In Africa, children have a number of malaria infections every year, it is common practice in Africa to treat all fevers with antimalarials without a diagnosis, and drug resistance to both artemisinin analogues and their partners may be accelerated. Another possibility is while treatment of malaria is more common in Africa; the fraction of parasites under drug selection pressure at one time could be lower than in Asia, as semi-immune patients in Africa commonly present with asymptomatic infections, which may encompass a large pool of malaria parasites that are not as likely to undergo drug exposure [442].

The future of artemisinin combination therapy in Africa is not easy to predict, and it may prove that artemisinin can protect its partner drugs for extended periods in Africa as in Asia or not as long or not at all. Accordingly, designs of the next generation of combination drugs should consider improvements in PK/PD matching, immunology, and epidemiology. The best choice for an ideal antimalarial partner drug will clearly require describing the selective windows of each drug and attempting to match them more closely than in first generation combinations. Understanding the patterns of drug resistance through use of molecular markers in Africa and Asia will be essential to detect the presence of emerging drug resistant parasites. One example of why this is necessary is the recently discovered disappearance of chloroquine resistance in Malawi 10 years after chloroquine was withdrawn from use [442]. This provides an opportunity to measure how well artemisinins and their partner drugs are capable of deterring the reemergence of resistance to chloroquine. Studies of changes in resistance to chloroquine may provide data to prolong the use other chloroquine analogues currently in use in drug combinations to include amodiaquine and piperaquine particularly given the success in using piperaquine to reduce the probability of new infections in regions with high transmission of malaria [378, 389].

6.6.2. The Impact of PK/PD Matching On ACT Efficacy

Selection of artemisinin doses in ACTs has historically been conducted empirically in the absence of PK and PD data. PK/PD matching of artemisinins with partner drugs has not been a topic of research particularly when artemisinins are administered as monotherapy. The treatment regimens for uncomplicated *falciparum* malaria have been based on trials designed to provide rapid symptom resolution, minimal adverse events, and prevention of recrudescent infections. In a study by de Vries *et al.*, the study authors suggest treatment of uncomplicated malaria in Southern Vietnam with quinine dosed for 7 days was efficacious [443]. The study did note a high rate of recrudescent infections, and the recrudescent infections were attributed to reduced sensitivity of malaria parasites to quinine. By adding one treatment with artemisinin to the quinine treatment regimen, both the cure rate and the parasite elimination rate were increased. To model this question, the authors utilized a nonlinear mixed-effect model to assess parasite population kinetics. The mono- exponential parasitemia decline observed was fitted to a model, and the average half-life of parasite elimination was shown to be shorter after artemisinin treatment (5.1 hours) than after quinine treatment (8.0 hours).

In this study, the model of recrudescence that was the best fit was a model showing a higher terminal parasitemia or P_{term} and a slower rate of parasite clearance. The patients treated in this study were classified using this model to groups based on P_{term}, and the outcome of their infections was shown to correlate with the model prediction in 78% of the patients. The data from this study show that *falciparum* malaria parasite with higher tolerance to quinine which is prevalent in Vietnam demonstrated higher rate of recrudescence and slower parasite clearance were rapidly cleared with a lower terminal parasitemia (P_{term}) by just one dose of artemisinin. This study also showed prevention of recrudescent infections is facilitated by treatment with quinine for at least 3 days after dosing with artemisinin [443]. In patients infected with severe *falciparum* malaria, Davis *et al.*, determined both their PK parameters and the PCT_{50} values (the duration of time required to clear 50% of infecting parasites) using serial parasite observations made after IV administration of artesunate. The data obtained from this study showed that the half-lives of DHA and AS were not altered by severity of disease, and the clearance of parasites was very swift, ranging from 6-9 hours, leading to recovery and clinical cure [347]. Patients presenting with AUC value <10 µmol/h/L were associated with a PCT_{50} >10 hours. This data does present a challenge for PK/PD modeling, and the failure of such models to describe clinical outcomes of antimalarial treatment in general and artemisinin treatment in particular is likely a consequence of the stage of parasite growth where they are active.

Using PK/PD modeling, Hoshen *et al.* hypothesized a small percentage of malaria parasites become cytostatic or dormant because of malaria drug treatment. At this stage, the growth and development cycle of the parasite is halted, which results in parasites that are not drug susceptible to further dosing until the dormant state ends. This hypothesis suggests that the antimalarial activity of AS would be slower in such cases which would result in a requirement of more frequent doses or extended treatment periods beyond the customary three days of ACT treatment. The authors derived a strategy to select appropriate models to describe antimalarial treatment [444].

In a further report, Hoshen *et al.* experimentally modeled PK data and treatment data derived from a variety of regimens utilized to treat Thai patients treated with AS combined with mefloquine. The model did not assume PD interaction between mefloquine and AS, however, the parasites in this geographic area had been shown in many studies to be mefloquine-resistant. The model demonstrated that AS or MQ monotherapy would fail to cure patients infected with *falciparum* malaria presenting with moderate parasitemia, however, the model suggested combination treatment with artesunate and mefloquine over a 3-day period would be successful. For patients infected with higher levels of parasitemia, the model suggested that 5 day treatments with the combination of mefloquine and AS would be required for cures. Simulations were conducted to examine a circumstance where decreased resistance to mefloquine was possible and re-infections would take place. Further simulations were conducted to model malaria infections in semi-immune patient populations in Africa. The predictions of this study were on target with clinical outcomes as shown in a variety of studies examining the efficacy of the AS-MQ combination. This study yielded some very useful data, and the results merit a broader use to model other ACTs [252].

Angus *et al.* studied the AS dosing regimens used to treat acute *falciparum* malaria in adult Thai patients. Patients in this study were treated with AS administered as a single dose orally, and then patients were treated with orally dosed MQ. Simulations were conducted to best fit the relationships between the dose administered, the concentrations of AS and its metabolite, DHA, measured in the plasma of patients, and the percent clearance of parasites observed (PC_{50}, PC_{90}, and PCT) to determine the proper PD model to be applied. A sigmoid inhibitory effect model was shown to provide the best fit, and considerable variation in the PC_{50} and PC_{90} values observed in patients treated with mefloquine monotherapy *versus* those treated with mefloquine and AS. A better model of the relationship between drug dose and PCT was obtained as shown in Fig. **18.** The EC_{50} required to achieve the half-maximal parasite clearance (PC_{50}) was shown to be 0.7 mg/kg, the dose required to achieve 90% parasite clearance was shown to be 1.2 mg/kg (the PC_{90}), and 1.4 mg/kg was required to achieve 100% parasite clearance (PCT). The lowest-dose extrapolated estimates for the maximum effect dose (E_{max}), however, were similar for all three variables at a dose of AS at roughly 2 mg/kg. The E_{max} was achieved at 28.6 hours, and the EC_{50} was estimated to be 1.6 mg/kg body weight. This data suggests no decrease in PCTs in patients treated with single oral doses of AS higher than 2 mg/kg, and this data reflects the average lower limit of a maximum effective artesunate dose [252].

It is not clear which PK parameter is most relevant to model the pharmacodynamic effects of artemisinin compounds. Possible parameters that may be most critical include the C_{max}, the AUC, or the time above MIC. Further studies in man will be required to understand the concentration-effect relationships of the artemisinin compounds. The current combination treatment regimen for uncomplicated malaria is to administer AS for three days at a dose of 4 mg/kg every day [78]. The available data on-hand suggests this dose provides adequate antimalarial efficacy with an acceptable safety margin. Additional studies are needed to understand the efficacy relationships between different pharmacokinetic parameters and the effects of various doses of artemisinin compounds on the period required for parasite clearance.

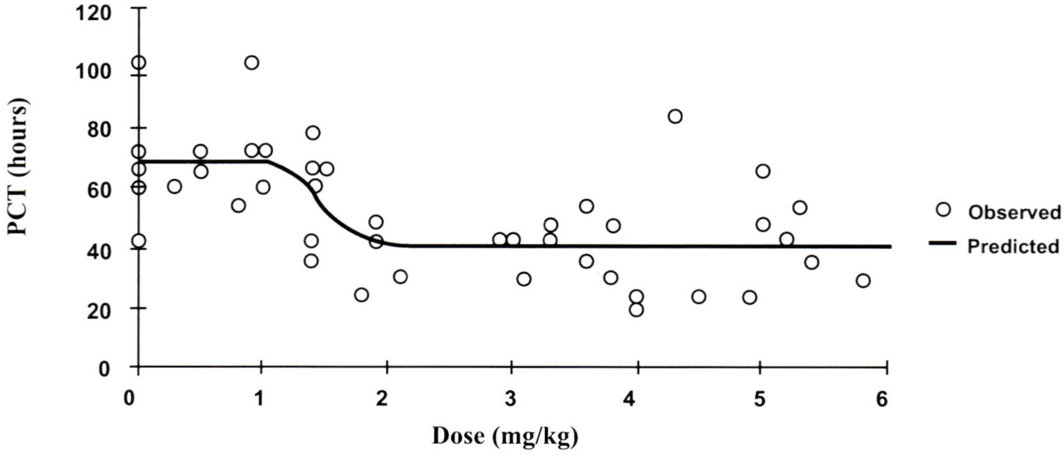

Figure 18: Relationship of oral artesunate dose to parasite clearance time (PCT) is shown [252].

6.6.3. PK/PD Matching of Artemisinins to Pick the Best Drug Partners for Combination Therapy

Studies of existing ACT combination drugs inform the PK/PD characteristics of what is available, and the next question is what PK/PD characteristics would be ideal if they were available in a next generation product. An ideal drug for malaria treatment would have enhanced activity against ring stage parasites, sustained, depot-like release, a short elimination half-life, and rapid clearance. This drug would be administered in combination with a partner drug(s) with a matching PK/PD profile to improve efficacy and deter resistance [422]. Such PK/PD characteristics would provide for rapid killing, a long period of action to facilitate administration at one encounter, and rapid clearance to avoid periods of persistent sub-lethal drug levels, which selects for drug resistant parasites.

Antimalarial compounds with longer half-lives such as mefloquine and piperaquine (half-life ranges from 2-4 weeks) are readily available but neither of these drugs offers the ideal PK/PD profile, which consists of intermittent levels of drug to "pulse" kill infecting parasites followed by rapid clearance to avoid selection of drug resistant parasites. Previous research on the use of polymers to release malaria vaccines in a pulsed release is one approach that could be applied to development of new drug products. Nanotechnology formulation may provide another method for formulating drugs possessing the ideal PK/PD profiles. Nanoparticle delivery of vaccines and drugs may offer the delivery of both products in a desired manner; however, one barrier for the use of nano-formulated delivery of drugs is the restriction in drug dose that can be delivered. Delivery of antimalarial drugs by nano-formulation will require very potent drugs delivered in a small dose. Subcutaneous implants similar to the Norplant device should also be considered.

In some epidemiological circumstances, drug with ideal PK/PD profiles may not be as important, particularly when antimalarial drugs are utilized in regions with limited malaria transmission. One case where this is relevant is mass drug administration to eradicate infectious reservoirs dosed in large numbers of subjects at the lowest malaria transmission period in areas with seasonal outbreaks of malaria. Given a low probability, a parasite would encounter sub-therapeutic drug levels in this kind of setting, there could be no problems encountered after administering a drug combination with a mismatching PK/PD profiles. This example illustrates why consideration of malaria epidemiology and settings is important when contemplating the desired drug characteristics for malaria eradication. This concept supports tailoring target product profiles (TPPs) for specific therapeutic indications based on properties of a parasite in a particular geographic area, different characteristics of human populations, and which stage of either malaria control or eradication is being targeted [436].

6.6.4. The Effects of Partner Drug Stereoselectivity on ACT PK/PD Matching

A number of drugs contain centers of structural asymmetry, and exist as enantiomeric mirror image twins, which possess non-superimposable structures. Enantiomers often have similar chemical properties, but can differ in pharmacokinetic and pharmacodynamic properties. Several of the known antimalarial drugs are chiral, and these drugs are often administered as racemates (mixtures of enantiomers). These drugs existing as racemates include quinacrine, chloroquine, mefloquine, primaquine, lumefantrine, tafenoquine, and halofantrine. Quinidine and quinine are also found as stereoisomers, although these drugs are given independently as opposed to dosing them together. The majority of these drugs have little stereoselectivity when the potency of these enantiomers are examined *in vitro*.

Mefloquine, by contrast, shows stereoselectivity *in vitro* against some isolates of *P. falciparum*, with a eudismic ratio (the ratio of pharmacologic activity of two enantiomers) of almost 2:1 in favor of the (+)-enantiomer. Additionally, for some of these drugs such as primaquine, halofantrine, and chloroquine administration of different chiral forms results in varying degrees of adverse effects. These antimalarial drugs display PK stereoselectivity leading to enantioselectivity in plasma concentrations. While the oral absorption of these drugs is not stereoselective, stereoselectivity is observed in the volume of distribution or the clearance of these drugs. Plasma protein binding of a number of antimalarial enantiomers has been shown to demonstrate a degree of stereoselectivity, which leads to stereoselective blood cell and tissue distribution.

Over the past twenty-five years, there has been increased focus on the stereoselective aspects of both the efficacy and disposition of chiral drugs as most chiral drugs on market have been shown to exhibit stereoselectivity in their PK and PD properties [445]. PK differences that result in altered blood or plasma concentration-time profiles of drug enantiomers may provide stereoselectivity in their PD properties *in vivo*. For the majority of antimalarial racemates, individual enantiomers are not readily available, and clinical trials of these enantiomers to determine a concentration-time relationship are not feasible due to the cost and effort associated with chiral separation of specific enantiomers from the racemates. The inability to test the efficacy of enantiomers of these drugs in man is one problem, which is enhanced by the differential sensitivity of parasites to antimalarial enantiomers. There are published studies on the anti-inflammatory response between different enantiomers of hydroxychloroquine when considering their concentration-effect or concentration-toxicity profiles after racemate dosing.

Tett and colleagues studied plasma concentrations of hydroxychloroquine enantiomers after racemate administration to 43 patients with rheumatoid arthritis [446]. A broad range of enantiomer drug concentrations were noted in blood samples, and determination of a therapeutic range was deemed not possible given the variability observed which were effective in treating the various symptoms of arthritis. Patients with severe arthritis, however, were shown to have higher blood drug concentrations of both enantiomers. This paradoxical finding was shown in a previous study using a non-stereo specific assay methodology [447]. This finding was caused theoretically by elevated a1-acid glycoprotein levels in these patients, which occur because of more severe inflammation, which in turn caused increased binding of hydroxychloroquine to protein, reduced drug clearance, and higher plasma and blood enantiomer concentrations in severe arthritis patients [448].

(+)-Halofantrine was shown *in vitro* to be more potent than the (-) halofantrine in inhibiting repolarizing currents when tested against feline ventricular myocytes [449]. In a follow-on study of 15 subjects dosed with 500 mg/day of (±)-halofantrine for 42 days, the connection between the QTc interval and the enantiomer concentration was assessed [450]. In 13 of the 15 subjects, a significant correlation was observed between the concentration of the (+) enantiomer and prolongation of the QTc interval. In 10 of the subjects, by contrast, a significant correlation between the concentration of the concentration of the (-) enantiomer and QTc interval prolongation was observed ($p < 0.05$). Plasma drug concentrations of enantiomers measured after administration of the racemate covaried, which led to significant difficulties trying to determine which enantiomer is associated with cardiotoxicity. The regression coefficients were noted to be higher for the (+)-enantiomer than for the (-)-enantiomer in 80% of volunteers, and the data seems to suggest a stronger association between the (+)-enantiomer concentration and prolongation of the QTc interval [576].

To date, the relationship between stereoselectivity of chiral antimalarial drugs and their associated PK and/or PD profiles is not well understood. Concerning antimalarial potency, with mefloquine as the exception, stereoselectivity has not been shown *in vitro*. PK differences may occur between malaria drug enantiomers, which can lead to stereoselectivity in their PD effects observed *in vivo*. In addition to the antimalarial effects that are noted for a particular enantiomer, the effects of stereoselectivity may also be responsible for other PD effects observed. Given a the small number of drugs on market, with the complications of drug resistance limiting use of certain antimalarials, understanding antimalarial drug enantioselectivity may be worthwhile to maximize use of drugs that exist now to enhance patient treatment outcomes and reduce emergence of drug resistant parasites. The data achieved by testing stereoselective drugs may enhance our understanding of drug mode of action and it could be used to optimize clinical efficacy and safety.

Chapter 7: PK/PD Modeling of Antimalarial Drug Combinations

CHAPTER 7

PK/PD Modeling of Antimalarial Drug Combinations

Abstract: The mass-action law, the equilibrium law, and the absolute reaction rate theory have all had an impact on the mathematical modeling of biological interactions, and these fundamental discoveries are the foundation for PK/PD modeling. These physicochemical approaches are very useful tools to help understand mathematically the interaction of drugs and combinations with biological systems. Theories have been developed that can be applied to understand a variety of biological applications based on these laws. Accordingly, the algorithms for computer- based analysis and simulation based on these principles been created. Modeling and simulation are important elements in decision making by regulatory agencies affecting both industry and the public. PK models exist to assemble all of the data derived from both nonclinical and clinical studies that have been performed in the drug development process, which provides a means to guide future studies with predictive models. Physiologically based PK (PBPK) models differ from classic PK models due to their incorporation of specific tissue compartments associated with exposure, biotransformation, toxicity, and clearance that are all connected through the flow of blood. The objective of PK/PD modeling as applied to antimalarial drug development is to develop and apply models to characterize pharmacokinetic parameters reflecting the concentration of drug over time and the pharmacodynamic relationships, which describe the effect of drugs with respect to drug concentration. PK modeling elements describe the distribution and clearance kinetics of a drug at the macro level. Adding a PD component to this model adds a drug effect element to characterize drug combination *in vivo*. These models can assist in choosing appropriate combination partner drugs or alternate first-line treatments for treatment of malaria in a given transmission setting, which may be relevant to malaria eradication efforts.

Keywords: Antimalarial policies, computerized simulation and analysis, drug combination, efficacy, mathematical modeling, model, modeling, modeling theory, PBPK/PD modeling, PD modeling, PK modeling, PK/PD modeling, resistance.

Nonclinical studies and clinical trials show drug safety, efficacy, and the PK/PD properties of a new drug tested under very well controlled circumstances in populations that are relatively homogeneous. These kinds of studies generally do not answer relevant questions about population variability in ways that predict PK/PD activity for larger groups, which affects safety and efficacy. Semi-physiological clinical PK/PD modeling and simulation offers the possibility of utilizing data obtained in the laboratory and the clinic to make accurate characterizations and predictions of PK/PD activity in the target population based on variability in predictive factors.

Qigui Li and Mark R. Hickman

Modeling and simulation have the potential to be important tools in all phases of drug development from preclinical through clinical and post-marketing phases providing scientific evidence upon which to base key decisions during all stages of a product's life cycle. Modeling and simulation are dependent on use of statistical models that provide simple descriptions of physiology that are actually quite complex. Although modeling and simulation have been carried out successfully within the pharmaceutical industry for some time, they were not implemented in clinical trials until the early 1980s when the notion of therapeutic drug monitoring became more widely used. FDA regulatory authorities began to notice some years ago that registration packages for new chemical entities lacked exposure and PK information in target patient populations, and they began requesting these types of data. Advances in the application of estimation methods including maximum likelihood and, in particular, nonlinear mixed effects modeling in the 1970s, enhanced the utility of PK/PD modeling and simulation, and demonstrated how they could be used as useful tools for new drug development. The release of the nonlinear mixed effects modeling software, NONMEM, in 1980 was a major milestone. Numerous successful applications have shown the utility of the NONMEM model for PK/PD data analysis, particularly for sparse data derived from a large number of people, which gave rise to the concepts of population pharmacokinetics or the population approach.

At the same time, methods to predict human pharmacokinetic parameters based on pre-clinical data were also being rapidly developed as new tools for down-selection of candidate drugs. In an environment of high throughput testing to identify compounds with potency, it is essential to have methods that can be used to predict human PK characteristics. Data such as ionization, lipophilicity, protein binding, solubility, metabolic stability upon exposure to liver microsomes, and membrane permeability can be utilized as data to be inputted to predict PK parameters to include the amount of drug absorbed, the fraction of drug metabolized and drug tissue distribution. These PK parameters are useful to make predictions on the concentration of drug over time for novel chemical entities, particularly, in the blood and tissue compartments. Physiologically, based pharmacokinetic (PBPK) models were actually being used in pre-clinical drug development to enhance understanding of the complex interactions of biological and physiologic parameters that affect drug behavior at the molecular level in multiple physiologic compartments. Compared to standard compartmental models, PBPK model are designed to simulate a more physiologically oriented description of the system under investigation. A PBPK system that simulates the PK environment in a physiological model has clear advantages over a PK model that does not [451].

7.1. THEORETICAL BASIS FOR MATHEMATICAL MODELING OF DRUG COMBINATIONS

The administration of drug combinations comprised of partner drugs with different modes of action can result in enhanced drug efficacy against a disease. An example of this is drug synergy where the combination of drugs has a greater effect than each component. The potential positive synergy outcomes include: 1) increasing therapeutic efficacy; 2) increasing or maintaining efficacy with a decreased dose to minimize toxicity; 3) minimizing emergence of drug resistance and 4) provide enhanced synergy selectively against a specific drug target or enhancement of efficacy (also known as efficacy synergism). An unfavorable outcome of a drug combination may also be synergism to antagonize the host where a drug combination has enhanced toxicity over the toxicity observed with each component. To achieve maximum therapeutic benefits, combinations of drugs have become widely used treatments for diseases such as cancer and infectious diseases such as HIV, TB, and malaria.

7.1.1. The Impact of the Law of Mass Action, Equilibrium Reactions, and Reaction Rate Constants on Mathematical Models

The law of mass action, the equilibrium law, and the absolute reaction rate theory can be used to conduct mathematical modeling of biological interactions. The equilibrium and steady state approaches, for example, when applied at a constant temperature and pressure, have been very useful for modeling enzyme kinetics and receptor-ligand interactions. These physicochemical methods are excellent tools to help understand mathematically the interaction of drugs with biological systems. Theories have been developed based on the principles that can be applied to describe a variety of biological systems, and algorithms for computerized modeling and simulation have been developed based on these theorems.

Most drugs used in man inhibit enzymes, receptors, or pathways. Enzymatic pathways provide a clear means of understanding the effects of drugs on pathway components, and the kinetics associated with each drug-enzyme interaction. Introduction of drugs that act as enzyme competitors affects enzyme kinetics and this, in turn, can lead to other equations to describe each enzyme kinetic interaction. The specific equations are more easily solved using the ratio of reaction rates measured when an inhibitor is present (v_i) and (v_0) when an inhibitor is absent. This ratio f_i/f_u describes the fraction of drug that is not inhibited (f_u). The ratio of f_i/f_u or $(1 - f_u)/f_u$ is equal to $[(f_u)^{-1} - 1]$ or $[(1 - f_u)^{-1} - 1]^{-1}$, where $1 - f_u = f_a$, and that provides a solution for the fraction of compound that is affected or inhibited. Taking this relationship further, the ratio of $(1 - f_u)/f_u$ (is equivalent to the ratio of $(I/IC_{50})^m$, (m is the kinetic order).

In addition, further derivation gives this relationship to define the amount of enzyme an inhibitor can combine with: $K_i/I_{50} = E_x/E_t$, (E_t is the total quantity of enzyme, and E_x is the fraction of enzyme available). This enzyme-inhibitor relationship will hold regardless of the total number of enzyme products or substrates or their mechanisms of reaction, and this relationship is not affected by the inhibition mechanism. Accordingly, this method will result in cancellation of kinetic constants like K_m, K_i, or V_{max}, which leaves only the relationship of dose and effect of the enzyme inhibitor [87].

A systematic analysis utilizing the classic kinetic enzyme-substrate-inhibitor interaction models showing enzyme-substrate interactions with a variety of inhibitory mechanisms and an array of mechanisms of reaction. For all of the enzyme systems analyzed, the fractional velocity (f_v) and fractional inhibition (f_i) when inhibited by an inhibitor (I) can be shown as follows:

$$f_v = [1 + (I/K_i)(E_x/E_t)]^{-1} \text{ and } f_i = [1 + (K_i/I)(E_t/E_x)]^{-1}, \qquad (0)$$

where K_i is the dissociation constant of the enzyme-inhibitor, E_t is the total enzyme amount, and E_x is the enzyme available for combination with an inhibitor. The ratio of E_x/E_t can be expressed mathematically using a distribution equation to describe each enzymatic mechanism of reaction and each enzymatic mechanism of inhibition. By definition, $f_v = v_i/v$ and $f_i = (v - v_i)/v$, where v_i is the reaction velocity in the presence of an inhibitor and v is the reaction velocity in without an inhibitor. Further derivation provides another relationship: $K_i/I_{50} = E_x/E_t$ (I_{50} equals the concentration of I, the inhibitor, required for 50% inhibition). Given this relationship, K_i cannot be greater than I_{50}, and the ratio of K_i and I_{50} defines the distribution of an enzyme in an enzymatic reaction conducted under a particular set of conditions.

The median-effect equation is a simple method of describing the relationship between dose and effect, which is given by $f_a/f_u = (D/D_m)^m$ where, D defines the drug concentration, f_a defines the percent inhibition or fraction affected and f_u is the fraction not affected calculated by subtracting f_a from 1. D_m is defined as the median-effect dose such as the ED_{50} or the IC_{50} which actually causes a 50% inhibitory effect, and m is a coefficient which defines the dose-effect relation curve shape (if m = 1, a hypberbolic curve is indicated, m > 1 indicates a sigmoidal curve, and m < 1 indicates a flat sigmoidal dose-effect curve). How well the data conforms to a plot of median-effect is assessed by using the linear correlation coefficient (r) where a coefficient of r = 1 equals the best conformity possible. Using the median effect principle to define the relationship between dose and effect is quite different from standard methods where an empirically derived curve is used to fit an array of scattered points. Empirically defined curves are not necessarily capable of drawing a curve for two well-determined data points, while drawing a curve between two points is readily accomplished using the median-effect principle. These empirical or statistical approaches can be enormously difficult to apply in complicated situations such as the evaluation of drug combinations [87].

7.1.2. Extension of the Mass-Action Law to Systems with Multiple Drug-Effects

1) Combination Drug-Effect Equations

The median-effect equation for one drug can be utilized for a number of drugs, and for a combination of two drugs in a first-order system (when m = 1), the following equation is derived:

$$\frac{(f_a)_{1,2}}{(f_u)_{1,2}} = \frac{(f_a)_1}{(f_u)_1} + \frac{(f_a)_2}{(f_u)_2} = \frac{(D)_1}{(D_m)_1} + \frac{(D)_2}{(D_m)_2} \qquad (1)$$

D is the drug concentration, f_a defines the percent inhibition or fraction affected), and f_u is the fraction that is not affected. D_m is defined as the median-effect dose such as the ED_{50} or the IC_{50}, which actually causes a 50% inhibitory, and m is the coefficient, which defines the dose-effect relation curve shape as discussed previously.

When $m \neq 1$, then

$$\left[\frac{(f_a)_{1,2}}{(f_u)_{1,2}}\right]^{1/m} = \left[\frac{(f_a)_1}{(f_u)_1}\right]^{1/m} + \left[\frac{(f_a)_2}{(f_u)_2}\right]^{1/m} = \frac{(D)_1}{(D_m)_1} + \frac{(D)_2}{(D_m)_2} \qquad (2)$$

Equations 1 and 2 are derived based on two drugs actually having the same mechanism of action with different effects, which is the same assumption, made when graphing a classic isobologram of the effects of two drugs dosed together. If it is assumed two drugs in a combination actually have dissimilar mechanisms of action and different effects, a third equation applies derived from the first two:

$$\left[\frac{(f_a)_{1,2}}{(f_u)_{1,2}}\right]^{1/m} = \frac{(D)_1}{(D_m)_1} + \frac{(D)_2}{(D_m)_2} + \frac{(D)_1(D)_2}{(D_m)_1(D_m)_2} \qquad (3)$$

Given cases that are not purely exclusively different mechanisms of action, equation 3 may underestimate drug interactions that are synergistic, and one might conclude that Equation 2 constitutes the foundation equation and a condition affecting synergy should be addressed using

Equation 2. Combinations of two drugs that are then diluted serially actually behave as a third drug when considering the relationship between dose and effect. Accordingly, $y = \log [(f_a)_{1,2}/(f_u)_{1,2}]$ *versus* $x = \log [(D)_1 + (D)_2]$ will give $m_{1,2}$, $(Dm)_{1,2}$ and $r_{1,2}$ [87].

2) The Combination Index Equations, Theorem, and Plot

Using Equations 1 and 2, Chou created a new term called the combination index (CI) to estimate synergy or antagonism for two drugs in a combination

$$CI = \frac{(D)_1}{(D_x)_1} + \frac{(D)_2}{(D_x)_2} = \frac{(D)_1}{(D_m)_1[f_a/(1-f_a)]^{1/m_1}} + \frac{(D)_2}{(D_m)_2[f_a/(1-f_a)]^{1/m_2}} \quad (4)$$

where $CI < 1$, suggests drug synergy, $CI = 1$ suggests additive effects, and a $CI > 1$ suggests drug antagonism. In the denominator, (D_x) defines D1 "alone" inhibiting a system by x%, and $(D_x)_2$ defines D2 "alone" inhibiting a system by x%. $(D)_1 + (D)_2$ in the numerator "in combination" describes inhibition of a system by x%. A combination index equal to 1 defines an additive drug effect, and a combination index value less than 1 suggests drug synergy. Combination index values greater than 1 suggest a drug antagonism effect.

Plots of the combination index on the y-axis with effect levels on the x-axis (f_a) are called f_a-CI plots or CI plots [87]. Combination index values for drug synergy extend from 0 to 1, and combination index values for drug antagonism extend from 1 to infinity. The plot of f_a-log(CI) helps handle off-scale points in a f_a-CI plot and also provides a symmetrical plot where additive effect are set at zero *i.e.*, $\log(CI) = \log(1) = 0$]. Accordingly, in the f_a-log(CI) plot, drug synergy is shown by a value that is negative [*i.e.*, $\log(CI) < 0$], and drug antagonism is reflected by values that are positive [*i.e.*, $\log(CI) > 0$]. Therefore as shown in equation 4, when the combination index = 1, the classic isobologram for two drugs at their ED_{50} is defined as:

$$\frac{(D)_1}{(D_m)_1} + \frac{(D)_2}{(D_m)_2} = 1 \quad (5)$$

and the ED_x isobologram for two drugs providing x% inhibition is defined as:

$$\frac{(D)_1}{(D_x)_1} + \frac{(D)_2}{(D_x)_2} = 1 \qquad (6)$$

Fig. (**19**) shows a classic drug combination isobologram and shows an isobologram normalized by dose. Isobolograms derived from drug combination studies that are typically obtained and are shown and interpreted in Fig. **20b** and **20c**.

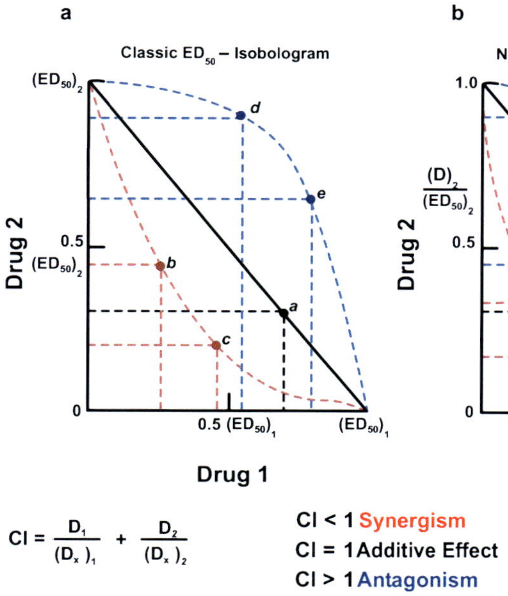

Figure 19: The ED_{50} isobologram is shown in figure a, classic isobologram for two drugs with actual doses on the x- and y-axis. b, dose-normalized isobologram for two drugs with normalization of dose with ED_{50} to unity on both x- and y-axis. In both cases, the ED_{50} can be extended to EDx for the X% inhibition. The isobol holds irrespective of the combination ratio or shapes of dose-effect curves and irrespective of the mechanisms of the drugs or the units the drugs. If the combination data points fall on the hypotenuse (*e.g.*, point a), an additive effect is indicated. If the combination data points fall on the lower left (*e.g.*, points b and c) or on the upper right (*e.g.*, points d and e), synergism, or antagonism is indicated, respectively. If the combinations are in a constant ratio, the classic isobologram (a) can be constructed with a stroke of the key using computer software [87]. If the combinations are in non-constant ratios, the normalized isobologram (b) can be constructed automatically (see Fig. **8, b** and **c**). The constant-ratio combination design [*e.g.*, at $(ED_{50})/(ED_{50})_2$ ratio] is recommended. Multiple dose-effect data points for each drug alone is a prerequisite for drug combination studies so that m_1, $(D_m)_1$, m_2, and $(D_m)_2$ values can be determined, whereas the number of the combination data points can be one or more [87].

Equations describing the effects of multiple drugs are derived from the median-effect principle, which leads to the equation defining the combination index. The equation describing a combination of 5 drugs which provide x% inhibition is as follows:

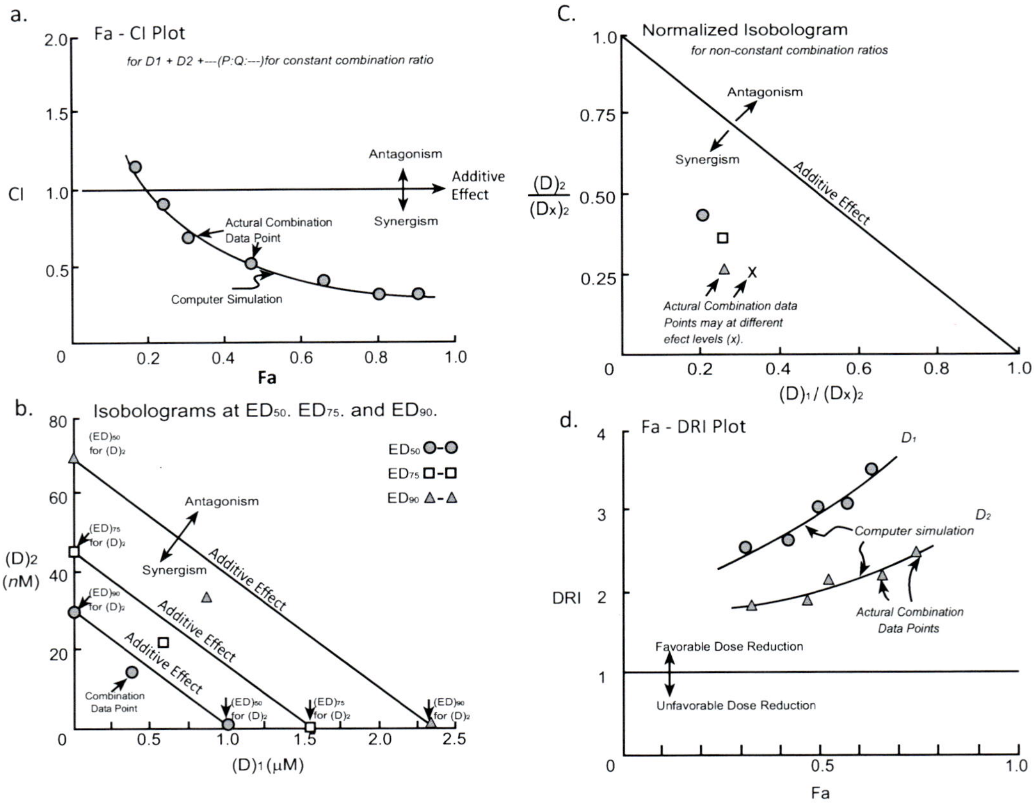

Figure 20: Typical examples of drug combination plots and their interpretations based on the Chou and Talalay combination index theorem. a, Fa-CI plot. b, classic isobologram at ED_{50}, ED_{75}, and ED_{90}. c, normalized isobologram for combination at different combination ratios, and d, the Fa-DRI plot. All of these plots can be generated automatically by using CompuSyn [87].

$$
\begin{aligned}
{}^{5}(\mathrm{CI})_{x} = {} & \frac{(\mathrm{D_x})_{1-5}[\mathrm{P}/(\mathrm{P}+\mathrm{Q}+\mathrm{R}+\mathrm{S}+\mathrm{T})]}{(\mathrm{D_m})_1\{(f_{a_x})_1/[1-(f_{a_x})_1]\}^{1/m_1}} \\
& + \frac{(\mathrm{D_x})_{1-5}[\mathrm{Q}/(\mathrm{P}+\mathrm{Q}+\mathrm{R}+\mathrm{S}+\mathrm{T})]}{(\mathrm{D_m})_2\{(f_{a_x})_2/[1-(f_{a_x})_2]\}^{1/m_2}} \\
& + \frac{(\mathrm{D_x})_{1-5}[\mathrm{R}/(\mathrm{P}+\mathrm{Q}+\mathrm{R}+\mathrm{S}+\mathrm{T})]}{(\mathrm{D_m})_3\{(f_{a_x})_3/[1-(f_{a_x})_3]\}^{1/m_3}} \\
& + \frac{(\mathrm{D_x})_{1-5}[\mathrm{S}/(\mathrm{P}+\mathrm{Q}+\mathrm{R}+\mathrm{S}+\mathrm{T})]}{(\mathrm{D_m})_4\{(f_{a_x})_4/[1-(f_{a_x})_4]\}^{1/m_4}} \\
& + \frac{(\mathrm{D_x})_{1-5}[\mathrm{T}/(\mathrm{P}+\mathrm{Q}+\mathrm{R}+\mathrm{S}+\mathrm{T})]}{(\mathrm{D_m})_5\{(f_{a_x})_5/[1-(f_{a_x})_5]\}^{1/m_5}} \qquad (7)
\end{aligned}
$$

The equation which describes a combination of n-drugs providing x% inhibition is as follows:

$$^{n}(CI)_x = \sum_{j=1}^{n} \frac{(D)_j}{(D_x)_j} = \sum_{j=1}^{n} \frac{(D_x)_{1-n}\{[D]_j/\sum_1^n[D]\}}{(D)_m)_j\{(f_{a_x})_j/[1-(f_{a_x})_j]\}^{1/m_j}} \tag{8}$$

Where $^{n}(CI)_x$ defines the combination index applying to n number of drugs providing x% inhibition. $(Dx)_{1-n}$ is the total dose provided by n number of drugs providing inhibition of x% when combined. $\{[D]_j/Sn1\ [D]\}$ defines the proportion of the dose provided by each of the n drugs providing inhibition of x% when combined. The equation $(D_m)j\{(f_{ax})_j/[1-(f_{ax})_j]\}^{1/mj}$ defines the dose for each drug by itself which inhibits by x%. D_m defines the median-effect dose, f_a defines the fraction inhibited at x%, and m defines the slope of the median- effect plot as previously described [87].

3) Algorithms for Determining Synergism and Antagonism

Effects of combination drug treatment are thus generally grouped into three categories. Synergistic effects are noted where a combination of drugs provide an effect that is larger than the effect of each drug by itself. Additive effects are noted where the combination of drugs provides an effect which is the same as their effects by themselves, and antagonistic effects are noted where the combination of drugs shows decreased activity compared to their effects when dosed alone. Chou [87] discussed strategies for assessing and simulating the effects of drugs in combination defined by the Combination Index as discussed previously and shown in Table **25**. In another method, the calculation of the effects of drugs e in combination can be defined by calculating a "Q" factor as shown in Table **25** [452].

Equations 4 and 8 defining the combination index can be used to define an algorithm to automate calculating combination index values for different levels of effect or f_a levels. Automated calculation of CI values has been defined using calculations shown in Fig. **(21)** [87].

4) Main Characteristics of the General Equation

The overall theory of dose and effect is defined in equation 9 and the combination index theory is shown in equation 8, including equations 1-6. Thus, for each drug entity, the units of report are canceled out and the derived value from these equations is without units which makes these equations so useful. As previously mentioned, fractional velocity (f_v) and fractional inhibition (f_i) involving an inhibitor (I) can be calculated as shown in Equation 9:

$$f_v = [1 + (I/K_i)(E_x/E_t)]^{-1} \quad (9)$$

where, K_i is the dissociation constant of an enzyme-inhibitor, E_t defines the overall amount of enzyme, and E_x is the amount of available enzyme for combination with an inhibitor. The ratio E_x/E_t is calculated using a distribution equation for each enzyme reaction mechanism and for each inhibitor inhibition mechanism. By definition, $f_v = v_i/v$ and $f_i = (v - v_i)/v$ and v_i is the velocity of a reaction when an inhibitor is present and v defines the enzyme velocity without an inhibitor. In addition, as the CI equation is without units, D_1 could be concentration of drug in micro-molar values, D_2 might be defined in units of mg/ml, D_3 could be in standard international units, and so on. Interactions between these drugs can be defined as drug synergy, antagonism or additive effect as long as the linear coefficient shows to the relationship conforms to the principle of mass-action (*e.g.*, r > 0.95).

Table 25: CI and Q Calculations to Determine Effects of Combinational Drug Therapy [452]

CI Calculation[1]	Combination Index[2]	Effects of Combination Drug Therapy
$^n(CI)_x = \sum_{f=1}^{n} \frac{(D)_j}{(D_x)_j}$	< 0.1	Very strong synergism
	0.1-0.3	Strong synergism
	0.3-0.7	Synergism
	0.7-0.85	Moderate synergism
	0.85-0.90	Slight synergism
	0.90-1.10	Nearly additive
	1.10-1.20	Slight antagonism
	1.20-1.45	Moderate antagonism
	1.45-3.3	Antagonism
	3.3-10.0	Strong antagonism
	>10	Very strong antagonism
Q Calculation	Q Value	Effects of Combination Drug Therapy
$Q = \frac{Ea + b}{(Ea + Eb - Ea \times Eb)}$	$Q \leq 0.85$	Synergism
	$0.85 \leq Q < 1.15$	Additive
	$Q \geq 1.15$	Antagonism

[1]Mass-action law based computer software: CalcuSyn (earlier version) and CompuSyn in Windows format. [2]Combination index (CI): A quantitative measure based on the mass-action law of the degree of drug interaction. n(CI)x: The combination index for n drugs at x% inhibition; Dose (D): Effective dose used in combinational drug therapy; n: Refers to numbers of drugs or compound used in combinational drug therapy; Dose X% (Dx): signify the potency of each drugs that inhibits a cell system x%; A: drug A; B: drug B; Ea+b: average effect of combinational treatment; Ea: average effect of drug A only; Eb: average effect of drug B only.

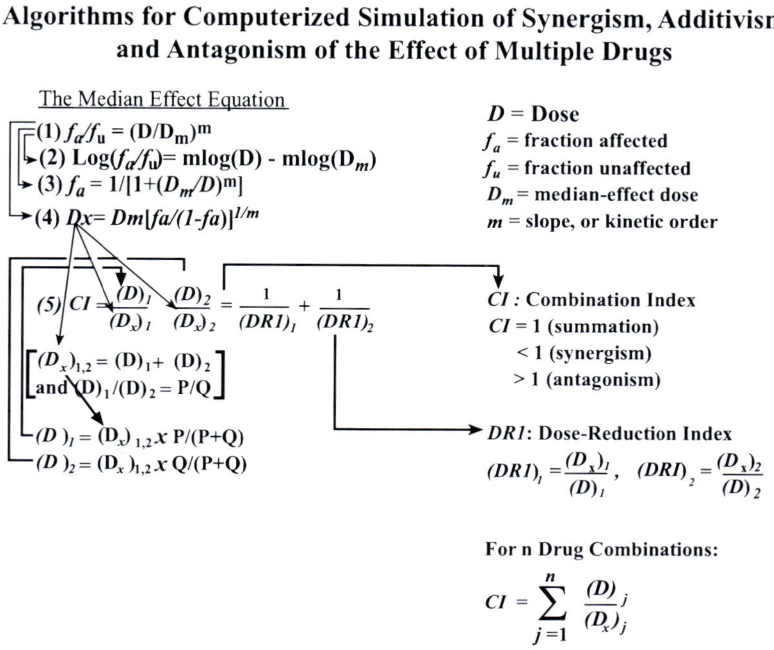

Figure 21: Algorithms for computerized simulation of CI plot and DRI plot at different effect levels (fa values). The combination ratio for $(D)_1$ and $(D)_2$ is designated as P/Q. Both plots are valid irrespective of the number of drugs combined, the combination ratios, the mechanisms of drugs, and the units of the drugs and irrespective of the nature of the targets. These algorithms are the basis for computer software such as CompuSyn that automates CI calculations [87].

These equations can also be used to calculate the effects of known compounds with novel chemical entities with unknown structures or mechanisms of action. It is also possible to combine mixtures of compounds with each other and determine a drug interaction. The applications of these equations have been extended to combinations of drugs administered for cytotoxicity studies where the combinations were studied under a variety of oxygen tension conditions. Using the combination index theorem, drug synergy or antagonism can be assessed with minimal data of as long as the parameters of m and D_m for each drug are defined by the median-effect plot. These equations provide for calculation of drug effects based on the simplest set of dose-effect situations which affords savings in the number of animals required for study, the effort involved, the time required, and the cost necessary [87].

5) The Drug Combination Index Plot and Isobologram

An isobologram is a graph showing the sum of equally potent doses, and this method was innovated approximately a hundred years ago. In past years, scientists were forced to graph dose effect curves on paper, however, today, isobol equation and the median-effect principle to quickly graph isobolograms showing different levels of effect ranging from a 50% inhibitory or effective dose up to a 95% inhibitory or effective dose for drug combinations in a matter of seconds (Fig. **19**).

The f_a-CI plot and the isobologram should yield identical results for drug combination research as both plots are derived from the same equation for a combination index; the isobologram is oriented toward dose while the CI plot is oriented toward effect. Isobologram plots and f_a-CI plots are closely related, however, the isobologram plot does have one critical limitation-plots in two dimensions can be shown easily, which works well for a combination of two drugs, however, plots of three or more drugs using an isobologram plot are difficult to perform and hard to interpret. CI plots, on the other hand, can be viewed at all f_a levels at the same time with any combination of n number of drugs desired [87].

$$\sum_{j=1}^{n} = \sum_{j=1}^{m} + \sum_{j=m+1}^{n} \quad (10)$$

Where $1 \leq m \leq n - 1$ and n and m are integers. Second, if two-drug isobolograms are shown at three or fewer effect levels (*e.g.*, at ED_{50}, ED_{70}, and ED_{90}), usually the graph will be readable by inspection, however, if an isobologram were to be constructed for four or more effect levels, it would usually be too messy to read because of data scattering or data point congestion or overlapping.

6) How Relevant are Calculated Predictions of Drug Synergism?

There are many reports in the literature of combinations of drug synergy when one drug is combined with another. This claim may well be valid based on certain experimental conditions to include the cell line used, the species of the cell line, the sequence of drug addition, the incubation temperature, *etc*. For some diseases, drug synergy or antagonism may be relevant at lower dose or effect levels, however, for infectious disease treatments; synergy at high levels of effect is more relevant to a treatment outcome. Accordingly, drug synergy or antagonism at varying levels of effect may be more or less relevant depending on which disease is being treated. In addition, drug synergy toward an infectious organism and drug antagonism against a host is clearly important, and the practical considerations on whether synergism can be achieved physiologically at non-toxic drug levels are important. In previously published work, Chou and Ghavami [87, 451] suggested a semi-quantitative technique to describe drug synergy or drug antagonism (Table **25**).

To provide relevant information regarding synergy and antagonism at different levels of effect, many publications require the CI and dose-reduction index (DRI) values to be shown for the ED_{50}, ED_{75}, ED_{90}, and ED_{95} levels.

7.2. THE USES OF PK, PD, AND PBPK/PD MODELING IN DRUG DEVELOPMENT

7.2.1. Advances in PK Modeling

Pharmacokinetics is focused on modeling underlying biological processes involved in drug disposition. Pharmacokinetics describes physiological processes associated with drug absorption, drug distribution, drug metabolism, and drug clearance or elimination (ADME). Characterization of these processes is essential to understanding patient-drug interactions, drug-drug interactions, and effects of environment and disease on exposure to drugs. Pharmacokinetic studies provide a holistic view of how drugs are processed by the human body aids us in the developing dosing regimens tailored to different subpopulations. Pharmacokinetic studies are enhanced by advances in computer technology, analytical methods, and pharmacogenetics. New computer systems with enhanced computational abilities coupled with more advanced software has provided new avenues to explore PK on an individual and population basis. A better analytical method gives a better concentration-time profile and allows pharmacokinetics of an individual drug to be thoroughly studied. Pharmacogenetics is a newer, related field, which provides tools to understand finally differences between individuals concerning drug disposition associated with genetic differences in metabolism or drug transport. The concentration-time relationship of drugs in plasma or at the site of effect is the most critical element in the study of pharmacokinetics. A drug PK profile includes identification of the most relevant model (compartmental *versus* non-compartmental) and estimation of PK parameters for the model. PK parameters including the drug half-life, absorption rate constant, volume of distribution, and clearance are a summary of relevant PK parameters of a drug and these parameters are criteria to down-select drug candidates in development [452].

1) Modeling Drug Absorption:

Drug absorption is defined as the physiological process through which drugs enter the body and become available for subsequent PK processes of distribution, metabolism, and excretion. This absorption definition is not applicable to administration of drugs intravenously as this means of drug administration by passes the normal processes of drug absorption which impact orally administered drugs. Drug absorption of orally administered drugs occurs through either active transport or passive diffusion. The most important parameters of the process of drug absorption are the extent of drug absorption, the order of drug absorption, and the rate of drug absorption. Absorption may occur through either a first order or a zero order process or through some combination [8]. Additional efforts may be required, however, to describe absorption for some drugs. Absorption of drugs across the GI tract might be discontinuous and variable in nature for some drugs, for example, and variable absorption is a process that can be described through modeling. Suttle *et al.* [453] modeled the absorption of ranitidine and cimetidine, which are H2-receptor agonists, using two separate sites of absorption in the gastrointestinal tract to address twin peaks in the profile of drug concentration *versus* time. The authors utilized LaPlace transforms to model the effects of different hypotheses of absorption such as spatially separated absorption sites.

Wright *et al.* [454] assumed multiple sites of absorption in the gastrointestinal tract to fit both oral and intravenous data of an antiviral uracil analogue (L- FMAU) simultaneously. To reach a final solution, the authors utilized differential equations to describe transfer of drug across a variety of compartments using simple non- linear regression. Other drugs have been shown to have much more complicated profiles of drug absorption, which require solutions that are more complicated. For example, cyclosporine (CsA) has a flat absorption profile with significant variability over time [455].

To model the absorption of cyclosporine, Debord *et al.* utilized a gamma model [456], which fitted the data as an asymmetric S-shaped curve accompanied by an early flat phase. This gamma model was later shown to be valid *in vivo* with data from renal, cardiac, and lung transplant patients. The authors predicted the kinetics of cyclosporine absorption using Bayesian forecasting with their own custom computer program [457]. Another model of cyclosporine absorption was created using the non-linear mixed effects model (NONMEM) [457], which provides a simpler, easier to use means to implement the algorithm used to develop individualized cyclosporine therapy.

2) Modeling Drug Distribution:

Understanding how drugs distribute to various organs of the body is essential. Different processes make diverse contributions to drug distribution including a variety of transport proteins and binding of drugs to proteins and body tissues. Prediction of drug concentrations at the site of effect gives useful information regarding the most optimal dose for drug administration and the drug efficacy profile.

Hybrid PK models are also available for predicting drug concentrations in tissues. Gallo *et al.* combined data from *in vitro* and *in vivo* experiments to predict concentrations of a variety of retroviral compounds in the brain. In a different study by the same authors, a physiologically based hybrid PK model was used to make predictions of cancer drug concentrations inside tumors [458]. Hybrid pharmacokinetic models can be modified to scale from rodents to man, and they are useful tools to understand the differences in drug disposition between experimental animal models and human beings. Drug transport between mother and fetus through the placenta can be difficult to study experimentally, and animal models of this process provide a means to understand drug distribution across the placenta Huang *et al.* [459] described a rat compartmental model for maternal to fetal transport of a retroviral drug, zidovudine. In this study, three different models of distribution were evaluated for maternal tissue and plasma compartments, amniotic fluid, the placenta, and the fetus. A number of different equations were fitted simultaneously to describe the drug concentration data over time, and the final model was chosen based on its ability to describe drug exposure in all compartments.

A number of PK models have been created to describe pharmacokinetics in the eye. Sakanaka *et al.* [460] described the ocular kinetics of bunazosin, a glaucoma drug, after the drug was injected into the eyes of rabbits. Concentrations of bunazosin in the cornea, tears aqueous humor and the ciliary body of the iris were quantitated. A two-compartment model was created to describe the pharmacokinetics of bunazosin in tears, and the drug concentration profile derived was associated with the drug effect of relieving intraocular pressure by using an aqueous humor flow model and an indirect response model.

Ranta *et al.* [461] utilized *in vitro* cell culture studies in combination with pharmacokinetic modeling to describe the ocular kinetics of six different beta-blocker drugs. Drug absorption and drug desorption through the corneal epithelial cells was assessed using a human corneal epithelial cell culture model. A simulation model based on business software called Stella was created and provided a prediction of the disposition of ocular drugs applied topically to the eyes of rabbits. The Stella software allows for production of a pharmacokinetic model without advanced knowledge of mathematics or computer programming. This software may be useful for screening new drug candidates and conducting formulation studies where there are no *in vivo* data available. Ezzet *et al.* [462] created a population PK model to describe the PK parameters of ezetimibe, a cholesterol-lowering drug known to undergo enterohepatic circulation.

Enterohepatic recirculation prolongs the mean residence time of drugs, and this recirculation may act to potentiate drug activity. The model derived in this study was created to describe the many peaks in the drug concentration profile over time produced because of enterohepatic recirculation.

3) Modeling Drug Metabolism:

Drug-drug interactions result in induction of metabolism or inhibition of metabolism. The metabolic changes triggered by drug administration over time are clinically relevant to model as these changes can affect dosing decisions made throughout treatment. Many drugs produce drug metabolites that have activity which contributes to the overall drug effect, and mechanistic pharmacokinetic drug models which are capable of incorporating kinetics of drug metabolites are quite useful. Yamano *et al.* [463] reported the use of a model to describe inhibition of metabolism of midazolam, a benzodiazepine seizure drug, by CYP3A inhibitors. The inhibition model of midazolam metabolism was derived by combining *in vitro* and *in vivo* experiments, and the model was utilized to make predictions on the rise of midazolam in the liver relative to the plasma after simultaneous administration of CYP3A inhibitors such as itraconazole, cimetidine, and erythromycin in man. This model was also used to predict how much the metabolism of midazolam would be inhibited after repeat oral administration of erythromycin. The midazolam inhibition model utilized a kinetic model of the CYP3A enzyme which was inactivated, kinetic parameters of the drug and the inhibitor, and the amount of active enzyme available. The AUC of midazolam was hypothesized to increase by 2.6 times after concomitant administration of erythromycin over the AUC observed with midazolam by itself. The predicted effect of metabolic inhibition of CYP3A was shown to correlate with the data observed in other reports.

Ward *et al.* [464] created a model, which fitted the drug disposition of valproate glucuronide metabolized in isolated perfused livers of rats, which were also treated with probenecid, a drug that increases uric acid excretion. The effects of probenicid on hepatobiliary disposition were modeled, and the results of the model suggested that probenecid acts to inhibit the formation, biliary excretion, and sinusoidal clearance of valproate glucuronide. The authors focused on accounting for those biologically relevant processes and avoided including models of theoretical processes, which made their model much simpler. Ten different models were created to find the best fit, and finally one model was selected which provided the most appropriate solution. Another model created by Svensson *et al.* [465] utilizing non-linear mixed effects modeling was created to fit *in vitro* data on the metabolism of artemisinin The authors tested patients for different CYP covariates (CYP 2B6, CYP2A6, and CYP3A4 activities) and incorporated the inter-occasion and inter-individual variability data to create constants of first-order formation of metabolites. This method can be very useful for selecting among different patterns of metabolism when metabolites are already known.

An enzyme induction model for artemisinins was created by Elsherbiny *et al.,* [466] to describe the auto-induction of artemisinin metabolism that has been noted in many studies previously discussed. This study was based on an assumption that the inductive properties of artemisinin antimalarials could be mimicked by using mephenytoin as a probe for the enzyme activity of CYP 2C19 and CYP2B6. The population PK of S-mephenytoin and its metabolites, S-4'-hydroxymephenytoin and S-nirvanol, to include models of enzyme turnover and enzyme induction were created using non-linear mixed effects modeling. A rich data set was obtained from 14 volunteers who were administered mephenytoin before administration of artemisinin and after administration of artemisinin for ten days. Sparse data were obtained from 74 volunteers administered mephenytoin before artemisinin analogue administration, during artemisinin analogue administration, and after administration of artemisinin, artesunate, DHA, artemether, or arteether, for five days. The aim of this study was to create a pharmacokinetic model of enzyme turnover to fit data on the induction of CYP2C19 by artemether, artemisinin, and arteether, and artemisinin induction of CYP2B6.

In the study of the sparse data set, the effect of artemisinin drugs on CYP enzymes suggested rapid enzyme induction. The NONMEM software utilized in this study predicted the subject phenotypes correctly who possessed CYP enzyme polymorphisms derived from phenotype data from the rich data pool or because of the inability to observe creation of mephenytoin metabolites in the sparse data pool. The model derived from this study showed that all of the artemisinin derivatives in this study, artesunate, arteether, DHA, or artemether, were shown to induce CYP2B6, but CYP2C19 was induced by artemether and arteether and artemisinin showed induction of CYP2C19 and CYP2B6. The induction effect observed in this study differed among the artemisinin analogues as artemisinin showed the most profound induction effect of CYP2C19 and CYP2B6 among all artemisinin compounds tested. The rate of CYP2B6 production was elevated by 16.9% by artesunate, 61.5% by arteether, 79.7% by artemisinin, 19.9% by dihydroartemisinin, and 76.1% by artemether and. The rate of production of CYP2C19 increased 4.9% by artemether, 14.8% by arteether, and 51.2% by artemisinin. The CYP inductive capacity varied among the artemisinin analogues, which is very significant when considering selection of partner drugs for antimalarial combination therapy to minimize the potential for drug-drug interactions. The author's model correctly described the population pharmacokinetics of response to S-mephenytoin and S-mephenytoin metabolites, S-4'-hydroxymephenytoin and S-nirvanol, and confirmed the induction of CYP2C19 by different artemisinin analogues [466].

4) Modeling Drug Elimination

Multiple processes in different organs to include the kidneys, liver, and biliary system play a role in drug clearance. These physiologic processes can observe first order or saturable (Michaelis-Menten) kinetics. A number of nonlinear clearance mechanisms can also be involved. For example, non-linear biliary and renal clearance of antiviral polyoxometalates was reported by Ni and Boudinot [467]. Polyoxometalates have been shown to bind plasma proteins in a nonlinear manner, and fitting this data correctly required modeling unbound drug concentrations to assess renal and biliary clearance processes. The authors utilized a tri-exponential equation to fit unbound drug concentrations over time. Two different renal drug elimination models were created to fit the profiles of drug concentration time of three polyoxometalates. The first model fitted glomerular filtration, nonlinear active drug reabsorption, and saturable tubular secretion, the second model fitted glomerular filtration, non-saturable tubular drug reabsorption, and active tubular secretion, and the third model described biliary clearance utilizing a Michaelis-Menten equation. All of the model equations were applied at the same time using the WinNonlin PK software package.

A mechanism-based model was created by Hansen and Balthasar [468] in a different study to fit data on elevated clearance of the antiplatelet antibody 7E3 produced after administration of IV immunoglobulin. A model was created for the 7E3 antibody in rats treated with and without IVIG. Studies in mice, which lack the FcRn receptor, which binds IV immunoglobulin, were also utilized as FcRn has been shown to be involved in clearance of IV immunoglobulin. The ultimate mechanistic pharmacokinetic model created used data from all of these studies. This mechanistic model can be used to identify novel therapeutic drug targets and understand how drug treatment affects the overall effect of 7E3. Other drugs exhibiting drug disposition that is target mediated have been reported [452], and receptor mediated endocytosis has been shown to be the primary elimination pathway for elimination of some drugs at moderate doses [469], or disposition has involved dose-dependent kinetics [470].

In conclusion, PK modeling today emphasizes the creation of mechanistic models applied to population data. Applying these models to study populations enables pharmacokineticsts to describe variability using both rich and sparse PK data. This enhances the data derived from preclinical research and clinical trials. Pharmacokinetic models are excellent tools to understand physiological processes contributing to drug effect and disposition, which can play a pivotal role in optimizing drug treatment therapy.

7.2.2. Physiologically Based PK (PBPK) Modeling

Physiologically based PK or PBPK models are different from classic pharmacokinetic models as PBPK models incorporate tissue-specific compartments playing a role in absorption, exposure, metabolism, toxicity, and elimination processes that are connected by the flow of blood (Fig. **22**). In a PBPK model, tissue compartments connected by flows of blood are modeled using factors derived from physiological processes, which permit extrapolation to other species by simply altering the factor properly [471]. A significant benefit provided by the use of a PBPK model is parameters that have an influence on ADME processes can be included in the model in a meaningful way that represents the mechanisms at work assuming the physiological process is well understood and data on the process are available. As the models are based on known physiological mechanisms, extrapolation to other species or other situations that differ from the experimental conditions used to collect the data used to fine-tune the model is appropriate. PBPK models based on physiological mechanisms can be used to examine questions associated with the use of different experimental designs, and they can play a role exploring possible reasons to explain unexpected results. PBPK modeling has been successfully used to extrapolate data between animal species and to predict human pharmacokinetic parameters using animal-derived data.

PBPK approaches have a number of advantages over classic PK models to include: 1) PBPK models are created using physiological, anatomical, and biochemical data which is distinct from the actual data derived from concentration time-course curves; 2) PBPK models allow for evaluating physiological mechanisms governing drug disposition of a number of compounds by comparing pharmacokinetic results with predictions made by models; 3) PBPK models utilize drugs to probe physiological processes to derive additional data on how compounds are absorbed and cleared through different transport pathways and compartments in the body; 4) PBPK models can be applied in safety assessments;

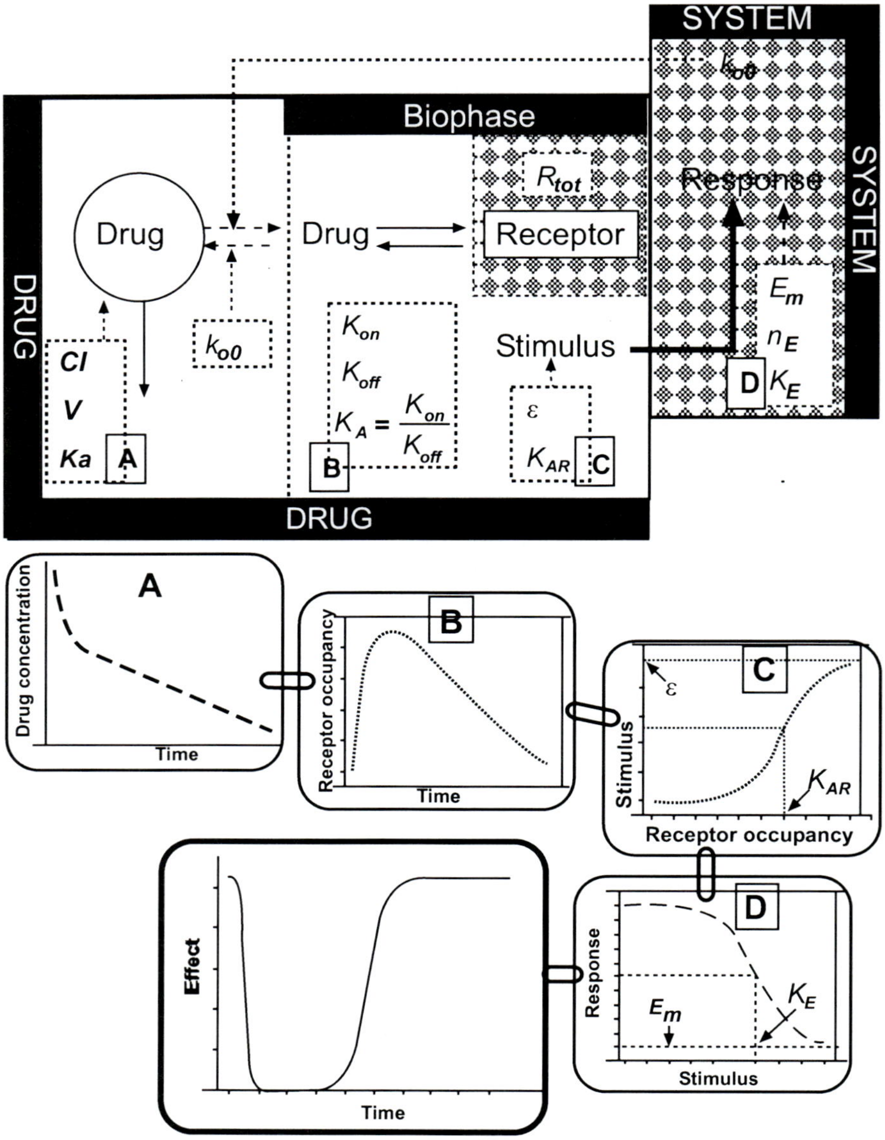

Figure 22: Processes in the causal chain between drug administration and the change in response over time, including the pharmacokinetics of a drug (process A), target site distribution and receptor (target) binding kinetics (process B), receptor activation (process C) and transduction (process D). These processes are characterized by receptor theory models incorporated in mechanism-based PK/PD models. These models explicitly distinguish drug and system specific properties, which are shown in the solid white and shaded area's respectively. *Cl,* clearance; *V*, volume of distribution; *Ka*, absorption rate constant; K_{e0}, biophase distribution constant; k_{on}, association rate constant; k_{off}, dissociation rate constant; $K_{A,}$ receptor affinity; e, intrinsic efficacy; K_{AR}, receptor occupancy resulting in 50% stimulus; E_m, maximum effect; n_E slope of stimulus-response relationship; K_E, stimulus resulting in 50% effect [87].

5) PBPK models utilize database annotation as a means of archiving data on pharmacokinetic parameters, kinetics, and toxicity of particular drugs. All of these advantages have driven broad innovation and use of PBPK models in the last decade particularly models pertaining to drugs [472].

The next section describes the historical development of PBPK modeling, and discusses the growing use of PBPK models in industry for drug development. There are a number of uses of PBPK models to describe the effects of small molecules that have not yet been widely explored.

1) Historical Perspective of PBPK Modeling:

PK modeling is used to describe both pharmacokinetic and toxicokinetic parameters, and the use of these models arose from a requirement to understand the concentration of compounds at the target site and relate that to the dose administered given both good and bad responses to compounds at the target site or elsewhere in the body are possible. Understanding the free concentration of drug in the tissues is more relevant than understanding the amount of drug at the site of absorption. Pharmacokinetic models are excellent tools to understand the dose delivered at target tissues for a broad array of different drug exposure circumstances.

The first physiological model was developed in the 1930s to understand drug disposition using equations to model drug absorption, distribution, and clearance. Given the lack of computer tools at that time, solving these equations was not feasible. Without robust computer tools, mathematically derived solutions were only available for very simple PK models derived using basic compartmental modeling Pharmacokinetic modeling efforts were directed toward describing concentration time curves simply and exactly rather than attempting to derive models with a relationship to physiology. Early efforts in this regard are described as data based compartmental modeling which reflected vast intricate data collection on drug concentration profiles over time. The drug concentration profiles over time were assessed and model parameters were estimated by curve fitting.

Physiologically based pharmacokinetic modeling was first innovated by pharmaceutical companies, however, the principal use of these tools was focused on making risk assessments of the environment. The use of PBPK models was not extensive due to the complexity of these models mathematically and the amount of data required for input. Further advances in understanding tissue distribution and hepatic metabolism using data from both *in vitro* and *in silico* sources have made PBPK modeling easier and more useful. This provides an opportunity to integrate a wealth of input data from a variety of sources to estimate concentration-time profiles for both tissue and plasma, PK parameters, and to gain valuable insight into compound mechanism of action. Given the growing utility of PBPK models, there has been increased interest in actually using these types of models to aid in drug development [472].

Utilization of a PBPK model requires biochemical, physiochemical, and physiological parameters. The physiological foundation of a PBPK model is strength and a weakness as PBPK models can take time and money to make. Over the last decade, general PBPK models have been created capable of simulating pharmacokinetic data for animal studies and human clinical trials utilizing a variety of physicochemical parameters couples with *in vitro* data. These general PBPK models have been created utilizing a variety of software tools to include acslX, MATLAB®, and Berkeley Madonna. These programming tools permit simple integration of preclinical animal PK data into a final PBPK model capable of predicting human PK parameters. While these tools simplify the use of PBPK models, end users must understand the models and the equations used to create the models to understand the model output generated. These new generic models provide a means of rapidly creating a PBPK model in a few hours where prior PBPK model construction would take a month to complete. The generic PBPK model is therefore a very useful tool for assessing PK properties in preclinical development [471].

2) Current Applications of PBPK Modeling in Drug Development

Given the growing popularity of this approach, Rowland *et al.* [471], counted the total publications per year which described the use of "physiologically- based PK" utilizing the online tool Web of Knowledge, and his review of these publications has shown an exponential increase over time in the number of publications incorporating PBPK modeling. PBPK models are useful from the early stage of drug development *in vitro* and in animals all the way through final drug development (Table **26**). Drug discovery in the modern era has evolved into an environment complete with a plethora of data derived from high throughput screening creating data on tens of thousands of compounds tested for drug efficacy and pharmacokinetic properties. A significant fraction of ADME data create in the course of early preclinical testing can be utilized to create a PBPK model. In contrast to allometry (the study relating body size to anatomy, shape, behavior and physiology), PBPK modeling can be used to make a wide variety of predictions including: predictions of drug absorption, drug distribution, drug clearance, the plasma drug concentration: time profile, drug-drug interactions, the effects of age, the effects of genetics, and the effects of disease [471].

Table 26: Role of PBPK modeling at various stages in preclinical and clinical development [471, 472]

Model Application	Impact
Lead optimization	
• Determining key *in vitro* data impacting absorption and PK	• Provides guidance to chemists and provides a basis for screening cascade
• Predicting PK with *in silico* and *in vitro* data as inputs	• Verifies the PK properties of a chemical series are understood, helps prioritize compounds for additional *in vivo* experimentation
• Understanding mechanisms impacting PK	• Compares the PBPK model to *in vivo* PK data to identify potential reasons for mismatch and to guide additional experimentation
Clinical candidate selection	
• Absorption modeling	• Predicts if a compound will exhibit a significant food effect
• Comparing exposure window for lead candidates	• Links human PK to PK/PD models for pharmacological and toxicological effects improves basis for choosing best candidate
• Identifying key uncertainties	• Allows for targeted experimentation
Entry into human	
• Predicting human PK and efficacious dose	• Determines if a compound will be efficacious in the clinic
• Understanding key sources of variability	• Provides important information for clinical trial design
• Simulate clinical trial results	• Uses the PBPK model simulation to optimize clinical trial design
Clinical development	
• PBPK/PD modeling	• Increases understanding of dose of active compound delivered to target tissues and its relationship to toxicological and efficacious effects
• Predicting PK for patient population	• Incorporates physiological changes from a disease state allows prediction of PK in the patient population
• Predicting PK for population of different age	• Incorporates age-specific physiological differences allows prediction of PK for a specific age group, *e.g.*, children or the elderly

3) PBPD Modeling

In plain English, pharmacokinetics is considered "What the body does to foreign chemicals", and pharmacodynamics is considered "What foreign chemicals do to the body". Physiologically based pharmacodynamic modeling (PBPD) is defined as computer simulation of pharmacologic or toxicological effects of drugs based on biology of chemical/drug-receptor interactions. This pharmacokinetic and pharmacodynamic continuum describes the entry point where a drug enters the body to the point of a pharmacologic or toxicological effect. When describing such a continuum, it is difficult to separate where pharmacokinetics ends and pharmacodynamics begins. When considering the toxicology or pharmacology of a drug, one must consider both pharmacokinetics and pharmacodynamics to understand the relationship between the two. To consider either PK or PD by itself only provides one component of the overall problem.

PBPK modeling came before PBPD modeling by a number of years due to the incomplete understanding of the mechanisms of action for many drugs. It is not surprising that PBPK models were derived first as they were developed from early studies of analytical chemistry, mammalian physiology, and principles of mass balance. PBPD modeling is entirely dependent on an understanding of how drugs interact with their receptors, and studies of the biology associated with drug-target interactions have taken more took time to come to fruition. PBPK modeling has now matured and research studies are focused on complex systems to include multi-chemical interactions, sub-compartmentalization of organs, and special models such as dermal uptake of drugs or reconstruction of exposure doses [473].

4) PBPK/PD Models

Human exposure to drugs is rarely limited to single compounds. Adverse drug interactions in patients are a topic of significant concern, and in excess of 2.2 million adverse reactions to drugs were estimated to have taken place in hospital patients in 1994 in the US with 106,000 of those interactions being fatal [474]. Patients in this in this study were given an average of eight different drugs over the course of their hospital stay. Compared with other causes of death, the investigators of this study [474] concluded adverse drug reactions ranked in the top six causes of death in 1994 in the US. Accordingly, having more robust and relevant interactive and more advanced PBPK/PD models is of great importance to decrease adverse drug reactions in the US and around the world.

To understand these ADRs more completely, PBPK models must be integrated with PBPD models. The two most important aspects of this interaction include PK interactions and PD interactions. Interactive PBPK models are the easiest to discuss in detail, as the number of PBPD models available for even single drugs is very small to date. The best method of conducting interactive PBPK modeling of multiple compounds is to insure each component drug in a mixture of drugs is modeled. Each drug should have its own respective established PBPK model, and there should be a number of PK data sets established in laboratory animals as well as in man available for each of the component drugs. By having a strong set of data on PK interactions from the start, an interactive PBPK model can be built on a firm foundation of a well- characterized database of known PK interactions. An interactive PBPK model can be used to sort out drug interactions between component chemicals.

One example of such an interaction that modeling could help understand is the interaction of two component chemicals to inhibit metabolism of both compounds. The individual PBPK models for each component chemical could be joined together at the liver compartment by introducing enzyme inhibition terms in the mass balance differential equation. In some cases, other data requirements are needed. One example of other data requirements could be a need for ultralow dose PK data of a component chemical in the perinatal developmental stages of laboratory animals. This data set would be necessary, for example, for PBPK modeling to extrapolate PK data from perinatal animals to human fetuses and babies. Such interactive models are in their infancy, and additional development will be needed for routine use.

5) How can PBPK Modeling be a Useful Predictive Tool?

To create a PBPK/PD model, time course experimental data sets are needed to compare computer simulations training data sets with computer simulations to help validate PBPK models. For model validation, it is important that data sets beyond the working sets be used for comparison to the simulation results of the model. For instance, assume a PBPK/PD model was developed derived from PK and PD data sets derived from IV dosing of two dose levels of a particular drug reported by a laboratory. The validation of this PBPK/PD model for this drug should be conducted using different PK and PD data sets following oral and dermal administration of the same drug reported by other laboratories. In general, the greater the number of sets of data used for validation, the more robust the PBPK/PD model.

Once a PBPK/PD model is validated, the model may be used for simulation of other compounds, however, PBPK/PD models are generally limited today in terms of predictive value to the exact compound the model was developed for. For example, one study used a PBPK model that predicted a drug-drug interaction in man between erythromycin and triazolam using *in vitro* CYP3A4 inhibition studies [475]. This drug-drug interaction actually resulted in 15 fatalities in patients in Japan in 1993, and the basis for this interaction was found to involve a mechanism-based inhibition or "suicide inhibition", where liver enzymes metabolized a chemical to a metabolite, which, in turn, irreversibly inactivated the liver enzyme required to metabolize macrolide antibiotics, such as erythromycin.

Once a liver enzyme is inactivated permanently, metabolism of other co-administered drugs is impaired, leading to a "drug overdose". With the present state-of-the-art PBPK/PD models, investigators should be able to use a PBPK model to predict toxicities associated with combination therapies involving other macrolide antibiotics and co-administered drugs that are also metabolized by CYP3A4 assuming some basic PK parameters are established for the drugs along with data on drug metabolism by human CYP3A4 [475]. When additional mechanism of action data is available for different classes of compounds, it is reasonable to believe setting rules for reactions may be possible molecular attributes, and network models of novel reaction may be joined to PBPK/PD models to establish a second-generation PBPK model capable of predicting drug toxicity [473].

PBPK models facilitate the best use of preclinical ADME data by creating a structured means of storing the data on the compound, a framework to generate hypotheses to test, and a platform for making predictions based on the data. PBPK modeling provides an excellent tool for drug development to aid in the understanding of factors affecting PK and PD findings in complex biological systems.

7.2.3. Advances in PD Modeling

The increasing popularity of PBPK modeling signals movement from simple kinetic models to physiologically and mechanistically relevant descriptions of a biological system describing how drugs are absorbed, distributed, metabolized, and excreted in man. Applying PBPK models to assess disposition of drugs over time in man utilizes a combined approach to describe systematically physiological processes, which have a role in drug delivery to a target tissue. A number of PBPK models have been created to integrate data across different levels to describe how a drug interacts with a target at the molecular level. One example of such an interaction is reversible binding of a ligand, for example, the binding of methotrexate to its receptor, dihydrofolate reductase. Per this example, PBPK models must integrate processes at a number of different levels to include the level of the drug molecule, the cell, the organ, and the level of the whole organism to account for disposition of drugs, metabolites of drugs, and drug-receptor complexes.

The use of PBPK models is focused on predicting drug concentrations in various compartments of the body *in vivo*; however, these models can play a significant role in assessing efficacy and safety as well. Given the extensible nature of these models, they are capable of describing the relation between the dose of drug provided, the concentration of drug target site, and the biological response to drug administration. Elements of dosing related to tissue, organ, and organism, tissue levels of response have customarily been thought of as PD metrics. PD models used to evaluate drugs are generally more empirical and utilize simple compartmental analysis, which have been associated with plasma or tissue concentrations of active drug. With the advances in systems biology, physiologically based pharmacodynamic (PBPD) models have been created that describe changes in biological systems by drug action and the exposures and dosing which lead to these changes creating a therapeutic outcome or a health risk associated with toxicity. PBPK/PD models have also been shown to be very useful to assess risk of drug toxicity. One example of this is a PBPK/PD model, which linked the metabolism of chloroform to cell damage, cell death, and new cell growth.

By taking a systems biology approach, model creation efforts focus on describing normal biological function and the changes related to drug exposure. These changes commonly lead to tissue toxicity (too much drug) or a desired therapeutic efficacy outcome (drug dose is just right), and the good and bad effects of drug exposure can be modeled through using PBPK methods that link through PBPD models of cellular response. Outcomes of efficacy and toxicity can then be defined by how a drug interacts with a biological system. The disciplines of pharmacology and toxicology are at the intersection of PK studies (chemistry) and PD studies (biology). Next generation models of PK and PD will involve advances in providing increasingly detailed descriptions of biological systems, which will provide the means to create models that are more sophisticated.

When a PBPK model is used, the PD effects of a drug are clearly described clearly, and these effects are likely related to the concentration of free drug at a target tissue where drug activity takes place as opposed to trying to understand indirect effects through quantitation of drugs in the plasma. Quantitative information on response to dosing for toxicity and efficacy for a drug provides the necessary data to create PBPK models that can be utilized to answer questions on the possibilities associated with changing the ratio of efficacy to toxicity of a drug through alterations in drug delivery. PBPK model development will continue to expand given the many advantages of PBPK models to organize and describe various data sets to help understand drug efficacy and toxicity [476].

The rapid developments of advances in genomics, combinatorial chemistry, and high throughput screening have enhanced early drug discovery activities and have focused attention on the field of "discovery toxicology" [471-473]. PBPK modeling can play a useful role in this process by adding new dimensions of modeling to answer questions of toxicology even at the earliest phases of drug development. Quantitative Structure Activity Relationship (QSAR) analysis is a useful tool for estimation of specific drug PBPK parameters while data at the genomic level describes drug mechanism of action that can assist with drug design and help model the relationship between dosing and a pharmacodynamic outcome. PBPK models provide a framework to integrate quantitative data on physical properties of a compound combined with data on compound toxicity and ADME constrained within the basic physiological processes observed *in vivo*. This approach may be very helpful during drug development as data derived from modeling one development candidate can be used to create new models for structurally similar or mechanistically similar compounds.

7.2.4. PK/PD Modeling in Different Stages of Drug Development

Pharmacokinetic and pharmacodynamic (PK/PD) modeling facilitates understanding of drug safety and efficacy, and these models are powerful tools in the paradigm of "learning and confirming" used in drug development. In translational research, PK/PD modeling based on drug mechanisms is widely used to provide insights into drug safety and efficacy during clinical development. These mechanism-based models are different from PK/PD models that are simply descriptive as they are capable of providing quantitative descriptions of different physiological processes that act on drugs from when they are administered to where they actually provide an effect. These processes include drug distribution to the drug target, drug target binding, activation of the drug target, pharmacodynamic interfaces, drug signal transduction and drug feedback mechanisms associated with drug effect (see Fig. **22**). Mechanism-based PK/PD models utilize receptor theory elements to describe binding of drugs to targets, and the activation of drug targets shows enhanced utility for prediction when compared to simpler, descriptive PK/PD models. Accordingly, receptor theory provides the framework for: 1) predicting drug concentration-effect relationships *in vivo* and 2) describing the kinetics of drug-target binding over the period of drug efficacy.

PK/PD modeling and simulation are important tools to enhance the efficiency of the drug-development process, which is facing high attrition rates. Over the years, the use of PK/PD modeling to understand drug efficacy and safety, and thereby improve the quality of drug development decision-making, has been advocated by pharmaceutical companies, academia, and regulatory agencies. When these insights are obtained in early development, they can be used to a better predict efficacy and safety in the later stages of clinical development. This will reduce the attrition risk during the very expensive phases of clinical development because of problems with safety or efficacy. In translational drug-research, mechanism-based PK/PD modeling has evolved as an essential tool to bring forward early insights, both from drug discovery and from early preclinical testing, to avoid problems in later clinical development where failure is even more expensive [477].

Mechanism-based PK/PD models do have differences (see Fig. **22**), however, from full mechanistic or systems biology models. Fully mechanistic models follow a data driven, top down approach starting at a very bare descriptive level followed by adding layers to advance toward a systems biology type model. Mechanism-based PK modeling lies in the middle of this spectrum maintaining a mechanistic focus while still embracing systems biology model elements. Consequently, changes in these processes due to disease progress can be considered.

The principles of receptor theory date back to the pivotal work of Clark and Gaddum in the 1930s, based on the earlier work of Hill [478] providing the basics of Black and Leff's operational model of agonism [479], and the principles and applications of agonism have been extensively reviewed by others [480]. New developments in mechanism-based PK/PD modeling have arisen through incorporation of receptor theory into these models to enhance the value of these tools for translational drug research. In traditional PK/PD modeling approaches, empirically derived models like the Hill equation are utilized to describe the shape of a drug concentration *versus* effect profile. The Hill equation is defined by three parameters: the maximum effect, the concentration resulting in 50% of the maximum effect and a Hill coefficient representing the steepness of the slop of the curve describing concentration *versus* effect.

The Hill equation combines all intermediate steps between the association of a drug to a receptor and the activation or stimulation of that receptor in one equation. Accordingly, the Hill equation does not explicitly distinguish drug specific parameters such as drug affinity for a certain receptor or the ability of a drug to activate the receptor based on parameters such as the receptor density or the transduction relationship between receptor activation and a pharmacological effect. For example, the concentration-effect relationship for a drug with a high affinity for a receptor but low efficacy can be described with the same set of parameters as a drug with low affinity but high efficacy.

In addition, the Hill equation assumes equilibrium conditions of the system. This important assumption might be valid in some cases, but definitely not in all cases.

Although the use of the Hill equation for illustrating concentration- response relationships under equilibrium conditions is well established, its descriptive nature limits use for extrapolation. For instance, the Hill equation for the concentration-effect relationship cannot be readily used to predict a drug-receptor relationship in a different tissue with a different receptor density or another stimulus-response relationship. This would require a mechanism-based model that separates the drug from a set of system- specific parameters. Classical receptor theory can be applied to make this separation, as the action of a drug arises from two independent components to include the agonist dependent component of a drug and the tissue dependent component. Accordingly, receptor theory provides the basis to predict *in vivo* concentration-effect relationships.

The system specific element is determined by the concentration of the receptor, which defines the receptor binding capacity and the stimulus response relationship or transducer function (process D in Fig. **22**). Receptor binding and activation determine the drug-specific component (process C in Fig. **22**). In all approaches to incorporate receptor processes into PK/PD models, the receptor or target-binding component is described with a hyperbolic equation, typically the Hill-equation. The stimulus-response relationship has been incorporated in different ways, which can be separated in semi- parametric and fully parametric approaches [477].

As mechanism-based PK/PD models are typically defined by having far more parameters compared to descriptive models, estimation of parameters requires combining data from a wide variety of experiments to distinguish between drug parameters and system specific parameters. For instance, Tuk *et al.* used one experiment to estimate benzodiazepine receptor binding and activation and a separate experiment to estimate the relationship of benzodiazepine stimulus response [481]. Fixing the system specific parameters of the stimulus response relationship to the values obtained from one experiment allowed estimation of the drug specific parameters while intrinsic efficacy and receptor affinity were defined in a separate experiment. While other descriptive approaches for modeling benzodiazepine failed, this approach allowed a description of the pharmacodynamic interaction between the benzodiazepine compound midazolam and its active metabolite, a1-OH-midazolam, using electroencephalogram (EEG) measurement as a pharmacodynamic endpoint in rats. Tuk *et al.* used an unknown, but monotonically increasing stimulus-response function to link receptor binding to the resulting effect [481]. This is a semi-parametric approach, since it used a parameter to model binding of drug to receptor and drug activation *via* a non-parametric function to model transduction of a signal [482].

In contrast to the semi-parametric approach, the full-parametric approach requires the actual shape of the transducer function to be known, since both the receptor binding and activation process and the process of signal transduction are described with a parametric function. The Operational Model of Agonism (OMA) is a full- parametric method, in which the receptor binding and activation is linked to a hyperbolic stimulus-response relationship, although, in principle, the stimulus-response relationship can be of any shape [482, 483]. The OMA can be applied for estimating receptor affinity of both agonists and antagonists, and, in addition, OMA can be used to estimate the intrinsic efficacy of partial agonists.

As with the semi-parametric approach, the OMA is also defined by a variety of parameters. As these parameters refer to different interrelated processes in the chain between drug administration and effect, they cannot be estimated simultaneously using data from a single exposure response relationship [484]. This would result in biased parameter estimates showing high uncertainty. Over the years, several methods have been proposed that allow adequate estimation of the OMA. Four different methods have been described in the literature that can be used to estimate the OMA: the comparative method, the inactivation method, the interaction method, and the prior method.

Method 1: Comparative

The comparative method uses concentration-effect data from a number of compounds with different target affinities and intrinsic efficacies [485]. This method assumes that the compounds share the same system-specific parameters for maximum effect (E_{max}), and the same parameter for the steepness of the stimulus response relationship (n), where E_m and n are defined by the intrinsic efficacy and slope of the Hill equation of the full agonist, respectively [485]. As a result, relative *in vivo* estimates of affinity of a receptor to a drug and its efficacy are available for partial agonists. The assumption in this approach, however, is that all partial agonists operate through the same receptor system, and this assumption might not be generally applicable, for instance, if some of the compounds bind to other receptors or subtypes also. This could result in biased parameter estimates, since the operational affinity and intrinsic efficacy would be, in that case, a composite of different receptor occupancy curves.

Method 2: Inactivation

Alternatively, partial agonism can be induced by reducing the total receptor number through irreversible receptor inactivation [485]. This method yields information on the effect of a full agonist without receptor inactivation, and yields information on a partial agonist where receptor inactivation takes place. This method allows for sharing the same system specific parameters for E_{max} and n. Accordingly, the inactivation method is the only method that allows estimating the target affinity and intrinsic efficacy of a full agonist. Nevertheless, Van der Graaf *et al.* showed that high statistical correlations are expected between affinity and efficacy [486]. This is inconsistent with the inherent feature of receptor theory models to distinguish between system and drug specific parameters, and these findings are independent of study design. A multiple curve design where two curves for the full and partial agonist are derived using the same tissue is not superior to a single curve design, which studies only one curve per tissue [487]. Garrido *et al.* reported similar issues in estimating the parameters of the operational model of agonism when applied to determining alfentanil concentration-effect curves in rats with and without irreversible blockade of the m-receptor with b-funaltrexaminen. Although these curves could be adequately described with a Hill equation, fitting the curves using the operational model of agonism did not result in unique estimates for affinity and efficacy. The authors argued that the main cause for the inability of the OMA to fit the data was due to the failure of an irreversible antagonist to produce a maximum response and eliminate the rat receptor reserve [488].

Method 3: Interaction

The interaction method uses concentration-effect data from a full agonist alone and when a partial agonist is present to estimate receptor affinity and relative efficacy of the partial agonist. In contrast with the comparative method, the interaction method actually confirms the assumption that the full and partial agonist bind to the same receptor. Although successfully applied to *in vitro* data, this method has not been used to estimate *in vivo* parameters [489].

Method 4: Prior

When using independently derived prior information to understand one or more model parameters, some of the model parameters can be fixed resulting in higher statistical power to estimate the remaining unknown parameters. For instance, *in vivo* receptor affinity could be fixed to values derived from *in vitro* receptor binding studies. This prior method has been used successfully to describe effects of the synthetic m- opioids alfentanil, sufentanil, and fentanyl on rats, and these experiments showed that the *in vivo* concentration-effect relationships derived from the use of EEG recordings as a pharmacodynamic endpoint could be predicted accurately using *in vitro* derived parameters for affinity and intrinsic efficacy. The preclinical estimates for affinity and efficacy in rats appeared to resemble closely the estimates for both values in man demonstrating the applicability of receptor theory models for inter-species extrapolation. The high *in vitro* and *in vivo* correlation observed for receptor affinity of adenosine A1 receptor agonists and GABAA modulators suggests that the prior approach would be applicable to modeling the interactions of these compounds also. Another example of the prior method is a recent study estimating the affinity *in vivo* of the ß1-adrenoreceptor to atenolol, which used a model based on the OMA to model effects of atenolol on isoprenaline-induced tachycardia [477].

The operational model for this study was extended with a term describing the competition of isoprenaline and atenolol for the ß1-adrenoreceptor in addition to adrenaline displacement. Using this pharmacodynamic interaction model, the *in vivo* affinity constant of atenolol could be estimated, while fixing the *in vivo* receptor affinity of the full agonist, isoprenaline, to the *in vitro* affinity constant Ki. The extension of this model resulted in estimating *in vivo* values, which were shown to be very close to the *in vitro* affinity constant data obtained from functional bioassays. Van Steeg *et al.* [394] were interested in estimating the *in vivo* affinity of an antagonist, but, in principle, their model could also be used to estimate the affinity and intrinsic efficacy of different full and partial agonists. In fact, this approach would be comparable to the receptor inactivation method with one difference being a competitive antagonist would be used rather than an irreversible antagonist to reduce the number of available receptors. It would be interesting to see if taking the competitive dynamic interaction between agonists and antagonist explicitly into account allows for estimation of affinity and efficacy parameters that are not confounded with system specific parameters. The combination of response surface analysis, looking at the drug effect as a function of two drug concentrations, and as recently proposed by Jonker *et al.* receptor theory could be a valuable tool for this analysis, as this approach can be applied to any type of interaction, either synergistic or antagonistic [490].

In conclusion, mechanism-based PK/PD modeling aims at describing the processes in the causal chain, which describes the path from administration of a drug-to-drug effect including distribution of target sites, kinetics of receptor binding, and the dynamics of receptor activation and transduction. Receptor theory plays an important role in this approach, since it forms the basis for predicting the *in vivo* relationships between drug concentration and drug effect. The main challenge in mechanism-based PK/PD modeling using receptor theory models is how to distinguish the estimation of the parameters of the processes in the causal chain. Estimating parameters with adequate accuracy and precision requires collecting data from *in vitro* and *in vivo* experiments that are specially designed to estimate parameters independently and subsequently combining these data from different sources in one comprehensive PK/PD model. This approach fully exploits the fundamental feature of mechanism-based PK/PD modeling to distinguish system parameters from parameters specific to a drug. One example of this combined modeling approach is using prior information on receptor binding kinetics derived from *in vitro* studies combined with target site distribution data, which provides independent information to distinguish causal steps in the kinetics of drug activity.

In this approach, mechanism-based PK/PD modeling is essential for combining all sources of information. In addition, it can be used to derive indirectly information about unknown process involved in the kinetics of drug action. As such, mechanism-based PK/PD models provide the means to describe drug safety and efficacy, and better descriptions of drug efficacy and safety will lead to improved efficiency for developing drugs with less attrition of compounds late in the drug development process [477].

7.3. IMPLICATIONS OF PK/PD MODELING ON DEVELOPMENT OF ANTIMALARIAL DRUG POLICIES

Modeling and simulation (M&S) are important tools for regulatory decision-making affecting both industry and the public. Given the rising tide of drug development failures in industry, the use of modeling and simulation provides a tool to avoid expensive drug development mistakes. Regulatory agencies have recognized and championed modeling and simulation as a drug development tool and such emphasis has encouraged use that is more widespread. There is a variety of initiatives that regulatory agencies have advanced to use M&S for clinical drug development.

The FDA, for example, has released a number of guidance to industry documents that have required M&S to advance drug development. The FDA has shown it wants to be part of the discussion on how to advance in drug development productivity and quality to provide effective, safe drugs to patients in the US. The End-of-Phase 2A (EOP2A) meetings mandated by the FDA were implemented to find opportunities to advance clinical drug development more rapidly and to enhance New Drug Application (NDA) quality by conducting meetings regularly with drug sponsors. In 2004, the FDA conducted a number of EOP2A meetings where all of the data at hand was modeled by the FDA to model the follow-on Phase 3 trial This modeling effort utilized data from all prior clinical studies to include disease changes, dose response, placebo effects, and baseline data. Simulation of clinical trials was conducted to assess the proposed designs of future trials to find other alternate designs to enhance the likelihood of a successful study. The FDA issued final guidance on End of Phase 2A meetings in September 2009, which clearly outlines the sponsor's responsibility to conduct EOP2A modeling to include model data in the meeting package. The guidance describes the elements required for an EOP2A meeting, which include electronic trial data sets and modeling files, detailed reports on modeling and simulation of the data derived from clinical trials, and interpretations of modeling data supporting the proposed trial design. Additional data to be provided includes appropriate data derived from nonclinical Phase 1 studies and associated modeling pertaining to PK variability as a consequence of other factors, both intrinsic and extrinsic [491].

The European Federation of Pharmaceutical Sciences (EUFEPS) routinely conducts drug development meetings to review these kinds of issues. The expectation for the use of modeling and simulation to make regulatory decisions is rising among a variety of regulatory bodies, and that does raise two relevant issues. The first issue is an expectation for creation libraries of disease models under the FDA's critical path initiative. Collaborations between academia, the FDA, and industry will likely be needed to develop disease model libraries. The issues associated with sharing data and models across all parties from industry to the FDA and to academia remain to be overcome but are not believed to be impossible to overcome. The second issue revolves around the question of how open European regulatory agencies may be to using modeling and simulation to reach regulatory decisions on drug efficacy and labeling. A variety of European national agencies has expressed interest in this issue, and it is likely that this interest will expand with time [492].

7.3.1. The Role of PK/PD Modeling and Simulation in Regulatory Decision Making

PK/PD modeling creates a mathematical model describing relationships between multiple variables to include time, dose, drug concentration, and drug response. PK/PD simulation is conducted by using a model to make predictions on possible outcomes, such as the efficacy of a drug with an altered regimen of dosing. PK/PD modeling and simulation (M&S) has been proposed as a tool to make drug development more efficient. The concept of modeling and simulation is hardly new, however, there is growing interesting in applying M&S to clinical trial design. Several Guidance documents issued by the FDA provide a snapshot of the

FDA's view on the proper use of these new tools to enhance both drug development and regulatory decision-making. Below, we have highlighted brief summaries of several important Guidance to Industry documents on key issues associated with the use of PK/PD models [493].

The Guidance for Industry on Dose-Response emphasizes describing desired and undesired drug concentration to affect relationships to help with providing individualized therapy, optimizing dosage regimens, and developing rational means to prepare dose instructions for product labeling. The guidance states understanding the relationship between dose and response provides a means for a variety of drug regulators to reach approval decisions based on a common data set. This guidance document was created by the Expert Efficacy Working Group of the International Conference on Harmonization of Technical Requirements for the Registration of Pharmaceuticals for Human Use (ICH).

The Guidance for Industry on clinical effectiveness of a drug or biological product re- emphasizes the requirement for having more than one adequate and controlled clinical study for drug approval, which reflects the FDA Modernization Act (FDAMA). A full section of this Guidance is titled 'Extrapolation from existing studies' and this section is focused on listing possible circumstances where added clinical trials are deemed unnecessary. The fundamental premise of this section is the risks and benefits of a drug are already established, and conducting additional studies would not be necessary to approve a product for use in a pediatric population or for other reasons to include modifications to release the drug in a different manner, additional formulations, or other drug regimen changes. In order to avoid additional clinical trials, the Guidance emphasizes how important it is to understand clearly the relationship between drug concentration and effect in the original New Drug Application (NDA). By engaging in planning prospectively, drug sponsors can utilize this guidance effectively to avoid additional expenses associated with clinical studies deemed not necessary.

Section 505(A) of the Federal Food, Drug, and Cosmetic Act gives sponsors a period of six months of marketing exclusivity for a pediatric therapeutic indication to incentivize industry to conduct actually studies in children. In a number of circumstances, a well-described PK/PD relationship is utilized in place of an actual study to investigate clinical drug efficacy. Accordingly, dosing recommendations for clinical use are routinely created PK/PD models and other clinical studies may not be necessary. Reports from two FDA advisory committees on antiviral and cardio- renal drug products showed half of the meeting was spent discussing PK/PD modeling for drug development.

The advisory committee on antiviral drugs spent considerable time discussing uses of M&S to explore various dosage regimens to understand the potential for drug resistance to HIV protease inhibitors and why patient drug compliance was very important. The same committee suggested the FDA develop Guidance for Industry on using PK/PD modeling to develop antiviral drug products. The cardio-renal advisory meeting explored the need to determine an exposure response relationship. In this meeting, the FDA presented retrospective studies of dose-effect relationships of over 10 antihypertensive agents recently approved for human use.

The point made from these retrospective studies is the dose-response range of the majority of drugs studied was insufficient to permit adequate identification of the 'optimum' dose. This data could affect a number of regulatory decisions, such as the approval of combination drug products (like ACTs) and claims of drug superiority. The cardio-renal advisory group suggested the following policies after reviewing this data: 1) use of model-dependent analysis to understand the shape of the exposure-response curve; and 2) the need for more innovative trial designs and models allowing frequentist (long term statistics of probability) and Bayesian (plausibility of a hypothesis based on incomplete knowledge) types of data analysis. With such a design, sponsors would have the best tools in hand to conduct adequate and well-controlled trials capable of establishing the exposure-response relationship to provide data on safety and clinical effectiveness.

The Guidance for Industry on population PK emphasizes the role of M&S for designing trials and analyzing data derived from trials. Guidance for Industry on exposure (PK)- response (PD) is underway, and this Guidance will add more support to the need for robust M&S. The exposure-response guidance available has focused on design and analysis of data from example PK/PD drug studies. The impact of all of these Guidance documents and advisory committee recommendations issued by FDA is very clear; sponsors can utilize these tools for efficient and cost-effective trials that minimize time and resources to accelerate the pace of drug development. Gathering data to understand the relationships between drug concentration, disease biomarkers, clinical endpoints, and surrogate endpoints while developing a drug for use in adults can provide useful tools to model study designs, analysis and dosage recommendations (labeling changes) for use of a new drug in pediatric patients. The utilization of concentration-effect relationships as a sole tool to support approval of a new dose/regimen not studied directly in clinical trials, has not being fully exploited by many companies in industry. The use of M&S for this purpose is actually one of the most powerful.

Typically doses/regimens that are 'directly' studied through clinical trials are used for labeling. M&S can be used as a very effective tool to explore whether intermediate doses not directly studied could potentially offer similar efficacy as other doses. Extrapolating outside the studied range, however, may or may not be feasible or accepted by regulatory agencies [493].

7.3.2. The Use of PK/PD Modeling and Simulation for Regulatory Applications

In this section, applications of M&S for regulatory submission will be discussed, however, due to the confidential nature of NDA submissions generalizations derived from real NDA review experiences will be discussed, as particulars are not available. Typical drug development strategies include deriving pharmacology data through dose ranging studies and bridging studies. Dose ranging studies are used to model drug concentrations or dose- effects and any desired/undesired relationships. Bridging studies are utilized to understand how other extrinsic or intrinsic factors may affect the PK of a new drug. These factors may include food intake, age, smoking, gender, or hepatic/renal impairment. Safety and efficacy data may not be collected in dose ranging or bridging studies, but these data could be simulated from a previously developed model. In one real-world example, the relationships between the dose of an analgesic drug, the pain relief provided, and the relationship between drug concentration and an undesired effect, an alteration in heart rate, were developed through meta-analysis of a number of clinical studies.

In other studies, patients treated with this drug who had severe renal impairment showed a 60% increase in the AUC (area under the curve) and a large increase in the C_{max} (maximum drug plasma concentration) compared to healthy individuals without renal impairment. Models of this drug were utilized to simulate outcomes in patients who had a 60% change in drug exposure on efficacy and e safety. Administration of a standard dose to patients with renal impairment was predicted to result in a very modest increase in the probability of pain relief and a 100% probability of increases in heart rate by 3 beats per minute. This kind of analysis would lead one to believe that the difference in exposure and C_{max} in these patients would have little to no adverse effects and no alteration in dosing would be needed. This example shows how M&S provides a powerful tool to integrate data across multiple studies supporting a single drug application. Simulating probability distributions of drug safety and efficacy for bridging studies would provide data for improved, scientifically sound processes of making regulatory decisions. Incorporating this data into a simulation will provide an excellent repository to access this data when needed for future use, such simulations can be very useful tools for determining exposure-equivalence intervals required to achieve approvals of any changes in the future in drug formulation.

One of the most frequently desired labeling changes for special populations are those alterations required for pediatric patients. M&S modeling can be applied to simulating dosing in special populations such as pediatric patients to address these kinds of questions. As previously described, if there is data to support the hypothesis that a disease process is similar for children and adults and similar efficacy data can be readily acquired, then pediatric studies measuring concentration and pharmacologic effects can be used to support changes to drug dosage in children. The question being posed in such pediatric modeling studies is "Can the PK/PD of a particular drug in children be predicted based on data acquired from adults?" Such a question is only answerable by understanding relationships between concentration and effect. Drug developers should be encouraged to utilize PK/PD modes derived from adult data to design trials for pediatric patients. Analysis of PK/PD data from trials in children may require reciprocally, data derived from trials in adults to describe PK parameters in this population.

A key goal of modeling is to identify intrinsic factors that may have an impact on PK parameters such as age, bodyweight, smoking, gender, or food intake. On example of the impact of such factors can be found in the disposition of nisoldipine. Nisoldipine is a channel antagonist of dihydropyridine calcium, and a daily controlled release formulation was approved for use in the US to treat patients with hypertension. Food intake was found to alter the rate of bioavailability (C_{max} of 2.75 μg/L without food intake *vs*. 7.5 μg/L with food intake) but decrease the extent of bioavailability (AUC 70.4 μg•h/L without food intake *vs*. 53 μg·h/L with food intake) of the controlled release product. The impact of the higher concentrations of available drug on blood pressure was evaluated using a concentration-effect blood pressure model. Simulations of the drug effect under a fed condition showed the increase in drug concentration would not cause a significant drop in blood pressure. The labeling of this formulation was altered to state that administration is recommended without food for optimal bioavailability. In another example, the PK/PD relationship of docetaxel in patients with cancer was studied and showed a subpopulation of patients with liver disease who are more susceptible to serious neutropenia. This finding led to changes in dose recommendation for patients with liver disease. The modeling and simulation of docetaxel shows the value added by the incorporation of modeling into prospective planning of clinical trials.

Identification of trial objectives and utilization of all currently available data on a drug are required elements for designing clinical trials. Modeling and simulation can provide a means to explore competing designs of clinical trials to achieve the objectives that have been identified. In general, Phase 3 trials are designed using sample size or power calculations calculated by conventional statistical software. PK/PD models, along with other data, provide better simulations to examine other design features such as dosage, sampling schedule, or trial duration. More innovation in trial designs, are required to take full advantage of M&S as a trial design tool.

M&S can also play a role in assessing the bioavailability/bioequivalence of modified release dosage forms. Relationships between *in vitro* dissolution and the rate of *in vivo* input expressed as the fraction of drug absorbed *versus* time is a method that allows for determination if a correlation exists between dissolution and absorption. A high- level correlation between dissolution and absorption allows for prediction of the plasma concentration profile for a certain drug formulation based on its *in vitro* dissolution. Accordingly, utilizing the *in vitro* dissolution data along with an *in vitro-in vivo* correlation model can be used to estimate bioavailability. Having a model available that connects data derived from *in vitro* drug performance and it's *in vivo* input rate would diminish the regulatory burden on industry by cutting back on the number of clinical studies required to attain market approval for a modified release dosage form. A waiver for *in vivo* bioavailability/bioequivalence studies is granted by FDA if plasma concentration-time profiles predicted for test and the reference data are not different by more than 20% in mean AUC and C_{max}.

In addition, the simulating plasma concentration profiles based on *in vitro* dissolution profiles would also provide data to help with quality control for drug product production by enabling manufacturers to set actually meaningful specifications for drug dissolution. By taking into account the exposure effect relationship, dissolution specification limits could be specified to insure no drug batches are released that might lead to plasma concentrations *in vivo* that are inadequate to achieve a full drug effect. One of the most commonly used application of modeling and simulation used in regulatory work, is to predict PK profiles for multiple dose regimens using single dose data. One example of this is dosing of compazine, which is used for treatment of patients with nausea, and vomiting. The FDA desired to characterize the steady-state performance of the sustained-release spansule dosage form relative to a capsule formulation.

A multiple dose study was not feasible because of safety concerns about testing the spansule formulation of compazine in healthy volunteers. By conducting deterministic simulations of the compazine PK profile at steady state, the FDA was able to support a regulatory decision regarding the bioequivalence of the compazine spansule and capsule formulations. Modeling and simulation activities ultimately must provide a means to understand how well the model actually mirrors reality. The phrase 'model validation' has been in vogue for many years, however, the word 'validation', implies a process of robustness that is likely not applicable to most PK/PD models found in the literature. In addition, given the fact that the true model of reality and its parameters are not yet known suggests not using 'validation' as a descriptor of the utility of a model's utility. A bettor descriptor is "model qualification" or "model credibility" which is better terms to describe how well a PK model/simulation may be working. A model and its parameters can be described as 'qualified' to accomplish specific task(s) if they satisfy pre-specified criteria, such as insuring the model and its parameter set are capable of passing a predictive check.

Modeling and simulation tools are used by FDA working group members in the process of developing Guidance to Industry documents to contrast various scenarios and to suggest policy changes. Simulations have played an important role in identifying data to support the hypothesis that studies utilizing single doses are more sensitive than studies conducted with multiple doses to identify differences in bioavailability between two drug formulations. Because of this work, comparisons based on single dose studies are now encouraged by FDA to test the bioequivalence of two formulations. Another example of the use of M&S modeling involves blood pressure monitoring. By using M&S modeling, data on ambulatory blood pressure monitoring (ABPM) discovered not to have a placebo effect in contrast to the significant placebo effect that has been shown with manual cuff measurements. In addition, M&S has also played an important role as a tool for designing and analyzing clinical trials measuring ABPM.

In conclusion, M&S has been shown to play a significant role in making regulatory decisions affecting industry and the public. The FDA has recognized M&S as an invaluable tool for drug development, which is easily shown by a number of regulatory initiatives. The use of M&S in the process of clinical drug development discussed here illustrates the wide array of drug submissions accepted by the FDA. The use of modeling and simulation provides a critical tool for integration of data across the entire spectrum of drug development programs. Models based on *in vitro* data, physicochemical properties, and animal efficacy data utilized in early drug development area important tools for planning later stages in drug development [493].

7.3.3. The Use of Drug Modeling to Support Regulatory Approval of New Antimalarials

Models and simulations are in use to help explore policy options of malaria drug, to evaluate treatment options. They are very well suited to explore outcomes research for both biologic and economic issues. Modeling is an important tool to help estimate the utility of policies on antimalarial drug resistance and to help evaluate the cost effectiveness of antimalarial drug policy courses of action.

Resistance to antimalarial drugs has resulted in unnecessary morbidity, mortality, and financial loss that could have been avoided through better reasoned drug use policies. There is no justification for continuing to use ineffective drugs given the array of effective drugs currently available. Delaying a decision to change drug policy due to perceived implementation difficulties will only result in increases in malaria morbidity and mortality because of malaria drug resistance. The longer the decision to phase out ineffective malaria drugs is delayed, the more deep-rooted the use of ineffective therapies will become, particularly monotherapeutic treatment with artemisinins and other vulnerable partner drugs. The lack of knowledge of the impact of delay is likely one reason for the reluctance amongst potential funders and some national governments to make necessary drug policy changes, and the commitment of both entities is essential for implementation of effective, successful drug policy changes.

Development of a bio-economic model incorporating data on antimalarial drug use, parasite drug resistance, host immunity factors, epidemiology of disease, behavioral, and economic factors will be a very helpful contribution of a useful tool to this debate. The development of this type of model will require clarifying key relationships between important variables to include variables associated with carriage of parasites with resistant genotypes, patient compliance with treatment, and treatment outcomes in terms of illness duration and metrics associated with achievement of final disease cures. Extensive sensitivity analysis will be needed to illuminate the significance of variable uncertainties and the weight to be accorded to such factors as drug coverage and adherence. The key objective of development of such a model is to provide a tool for evaluation and planning changes in malaria drug policy and implementation. We believe that development of such a model will provide an effective tool to support rational decision-making on future deployment of ACT drugs [494].

The evolution of parasite drug resistance to *falciparum* was against standard antimalarial drugs such as sulfadoxine-pyrimethamine (SP) or chloroquine (CQ).

Through novel approaches based on evolutionary genetics and population biology will provide tools for understanding drug resistance to future antimalarials. Despite great advancements in malaria treatment that have been achieved over the past decade, full understanding of how the complex interactions of mutations conferring drug resistance *falciparum* malaria will require an approach that takes into account the structure of the parasite population among other demographic variables.

One approach that could be used to understand the spread of antimalarial drug resistance is to dynamically resistance mutations of model drug at different temporal and spatial scales with some simple outputs like malaria epidemiology or population metrics. Instead of developing one intricate model, that considers malaria infections globally with a wealth of associated complexity, rapid progress could be made on a family of related models interacting *via* common or related parameters to make specific predictions at one scale in one location. Some of these parameters may allow planning for the long-term effect of a drug policy decision at a regional level but may not be useful in describing development of resistance at a local level. Other models applied to single populations may be useful to make decisions over a limited time horizon if other factors such as the population structure can be considered of negligible impact.

These kinds of models might be developed by initially using a set of preliminary models capable of exploring the sensitivity of model dynamics to changes in simple common parameters at a given spatial or temporal scale. Then, such preliminary models could be further developed to make more realistic, data-driven models capable of making useful predictions. By considering processes that are non-deterministic or effected by chance in complex models, simulated data could be generated and then compared with real data. Through such a development process, models could become tools where scenarios can be tried and evaluated to describe model fit to real data. This kind of modeling approach may allow definition of what is 'a population' and how that population relates with other populations, which may provide operational units to manage drug resistance. Whatever modeling is finally applied to assess how drug resistance emerges could be substantially improved by combining molecular data with epidemiological investigations [495].

Many malaria-endemic countries frequently contemplate change in antimalarial drug policy to understand the impact of therapy, from deciding to implement ACT treatment or deciding which ACT treatment is best. With an appropriate dynamic data-driven model, decisions of malaria drug deployment, and the impact of a drug deployment decision can be reached quantitatively. A comprehensive model was constructed by one group to incorporate important biological and epidemiological factors of the insect vector, the malaria parasite, the human host and a proposed treatment regimen. This model was developed iteratively to identify the required parameters and the data needed to link this model to empirical evidence. This model provides quantitative outcomes metrics to include malaria incidence, malaria prevalence, treatment failures, and resistance spread in both high and low transmission settings. Accordingly, this model was used to assess different antimalarial treatment options associated with deployment of ACTs.

The model predicted robustly that drug resistance spreads much faster in low transmission areas than in high transmission areas, and failures to treat effectively disease are the driving force enhancing the spread of drug resistance. In low transmission areas, deployment of ACTs slows down the speed drug resistance emerges to partner drugs, particularly at high coverage rates. This effect decreases exponentially with longer delays in deploying ACT regimens and corresponding decreases in rates of coverage. In high transmission areas, however, drug resistance is primarily driven by the fraction of the population with residual drug levels present, which provides resistant parasites a survival advantage over non-resistant parasites. The emergence and spread of parasite drug resistance in both low and high transmission areas could be further slowed down by stopping the presumptive distribution of malaria drugs without a diagnosis, combination therapy drugs with significant mismatches in their half-lives, and reductions in transmission of malaria through bednet distribution, indoor residual spraying, and outdoor vector control. This model is a useful tool for understanding changes in treatment policies, *falciparum*. The outputs provided by this model make a strong argument for switching current drug regimens to ACTs in malaria endemic areas [496].

7.4. PK/PD MODELING: IMPLICATIONS FOR RESISTANCE OF ANTIMALARIAL COMBINATIONS

7.4.1. A Common Mathematical Model of Antimalarial Drug Resistance

Distinguishing between drug resistant and drug susceptible parasites is based on a black and white scenario where infections respond to antimalarial treatment or does not respond to treatment. Response to treatment is dependent on both patient and parasite factors. From a microbiology perspective, antimalarial resistance is not black and white but rather a continuum. Mathematically, antimalarial resistance has been modeled including data derived from various parasite subpopulations with different levels of drug susceptibility. As a population of infecting malaria parasites consists of both resistant and susceptible subpopulations, these subpopulations can be mathematically modeled separately.

Modeling changes in drug resistance state (from resistant to susceptible or from susceptible to resistant) has been one of the challenges of modeling parasite subpopulations. A change in state from drug susceptible to a drug resistant or temporarily not susceptible state during treatment has been modeled compartmentally using a functional space where parasites are "protected" from the antimalarial drug. Appearance of new drug resistant mutants during treatment has been modeled by adding a stochastic or chance event component. Selection of pre-existing less susceptible parasite subpopulations is a very relevant aspect of infection when strains emerge as resistant *in vivo* to antimalarial drugs. Pre-existing drug resistance can be suppressed through treatment with drug doses high enough to kill less susceptible subpopulations.

New mutations leading to antimalarial drug resistance noted to appear more frequently when the number of parasites is considerably larger reflected by the inverse of the frequency of mutation. Accordingly, clinical appearance of drug resistance is dependent on the initial burden of parasites present when antimalarial therapy is started. Delays in initiation of treatment or under dosage situations facilitate further replication of parasites and likely increase the probability of resistance. Various mechanisms are believed to be responsible for emergence of resistance to antimalarial drugs. In theory, the presence of efflux pumps to pump drugs out of the parasite and mutations render parasite enzymes immune to drug de-activation should be shown by an increased EC_{50}, increases in the half-maximal effective drug concentration. While alterations in the drug target site should reflect a reduced maximum effect or E_{max} (shown by the equation E_{max} = k_{kill} max/k_{death0}). Situations where the EC_{50} increases but the E_{max} is unchanged suggest that resistance to drugs can be overcome by boosting drug concentrations.

Meagher *et al.* [497] modeled the microorganism subpopulation kinetics using different susceptibilities to an antimicrobial drug, and all of the parameters, except the EC_{50}, were the same for all subpopulations. These authors used equation 11 (derived from the common model (Eq. 12), which reflects no inhibition of replication, includes nonlinear, capacity-limited, microorganism replication, and empirically modifies drug concentration through a susceptibility factor (1/MIC).

$$\frac{dN}{dt} = \frac{VG_{max}}{N_{50} + N} \cdot N - \left[1 + \frac{E_{max} \cdot \left(\frac{C}{MIC}\right)^H}{EC_{50}^H + \left(\frac{C}{MIC}\right)^H}\right] \cdot k_{death0} \cdot N \tag{11}$$

$$\frac{dN}{dt} = k_{replic0} \cdot E_r(C) \cdot N - k_{death0} \cdot E_d(C) \cdot N \tag{12}$$

A population pharmacodynamic approach has also been used to model the effects of antimicrobial drugs on multiple microorganism strains with varying levels of drug susceptibility. This approach models the IC_{50} as a hybrid parameter dependent on the mixture of subpopulations and allowing the EC_{50} or k_{kill} max factors to change when the population composition changes. Time-variant parameters can also be used to model adaptive resistance [497].

7.4.2. Use of PK/PD Modeling to Describe Antimalarial Drug Resistance

Antimalarial resistance models are focused on describing malaria epidemiology to predict effects of potential drug policy changes based on a thorough representation of underlying biology. The predictions of such models based on malaria prevalence and the fraction of infections resistant to treatment are used to calculate efficacy and cost of different treatment options. Previous mathematical models of malaria have focused on isolated aspects of malaria epidemiology, host dynamics, or drug resistance. A more recent holistic model by Hastings examines effects of drug PK and PD properties on drug resistance and evolves resistance in a more realistic manner by simulating gradually increases in drug tolerance [64]. The authors have aimed to a wide variety of factors to include epidemiological, parasitological, drug, host, vectorial, economic, and behavioral factors using available data [494, 498].

1) Outline of the Hastings Model:

The Hastings model is a time iterative model developing resistance in two stages as described previously through *de novo* emergence and spread. This model focuses only on emergence and spread of drug resistance, which allows assumptions on resistance to be made for a variety of drugs and drug combinations. These assumptions can be specified or explored in detail in a separate resistance emergence model, which also includes parasite mutation frequencies and host immunity factors, which affect a parasite's probability of survival. To utilize the Hastings model, a set of initial data inputs is necessary. The model is based on a population of patients with a given frequency of malaria infections and a percentage of infections caused by resistant parasites. The model assumes a single resistant parasite can expand in numbers and cause a resistant infection *in vivo*, and that this initial resistant infection is transmitted and the results of transmission include one or more than one resistant infection(s) in a subsequent host in the next cycle. Transmission in this model is modeled to occur at random in a host population, and at conclusion of each model cycle the number of total infections and the fraction of parasites that remain susceptible or the fraction that have become resistant are calculated. These intermediate cycle outputs are fed back into the model and the next model cycle begins with updated data on infection frequency and proportion of sensitive/resistant parasites. The cyclical process is repeated until a cycle time limit is reached, malaria eradication is achieved, or 100% of the remaining parasites are drug resistant (Fig. **23**).

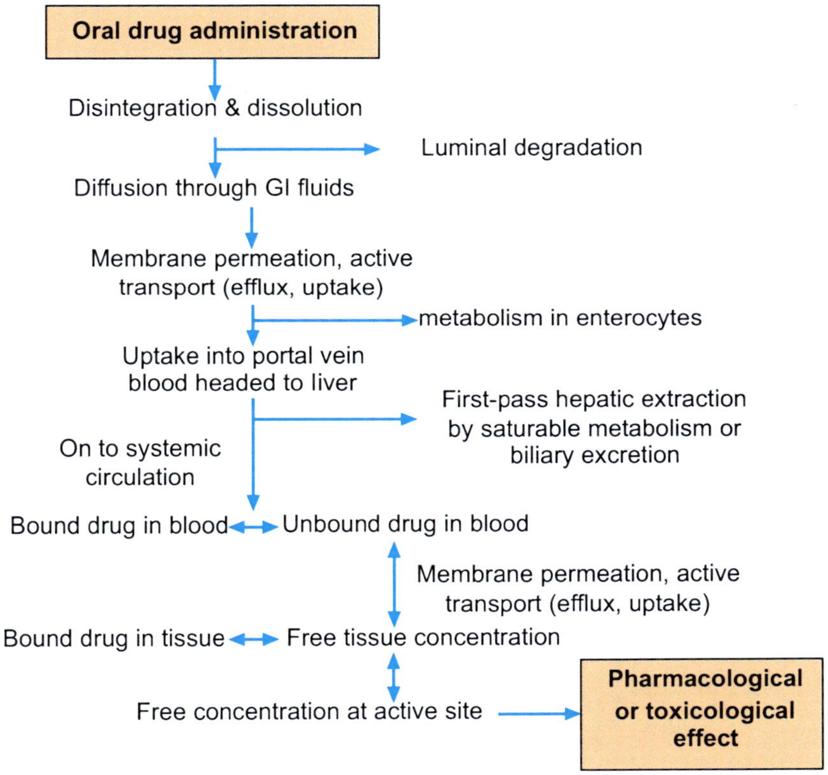

Figure 23: A schematic diagram of the processes impacting the free concentration of drug at the target. Reference cited from [8].

2) Impact of Immunity on the Hastings Model

The effect of immunity in the host on an infecting parasite is central to this model, and immunity impacts on transmission of parasites and emergence of drug resistance. Accordingly, this model also includes effects of immunity including a reduction in parasite numbers, reduction in symptomatic infections, an increase in the probability of self-cure, an increase in the rates of cure for treated infections, and reductions in the reproductive rate of parasites because of decreases in the length of infection and the diminished probability of treatment failure. Host immunity can affect emergence and spread of drug resistance in a variety of ways, which do influence the probability that an infected person may actually have malaria symptoms and seek treatment. The relationship between immune patients and non-immune patients is an oversimplified binary description of immunity; however, there are differences in the proportion of patients. Those patients with symptomatic infections are treated actually for malaria in low and high transmission intensity areas.

In a low transmission area, the level of innate immunity in the population is low and the majority of potential patients will almost certainly be symptomatic seeking treatment after a malaria infection. In high transmission areas, a high level of innate immunity exists and majorities of patients with parasitemia are asymptomatic and, likely, not all will seek treatment. They expose fewer parasites to antimalarial drugs (quantitatively, there will be higher numbers of infected patients in high transmission numbers than in low transmission areas, but a larger fraction of patients in high transmission areas will not seek treatment than in low transmission areas). In this high transmission/high immunity circumstance, selective pressure is lower as the resistant parasites do not have a transmission advantage given they are equally likely to be carrying non- resistant malaria parasites which can also be transmitted.

In each population, transmission of parasites occurs both within and across groups. Transmission in this model is measured by basic rates of reproduction, for drug sensitive parasites, the reproductive rate is lower in patients with treated malaria than in untreated malaria and the lowest if the malaria treatment administered is an ACT. The rate at which resistant parasites spread in the Hastings model is a function of the ratio of the reproductive rates of drug resistant infections to drug sensitive infections in each treatment group. Initially, a relative reproductive rate of four was implemented for the Hastings model. This factor was derived from a study showing patients who suffered malaria treatment failures after mefloquine treatment carried gametocytes for a period four times longer than patients with drug sensitive parasites did.

3) Incorporating Immunity into the Hastings Model

The mechanism by which immunity to malaria is acquired is complex in nature and the question of whether the age of the infected patient has an effect on how quickly immunity develops independent of exposure to malaria is still under debate. To make the Hastings model realistic, an immunity function was necessary to model effects of the frequency of infection on immunity, and, in addition, changes in immunity need to be fed back into the model. In order to do this, immunity functions were calculated based on a number of factors to include parasite density, age categorized rates of parasitemia, the incidence of severe malaria at different intensities of transmission, and malaria morbidity. These functions are implemented at each model cycle to determine the fraction of treated *versus* non treated infections, parasite density, and the parasite reproductive rates in age group related to parasite reproduction in a non- immune one-year old host. As infection frequency is altered over subsequent model cycle, the population "immunity profile" is allowed to change; these updates are possible through adjustments made to the level of immunity incorporated in the immunity function in the model based on a new value for the intensity of parasite transmission.

4) Model Inputs

The Hastings model requires value input for a number of key parameters. Where these values are measured, these values should be obtained from published data. Where no published data exists, these input values have been obtained from observations made in the field, and these model assumptions have led to different sensitivity analysis outcomes. The key initial inputs to the Hastings model are as follows [494]:

- Population size;
- The mutation rate of the parasite population can be set from a probability of 1 in 10^9 to 1 in 10^{18}; initial resistance level to a non-artemisinin partner drug;
- Initial estimated Entomological Inoculation Rate (EIR), which represents the malaria transmission intensity in certain geographic areas;
- The basic rate of reproduction (R0) of an untreated, sensitive infection ranging from a value of 1 to 10;
- The relative rates of reproduction of treated sensitive and resistant infections set in relation to the basic rate of reproduction (no cost to parasite fitness is assumed to resistant parasites with mutations;
- The maximum density of parasites is assumed in a non-immune patient to be 10^9 to 10^{12} parasites per person);

- The maximum percentage of infected patients treated with antimalarials can be inputted ranging from 50-100%;
- The ACT coverage rate, which can be inputted to range from (0-100%).

5) Using the Hastings Model to Estimate Drug Cost-Effectiveness

Once initial model inputs are made, the Hastings epidemiologic model can be used to estimate the cost effectiveness of ACT drugs over the long term under different conditions of implementation. Costs to both patient and provider are built into the model, which does provide a social perspective. One of the more fundamental concerns regarding use of ACTs has been the increased cost of drugs *versus* standard antimalarials, and the initial treatment cost with first-line drugs has been calculated separately from costs of treatment failure, which will increase exponentially over time due to increasing malaria drug resistance. The cost of initial patient treatment to a provider includes the cost of drugs, the cost of diagnosis and consultation, and inpatient treatment costs for a small percentage of patients who need hospital treatment. The cost of treatment failure includes antimalarial drugs (including second- and third-line drugs), the cost of diagnosis and consultation, costs associated with inpatient care, and costs associated with treatment of malaria complications to include cerebral malaria, renal failure, severe anemia, and low birth weight babies.

For patients who are admitted to public clinics and hospitals, costs associated with treatment include user fees for care, costs of transportation and food. User fees in the Hastings model do not represent an overall alteration in costs to society, however, so these fees are not included in the overall calculation. For patients receiving outpatient treatment or obtaining treatment through a non-public provider, direct costs paid by patients for treatment, diagnosis, consultation, and diagnosis can be included along with transportation and food costs. Along with direct costs, patients and society suffer indirect impacts due to loss of productivity, which can also be estimated in this model. This loss of productivity can be represented as an actual number of productivity days lost and costs associated with the loss of productivity. Estimate of actual costs associated with lost work must be calculated separately as there are methodological difficulties in estimating lost work costs associated with the agricultural calendar, the time of year, and in the context of family and society.

Each outcome derived from the Hastings biological model is then assigned a likelihood of treatment outcome of cure or failure depending on the level of parasite drug resistance and patient compliance. As the actual rates of cure for non- compliant patients is not known, estimates have been calculated using data derived from drug efficacy studies testing drug regimens with shorter durations than those currently on market. Over a period ranging from 5-10 years, the numbers of patient cures, failures and the costs of treatment can be combined. By changing input parameters, the effects of changing drug regimens, at varying rates of coverage, their costs, and their effectiveness in both patient care and in terms of social cost can be compared and contrasted. By including the efficacy and cost of different drugs with varying levels of compliance, overall cost-effectiveness associated with changes in policy and implementation can be compared. These costs might include specific packaging of combination therapy of drugs not co-formulated into one pill to increase adherence, for example, or increasing the percentage of malaria cases with a definitive diagnosis prior to initiation of treatment [494].

7.4.3. Modeling Practices to Estimate Drug Resistance of Antimalarial Drugs and Their Combinations

1) Intra-Host PK/PD Modeling of Artemisinin Drug-Resistance

Resistance to artemisinin drugs has been noted in patients infected with *falciparum* malaria has been shown in western Cambodia [4-6]. The resistance to artemisinin drugs has been associated with prolonged parasite clearance times (PCTs) after artemisinin treatment. While a new molecular marker has been associated with artemisinin resistance (the K-13 propeller mutation) [5], the biological cause of artemisinin resistance is not clear; however, one hypothesis to explain the delayed parasite clearance phenomenon is based on the premise that there is a reduction in stage-specific artemisinin sensitivity of young, circulating asexual ring stage parasites. A mathematical model has been developed to describe the parasite stage-specific PK/PD relationships in the host. Model parameters were estimated using detailed data derived from PK and parasite clearance data obtained from 39 patients from Pailin in western Cambodia (an area of artemisinin resistance) infected with uncomplicated *falciparum* malaria that were treated with artesunate and 40 patients from Wang Pha in northwestern Thailand where no artemisinin resistance has been observed.

A deterministic model for parasite multiplication and maturation during asexual blood stages has been developed to describe the relationship between parasite stage and artemisinin sensitivity or resistance. The basis for this model is the assumption that after infection with acute *falciparum* malaria the age distribution of asexual stage parasites conforms to a Gaussian distribution ranging from 1 to 48 hours. In *falciparum* malaria, only young un-sequestered parasites are in the peripheral circulation available to be counted in a peripheral blood smear. This model incorporates individual pharmacokinetic data derived from the concentration-time profile of dihydroartemisinin (DHA) (Fig. **24**) and stage-specific PK/PD relationships to provide a prediction of the numbers of young, circulating parasites that can be observed in peripheral blood smears over time for each patient. This stage- specific PK/PD relationship in this model is based on a hypothesis that antimalarial activity of artesunate and DHA, its principal metabolite, varies depending on the developmental stage of asexual blood stage parasites, which, in turn, suggests there is a different concentration-effect relationship associated with each developmental stage. This model outputs a specific concentration time curve for each stage of the sequential three life cycle stages of an asexual parasite - rings, trophozoites, and schizonts.

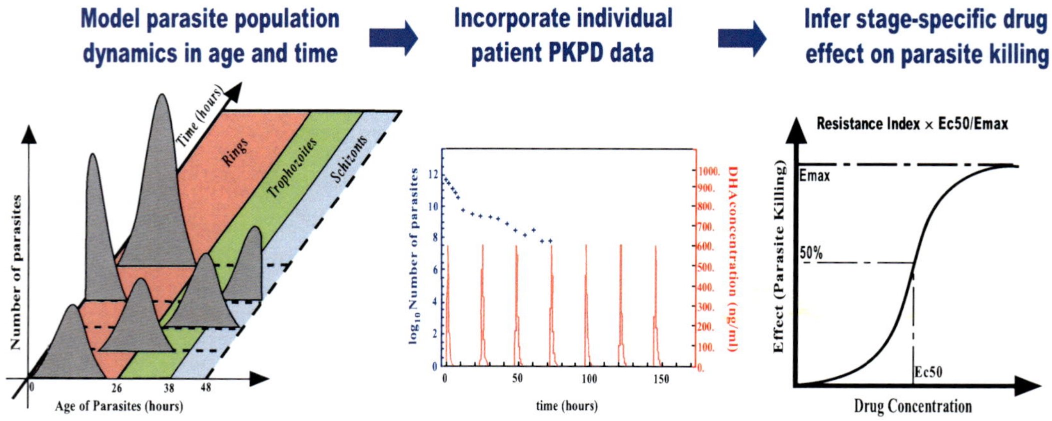

Figure 24: Illustration shows a model of parasite population, to include model structure, inputs, and outputs. An initial population of parasites (Left) is distributed normally over age and moves to the right over time. The concentration of the drug over time (Center) is incorporated into the model by assuming that subsequent doses have the same concentration profile as the initial measured dose for each patient. The model then combines a dose-effect relationship with the drug concentration to determine how many parasites at each stage are killed by the drug at each time point. The total number of circulating parasites predicted by the model is fitted to the observed parasite density data (Center) and the resistance index for each stage is inferred from the dose-effect curve (Right) [50].

Definition of a single parameter that defines the level of resistance is necessary to determine statistically significant changes in resistance associated with different life cycle stages and different geographical settings to help describe comparisons of the different concentration-effect profiles. For each parasite stage modeled, the concentration-effect relationship was further simplified into a single value called the resistance index (R.I.) based on the shape of the curve. High R.I. values correspond to high levels of drug resistance while low values correspond to lower levels of resistance [50]. Fig. **24** shows the outline model structure with its inputs and outputs.

This model was shown to predict that reduced concentration dependent killing of young, ring stage parasites that is the most likely factor causing the delayed parasite clearance observed in Pailin. In acute malaria, diminished parasite clearance after artemisinin treatment might result from reduced drug susceptibility of any parasite stage, but early, quick reductions in parasite density is associated with parasite sequestration or ring-stage killing. The principal difference between the artemisinin compounds and other antimalarial drugs is artemisinin compounds kill ring-stage parasites quickly. Changes in ring-stage killing alters the parasite clearance curve, and the curve then looks very similar to curves associated with other antimalarial drugs like quinine that have no effect on circulating ring stages.

A reduced effect of artemisinin drugs on circulating ring stage parasites explains current observations seen in the border regions of Cambodia. This model of artemisinin resistance is based on two assumptions. The first assumption is the majority of natural infections are normally distributed and the minority of infections presents with multiple parasite "broods" possessing different stages of development. The second assumption is that the asexual life cycle of the malaria parasite takes 48 hours to complete. While an asexual life cycle of 48 hours is often found in the classical malaria literature, and the 48-hour number is a reasonable assumption fitting observations made in patients, it is clear from a number of *in vitro* studies that variability in the length of the malaria life cycle can be observed under different conditions.

The parameters calculated from Pailin and Wang Pha did not show complete separation, and recent genotyping of the parasites from Pailin suggests that approximately 20% of malaria infections there are sensitive to artemisinin [6].This data may explain why the data was not completely separated between these two sites. These results may also explain discrepancies noted between *in vivo* findings of markedly delays in parasite clearance rate while the *in vitro* IC_{50} determinations of the same parasites showed them to be susceptible to artemisinin [5, 6]. Conventional methods of *in vitro* potency testing expose parasites to constant drug concentrations over the entire parasite life cycle. If only the ring stage is artemisinin resistant and the trophozoite or later schizont stages remain artemisinin sensitive, standard *in vitro* drug potency determinations will not detect an *in vivo* stage-specific resistant phenotype.

Artesunate and DHA have plasma half-lives in man of approximately 1 hour. This time equates to an effective plasma concentration above the IC_{99} of approximately 6 hours/day when dosed once daily. Despite the short plasma half- lives of the artemisinins, a once-daily dose is the current drug treatment recommendation. The artemisinin dose and dosing regimen of once per day is effective only due to the broad efficacy of the artemisinin drugs across multiple parasite stages. If ring-stage parasites become resistant to artemisinins, the timing of drug administration relative to parasite developmental stage becomes more important, and a single daily dose of artemisinin might not kill the parasite population at the most sensitive stage. As most uncomplicated *falciparum* malaria infections arise with a predominance of ring stage parasites, the first dose of an artemisinin drug would be predicted to have a sub- maximal effect.

This model was implemented to model alternative dosing regimens for artemisinins, and the model predicted doubling the frequency of artemisinin drug dosing to twice per day is more likely to reduce parasite clearance times than increasing the dose of artemisinin drugs dosed once per day. The shape of the concentration-effect relationship curve calculated from this model suggests that increasing individual doses would not alter the parasite clearance time. Increasing the frequency of drug dosing to twice per day doubles the length of time parasiticidal drug concentrations are found in the blood while doubling the drug dose actually results in a shorter length of drug exposure as a consequence of first order drug elimination. A shorter length of drug exposure increases the risk of treatment failure when parasites are refractory to drug treatment. A clinical trial is underway to test this question utilizing a multiple-dose artemisinin-dosing scheme.

Other mechanisms to explain artemisinin resistance have been proposed to include dormancy of ring-stage parasites [47]. Under typical conditions of artemisinin exposure observed in natural infections, small proportions of ring-stage parasites have been shown to stop maturing but are not killed by artemisinin drugs [46]. The presence of these dormant parasites is believed to be responsible for the recrudescence, which can range as high as 10% observed in patients treated with 7-day courses of artemisinin derivatives administered as monotherapy or artemisinin combination therapy where the partner drug is rapidly eliminated. In order to explain the slow rate of parasite clearance observed *in vivo*, however, a very high percentage of parasites would have to enter a dormant stage. These same dormant parasites would have to be rapidly cleared or the parasite elimination curve would be markedly biphasic in nature. The parasite-time profile curves observed in clinical trials do not show a biphasic curve, which does not support this hypothesis. Artemisinin resistance may be associated with parasite dormancy, but an increased fraction of parasites that are dormant does not explain observed profiles of parasite clearance.

In conclusion, Saralamba *et al.* [50] developed an intra-host mathematical model to describe parasitological responses after treatment with artesunate for uncomplicated *falciparum* malaria. The mathematical model produced was capable of describing parasite clearance for each patient modeled with a very accurate goodness of fit. The parameter sets that resulted in the best model fits to observed *in vivo* data are composed of much conserved concentration-effect relationship for trophozoites and schizonts parasites, but a variable relationship for ring stage parasites. This modelling effort suggests that artesunate efficacy in western Cambodia is reduced for ring stage parasites. This modeling result does support the hypothesis that artemisinin resistance is a function of ring-stage parasite resistance, and this model supports the hypothesis that increasing the frequency of artemisinin treatment will enhance clearance of parasites that are resistant to artemisinin drugs [50].

2) PK/PD Modeling of the Elimination Half-Life of Antimalarial Drugs Administered to Drug-Resistant Parasites

There are only a few classes of antimalarial drugs, and there is an ongoing debate on the most effective means to use them [9, 156]. The definition of the best use of drugs with very different PK properties is an unresolved question. Drugs possessing long half-life have two advantages when used for treatment. First, they provide a post- treatment prophylactic effect which guards against re-infection. This post treatment prophylactic effect is very important to aid recovery from anemia, a significant cause of malaria morbidity and mortality. Long half-life drugs provide a benefit to populations in areas with epidemic, seasonal malaria where the season is short and attack rates approach 100%. Second, long half-life drugs require reduced dosing regimens, which eliminates problems with patient compliance and reduces the risk of under-dosage. Slowly eliminated drugs will persist *in vivo* after the malaria infection has been cured, and the residual drug levels will select for drug resistance. Therefore, while drugs with long-half lives are beneficial for individual treatment, they can cause long-term problems at the level of the population.

A study was conducted to describe the role of drug half-lives in the emergence and spread of antimalarial drug resistance [153]. As described previously, there are three classes of drug susceptibility observed in *falciparum* malaria: *Res0,* susceptible parasites; *Res1,* a percentage of parasites that have intermediate susceptibility that can still be treated and killed; and *Res2*, a proportion of parasites that are completely drug resistant. The outcome of this study showed that *Res1* and *Res2* parasites evolve at a faster rate if the antimalarial drug used for treatment has a long half-life.

Previous models of drug resistance failed to take into account the effects of drug half- life, and this omission likely resulted in underestimation of rate of Res2 parasite evolution [156]. In addition, these earlier models assumed there were only two possible phenotypic classes in the population; fully sensitive or fully resistant. Clinical studies in the field have shown this assumption is not true with one exception being the resistance of atovaquone, which is caused by a single base pair mutation in the cyt b gene, which results in complete resistance. The rapid evolution of resistance to atovaquone is countered by inclusion of proguanil to achieve drug synergy to avoid drug treatment failure. Drug resistance progresses gradually, as seen in mefloquine resistance, or in a systematic manner beyond baseline sensitivity, to a fully drug resistant form, as seen in pyrimethamine resistance. By providing definitions of three types of resistance, a model of malaria drug resistance hews closer to the available biological evidence and the resultant predictions should provide a better fit to observed data.

Stringent definitions of drug resistance are required to make the mathematics solvable, and these definitions are employed in genetic models of drug resistance to population malaria [156]. The mathematical results derived from such models provide insight into the factors, influences, and population dynamics driving drug resistance evolution. To enhance the validity of these models, the range of clinical outcomes must be reconciled, with different levels of modeled drug resistance. Parasites disappear from the peripheral circulation in cases of successful treatment, which can be attributed to killing of *Res0* and *Res1* parasites. In patients who fail treatment, parasitemia remains elevated, the patient does not improve clinically, and the parasites are likely primarily from the *Res2* population. In cases of infections with 'parasitological' resistance, clinical improvements are often associated with persistence of parasites with borderline susceptibility at low levels.

Parasitological resistance is often observed in early drug resistance stages, and this phenomenon is a predictor clinical resistance in the future. Population models like those that the one discussed here do have a category of borderline susceptibility; parasites are either killed (*Res0*) or *Res1*, or they are not killed at all (*Res2*). To model this more closely, parasites must be permitted to show degrees of behavior associated with *Res1* and *Res2*, which is commonly observed in cases of sulfadoxine-pyrimethamine (SP) resistance. Under this modification, in some circumstances, parasites will be killed and cleared and in others, they will not be killed and cleared.

Response to malaria treatment is complex in nature as shown in Fig. **25**, and treatment response is a function of parasite drug sensitivity and drug concentrations in the blood, which vary because of drug half-life. This example shows the kinetics of SP *versus* drug resistance, which is very well characterized, however, these features are generally universal. All antimalarial drugs, except some artemisinin compounds, are absorbed more rapidly than they are cleared which provides a classic concentration/time curve composed of a maximum plasma concentration shown a few hours after drugs are administered followed by a quick decline at a defined rate. Variations in drug absorption and volume of distribution are known to cause differences in blood drug concentrations are not dealt with in this model, and this variability in ADME properties can play a role in emergence of drug resistance.

Mathematically, the time required for antimalarial drug concentration to decrease by half (elimination half-life: $t_{1/2}$) is related to the relationship $t_{1/2} = \ln 2/k_e = 0.693/k_e$. For a variety of drugs, modeling blood concentration profiles using compartment models with two or three different compartments may be needed, however, the majority of drug elimination is a consequence of terminal drug elimination describe by the terminal rate constant ß and the terminal half-life, which is described by $t_{1/2ß}$. The residual concentration of drugs in the blood of the host is adequate to prevent re-infection up to the point where drug concentration falls below the minimum parasiticidal concentration (MPC) for a particular population of parasites (Fig. **25**).

This period of time where residual levels of antimalarial drugs provide protection against re-infection is defined as the 'period of chemoprophylaxis' (PC). When more parasites that are resistant are more frequently encountered, the average PC decreases. For sulfadoxine -pyrimethamine, the average PC has been modeled to be 52 days for *Res0* genotypes and 15 days for the first *Res1* parasites, which appear. For *Res2* parasites the period of chemoprophylaxis is, by definition, zero. Drugs with shorter half- lives exhibit similar dynamics but the time-scale (as shown on the x-axis of Fig. **25**) is clearly shorter with a shorter PC. Given rapid clearance of artemisinin compounds and their active metabolites suggests even completely drug susceptible parasites are only affected by drug for limited periods only slightly beyond the period of treatment [65].

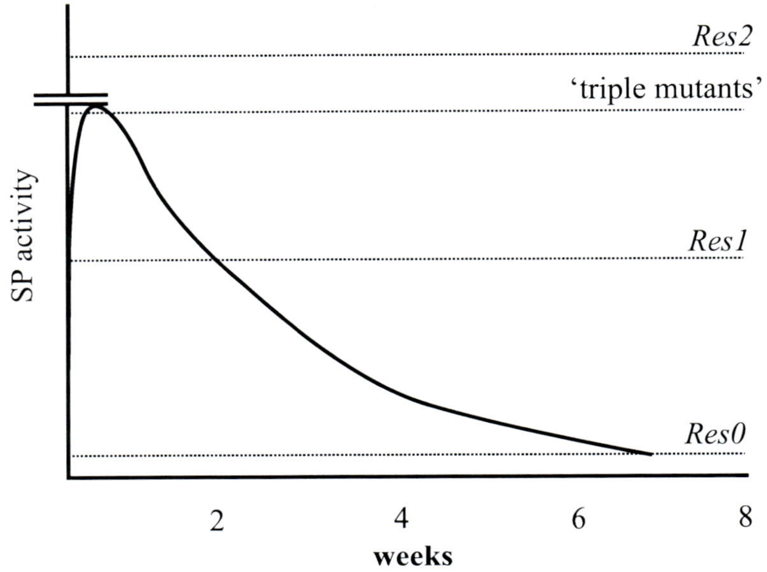

Figure 25: Pharmacodynamics and pharmacokinetics of SP. SP is administered orally at time zero and its concentration in the blood is represented by the solid line; it is rapidly absorbed, reaching peak concentrations within 12 h, after which both drugs are gradually eliminated at rates defined by the respective elimination rate constant (k) (from the first-order equation, 'half-life' is equal to 0.693/k). Drug concentration is represented by 'SP activity' on the left-hand axis, rather than the more usual stoichiometric concentration, because pyrimethamine and sulphadoxine exert synergistic activity against the parasite. Three classes of genotype are considered: *Res0, Res1* and *Res2. Res0* and all *Res1* subclasses except the triple mutant in dihydrofolate reductase (DHFR) are eliminated by drug treatment. This is because SP activity exceeds their respective minimum parasiticidal concentration (MPC; represented by the dotted lines) for a sufficient time-period. The DHFR 'triple mutant' is of borderline susceptibility. Given variability in SP activity profiles between treated individuals some of these infections will be eliminated, others will not. *Res0* parasites can infect a host only after 52 days have elapsed since treatment (by which time SP activity has decayed to below the *Res0* MPC), while *Res1* parasites can re-infect 15 days after treatment. The quadruple mutant (*Res2* resistance level) is completely unaffected by SP [65].

This method has been used to model the effects of drugs in combination most notably when drug partners have different half-lives, and development of resistance to pyrimethamine- sulphadoxine. An important element of this model is development of resistance to antimalarial drugs in two different phases. In phase A, *Res1* parasite drug resistance spreads and these parasites replace the *Res0* drug sensitive forms while *Res2* parasites are few I number. Phase B begins when parasites with borderline susceptibility are selected that are capable of escaping drug action and becoming *Res2* parasites. Selection of *Res2* parasites is rapid in nature from borderline *Res1* parasites and this selection in a population of patients leads to broad treatment failure. Drug treatment of patients is clinically possible during phase A, and providers may not be aware of significant changes in the genotype of the parasite population that signals onset of phase B. Surveillance programs on the ground are therefore essential after a new drug is introduced, to effectively monitor changes in drug efficacy and provide warning of pending drug failure.

Given that this model of drug resistance has added two new factors of drug half-life and partial drug resistance, it seems reasonable to consider implications for use of malaria drugs in the field. These model results and the results of other drug resistance models, all suggest antimalarial drug use should be as minimal as is possible. This leads to a conflict between what an individual needs and a population needs. Malaria can rapidly progress from unpleasant to deadly, and prompt access to inexpensive drugs is important to minimize morbidity and mortality. The downside to expanded access to drug treatment is excessive use of antimalarial drugs to treat fevers that are not due to malaria. This scenario will expand the emergence and spread of malaria drug resistance. There is no clear answer to this problem that would limit access to antimalarial drugs just to treat malaria, although broader use of inexpensive rapid diagnostic tests are a step in the right direction [153].

3) PK/PD Modeling of Mefloquine-Resistant Malaria Parasites

Mathematical modeling of mefloquine utilizing population pharmacokinetic and *in vivo* and *in vitro* PD data from the field has been conducted to examine questions of dose and the appropriate time point for monitoring the evolution of resistance. Mefloquine's long half-life of 2 to 3 weeks in infected patients drivers many questions of what dose is best to avoid emergence of resistance and what duration of time is best to examine patient outcomes to assess the emergence of mefloquine resistance. The elimination phase of mefloquine is bi- or tri-exponential, with a slow decline in blood drug levels in the terminal phase, which provides a long period when declining concentrations of mefloquine ranging from 20-80% of the original therapeutic level are associated with intermediate inhibitory activity against *P. falciparum*. Thus, as seen in bacteria, an important factor that may be relevant to predict the probability of developing drug resistance may be related to the time required drug concentrations to fall to a level 20-80%

of the therapeutic concentrations where these drugs exhibit their maximum inhibitory effects [499].

A mathematical model was derived to model emergence of mefloquine resistance based on data derived both *in vitro* and *in vivo* to compare development of mefloquine resistance with either lower or higher antimalarial doses of mefloquine. The work that defined this model was the derivation of a mathematical equation describing changes in parasite burden with time in the presence of mefloquine. For *de novo* selection of resistant parasite mutants, if one malaria parasite for every 10x parasites possesses a mutation conferring drug resistance, the probability a patient has such a drug resistant mutant is $(1/10^x) \cdot P_t$, where P_t is the total number of parasites at time t.

The total number of parasites present in a patient at a particular time (P_t) balances the mean parasite multiplication rate and the fraction of parasites killed and cleared by antimalarial drugs and host defenses. Accordingly, changes in parasitemia can be described as $(dP/dt) = a \cdot P - f(C) \cdot P - f(I) \cdot P$ where a is a parameter representing the growth rate constant of the parasite, $f(C)$ is a function, dependent on the concentration of the drug (C), that represents the killing of the parasites. $f(I)$ is a function that represents the host's background immunity to malaria.

The contribution of host immunity contributes little to drug effect at high mefloquine concentrations, but this factor does become more relevant at low concentrations of mefloquine. This factor is not relevant in most cases, although in regions with high rates of malaria transmission where drugs that are either partially effective or ineffective are used, host immunity can be the main factor associated with therapeutic outcome. Thus, $(dP/dt) = a \cdot P - f(C) \cdot P$.

Parasite killing is considered in this model to be a first-order process continuing without change during the period of parasite clearance. This assumption is because the pathogenic processes of malaria infection are all intravascular and antimalarial drug activity is associated with concentrations of unbound drugs present in plasma. Parasite killing is e described by a sigmoid E_{max} model:

$$f(C) = k1 \cdot \frac{C\gamma}{C\gamma + C_{50}^{\gamma}} \tag{13}$$

Where k_1 is the first order rate constant describing killing of parasites, γ is the slope of the concentration-effect curve, C is the drug concentration, and C_{50} is the drug concentration capable of killing 50% of the parasites. The concentration of antimalarial drugs in patient plasma is not constant, and the concentration rises as drug is absorbed and declines over time as drug is distributed throughout the body and eventually eliminated. Concerning mefloquine, the phase of drug elimination has been shown to be bi-exponential or tri-exponential and assuming intermediate concentrations of mefloquine are selective only during the terminal elimination, a mono-exponential elimination phase that corresponds to the terminal elimination phase of an antimalarial drug could be used. Therefore, $C = C_0 \bullet e\text{-}k \bullet t$ where t is time (in days), k is the terminal elimination rate constant of mefloquine, and C_0 is the C_{max} or maximum mefloquine concentration.

P_t was determined by integrating (dP/dt). The following solution results:

$$P_t = P_0 \cdot e^{a \cdot t} \cdot \left[\frac{(C_{50})^\gamma + \left(C_0 \cdot e^{-k \cdot t}\right)^\gamma}{(C_{50}) + (C_0)^\gamma} \right]^{k1/(k \cdot \gamma)} \tag{14}$$

where P_0 is the total parasite burden at time zero before addition of drug.

The speed resistance develops to malaria drugs is varies considerably with patterns of drug use. Uncontrolled self-medication associated with insufficient treatment will provide pressure to select for development of resistance as this practice exposes many parasites to ineffective concentrations of antimalarial drugs. In this study of mefloquine drug resistance, the effects of two different treatment options can be tested. This is a very relevant example given the rise of resistance to mefloquine in Southeast Asia. This rise in resistance could have been delayed further or prevented.

In the PK/PD models presented here, dose linearity was assumed for mefloquine, but recent studies have shown that acute malaria infection reduces the bioavailability of orally administered mefloquine. If a dose of 25 mg/kg of mefloquine is split (15 mg/kg initially followed by 10 mg/kg later) to avoid adverse events such as neurotoxicity or gastrotoxicity, the second element of the dose is associated with a disproportionate elevation in the blood drug level and a 50% increase in the area under the concentration-time curve. Accordingly, splitting the dose of 25 mg/kg of mefloquine results in greater drug bioavailability, and increased drug bioavailability is less likely to select for resistance. The relationship between the EC_{90} (*in vivo*) and the EC_{90} (*in vitro*) for mefloquine is unknown. The concentration-effect curve *in vivo* is shifted to the right of the concentration-effect curve *in vitro* due to the binding of mefloquine to plasma proteins, which decreases the concentration of free drug. Only the free drug that is not bound to plasma proteins is capable of crossing membranes and killing intracellular malaria parasites. *In vitro* assays of plasma protein binding to mefloquine are also confounded by a tendency of mefloquine to stick to plastic and other laboratory hardware. The level of protein binding is generally considered to be very high, approximately 98%.

The level of drug resistance in the population is consistently underestimated. *In vivo* models have shown malaria recrudescence can take place 4 weeks after treatment. In addition, the process of evolving mefloquine drug resistance typically presents few early episodes of recrudescence, and a larger fraction of recrudescence actually occurs after 28 days. This data confirms the hypothesis that conventional assessments of treatment response at a time 28 days after treatment underestimates the real level of drug resistance, and longer periods of follow-up are necessary. Such models suggest initial administration of mefloquine at doses of 15 mg/kg, for example, would provide an increased probability for drug resistant parasites to be selected and treatment with mefloquine at this dose is more likely to result in rapid drug resistance than simply using the higher mefloquine dose (25 mg/kg) [499].

The modeling outputs described here provide the means to conduct pharmacoeconomic assessments of drug policy changes. The extrapolations from the models discussed here are still pertinent to artemisinin combination treatment, however, the quantity of parasites actually exposed to sub-therapeutic drug levels are significantly diminished after ACT treatment as the vast majority of parasites are killed after exposure to artemisinin compounds [62]. With regards to mefloquine, treatment should involve administration at a dose of 25 mg/kg, not 15 mg/kg combined with an artemisinin compound for maximum effect and minimum probability of developing drug resistance [499].

4) Considerations for Proper Design of ACT Resistance Models

The scientific basis for implementation of malaria drug policies comes from empirical data and from mathematical models on emergence of resistance to standard antimalarial drugs such as sulfadoxine-pyrimethamine, chloroquine, and other historic antimalarials administered as monotherapy. Unfortunately, there are a number of problems with modeling based on this data as part of the empirical data derived from monotherapeutic treatment cannot be included in these models and some of the models have failed to account for the complex evolution of *falciparum* malaria in man. *Falciparum* drug resistance has been modeled using either dynamic population epidemiological models or approaches based on population genetics, however, other more intricate models have also been designed. The basic population theories of genetic mutation, recombination, and selection have been utilized to describe the dynamics of the evolution of drug resistance forward in time. Population genetic modeling has been used to describe the parasite fitness costs associated with drug resistance by modeling the intensity of malaria transmission, human immunity, and multiplicities of infection (MOI). Neither of these two approaches have tools to assess the evolution of drug resistance through antimalarial drug selection nor do they address how the effects of drug resistance caused by parasite population structure. These two model approaches, the epidemiological model and the population genetic model do yield consistent outputs. Both models have predicted that the rising prescription of antimalarials would lead to emergence of parasite drug resistance [500].

The population genetic model has provided useful retrospective analyses of drug resistance to antimalarials utilizing genetic footprints of parasites acquired through selective collection studies. This approach is based on coalescent theory, which describes evolution of parasites at neutral loci under different demographic scenarios, and selection, which includes intricate patterns of a population structure. Coalescent theory attempts to trace all forms of a gene shared by population members to a single ancestral copy, known as the most recent common ancestor, also known as the co-ancestor. The inheritance relationships between alleles noted are represented as a gene genealogy known as the coalescent, which is similar to a phylogenetic tree. Understanding statistical properties of the coalescent under varying assumptions is the foundation of coalescent theory.

Together, models of population dynamics and population genetics can be used together in a complementary manner through consideration of various levels of time, space, and complexity. The goal of using both models is to build a framework where each approach enhances the other. Instead of developing, a grand complex model that considers all aspects of malaria infection, a family of models that are related can be created based on predictions required interacting through common parameters. Such models might be developed through use of preliminary model sets allow exploration of model sensitivity to make an initial evaluation based on differences in common parameters at a similar temporal or spatial scale. Preliminary model efforts will lead to more intricate, predictive models by incorporating the effects of chance or stochastic processes in complex models. This type of effort could create models of real experimental design capable of testing specific scenarios with real data [495].

7.5. PK/PD MODELING: IMPLICATIONS FOR EFFICACY OF ANTIMALARIAL COMBINATIONS

7.5.1. Common Mathematical Models of Antimalarial Drug Efficacy

The objective of PK/PD model development is the application and development of mathematical models to predict and describe PK (dose to concentration relationships) and PD (concentration to effect relationships) of drugs used for treatment of disease. The PK modeling element of a PK/PD model describes the macro-distribution of the drug while the PD or effect-compartment of a PK/PD models adds a hypothetical effect compartment, which describes delays associated with drug action. In compartmental models, the profiles of concentration *versus* time are modeled through exchange of drugs between hypothetical connected compartments, each with their own rates of drug absorption, distribution, and elimination. Drug distribution to the target tissue is modeled using a plasma effect-site equilibration constant (ke_0; or its half-life [$t_{½}$ k_{e0}] = $\ln 2/k_{e0}$). Concentration-effect relationships are often modeled using the sigmoid maximum effect (E_{max}) as follows: E_{max} model [$E = (E_{max} \text{ x } C)/(EC_{50} + C)$],

where, C is drug concentration at the receptor site and EC_{50} is the concentration of drug

where the effect = $E_{max}/2$.

The first order rate constant derived to model the exchange between the plasma and effect compartments was described in 1968 by Segre. Segre modeled the transfer of norepinephrine through the circulation and predicted a time delay of 15 seconds between the change in the concentration of norepinephrine in the plasma concentration and alterations in blood pressure in a cat, which showed the target site of epinephrine is not in plasma. This model was further developed in two separate studies by Hull and Sheiner published in 1979. Effect-compartment models are empirical in nature, and they do not describe the mechanism or physiology of a drug. Modern mechanism based distribution models have been created to make such descriptions [482]. For example, a mechanism-based PK/PD model can be developed to include receptor theory concepts, which describe interactions between drugs and receptors to quantify the rate-limiting factors in drug effect associated with drug distribution as opposed to receptor kinetics [501].

PK/PD modeling studies are now conducted simultaneously on a population basis rather than through analysis of individual PK/PD profiles. A population approach provides estimates of population PD and PK estimates, assesses variability sources influencing PD and PK describes the level of inter and intra-subject variability, and provides estimates of variability associated with effects, which are random. Nonlinear mixed-effects modeling is necessary to actually separate random parameters from PD and PK parameter estimates that are fixed. A variety of statistical packages can be used to conduct nonlinear mixed-effects modeling, and the NONMEM® package is most widely used for this purpose. Particularly for pharmacology studies of anesthetics and analgesics, population PD and PK analyses, PK/PD analyses and drug-drug interactions [501].

7.5.2. Mechanistic Within-Host PK/PD Efficacy Models

Mechanistic within-host models relate concentrations of antimalarial drugs with a profile of parasite number over time to assess dosing regimens and antimalarial partner drug choices. A complete simulation was conducted to evaluate a stage-specific PK/PD model designed to predict within-host responses of parasites to drug treatment. Three antimalarial combination therapies, AS-MQ, DP, and AL, were selected for evaluation in this model. This PK/PD model included the evaluation of the initial parasite burden, drug concentration-time profiles, a parasite, and drug distribution throughout the life cycle of the parasite. Additional elements of this model include the EC_{50}, the drug concentration *in vivo* associated with 50% of the parasite killing effect (assessed through use of the *in vitro* IC_{50}), the maximum drug kill rate, the plasma protein binding of each drug, and the partition ratio of whole blood to plasma for all of the drugs evaluated. All stochastic or chance effect simulations were conducted utilizing a Latin-Hypercube sampling approach. This within-host PK/PD simulation-based method was used previously to model dosing schemes of artesunate, mefloquine, chloroquine, and the ACT combination of mefloquine and artesunate. A more recent within host PK/PD model incorporating the specific time a parasite resides within a particular parasite stage has been innovated, and a chance or stochastic effect model was utilized to assess artesunate dosing regimens [103].

This PK/PD model was derived from the work of Saralamba *et al.* [50], who innovated a discrete-time model incorporating dispersal of parasites by age within a parasite population infecting a patient. This model determines how parasite age distribution alters after treatment and exposure of the population to antimalarial drugs. The discrete time model [50] and the PK/PD parameter values used for simulation of individual parasitemia -time profiles modeled to reflect effects of antimalarial drugs are described in equations 15, 16, 17, and 18. The parasite load for each patient (P_{0i})i) is dispersed prior to drug administration into periods of 48 hours to incorporate the asexual blood stage growth of *P. falciparum* using a Gaussian distribution described with an average age of μ hours and standard deviation of s hours.

$$N_i(a, t) = N_i(a-1, t-1)e^{-k_i(a-1,t-1)} \text{ for } 1 < a \leq 48 \quad (15)$$

and

$$N_i(1, t) = PMF \times N_i(48, t-1)e^{-k_i(48,t-1)} \text{for } a = 1. \quad (16)$$

In (15) and (16), $k_i(a, t)$ is expressed as a constant kill rate for drug treatment of parasites aged *a* hours at hourly time point t, and in Eq. (16), the parasite multiplication factor or PMF is expressed as the quantity of merozoites created by each blood stage schizont in a 48 hour life cycle which reinvades erythrocytes. The kill rate constant for combination therapy is modeled as follows:

$$k_i(a, t) = k_{drug1,i}(a, t) + k_{drug2,i}(a, t) \quad (17)$$

where drug_j, for j = 1, 2, is one drug in a combination treatment. The kill rate constant in equation (17) makes the assumption that the effects of $drug_1$ and $drug_2$ on a parasite population *in vivo* are distinct. The kill rate constant and drug concentration relate as follows:

$$k_i(a,t) = k_{max}(a) \times \left[c_i(t)^{\gamma} / \left(c_i(t)^{\gamma} + EC_{50}^{\gamma}\right)\right] \quad (18)$$

where $c_i(t)$ is drug concentration in plasma at time *t* for patient *i, γ* is the concentration-effect relationship slope, the EC_{50} is the drug concentration *in vivo* which results in the death of 50% of parasites and k_{max} is the maximum kill rate for each drug which is assumed constant across parasites of ages '*a*'. The drug concentration-time curve $c_i(t)$ for each drug is created as a one or two compartment PK model with first-order absorption and elimination from a central body compartment. This simulation was created to be as complete as possible with random use of data derived from six PD parameters with Latin-Hypercube-Sampling (LHS), and PK inter-patient variability estimates for each antimalarial were included. The percentage of "patients" that were cured (95%) correlated with the *in vivo* EC_{50} and rate of killing (k_{max}) of partner drugs dosed with an artemisinin partner. Cure rates of 95% are consistent with outcomes of a number of different ACT drug trials.

The EC_{50} values that were shown to correlate with cures were surprisingly higher than EC_{50} values that have been derived from *in vitro* potency data obtained from *in vitro* IC_{50} testing despite elements of the model designed to model differences in protein binding of drugs *in vitro* with protein binding *in vivo*. *In vitro* potency testing evaluates anti-malarial drugs assessing growth inhibition of parasites in elevated concentrations of free drug in a 48-hour period, the length of a parasite growth cycle. One possible explanation for these differences is the length of *in vitro* testing which only lasts for 48-72 hours. This duration is likely acceptable for comparing the potency of one antimalarial compound to another, however, this period may not be long enough to describe *in vivo* outcomes.

Another explanation may be that *in vitro* potency assays do not describe the rate of killing of an antimalarial compound. Atovaquone, for example, has one of the slowest rates of killing while artesunate one of the fastest. Both drugs have excellent IC_{50} values when tested *in vitro* against susceptible parasites. Both of these limitations of *in vitro* testing may explain why *in vitro* assays do not agree well with the observed pharmacodynamic effects *in vivo*. There is evidence from field studies that the proportion of cured patients has been shown to decrease if patients who were infected with asynchronous parasites were treated with AL; however, parasite synchronicity was not shown to affect the percentage of cured patients after treatment with AS-MQ or DP. The parasite clearance times (PCT) for the three ACT drugs evaluated (AL, AS- MQ, and DP) were noted to be longer in patients whose infections were asynchronous and shorter in patients with an initial parasite burden composed of parasites whose average age was increased. The model prediction that asynchronous infections are slower to clear is plausible given the fact there will be parasites in early ring stage or in late schizont stage that are outside the kill zone during periods when patients are only exposed to the ACT partner drugs which is approximately 7-24 hours for piperaquine or mefloquine.

This modeling approach has a number of advantages, and one of the most important elements is the Latin Hypercube Sampling method, which randomly selects and combines 5,000 sets of PD parameter values, with 100 different PK profiles of 100 for reach drug modeled to understand inter-patient variabilities in drug exposure. In addition, this model was used to compare an alternative dosing regimen, which highlights the use of PK/PD models used to assess dosing regimens. This particular model has the means to assess associations between a wide variety of PK parameters such as the C_{max} the AUC, the time above the therapeutic concentration, and parasitological outcomes. There were a number of limitations noted in this study, which include model assumptions that background immunity of patients was low. There were no drug synergisms between the partner drugs in the ACTs evaluated, and the model assumes, that the maximum kill rates of both artemisinin and partner drugs must remain the same for parasites of various ages within defined particular kill zone period (for example the kill zone for artesunate ranges from 6 to 44 hours).

In addition, the parasite clearance times in this simulation study were approximately 24 hours in length while PCTs of approximately 48 hours have frequently been observed in other studies. This difference in PCT values may be due to one single factor or multiple factors in combination to include: 1) assumptions of no drug synergy between partners which may not be true; and 2) maximal kill rate of piperaquine was derived from *in vitro* data. The actual kill rate may be different from the kill rate noted *in vivo,* and the actual quantity of circulating parasites was derived from calculations conducted at intervals of one hour after treatment while actual clinical studies determine PCT values derived from microscopy conducted daily not every hour.

In summary, this simulation approach showed of the implementation of a mechanistic within-patient PK/PD model to compare outcomes after treatment of hypothetical "patients" with a variety of dosing regimens for malaria treatment. The data from this study does suggest parasitological outcomes should be assessed for a variety of different pharmacodynamic parameter value scenarios, particularly the unknown *in vivo* EC_{50} values. These simulation studies cannot be used to replace clinical trials however, these studies should be used to aid in devising the most appropriate dosing regimen, and the best potential partner drugs for combination drug treatment. Simulation approaches have potential to cut down on the number and extent of Phase 2 and 3 clinical trials for antimalarial drug development leading to reductions in time and money to develop new drugs [103].

7.5.3. Mathematical Efficacy Models of Artemisinin and its Derivatives

Artesunate is already in use in the field; however, the dosing regimens and durations for artesunate treatment of malaria have been developed empirically through clinical trials, not by using PK/PD modeling. The PK parameters of artemisinin derivitives have been evaluated in malaria infected and healthy subjects. Artemisinin has been shown to induce its own metabolism, which results in declining drug concentrations after repeated dosing. A few models provide a basis to choose dose or length of artemisinin treatment *in vivo* [502, 503]. A PK/PD modeling of artesunate is not straightforward as artesunate undergoes extremely fast drug disposition, and the stage specificity of artesunate action must be modeled explicitly. In addition, use of standard PK/PD modeling of artesunate frequently fails to explain clinical outcomes. One PK/PD model of the activity of artesunate has led to a hypothesis of parasitological dormancy after drug treatment. Under this hypothesis, the parasite maturation cycle stops and they are resistant to artesunate until they "awake". One study of artemisinin-induced drug metabolism was conducted by modeling salivary artemisinin concentrations obtained on 4 out of 6 days of drug administration providing a comprehensive investigation of the PK of artemisinin after multiple doses.

Elevated quantities of artemisinin in the liver were shown to induce production of a CYP enzyme precursor in a linear manner, which resulted in elevated quantities of CYP enzyme produced. In this study, the authors collected enzyme samples on the first day of drug administration and the last day of drug administration. Accordingly, the sampling limitations in this study cannot be used to derive PK/PD parameters, the enzyme half-life, and the absorption lag time of artemisinin accurately, and thus these parameters were kept fixed. The half-life of the liver enzymes induced is a system level parameter modeled to be independent of artemisinin concentration, and therefore, the enzyme half-life was assumed constant. The absorption lag-time was fixed due to insufficient data on hand for parameter estimation. In this model, inclusion of compartment for the enzyme precursor did not improve the model fit. In addition, the authors characterized the saturation of metabolic induction. The authors also assumed the half-life of the liver enzyme based on previously published data, and the induction of liver enzymes was assumed similar in malaria infected and healthy subjects.

This proposed model features compartments representing various parasite life cycle stages. The quantity of parasites was estimated to incorporate a drug resistant pool, a drug sensitive pool, and an injured parasite pool. The injured parasites were cleared more quickly than the rate of parasite injury. The final model incorporated a non-detectable pool of replicating parasites from which parasites were transferred into circulation. There are varieties of opinions on whether artemisinin is active against all or some blood stage of *falciparum* parasites. This proposed model includes a compartment that is resistant to artesunate composed of early ring stage parasites. The average duration of the parasite asexual life cycle was assumed 48 hours, and the mean time for parasites to transit from the invisible, sensitive stage to an early ring-stage parasite form was modeled to be the longest transit time possible in the life cycle. A fixed replication factor of 15 was utilized for the final model, which translates into a shorter mean transit time for parasites to move from the invisible to visible life cycle compartment. This model outcome is supported by *in vitro* studies of parasitological dormancy, and it merits further exploration *in vivo*. The expected parasitological outcome *in vivo* would include slower antimalarial activity, leading to frequent dosing possibly over a longer period of time and extended surveillance after treatment is finished.

The proposed semi-mechanistic PK/PD model was shown to estimate the time course of salivary artemisinin concentrations after repeated drug dosing and quantity of parasites per treated patient. While the parasite life cycle was derived from data from patients treated with artemisinin monotherapy, the structural model of the parasite lifecycle is independent of antimalarial drug used for treatment and this model component can be used to assess concentration data effects derived from other antimalarials or ACT treatments [17].

7.5.4. Mathematical Efficacy Models of ACTs

The combination of artesunate-mefloquine has been used to treat patients infected with uncomplicated *falciparum* malaria in various regimens in Southeast Asia. The combination was modeled utilizing experimentally determined PK data from clinical studies of this combination assuming no PD interaction between the two drugs, but the model did assume the parasites were mefloquine resistant. The predictions derived from this model agreed well with experimental data derived from clinical efficacy studies. The model showed artesunate or mefloquine monotherapy would fail to achieve cures at moderate parasitemia, however, the same "patients" could be treated with a combination of AS-MQ administered for 3 days. To treat infections presenting with high parasitemia levels, 5 days of AS-MQ treatment were predicted to be necessary. Simulations were conducted to model conditions of lower levels of resistance to mefloquine in semi-immune patient populations. Given the strong correlation between model predictions and clinical observations, this study supports the using modeling and simulation to assess the outcomes of drug combination use and dosing in various settings [504].

A second mathematical model was created to predict transmission outcomes in six regions of Tanzania with varying degrees of transmission after a hypothetical implementation of ACT treatment as first line therapy in place of antimalarial monotherapy with standard drugs. The reason for establishing this model was to understand properly the impact on malaria transmission in areas where patients are treated with ACTs and other antimalarial drugs [505]. This study estimated a reduction in parasite transmission could be achieved by implementing various drug combination treatments for *falciparum* malaria in malaria endemic regions.

The authors used this model to estimate impacts of malaria treatment with drugs of varying efficacy, different periods of prophylaxis, and effects on gametocytes. Treatment rates, impacts on symptomatic and asymptomatic infections in the six Tanzania study areas were also modeled including data derived from a survey of 5,667 patients conducted in a period before the policy change from the use of sulfadoxine-pyrimethamine as first-line treatment to ACT treatment. This model estimated that antimalarial treatment with an efficacious drug possessing a long prophylactic period but no gametocyte activity in an area with high transmission is more effective in reducing parasite transmission than ACT drugs that are short acting. This model illustrates the potential for significant impact by ACTs on malaria transmission. This analysis demonstrated that the gametocytocidal antimalarial drugs have the biggest effect in areas with low malaria transmission, while the post treatment prophylactic effects of antimalarials have a larger impact in high malaria transmission regions with high transmission.

An ACT possessing the anti-gametocyte activity associated with an artemisinin coupled with the prophylactic effect partner drug possessing an extended half-life was modeled to have the most significant transmission impact in all of the study areas in Tanzania. ACTs with long-acting partner drugs such as AS-MQ and DHA- piperaquine are in use in some areas. If DHA- piperaquine were used broadly in areas with high malaria transmission, the post-treatment prophylactic effect of piperaquine would have to be weighed against providing selective pressures to develop piperaquine resistant parasites [153].

Careful resistance surveillance will be important to assessing the impact of drug policy changes on drug resistance. The findings of the authors that a long-acting non- gametocytocidal treatment had an effect on gametocyte transmission similar to that of short-acting ACTs in areas with high malaria transmission should be carefully assessed in the context of development of resistance. A drug regimen of this nature would have to consist of multiple efficacious antimalarial drugs. Current non-artemisinin combinations such as AQ - SP and CQ -SP have limited efficacy today due to broad drug resistance in many areas [23].The impact that might be predicted for use of treatments that are longer acting is relevant when considering development of non-artemisinin combinations in the future and given the emergence of artemisinin resistant this makes ACTs less attractive. The development and deployment of drugs with enhanced gametocytocidal activity would be predicted to provide a benefit for malaria control by reducing transmission. Primaquine is an existing drug with known gametocidal activity, however, there is evidence that low-dose primaquine does not provide an advantage over use of artemisinin compounds for reduction in malaria transmission [505].

Clinical studies of ACT treatment conducted in areas where malaria transmission is low have shown a 50% to 75% reductions in episodes of malaria, however, reduced levels of vectors during the same period were also noted [68]. In a study conducted on Zanzibar which had levels of malaria transmission that were very low, no clear changes in malaria incidence were observed during 2004 after introduction of ACTs. This is a time when 34,724 treatments of artemether-lumefantrine were provided to treat patients in an overall population of 85,000 people. The authors were not sure what level of ACT coverage was achieved, but in equivalent settings, this would equate coverage of 30% of the population at risk with a concomitant reduction of clinical malaria by 16%, which might mask seasonal malaria trends in Zanzibar or decreased by poorer patient adherence. The results of this modeling and outcome study on ACT impact are useful for comparison purposes particularly comparisons with long acting non- artemisinins. This model suggests SP introduction many years ago in place of chloroquine, which was failing due to drug resistance and resulted in reduction of 20%-30% in clinical episodes of malaria. Decreases in clinical episodes of malaria by 40% have been shown to coincide with the introduction of SP in regions with high malaria transmission in southern Tanzania [505].

In Kenya, these studies were structured to be observational in nature and they were conducted at the same time efforts were made to enhance vector control. Cluster- randomized trials, which actually measure the impact on malaria transmission by using different antimalarials for first-line treatment, would be of use to support or refute the findings of this model. Given ongoing interest to reduce transmission of malaria eliminate the parasite, this data does suggest ACTs might be useful tools for malaria intervention and control efforts particularly in areas with low transmission. Reductions in malaria transmission should be a lead quality attribute considered in development of future antimalarial drugs, and deployment of such drugs may well provide benefits in reducing transmission and correspondingly achieve decreases in malaria morbidity and mortality in endemic countries. Those results also suggest that ACTs may provide transmission reduction at a level similar to deployment of insecticide-treated nets in areas with low malaria transmission. ACT partner drugs and non-artemisinin regimens with longer half-lives and post treatment prophylactic effect could provide considerable impact on transmission in high transmission areas however, the potential for use for malaria control and elimination efforts must be considered with the risk of selecting for parasite resistance [505].

Chapter 8: Population PK/PD of Antimalarial Combinations

CHAPTER 8

Population PK/PD of Antimalarial Combinations

Abstract: Population PK studies are integral components of clinical trials with many patients, such as a Phase 3 trial, and these studies involve collection of a few blood samples from each trial participant or from a smaller subgroup of participants selected at random. Computer simulation studies are conducted in advance to describe the number of samples that will be collected from participants and the collection time and frequency of blood sample collection. Population PK studies do not require extensive criteria for design compared to other methods, and these studies are readily adaptable to clinical settings. Population PK modeling provides a means to obtain PK data after administration of a drug from a limited amount of data collected from a population of treated participants. Population PK modeling provides a capability in excess of statistical modeling of sparse data, and it is a powerful tool that can be used to investigate variables affecting inter-individual PK parameter variability. PK data derived from populations can be used to derive the most efficacious and safe dosing regimens. The advantages of population PK/PD modeling and simulation for drug combinations include: 1) clinical trial design optimization for efficacy assessment of drug combination partners; 2) population PK/PD model development validation using limited internal data; 3) PK/PD model external validation utilizing data derived from independent studies; and 4) prospective clinical drug evaluation. PK/PD model outputs can be used to optimize specific drug dosing regimens that can be used to develop guidelines for dosing other drugs, either on market or newly developed, with similar drug mechanism of action or disposition. While the need to conduct modeling to describe drug disposition through profiling PK parameters is clearly established as an essential tool, there is also a need for population level modeling, particularly incorporating effect pathways of drug combination.

Keywords: Children, drug combination, phase 2 clinical trials, phase 3 clinical trials, population, population evaluation, population PD, population PD modeling, population PK, population PK modeling, population PK/PD, population PK/PD modeling.

Drug development for infectious disease treatment is not popular in the pharmaceutical industry due to the costs associated with this effort and limited opportunities to make a profit particularly for tropical diseases not found in the developed world. Antibiotics and other drugs for treatment of infectious disease are administered for brief periods during illness and then discontinued, unlike the administration of drugs for treatment of chronic diseases in man such as heart disease, diabetes, or mental health problems. Even infectious diseases due to bacteria or viruses found in the developed world are not popular targets of drug development given the limited profit to be made in this therapeutic area.

Qigui Li and Mark R. Hickman

Development of drugs for tropical diseases not found in the developed world is even less popular as it affects people who cannot pay for drugs developed. Of the 1,393 new drugs developed between 1975 and 1999, less than 1% of those drugs were intended for treatment of tropical diseases, and only 4 drugs with antimalarial activity moved forward [139, 391].

While there is a requirement for drug development of new compounds that are inexpensive and efficacious for treatment of tropical diseases, this therapeutic area has little profit and there is no incentive to interest drug manufacturers to develop drugs for use primarily in third world countries with limited resources which is where tropical disease occurs. Drug development for tropical diseases is much slower compared to drugs developed for use in first world countries. Given there are very few new drugs being innovated to treat malaria, much can be gained by clinical studies to optimize the drugs already on market for malaria treatment. Pharmacokinetics is the mathematical description of all of the parameters affecting the concentration-time profile of a drug *in vivo*. PK models provide a quantitative means of describing drug disposition through the processes of drug absorption, distribution, metabolism, and excretion. Pharmacodynamics describes the concentration-effect relationship over time along with other effects that may be either beneficial or harmful. PK and PD property characterization of a novel chemical entity or an existing drug can be a powerful tool to accelerate approval of a new drug or enhance the use of an older one.

The PK properties of most drugs are typically conducted using a standard method of intensive sampling of a limited number of healthy subjects. These labor-intensive studies are focused on describing PK/PD effects in very few people who are not necessarily representative of an actual patient population to be treated. Larger studies actually conducted with the proper target population have significant advantages. Patient characteristics such as disease severity, gender, weight, ethnicity, or impairment of kidney and liver function, which can alter drug disposition, can be described in detail. Intensive sampling of blood from a large numbers of subjects over time is not generally feasible. Intensive sampling may be medically contraindicated for some subjects, who are very ill, such sampling is not feasible for infants or the elderly, and it may not be logistically possible. In addition, intensive sampling is expensive in developing countries where tropical diseases occur. Population PK studies use PK data obtained from a small number of samples or only one sample from each subject and the data derived from these few samples can be analyzed using population methods [506]. The population-based approach utilizes statistical methodology to make estimates for mean PK parameters such as drug half-life, distribution, and clearance, and to help identify characteristics of the disease or patient that can explain inter-patient PK parameter variability [507]. If these variables can be characterized, then predictions for drug concentrations over time in a treated individual will be more accurate [508].

8.1. POPULATION PK MODELING

8.1.1. Traditional Pharmacokinetic Methods

Clinical development of drugs progresses in studies in three phases. Phase 1 studies describe PK parameters and safety in a small group of volunteers who are healthy. Phase 2 studies describe safety, efficacy, and PK parameters in a small group of ill patients who must be treated. Phase 3 trials evaluate safety and efficacy of drug treatment in large populations of sick patients needing treatment. PK profiles have been created in most drug development studies only in Phase 1 or Phase 2. Phase 1 and 2 PK analysis data is composed of serial sampling of plasma, serum, blood, or urine, and these samples have been traditionally analyzed in a two-step approach. The first step of traditional PK analysis is separate estimation of PK parameters for each individual using either non-compartmental or compartmental modeling. The second step involves utilizing the distribution, variability, and median values for individual PK parameters to estimate PK parameters for the entire population. This method is simple and PK parameters are easily calculated for a population of subjects, but the disadvantage of traditional PK methods is the number of samples required for each subject to obtain data.

This becomes a significant problem when considering special populations such as pregnant women, children, the elderly, and patients with venous access problems.

- The majority of Africans presenting with severe malaria are young, anemic children who cannot be repeatedly sampled safely. The inability to obtain samples from children, the elderly, and those with impaired venous access results in exclusion of subjects, reduced sample numbers, and potential introduction of sample bias.

- In addition, loss of samples due to failures in maintaining the cold chain during sample storage and transport activities (a constant problem in the tropics) will lead to subject exclusion and reductions in sample numbers. Inadequate sampling due to patient unwillingness to undergo phlebotomy multiple times to obtain serial samples is another factor, which may limit subject numbers and introduce bias.

- The costs associated with drug quantitation across large numbers of patient samples can be prohibitive which may also lead to decreases in the numbers of subjects with full PK profiles. This type of individual focused approach will lead to systematic overestimation of inter-individual variability, which also is a source of bias. Individual PK parameters are estimated from a drug concentration-time profile with some level of analytic error, which will add variability to estimates of PK parameters, which will increase inter-individual variability.

- PK estimates using the two-step process described must be conducted for all individual using the same PK model. If half the data derived from subjects is fitted using a one- compartment model and the other half is fitted using a two-compartment model, combining parameter data will not be possible [508].

8.1.2. Population Pharmacokinetic Methods

Population based PK analysis methods only need a limited number of samples from each subject. With fewer samples per subject in a population PK study, more patients can be studied and studies can be conducted with patients who cannot be involved with extensive serial collection of blood samples. One good use of a population PK study is incorporating population sampling as part of a Phase 3 clinical trial, which would provide more subjects who are likely more representative of a larger population (Fig. **26**). The data for all of the individual subjects are analyzed at the same time, and the population PK model is structured to take into account data with variance sources, both inter-individual and intra-individual.

Population PK methods have a number of advantages: 1) All subjects are included in a population analysis, and subjects with a missing sample are still included; 2) Samples for a population PK study can be obtained at different times, and variation in sample collection time is actually a desired feature of the population PK approach; 3) Population PK studies compile more data as more subjects are studied for the same level of effort; 4) Estimates of intra-individual, inter-occasion, inter-individual, and intra-occasion variability are possible in a population PK study; 5) Population PK approaches permit identification of patient subgroups who present differences from the rest of the population and dosing information on these subgroups can be obtained; 6) The relationship between efficacy and PK can be explored to determine risk-benefit relationships; 7) It is also possible to obtain PK parameters for individuals from an analysis of a population.

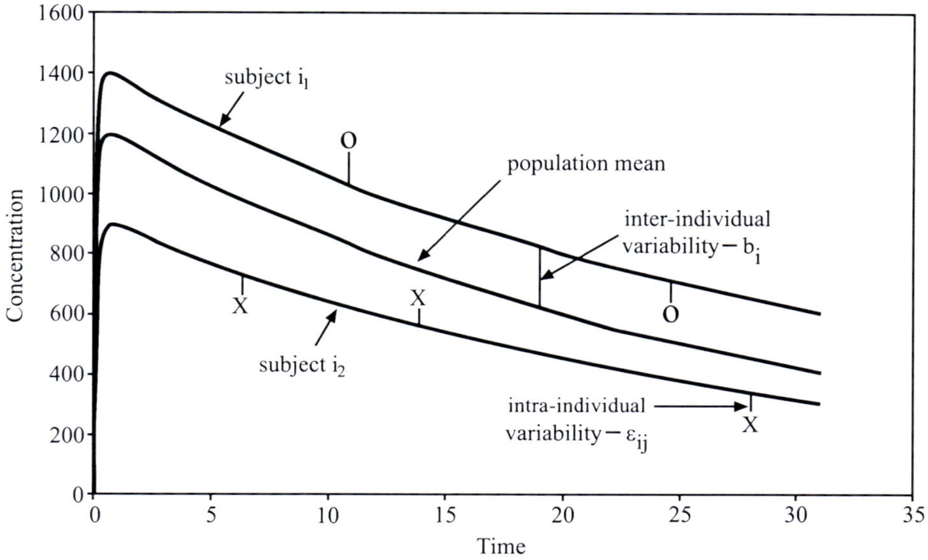

Figure 26: Sources of population pharmacokinetic variability. The black (middle) solid line represents the population mean. The outer solid lines represent the individual profiles "for subject i_1" and "subject i_2". The difference & between an individual profile and the population mean profile is due to inter-individual variability while the difference between the observed data and the individual profile is due to intra-individual variability. The values of the y and x axes represent arbitrary units [508].

The disadvantages of population PK methods are follows: 1) Initial PK data is required before a population PK study is undertaken (which can readily be obtained in a Phase 1 study); 2) Population PK studies are logistically more complex than traditional, individual PK methods, although sample collection in a Phase 3 study could be conducted at the same time as collection of efficacy samples; 3) Population PK studies require statistical and mathematical expertise, use of complex simulation software, and knowledge of the theory of population PK; 4) The limited data obtained from a population PK study may be insufficient to create a reasonable PK model [508].

Given population PK studies are relatively new, computer based simulation models to estimate subject number, number of samples, blood sample timing and frequency are being developed to provide a method to insure enough samples are collected with the proper frequency at the most appropriate time to provide the best PK parameter estimates. Study investigators are provided a window for sampling which defines a time range for sample collection as opposed to one specified time. Subjects in a population PK study should be sampled at different periods throughout the study to assess any changes in PK parameters. Population

PK sample protocols do not have to be complex in nature, and sampling times can be devised for the convenience of both the subjects and the staff. While flexibility in sampling collection times is an attractive benefit of population PK study methods, it is important that the actual sample collection time be accurately recorded. Population PK studies allow for considerable flexibility regarding blood sample collection and patient inclusion criteria. Fewer design criteria are needed for a population PK study than traditional PK studies, and population-based approaches can be readily fitted into clinical settings. Practical issues that must be solved include integration of a population PK study in the context of a protocol for a large clinical trial, data quality control, and the additional cost, expertise, and time, necessary for laboratory analysis of samples and statistical analysis of data [508].

8.1.3. Population Pharmacokinetic Methods for Antimalarial Combination Drugs

Drug combination studies using population pharmacokinetic approaches have been conducted, and one example is a population PK study of artemether-lumefantrine that was constructed in three steps [509]. The first step-involved selection of a compartmental model to fit dense, intensive sampling of drug concentration data obtained from patient's plasma in a hospital setting. These data were then refitted using all of the plasma drug concentration data available both dense and sparse, and the final models for a population created were then used to describe the effects of a variety of disease specific and demographic variables on pharmacokinetic parameters. Population PK data on artemether were available for one study, and lumefantrine data were available for several studies. Given fluctuations in the plasma concentration values obtained for artemether, the authors decided to fix the volume of distribution (Vd), the absorption rate constant (ka), and the total body clearance (CL) at an estimated average value after initial fitting was completed to obtain a good model fit [509]. A two-compartment model was observed to provide an adequate fit for lumefantrine, and a one-compartment model was utilized for DHA and artemether. The next step was to fit the impact of demographic variables and clinical characteristics and *versus* parasite count over time against pharmacokinetic parameters. A lag-time of two hours from drug administration to drug absorption was accepted to estimate how quickly lumefantrine is absorbed. The estimate of the lumefantrine absorption lag-time was acquired from prior studies in patients infected with acute malaria. Plasma concentrations of lumefantrine were modeled as:

$$C_j(t) = C_{pred,j}(t) + \varepsilon_j(t) \qquad (19)$$

where $C_j(t)$ defines the actual drug concentration and $C_{pred,j}$(t defines the predicted concentration for the jth patient at time t. The intra-patient errors for the drug concentrations in the plasma include assay or measurement error defined as $\varepsilon_j(t)$, were assumed to arise from a normal distribution characterized with mean 0 and variance $\sigma^2\varepsilon$ [509]. The inter-patient PK parameter variability was fitted as a proportionality term. Accordingly, the clearance (CL) for the jth patient was assumed a fixed effect by the following equation:

$$CL_j = CL \cdot \exp(\eta_{j,CL}) \tag{20}$$

where CL is the estimate for the population, and exp ($\eta_{j,CL}$) is defined as the deviation in clearance (CL) for the jth patient. The random effects $\eta_{j,CL}$ were assumed to arise from a normal distribution (with mean 0 and variance σ_{CL}). The inter-patient coefficient of variation (CV) in clearance (CL) is assessed by the estimate σ_{CL}. Patient characteristics such as bodyweight (Wt), was defined as a fixed effect, and these characteristics were incorporated in the clearance model as:

$$CL_j = [CL + \theta \cdot (Wt)] \cdot \exp(\eta_{j,CL}) \tag{21}$$

where θ is the coefficient of bodyweight. Observed bodyweight and other continuous covariates (demographic and pathophysiologic variables) were centered using median values to insure the estimates for the population would be consistent with values for an average patient. The η values for different PK parameters were assumed independent. Since the Vd of the central compartment (Vc) and the bioavailability fraction (F) cannot be assessed independently, F1 (the fraction of the first dose) was fixed as equal to 1 to allow estimation of the Vd (Vd/F). The bioavailability fractions of the subsequent doses (F2.Fn), where n = 8, could then be estimated relative to F1 in order to approximate changes in bioavailability over time assuming constant Vd. Under this parameter specification, the estimated inter-patient variability in Fi is the combined variability in Fi and Vc. The terminal slope (β) and the transfer rate constant from the peripheral compartment to the central compartment (k_{21}) did not vary to any significant degree between subjects, and therefore the variance term for terminal slope and the transfer rate, σ^2_β and σ^2_{k21}, were set to zero.

A likelihood ratio test was utilized to assess whether the fixed effects were significant. A new model was preferred to a previous model if the change in -2log likelihood was greater than $\chi2\ \alpha,\upsilon$, where α (= 0.05) is the significance level and υ

is defined as the number of new parameters in the successor model. Models with dissimilar covariance structures such as models with a different number of random effects were compared using Akaike's Information Criterion (AIC). Models possessing the highest AIC were considered to be superior. Assumptions for drug distribution were assessed utilizing graphical methods and normality tests. Model goodness-of-fit was tested through residual analysis, and food intake data were analyzed to examine the effects of eating on lumefantrine PK parameters. The type of food intake was recorded prospectively as no food intake, liquid intake only, intake of a light meal, or intake of a normal meal. The times when food was consumed were not recorded just the type of food and whether it was consumed prior to drug administration. Using the estimated F1-F8, a mixed effect model was created using the mixed effect procedure of the SAS statistical software program (SAS Institute Inc., Cary, NC, USA). Patient-specific effects were modeled as being random, while the time of food intake and the type of food intake were fixed effects [61, 509].

8.1.4. Role of Population Pharmacokinetics in Drug Development

Population PK modeling methods provide the means to collect data on drug PK parameters using limited data derived from the population as a whole. Population PK modeling provides more capabilities than complex statistics to assess limited, sparse data, and additional questions on inter-individual PK variability can be assessed. The output from a population PK model can be utilized to tweak drug-dosing regimens to make them safer and more efficacious particularly in patient subpopulations that are rarely studied in traditional PK testing such as pregnant women, children, and the elderly. Population PK modeling does not replace traditional, intensive, PK assessments conducted during Phase 1 and 2 trials, but this method dose provide a very useful tool to assess the drug PK parameters in a larger, more representative population of subjects or in discrete patient populations that cannot be intensively sampled such as the very young or the elderly. Population PK modeling requires more effort than traditional PK modeling, significant expertise in statistics, and more time to develop an appropriate population PK model. Given the need to optimize dosing with existing drugs to treat tropical disease we must get the most out of existing drugs through the most appropriate drug regimen possible particularly for patient subpopulations whose PK parameters are intrinsically different from the rest of the population. Population modeling characterizes PK variability and therefore gives an evidence-based model for treatment optimization. Researchers developing antimalarial drugs should consider designing Phase 3 studies directed toward obtaining population PK data [508].

8.2. POPULATION APPROACH TO ANALYZE PK/PD OF ANTIMALARIAL DRUGS AND COMBINATIONS

8.2.1. Early Experience Using Population PK/PD Analysis on Antimalarial Drugs and ACTs

Modeling PK parameters provides valuable information on drug disposition, and there is a need to model drug effect (PD) pathways, particularly when evaluating the efficacy of antimalarial drugs. Antimalarial drug treatment of patients with uncomplicated malaria is focused on clearing parasites and curing the malaria infection. Artemisinin compounds used as partner drugs in ACTs have well-known effects on clearing ring-stage malaria parasites. Rates of parasite clearance can serve as effective PD measures for antimalarial drugs. For combination partners such as the quinolines (mefloquine, lumefantrine, *etc.*) the effects of drug clearance of parasites are minor compared to those of the artemisinins, and the principal measure of their drug effect is made by assessing malaria cure rates.

1) Mefloquine and AS-MQ

One modeling example to describe the PK and PD characteristics of an antimalarial drug combination was shown in a modeling study of data derived from a large study of AS and mefloquine used in combination to treat uncomplicated *falciparum* malaria. This modeling study was retrospective in nature conducted using population models to estimate the population PK parameters of mefloquine. The population PK analysis of mefloquine and AS in combination was conducted to evaluate potential drug regimen changes in mefloquine dosing as monotherapy and when used as part of an ACT. The study population used for this work was comprised of patients in western Thailand infected with uncomplicated *falciparum* malaria receiving therapy with mefloquine in various doses or mefloquine and AS in combination. The pharmacokinetic properties of mefloquine were evaluated by use of nonlinear mixed-effects modeling. In this study, two different drug regimens were tested. 1) 159 patients were given a split oral dose of 15 mg base/kg followed by administration of mefloquine at 10 mg/kg 24 hours later. 2) 98 patients administered a single mefloquine dose of 25 mg/kg (n = 98). 3) 105 patients were treated with oral mefloquine combined with artesunate. 74 patients received a split dose of mefloquine, and 31 patients were given a single dose of mefloquine.

Splitting the mefloquine dose enhanced the area under the concentration-time curve (AUC) by 50% for monotherapy and by 20% for combined therapy. The apparent volume of distribution (V/F) was much lower in patients who received split doses of mefloquine monotherapy compared with a single dose of mefloquine. Patients receiving mefloquine as monotherapy who cleared their parasites in less than 48 hours also presented with a significantly higher AUC compared with patients who showed slower clearance of parasites. The PK parameters for infected patients treated with mefloquine were not affected by any demographic variables beyond body weight or severity of disease. Assuming the volume of distribution and clearance are unaffected by a particular dose regimen, then splitting the mefloquine dose of 25 mg/kg should improve both mefloquine oral bioavailability and *falciparum* treatment efficacy.

The mefloquine PK parameters were not significantly influenced by demographic factors including sex, age, or severity of disease. By splitting the dose of mefloquine used as monotherapy from one dose of 25 kg/mg to an initial 15 mg/kg followed by treatment dosed at 10 mg/kg the next day, the oral bioavailability of mefloquine increased by 50%. The bioavailability was enhanced by 20% in patients who were treated with mefloquine administered as a split dose along with artesunate administered as a combination treatment. The increase in oral bioavailability correlated with faster clearance of parasites, which has been used as a substitute outcome measure for malaria cure. Through this population clinical trial PK study conducted retrospectively, a therapeutic benefit of mefloquine dose splitting was demonstrated by a population PK analysis of limited, sparsely sampled data derived from a large population of patients [510].

2) Lumefantrine and artemether-lumefantrine (AL)

In a second study of artemether-lumefantrine, 260 patients were enrolled in a dose-finding study. AL was administered orally as: A: 4 x 4 tablets administered in a 48 hour period, B: 4 x 2 tablets administered in a 48 hour period or C: 3 x 4 tablets administered in a 24 hour period. Each tablet was comprised of 20 mg of artemether and 120 mg of lumefantrine. The pharmacokinetic profiles were assessed using a population PK model, which combined full PK profiles from 42 patients with limited, sparse data from 218 patients. The median absorption half-life for lumefantrine was shown to be 5.3 hours, and a drug half-life of 4.5 days was observed with a T_{max} of 10 hours. The absorption half-life of artemether and DHA was shown to be 1.9 hours, the T_{max} was shown to be 1.8 hours, and the drug half-life was shown to 0.84 hours. There was significant variability noted in bioavailability assessments for both artemether and DHA both between doses and between patients, however, the variability in bioavailability was shown to be lower for lumefantrine. The bioavailability of lumefantrine increased over time by three times after the third dose when compared to the bioavailability noted after the first dose. A higher AUC for artemether or DHA was shown to be associated with decreased parasite clearance times, and a higher lumefantrine AUC was shown to be associated with significant increases in the probability of patient cure.

Using a population PK modeling approach, the PK/PD properties of lumefantrine and artemether were shown to be very different. The AUC of lumefantrine was linked to overall cure, and lumefantrine co-administered with artemether was shown to help preclude recrudescent infections. The short-duration therapy with artemether was shown to be quickly absorbed with a brief drug half-life, and artemether treatment in this group was associated with clearance of parasites. The complementary PK/PD properties of lumefantrine and artemether were the sum total of the reasons why a fixed-dose combination of these two drugs was developed. While the 4 x 4 drug treatment regimen was shown to be efficacious in most areas with endemic malaria, drug combination absorption has been shown to be poor in some Asian patients, roughly 2.5 times lower than Chinese subjects. The prevalence of parasites that are drug resistant in Thailand is much higher than in China, and cures of disease do require higher drug doses [509].

Another prospective PK/PD evaluation of lumefantrine was conducted in 266 Thai patients with uncomplicated infections with multi-drug resistant *falciparum* parasites who were administered blinded comparisons of different drug treatment regimens of artemether-lumefantrine. Three different AL drug treatment regimens were tested. The first regimen contained an average adult dose of lumefantrine of 1,920 mg administered as four doses over a 3-day period (regimen A). The second regimen was comprised of 2,780 mg of lumefantrine administered as six doses over a period of 3-day period (regimen B), and the third regimen included 2,780 mg of lumefantrine administered as six doses over a 5 day period (regimen C). Detailed PK data was obtained for 51 adults who were hospitalized, and limited, sparse data was obtained for 215 other infected patients of different ages treated on an outpatient basis. The absorption half-life of lumefantrine for the overall population was shown to be 4.5 hours, and the median peak concentration of lumefantrine was shown to be 6.2 μg/ml in patients received 1,920 mg in four doses over 3 days (regimen A). 9.0 μg /ml in patients who were given 2,780 mg in six doses over 3 days (regimen B), and 8.0 μg/ml in patients who were given 2,780 mg in six doses over 5 days (regimen C). For patients with malaria disease, significant variability in drug absorption was noted illustrated by the high coefficient of variation of 150%.

The absorbed drug fraction rose and variability in absorption declined when these patients recovered principally due to the resumption of food intake. Eating a normal meal at a time close to the administration of drug increased the oral bioavailability by 108% (90% CI ranged from 64%-164%). The treatment regimen of 2,780 mg administered over 3 days resulted in a 60% higher AUC while administration of 2,780 mg over 5 days resulted in a 100% increase in the AUC. The different lumefantrine treatment regimens resulted in different median periods of drug exposure above the estimated MIC of 280 µg/ml. The estimated MIC for regimen A was 204 hours (1,920 mg in 4 doses for 3 days), 252 hours for regimen B (2,780 mg in six doses for 3 days), and 298 hours for regimen C (2,780 mg in six doses for 5 days). The oral bioavailability of lumefantrine is highly dependent on food intake, and food intake in patients infected with malaria is poor during the symptomatic period of infection, however, food intake has been shown to improve substantially as symptoms subside. Higher rates of cure were observed for groups B and C, and the higher cure rates observed in this study with administration of 2,780 mg in six doses for either 3 or 5 days likely were a result of increases in AUC and increased time above the *in vivo* minimum inhibitory concentration [511].

Bioavailability differences in this study were noted between samples taken in two different field sites, Mae La and Bangkok. Bioavailability differences are likely due the timing of drug administration as drugs were administered in Bangkok after lunch, while in Mae La, lumefantrine doses were administered a few hours after breakfast. A previous prospective population PK and PD study showed the area under the curve (AUC) is the most important predictor of lumefantrine antimalarial activity [509]. Given the results, the authors recommended the 6-dose regimen of 2,780 mg administered over 3 to 5 days to achieve drug exposure above the MIC, which was the most efficacious treatment of *falciparum* malaria in patients with no immunity to disease.

3) Artemisinin, Artemether, and Dihydroartemisinin

A PK/PD study was carried out in 56 Vietnamese patients infected with uncomplicated *falciparum* malaria. The patients included 23 pediatric patients who ranged in age from 2-12 years and 31 adult patients who ranged in age from 16-45 years treated with oral artemisinin dosed at 10 mg/kg/day over a 5-day period. Artemisinin concentrations were assessed by HPLC for 107 plasma samples on the first day and 33 samples collected on the last day. The population PK/PD model for this study was developed using NONMEM, and the model incorporated inter-occasion variability and accounted for an artemisinin PK change over time modeled as differences in oral bioavailability. The efficacy of artemisinin for malaria treatment was monitored by fever clearance and parasite clearance times, which were comparable between adults and children [512].

The disposition of orally administered artemisinin in this trial was fitted best using a one-compartment model with separate PK estimates for children and adults. In this study, oral availability of artemisinin for both adults and children was estimated to decrease over the period from Day 1 to 5 by a factor of 6.9, which was attributed to auto-induction of hepatic enzymes [284]. Artemisinin PK data was successfully accumulated for both adults and children using 2-3 capillary blood samples along with a small sample for parasitemia monitoring. The PK parameters obtained from this population PK study were found to be comparable to those derived from intensive PK studies of adults. This reduction in bioavailability noted in this study was similar in both adults and children, which suggests that artemisinin PK is time-dependent in both adults and children. Given the sample volume required for intensive PK evaluations, this kind of study could not be conducted in children. The use of capillary sampling coupled with a population PK model approach provided the means to conduct a study that could not be conducted otherwise. The parasitemia measurements taken were timed to occur at the same time as PK blood sampling to see if a relationship could be determined between the PK of artemisinin and the PD outcomes such as fever and parasite clearance times. However, no associations between PK and PD parameters could be made [508].

These authors of this study concluded that artemisinin dosing of children should be done based on bodyweight and adults should be dosed with a standard dose [512]. The sampling schedule for PK studies of the artemether-lumefantrine combination has left questions regarding the true value of PK parameters for each drug in a population. Data derived from AL dosing of 34 adult patients infected with *falciparum* malaria serially sampled during treatment and 114 patients also infected with *falciparum* malaria sampled occasionally during treatment was modeled, and the PK parameters derived suggested an absorption half-life of 1.9 hours with an inter-patient coefficient of variation (CV) of 63% [509]. The elimination rate constant was estimated to be 0.83 per hour, giving a $t_{1/2}$ of 0.84 hours with an inter-patient CV of 50%. The mean T_{max} for artemether was achieved at 1.8 hours after drug was administered. The apparent clearance (CL/F) was calculated to be 180 L/h with an estimated total apparent volume of distribution (Vd/F) of 217L. Either these estimates varied both up and down after subsequent doses, which suggest differences in PK properties, or, more likely, alterations in the fraction of drug absorbed (F).

Artemether is metabolized *in vivo* to the active antimalarial metabolite, DHA. The mean k_a, which is the conversion rate of artemether to DHA, was calculated to be 0.37/hour with an inter-patient CV of 45%. Clearance of DHA was shown to be more rapid than artemether, and the t½ was estimated to be 0.43 hours with an inter-patient CV of 30%. Significant intra and inter-patient variability was observed for DHA similar to artemether. If the pharmacokinetic properties of DHA were modeled as being fixed during dosing, then the CV for the absorbed and converted drug fractions likely varied widely as the CV for the third dose was shown to be 165% (130% for artemether) [61].

This type of study demonstrates the use of population PK models built on intensive sampling of a small number of patients supplemented with scarce data from many patients. Population PK has also been performed for the non-ACT combination of proguanil [284] and atovaquone [239]. The two separate PK population studies of these two drug partners were conducted based on retrospective population PK data analysis using data compiled from different Phase 2 and 3 clinical trials conducted in Thailand, Kenya, Zambia, and the Philippines of patients with *falciparum* malaria administered atovaquone-proguanil or atovaquone monotherapy. The goals of this retrospective population PK study were focused on estimating population PK for adults and children from three distinct ethnic groups. Atovaquone absorption is known to be dependent on and altered by concomitant food consumption; therefore, this variable was eliminated as subjects were dosed with atovaquone administered with fruit drink or milk.

The PK effects of dosing proguanil with atovaquone were also investigated. Based on the parameters modeled, the investigators concluded the data from this retrospective population PK study supported the hypothesis that dosage of proguanil could be conducted on patient bodyweight alone, and the authors also concluded that patient bodyweight was an important element in determining patient dose. The oral clearance of atovaquone was found to be the same for Malay and Oriental patients but 58.5% lower in black patients. The pharmacokinetic parameters of atovaquone were unaltered by co-administration with other antimalarial drugs or by dosage [508].

8.2.2. Recently Conducted Population PK/PD Analyses

1) Intramuscular Quinine Administered to Children

Although artesunate is clearly superior for treatment of severe malaria, parenteral quinine is still widely used for therapy. For the past 30 years, the recommendation for quinine treatment has involved a loading-dose regimen; however, this regimen is not often used for patient treatment. A population PK study was conducted using samples derived from 75 Tanzanian children ranging in age from 4 months - 8 years infected with severe *falciparum* malaria receiving intramuscular quinine. 69 patients were administered a 20 mg/kg quinine loading dose, and 21 of these patients showed detectable plasma quinine levels at the beginning of the study. A zero-order absorption PK model with one-compartment disposition was used to describe adequately the data obtained from this study.

Body weight was found to be the only covariate that was significant, and therefore body weight was utilized as an allometric function for calculation of the clearance and volume parameters. The data from this population PK study showed the C_{max} noted after the loading dose of quinine was not affected by body weight, and there were no adverse events noted in patients who were administered a quinine loading dose. Intramuscular quinine is quickly absorbed when administered by injection to children infected with severe *falciparum* malaria. Given the population PK data, administration of a quinine-loading dose at 20 mg/kg was recommended by the authors assuming no other loading dose would be injected in the first 24 hours after admission and no other quinine dose would be injected in the first 12 hours after hospital admission.

2) Method for Analyzing Quinine Population PK/PD

The concentrations of quinine in this population PK/PD study were transformed by calculating the natural logarithm of each value and modeling the logarithms of quinine concentration using Version 7 of NONMEM. The PK/PD interaction model created used a first-order conditional PK estimate and a Laplacian PD model method. The difference in the objective function value (ΔOFV) was calculated using NONMEM as -2×, and the logarithm of likelihood was utilized for statistical criteria to evaluate hierarchical models (an ΔOFV of >3.84 was viewed by the authors to reach statistical significance a P value of <0.05, with a difference of 1 degree of freedom). The objective function value is defined as the square of the variance calculated between the predicted and observed values. Model evaluations were conducted using simulation diagnostics and goodness-of-fit plots.

The population PK model parameters for this study were calculated using a first-order rate constant (k_a) or by using the duration of zero-order absorption (DUR) to estimate the apparent volume of distribution (V/F), the elimination clearance (CL/F), and the inter-compartment clearance (Q/F). Given there was very limited data available to model the absorption phase, the sites of injection were modelled as a single-depot compartment, and the bioavailability (F) at the site of injection was assumed 100%. A number of models were used to attempt to estimate absorption at the site of injection including first and zero-order absorption either with a lag time or without a lag time and a flexible model of transit compartment absorption. Estimation of pre-dose concentrations in patients who were given a loading dose were conducted by flagging patients who were pre-dosed to permit calculation of baseline quinine concentrations for these individuals. Between-subject variability (BSV) and between-dose occasion variability (BOV) were modeled exponentially. Drug disposition was modeled using a variety of different models to include one and two-compartment models, a first-order elimination model, and a Michaelis-Menten elimination model.

NONMEM was used to model survival data with a time-to-event analysis, and patients were assessed for survival 12 hours after their last IM injection of quinine. The survival data was assessed using an exponential hazard function, a constant hazard function, and a Weibull distribution hazard function. 13 patients died among the 75 patients treated with quinine in this study, which is too small a number to model covariate analysis of time to event. Evaluation of drug concentration-response relationships were modeled as a direct effect related to plasma quinine concentrations or a delayed effect driven by cumulative exposure of quinine over time [513].

3) Quinine Population PK/PD Analysis Result Evaluation

Each subject provided plasma samples ranging between 1 and 5 yielding 341 concentration-time samples randomly distributed throughout the initial 24 hours, and all of the samples were used to conduct a population PK study of IM quinine. Post-dose plasma concentrations were highly variable ranging from 0.85 to 33.8 mg/liter. Four patients presented with elevated plasma quinine concentrations (>25 mg/liter), however, the high concentrations of quinine did not result in serious adverse events or death.

A one-compartment disposition model with zero-order absorption provided the best fit to the data obtained, and the zero-order absorption model proved the best among those tested. There was no significant difference in between-dose occasion variability in any of the population PK parameters, and the between subjects variability could not be reliably estimated so neither element was part of the final model. Model fit was improved by adding an off-diagonal element for the covariance matrix used to model elimination clearance and the apparent volume of distribution. The only covariate that had a significant effect was body weight, and patients with lower body weights were shown to have reduced quinine exposures in the 24 hours after quinine was first administered based on weight. Simulated exposure to quinine showed an average reduction of 7.19% in the first 8 hours in patients who weighed 5 kg compared to those patients who weighed 20 kg.

The reduction in quinine exposure was shown to accumulate after each dose of 10 mg/kg of quinine yielding a total average difference of 15.4% between patients who weighed 5 kg *versus* 20 kg. The peak concentrations of quinine observed after the initial dose were not altered by differences in body weight, however, average difference of 15.9% in peak quinine concentration were observed between patients who weighed 5 kg or less when compared to subjects weighing 20 kg after the third quinine dose. Given a difference of less than 20% in concentration and exposure, this phenomenon is unlikely to alter the clinical outcome given 85% of patients regardless of their weight will reach the therapeutic threshold of 8 mg/liter after initial loading. In addition, in excess of 95% of patients were shown to reach the therapeutic threshold within the 24-hour period after maintenance dosing. Without administration of a loading dose, less than 30% of patients reached threshold levels after the first dose and 89% reached the therapeutic threshold within the first 24 hours.

The best model to explain patient survival over time in this study was a constant hazard function model where the cumulative drug exposure is modeled as a function of maximum-effect (E_{max}). The median time required to achieve a 50% hazard reduction was roughly 6 hours, however, there were no significant differences in the post hoc estimates of total exposure ($P = 0.1358$) or maximal concentrations ($P = 0.1786$) when comparing the outcomes from the first dose in those children who survived to those children who died. The relationship between exposure and effect may illustrate the delayed antimalarial effects of quinine; however, a bigger set of data will be required to conduct analysis of drug concentration *versus* effect [513, 514].

In conclusion, this study showed that IM quinine was absorbed quickly and consistently, and a loading dose lead to quinine concentrations in the plasma that quickly attained the treatment threshold in African children infected with severe malaria. Despite broad array patient covariates, only one, body weight, had a significant effect on PK parameters, which does suggest this IM quinine treatment regimen can be used to treat all forms of severe malaria in children regardless of age. In this study, the authors conducted blood sampling in the first 24 hours, which may have had an effect on in the structural model chosen. Accordingly, a two-compartment model might actually have been a better structural model to estimate PK parameters if enough data were collected to differentiate between the phases of distribution and terminal clearance. The elimination half-life estimate for quinine that has been previously reported in the literature by Krishna *et al.*, however, is similar to the half-life reported for adults infected with severe malaria, however, the preponderance of data published suggest quinine is eliminated more quickly in children compared to adults. Body weight has not been shown in published data, to be a covariate for quinine PK, however, in this study, body weight was a significant covariate. This finding is consistent with other published work, as children with lower body weight have been shown to have an increased rate of elimination when treated with other antimalarials [515].

IM quinine treatment was shown to be successful in this study even in patients presenting with shock, severe anemia, and impaired perfusion. In this study, no laboratory or clinical findings, like diminished renal function, coma, or acidosis, were shown to have an effect on the PK of quinine. Accordingly, treatment with quinine does not need to be changed with different manifestations of severe malaria. Administration of IM quinine should include a loading dose as the risk of dying from severe malaria is most great and the potential for systemic toxicity is the least in the first 24 hours. Initial administration of the first routine dose should only be conducted in children already treated with a loading dose administered during the 24-hour period after admission [513].

4) Population PK/PD Analysis of Piperaquine Combinations

Dihydroartemisinin-piperaquine (DP) has become a more popular choice for malaria treatment in many countries. DP is well tolerated, provides excellent efficacy for treatment of blood stage *falciparum* and *vivax* malaria, and no serious adverse effects have been reported. Piperaquine has also been evaluated for seasonal malaria chemoprevention in children and adults. While piperaquine has been extensively used over the last decade, there is a dearth of data on piperaquine PK in Africans, and very little data on piperaquine PK in children. Historically, dosing of antimalarial drugs for children has been derived empirically based on data in adults scaled linearly based on body weight, however, there are a number of physiological processes such as drug elimination that don't scale linearly with body weight.

Accordingly, an accurate, evidence-based PK/PD description of a pediatric treatment regimen is an unmet need. To help address this unmet need, a PK/PD study was conducted in Burkina Faso in 236 children with uncomplicated *falciparum* malaria who were treated with DHA piperaquine. The patients in this study were given a body-weight based fixed-dose DP regimen over a 3-day period. Drug concentrations were determined by collection of capillary plasma samples and the data was fitted using a nonlinear mixed-effects model created using NONMEM Version 6 (ICON Development Solutions, Hanover, MD). The population PK of piperaquine was fitted best using a two-transit compartment absorption model and a three-compartment model of drug distribution. Body weight was noted to be a significant covariate, which affected both the volume of distribution and elimination clearance.

The model of transit compartment absorption performed well to fit the study data, and the final model permitted estimation of inter-individual variability for the relative bioavailability and absorption transit time, which yielded an absorption model, which fitted the extensive variability in absorption well. Piperaquine is well known to have poor oral bioavailability based on studies in rats with considerable variability in total exposure even when taken with food. As intake of food was controlled in this trial, considerable intra-individual variability in absorption was noted which may well be explained by differences in what foods were eaten concomitantly with drug administration. Children ranging in age from 2-5 years were given a higher dose normalized to their body weight than the children who were older ($P = 0.025$). These children demonstrated lower concentrations of piperaquine by day 7 ($P = 0.024$), however, combined with lower total exposure of piperaquine ($P = 0.021$), which suggests an increase in the piperaquine dose regimen for young children is both possible and necessary.

A previously published population PK study of piperaquine showed body weight is a significant covariate for both volume of distribution and clearance. Only 2 children had PCR-confirmed recrudescence of infection by day 42 of follow-up which demonstrates the excellent efficacy of this ACT even at a non-optimized dose. The day 7 concentration of piperaquine was shown to predict recurrence of disease after treatment ($P < 0.0001$). Population simulations derived from this study showed young children have decreased day 7 piperaquine levels than older children administered weight-derived doses, and boosting the dose of piperaquine administered to young children may be needed to achieve sufficient exposure of drug. Given this data, the authors of this study proposed a dose of piperaquine to provide drug concentrations such that at least 25% of children for each body weight had drug concentrations in excess of the 7-day piperaquine concentration target of 57 ng/ml. The dose of piperaquine predicted to achieve this goal is 30 mg/kg/day combined with 3.75 mg/kg/day of DHA, which is much higher than the piperaquine dose of 18 mg/kg day, which has been recommended. For DHA, the median dose of 2.78 mg/kg/day is similar to the modelled dose of 4 mg/kg /day. Some might argue given the outstanding performance of DHA-piperaquine at the original dose level, changing the dose is not necessary, however, elevated plasma drug levels will not only enhance efficacy, but also reduce selective pressure to develop piperaquine resistance through prevention of under dosing and higher drug levels will enhance the length of time piperaquine provides post-treatment prophylaxis.

The increased dose regimen suggested would only increase the dose of DP by 10%, which would likely be well tolerated. Other studies have been conducted with DHA piperaquine where dihydroartemisinin was dosed at 4 mg/kg/day, which was combined with piperaquine at a dose of 16 mg/kg/day to 241 adult Thai patients infected with uncomplicated *falciparum* malaria. This dose of DP was well tolerated with no serious adverse events. A DHA formulation of 5.3 mg/kg was tolerated well when dosed at one time to Thai volunteers, however, this increased DHA dose was associated with transient decreases in hematocrit and hemoglobin. Any changes in DP treatment regimens must be evaluated further for safety and tolerability to support changes in dosing of children [514].

5) Population PK/PD Modeling of Tafenoquine for Malarial Prophylaxis

The population PK of tafenoquine (TQ) was evaluated in soldiers from Australia administered tafenoquine for malaria prophylaxis. The 476 male and 14 female subjects were initially administered a loading dose of 200 mg of TQ every day for 3 days. These subjects were then administered a maintenance dose of TQ of 200 mg every week thereafter for 6 months. Blood samples for the PK study were obtained after the patients received their last loading dose and additional samples were collected at 4 weeks, 8 weeks, and 16 weeks. Tafenoquine drug concentrations were quantitated using LC-MS, and PK modeling of the population was conducted with NONMEM utilizing a one-compartment model. The inter-subject variability coefficient of variation (CV) for CL/F was 18% and the CV for V/F was 22%. The inter-occasion variability in CL/F was shown to be 18%, and the average drug half-life was shown to be 12.7 days. A correlation was noted between weight and the CL/F and V/F parameters; however, this correlation was not significant enough to merit a change in dose.

The model robustness for this TQ study was evaluated using a nonparametric bootstrap based on data from 200 samples. Individual tafenoquine PK estimates could not explain the relapse of 4 patients with *vivax* malaria who took tafenoquine for prophylaxis whose PK profiles were similar to those patients who were not infected with malaria. This may be a consequence of the dependence on CYP2D6 for metabolism of 8-aminoquinolines that has been noted in both human and animal studies. No association was noted between tafenoquine levels in the plasma and PK parameter values for either patients who showed adverse events or those that did not.

The population PK of tafenoquine was determined with double precision by using NONMEM, and the data was fitted with a one-compartment model comprised of first-order absorption and elimination that implemented first-order conditional interactive estimates. The preliminary data examination was done by using NONMEM to estimate PK parameters without covariates. The effects of variables such as weight, age, and the estimated creatinine clearance (CL_{CR}) were calculated through stepwise addition of these parameters to the initial model one at a time. After each variable was added, alterations in the objective function value were noted. The final tafenoquine model was evaluated by reviewing plots of the detected tafenoquine concentrations against the predicted tafenoquine concentrations shown by the population PK model, screened covariates, elapsed time, and discrete plots of the weighted residual concentration plotted against the concentrations predicted by the model. The 50th percentile tafenoquine concentration which serves as an estimate of the concentration predicted for the population and the 5th and 95th percentile tafenoquine concentrations were assessed using Active Perl and plotted against the elapsed time for the four sample windows at weeks 1, 4, 8, and 16 [515].

The tafenoquine population model produced showed that the data did not lead to adding an absorption lag time in the PK model. Examination of the influence of variables such as age, sex, or creatinine clearance (CLCR) on CL/F did not enhance model fit. Both sex and age variables altered V/F showing significant but small reductions in the objective function value (OFV, the sum of squared deviations between predictions and observations). The use of an allometric size model to calculate CL/F (power, 0.75) and V/F (power, 1.0) did not enhance the OFV in this model (OFV = +37), and including centered linear weights for both V/F and CL/F significantly reduced the OFV, from 22,177 to 22,138. The final population validated population model showed an estimated time (T_{max}) of 21.4 hours for peak tafenoquine concentrations after dosing. The T_{max} was estimated from conditional estimates for each subject's K_a and K_e ($T_{max} = \ln (K_a/K_e)/(K_a-K_e)$) for a one-compartment extra-vascular model. The average peak tafenoquine concentration observed was 321 ng/ml, and this value was quantitated using samples obtained from 42 subjects at weeks 4, 8, and 16, drawn within a time window close to the estimated mean population T_{max} (within 5%)of 21.4 hours.

The population PK model for tafenoquine was well validated, and the PK parameters derived clearly described tafenoquine disposition in a large cohort of deployed military subjects under long-term malaria prophylaxis. The population PK parameters derived for tafenoquine do support the hypothesis that tafenoquine can be administered weekly for extended prophylaxis for malaria. While body weight was shown to have an influence on CL/F and V/F, these factors did not have sufficient impact to merit changes to the loading or maintenance doses for individuals in the study. Changes in dose may be merited for subjects who are either very overweight or very underweight related to this soldier population. Dosing modifications for patients who are significantly overweight is likely a consideration for other malaria prophylactic drugs beyond tafenoquine. This population of predominantly Caucasian soldiers was quite homogenous, and additional PK studies may be needed to model tafenoquine administration to other populations. As GSK is currently pursuing licensure of tafenoquine for radical cure of *vivax* malaria, the multi-site Phase 3 trials required will provide a large body of data to support PK modeling of tafenoquine in non-Caucasian populations [515].

6) Artemisinin Based Combinations Used for Treatment of Malaria Infections in Children

PK modeling of artemisinin-based combinations is an important tool to design rationally dosing for these drugs, which, unfortunately, have been administered using empiric data rather than the best scientific tools available, particularly for special populations. PK data for artesunate and amodiaquine are sparse for children who are at high risk for malaria given their non-immune status. To help close the gap in knowledge regarding PK parameters of AQ and AS in children, a population PK study was conducted on patients administered a newly registered ACT comprised of AS and AQ administered as a fixed dose combination. Fixed dose combination drugs are believed to be the best therapeutic approach for treatment of diseases treated with combination drugs as patient compliance is improved *versus* loose drugs administered separately.

In order to compare efficacy data, understanding the comparability of bioavailability between a newly developed FDC and an established loose drug combination is important. For the AS/AQ fixed drug combination, a prospective population PK study was carried out in children ranging in age from six months to five years infected with uncomplicated *falciparum* malaria. Study participants received artesunate combined with amodiaquine in a fixed dose combination or were administered loose tablets of artesunate and amodiaquine. Each study arm contained 35 children to assess the PK properties of AQ and AS dosed as an FDC or as loose tablets. Population PK models for the two principal active metabolites of AS and AQ, desethylamodiaquine and dihydroartemisinin, and total artemisinin antimalarial activity (the sum of the plasma concentrations of AS and DHA) were created using a non-linear mixed effects model.

The two regimens tested were shown to have the same PK properties in children infected with *falciparum* malaria. The ratio of the AUCs for desethylamodiaquine comparing the loose tablets to the fixed dose combination was calculated to be 1.043. The ratios of the AUCs for DHA and total artemisinin activity comparing the loose tablets to the fixed dose combination were shown to be similar. Both regimens were well tolerated, and antimalarial efficacy was no different in the two different treatment groups, and rates of cure for the AS-AQ fixed-dose formulation group were shown to be 94.6% and 89.2% for the AS-AQ loose drug formulation group. Four of five patients exhibited malaria recrudescence confirmed by PCR, and they received AQ doses less than 10 mg/kg. The bioavailability of the fixed dose combination formulation of AS-AQ was shown to be similar to the bioavailability observed in patients administered loose tablets of AQ.

Amodiaquine is metabolized rapidly to desethylamodiaquine by the liver, and this metabolite contributes the majority of the anti-malarial activity of amodiaquine. This study yielded a half-life for desethylamodiaquine of 9 days similar to estimates of half-life from other studies of amodiaquine conducted in young children infected with malaria. By using sparse sampling and a population PK modeling approach, the PK parameters of two different AS-AQ treatments, one with a fixed dose combination and the other with loose tablets, were estimated in young children infected with acute malaria. Without the use of population PK modeling, this study could not have been ethically done given the heavy phlebotomy schedule imposed by traditional intensive PK sampling schedules.

The outcome of this population PK modeling study showed both AS-AQ treatments had similar PK properties in this special population infected with malaria. This data supports the hypothesis tested that a fixed dose combination would yield similar PK properties as the traditional loose drug treatment. The PK estimates of DHA and the total antimalarial activity of artesunate and DHA combined showed rapid drug absorption and elimination. DHA plasma levels were shown to be much higher after the first dose during the period of acute illness than after follow-on treatment administered during the asymptomatic recovery period. The DHA AUC and half-life values after the third dose were 50% lower than the values obtained after the first dose. The result is consistent with other findings of auto-induction of hepatic enzymes associated with DHA and artesunate metabolism.

Population analysis of sparse data usually results in tighter estimate ranges as the estimates on the high and low end from individuals are shifted to the mean of the population. Estimates derived from population PK models using sparse data may underestimate extended drug elimination at low concentrations (one example of this in antimalarials is found with chloroquine). While the kinetics of elimination estimated from this population PK model derived from sparse data may have underestimated the drug clearance phase, this underestimate is not likely to be significant to clinical outcome. The most important elements of this study was the estimates of bioavailability derived for both drug products which were shown to be similar which supports the replacement of a loose drug regimen with a fixed dose combination. Fixed dose combination treatments are generally associated with better patient compliance, which leads to better outcomes, diminished recrudescence, and a decreased probability of selective drug pressure on parasites due to a failure to complete full drug treatment. The fixed dose combination tested in this study is well tolerated, simple to administer, very stable with a shelf life of 3 years, and inexpensive with a cost of US $0.50 for children and $1.00 for adults for a 3 day treatment. This all adds up to a combination treatment that provides an enhanced operational advantage over treatments with separate loose drug tablets, and these data suggest this new fixed dose AS-AQ formulation is efficacious for treatment of children infected with uncomplicated *falciparum* malaria [516].

8.3. SPECIAL CONSIDERATIONS ASSOCIATED WITH POPULATION PK/PD MODELING

In this section, we will review the PK/PD equations, their approximations, and applications, with special focus on the questions of model stability, model parameter identification and application to population PK and PK/PD modeling.

8.3.1. Determining Optimal Designs of Population PK/PD Models

ACTs are in broad use worldwide for treatment of uncomplicated *falciparum* malaria; however, one issue that has arisen in Southeast Asia is the phenomenon of artemisinin resistance characterized by increases in the parasite clearance time. This increase is worrisome as delays of parasite clearance associated with artemisinin treatment may result in diminished efficacy and recrudescence in cases where the delay in parasite clearance exceeds the ability of the partner drug in an ACT combination to kill the remaining malaria parasites. This potential reduction in artemisinin efficacy underlines the importance of a good partner drug in an ACT and provides a strong impetus to understand fully the PK properties of ACT partner drugs using population PK studies. Population PK design methods have been developed over time for population PK studies resulting in sampling schedules that are statistically valid and clinically possible, and these new design methods have been shown to result in valid estimates of PK parameters. By utilizing such optimal design methods, sampling designs can be created for population PK trials using existing ACT partners such as amodiaquine, piperaquine, mefloquine, and lumefantrine co-administered with artemisinin compounds.

These optimized population PK study designs for these drugs were created using publicly available software using structural PK models obtained from published literature coupled with design specifications derived from a prototypical study of 100 patients administered different antimalarial partner drugs that provided five samples each to include a day 7 post-treatment sample. These optimal designs were then assessed using a procedure to simulate the PK estimate. For the ACT partner drugs evaluated, designs composed of two different sampling schedules with 50 patients in each schedule each of whom was sampled five times were modeled. The result of this study was a set of model parameter estimates with acceptable precision. The sampling schedules suggested from this study are of value and are worthy of consideration in other population PK studies that cannot accommodate intensive patient sampling.

Population PK/PD modeling provides a statistical basis for borrowing information from individual results to estimate population parameters, and study designs can be created with far fewer samples for each patient and an overall larger patient group. The most important element of population PK design is collection timing of blood sample as sampling times must result in enough information for model parameter estimation. Optimal designs for lumefantrine, mefloquine, piperaquine, and amodiaquine were created for a combined study that included children, adults, and utilizing a D-optimal design. A D-optimal design incorporates a maximal Fisher Information matrix (the Fisher Information matrix is used to forecast the precision of future experiments while they are in the design phase) in order to obtain the smallest possible standard errors. The designs were created using the

WinPOPT software [517], which includes the D-optimal design method for population PK studies. Accordingly, for each partner drug design, the following steps were conducted:

- Population PK models including parameter values for children, adults, and pregnant women were found in the published literature and entered into POPT;

- Key constraints were specified for the data derived from sampling 100 patients who provided five plasma samples each, one of which was fixed to occur on the 7th treatment day and two sampling designs;

- The best times to sample a population of children, adults, and pregnant women, were determined; and

- The sampling windows, the duration of time that a sample can be taken without affecting error rates of any parameter calculation, were calculated. For all of the designs tested, the sampling windows were created to achieve, in the worst-case scenario, nor more than a 20% increase in standard errors for any parameter when compared to the standard errors obtained by the best sampling times.

The rationale for using a subject set of 5 samples from 100 patients was derived from a survey given to 22 malaria researchers who had previously conducted PK studies in Africa and Asia [518] and from WHO guidelines. Obtaining a sample on the 7th day after drug administration was implemented as day 7 plasma drug concentrations have been determined to be important determinants of antimalarial treatment failure [519]. The two sampling designs tested with two groups of 50 patients per design were included to provide adequate coverage of PK profiles given the limited sampling conducted per patient and sample flexibility given one schedule might be too restrictive for an outpatient group. The drug doses for this study were specified based on WHO guidelines for malaria treatment [519, 520]. The study design for mefloquine was conducted using a one-compartment model provided an expected precision for the target populations. The designs were created in POPT with the assumptions that 100 patients were in the study, which leads to a calculation of the expected relative standard error based on the participation of 100 patients for all models evaluated. After evaluations of a number of different models, a two-compartment model was found to yield acceptable estimates for adults, and with more data, a two-compartment model can be estimated for populations.

The lumefantrine design provided a very good estimate of the published two-compartment model parameters that have been established for pregnant women. A two-compartment model was initially estimated for non-pregnant adults; however, unacceptably high relative standard errors were noted. This question was examined further in POPT by raising the sample number to eight per subject instead of five; however, the relative standard errors were high for a number of PK parameters. Varying the sample windows for this population may be one means of attaining a two-compartment model with acceptable relative standard errors for PK parameters. For children, a one-compartment model provided adequate information for most PK parameters, however, the model was estimated from published work where concentration determinations where to 72 hours, which does not provide enough data on the drug distribution phase of lumefantrine. Varying the sampling window for lumefantrine may be one method of exploring different structural models for this population.

While the design for desethylamodiaquine was found to yield acceptable precision for children and pregnant women, the adult model was derived from data obtained from pregnant or post-partum women infected with *vivax* malaria. Adult patients infected with *falciparum* malaria may present with PK profiles that are different from the simulated profiles, and men may have different PK profiles than non-pregnant women. Accordingly, the sampling schedule for desethylamodiaquine derived from this study may be an initial design, and, like the other partner drugs, varying the sampling window may provide alternative models that yield better PK parameter estimates. In addition, obtaining more samples may provide better estimates. This study provided an optimal design methodology to determine an initial optimal blood-sampling schedule for different antimalarial partner drugs utilizing the best current PK knowledge of and some of the practical limitations associated with obtaining blood samples from patients. These designs provide an efficient, economical means of conducting population PK studies of ACT partner drugs when intensive sampling over time is not feasible. These sampling designs provide a prototype for future population PK study designs for other investigators conducting PK studies [520].

8.3.2. Simultaneous Population PK/PD Modeling of Both Parent Drugs and Drug Metabolites

The WHO endorses ACT use to treat pregnant women with uncomplicated *falciparum* malaria in the second and third trimesters; however, the pregnancy effects on PK parameters of patients who have been administered artemisinin compounds are not well understood. In order to address this unmet need, a population PK study of oral AS and DHA, its metabolite, was conducted in 26 pregnant women in the second or third trimester and 25 non-pregnant women who were administered 200 mg of oral AS. Plasma DHA and AS concentrations were measured using LC-MS, and PK parameter estimates were made using nonlinear mixed effects modeling.

A model that simultaneously estimated both the parent compound, AS, and the metabolite, DHA, was created comprised of a mixed zero-order, lagged first-order absorption of AS, a one-compartment model for AS, and a one-compartment model for DHA. The model assumed AS would be completely converted to DHA, and the model was found to provide goodness-of-fit, stability, and showed good predictive ability. The apparent volume of distribution relative to bioavailability (VZ/F) for AS was estimated to be 195 L and for DHA, 914 L, and the clearance relative to bioavailability (CL/F) was shown to be 895 L/h for AS and 64.0 L/h for DHA. Effects of pregnancy on the clearance relative to bioavailability were shown to be significant and the CL/F for DHA in pregnant women was 42.3% higher in this population. In this analysis, population PK modeling provided data suggesting pregnant women administered oral AS clear DHA more rapidly than non-pregnant women did. These findings along with a previously published non-compartmental analysis of the modeled data, supports the hypothesis that increased doses of AS are necessary to provide DHA levels in pregnant women that are similar to non-pregnant women.

1) Population PK/PD Modeling of AS Administered to Pregnant Women and Controls

To model the data from the previously mentioned AS study in non-pregnant and pregnant women, the NONMEM version 7 software packages was used to conduct nonlinear mixed effects model building. Monte Carlo importance sampling with an interaction estimation method was utilized to fit PK models; Pdx-Pop 4.0 and Xpose version 4.1.0 were used to process the NONMEM 7 output. Model selection was conducted using a number of different criteria. An initial model was created with a total data set including data from patients who were pregnant, post-partum or controls, however, a model capable of fitting data from controls, pregnant women, and post-partum women was not obtainable. The portion of the data set with the most variability was noted in the post-partum patients, so the data set was divided into one set containing pregnancy and control groups and another set with post-partum patients. With the division of the data set into two groups, an adequate structural model was identified for the pregnant/control group only.

Modeling of the data set comprised of control and pregnant patients was first attempted with AS data only, and first-order absorption with one-compartment and two-compartment models were utilized to fit the data. Alternative absorption processes were examined to include zero-order absorption with lagged first-order absorption, first-order absorption, first-order absorption with lagged zero-order absorption, parallel dual first-order absorption, transit compartment absorption, and single Weibull absorption. DHA data from pregnant and control patients were first modeled independently to answer the question if a one or two-compartment model provided a superior fit of the data. A variety of models was tested to fit the metabolism of the artesunate parent and the DHA metabolite to include one-compartment models for both with various absorption types for artesunate. AS conversion to DHA was modeled as complete for all of the models tested, synchronized AS/DHA models were created using ADVAN 5, and inter-individual variability (IIV) of PK parameters was modeled using a lognormal distribution:

$$Pi = P_{pop} \cdot \exp(\eta j) \qquad (22)$$

where Pi is the parameter estimate for individual i, P_{pop} is the population estimate for the parameter, and ηi represents the deviation of Pi from P_{pop}. Residual variability (RV) was modeled with an additive model for log-transformed data:

$$\ln C_{ij} = \ln C_{pred}, \text{ if} + \varepsilon_{ij} \qquad (23)$$

where C_{ij} represents the jth observation for individual i, $C_{pred,\ ij}$ represents the predicted AS or DHA concentration for individual i, and ε_{ij} represents the residual random error for the jth observation of individual i.

2) Covariate Model Building of AS Administered to Pregnant Women and Controls

After completion of the base model, covariate analysis was conducted to determine if any covariates were present, which could explain the observed inter-individual variability. The covariates assessed included body max index, weight, age, albumin at baseline, pregnancy status, alpha-1-acid glycoprotein at baseline, and the window of pregnancy. The covariates investigated represent variables which could affect the PK of AS or DHA. The most relevant covariates to this study were identified by plotting the covariates against the PK parameter estimates and by plotting the covariates *versus* inter-individual variability. In addition, the Xpose software package was used to identify relevant covariates in this study. Evaluation of covariates that appeared to be affecting the PK of AS and DHA was conducted by evaluating the statistical significance of covariate plots through forward addition and backward elimination. To retain a model in the process of forward addition, the statistical probability threshold had to be $p < 0.05$, and for backward elimination, the statistical criterion was set at $p < 0.001$.

Categorical covariates were modeled using a proportional function:

$$P = \theta_1 \cdot (1 + \theta_2 \cdot COV) \quad (24)$$

where θ_1 is the estimate of the parameter in subjects with a covariate listed as 0 and θ_2 is the parameter alteration that is linked to the covariate being examined. Continuous covariates were centered on their median value, and they were modeled using a linear function:

$$P = \theta_1 + \theta_2 \cdot (COV - COV_{median}) \quad (25)$$

where θ_1 is the parameter estimate for a subject with a COV that is equal to the COV_{median}, and θ_2 is the alteration in the estimate of the parameter linked to the difference between the COV and the COV_{median}.

The final derived model for this study was composed of a one-compartment model for AS and a one-compartment model for DHA, with AS absorption estimated by a mixed zero-order, lagged first-order absorption process. After absorption, AS is swiftly converted to DHA, with half-life of roughly 9.1 minutes. The model showed the clearance of DHA was estimated to be 42% higher in pregnant women than in non-pregnant patients, and the half-life of DHA was estimated to be 45 minutes for women who are pregnant and 59 minutes for women who were not pregnant.

A number of diagnostic plots were utilized to examine the goodness of fit of the model, which included plotting the population predicted concentrations *versus* the measured concentrations, the conditional weighted residuals plotted against the population predictions, the measured concentrations compared to the individual predictions, and the conditional weighted residuals plotted against time. Population predictions were made using NONMEM7 using the EPRED option. One thousand bootstrap runs were performed using Perl-Speaks-NONMEM version 3.1.0 to evaluate the precision of the estimated parameters. Model stability was judged by condition number, and a condition number under 1000 was deemed suggestive of model stability. The predictive ability of the model was assessed through 1,000 simulated virtual observations each time point samples were taken. The measured drug concentrations were graphed with the 5th, 95th, and 50th, percentiles of simulated data above the lower limit of quantitation. The 90% prediction interval for AS and DHA concentrations was used to define the percentage of observed concentrations outside this interval which was defined by the e 5th and 95th percentiles [516].

A number of PK studies have shown problems in predicting AS absorption in post-partum women, which translates into failures to identify a proper PK model for the data derived from these patients. AS is rapidly converted to DHA after it is absorbed, and variability in AS absorption would be expected to lead to DHA concentrations that do not model well. The variability in absorption in post-partum women may be related to breastfeeding, and to properly assess the impact of breastfeeding on AS absorption, the women in this study were asked to take along their children on the day of their study appointment and breastfeed their children prior to administration of AS. A number of trials have been conducted to assess the impact of lactation on metabolism of ethanol, however, there is no data on the effects of lactation on AS metabolism. The studies on the effects of lactation show changes on ethanol metabolism in PK parameters, which could be related to variability in ethanol absorption or due to changes in physiology associated with lactation in general or due to the effects of breast pumping or infant suckling. Infant suckling has been shown to trigger release of hormones regulating digestion, and these hormones may function to change the digestive rates concerning processes such as gastric emptying.

Accordingly, the unpredictable nature of AS absorption in post-partum women could be due to the impact of infant suckling and lactation. The only covariate that was shown to be significant in this study was the impact of pregnancy on clearance of DHA, and the variability associated with pregnancy was calculated to result in a 42.3% rise in DHA clearance in pregnant women over non-pregnant women. The clearance parameter was not significantly different when comparing the two pregnancy windows, however, more subjects in each trimester is likely necessary to detect a significant difference between trimesters. The clearance parameters of DHA for pregnancy and control subjects in this study were similar to the DHA clearance values calculated by non-compartmental methods, however, the volume of distribution of DHA was reduced in the population. In this study, the DHA volume of distribution was increased in pregnant women, however, there was no significant association between the covariate of pregnancy status and volume of distribution. As this linkage was deemed statistically significant in the first step of covariate modeling, the relationship between pregnancy status and volume of distribution would likely be significant if a larger number of subjects were assessed.

This work described a predictive population PK model for DHA and AS in both women who were pregnant and women who were not pregnant in the Democratic Republic of the Congo. One central finding of this analysis is that an increase in oral clearance of DHA is linked with pregnancy status. The previous non-compartmental analysis of data modeled in this study noted a difference in clearance between women who were pregnant and women who were not pregnant, but no difference that was statistically significant was observed between these two groups. The outcome of this study supports the hypothesis that pregnant women may require a higher AS dose to obtain adequate levels of DHA in their blood similar to those achieved by non-pregnant patients who are administered a standard adult dose. While a larger analysis would be necessary to determine definitively the most appropriate dose of AS dose to be administered to pregnant women, the significant rise in DHA clearance in pregnant women described in in this study demonstrates the need for further work [521, 522].

8.3.3. Population PK/PD Modeling in Different Stages of Drug Development

PK/PD modeling and simulation (M&S) are powerful tools essential for learning-and- confirming data in drug development. The impact of PK/PD M&S on risk management and decision associated with drug development is always a function of the nature of the questions being addressed and the data available to answer those questions at different stages of drug development. For example, M&S methods are useful tools to understand biological inter-individual PK/PD variability in data from preclinical animal studies to help estimate reasonable clinical doses. Clinical trial simulations can also be utilized to predict the likelihood of successfully obtaining a response from patients given data from early drug development phases. Each phase of drug development is focused on obtaining sufficient information to understand the probability of future development of a new drug. Adding to the base of knowledge prospectively, helps define the critical path of drug development resulting in a new drug application. A paradigm of "learning-and-confirming" has been suggested as a useful method of conducting development of new drugs. Modeling and simulation tools can be powerful aids to implement this paradigm. Asking the best questions and understanding relevant assumptions are important elements of the "learning-and-confirming" model and both asking questions and understanding assumptions are essential components to obtaining the best M&S results. Some selected examples of PK/PD modeling and simulation utilized during drug development from the preclinical phase to Phase 3 are shown here in this section as case study examples.

New software has enhanced the application of modeling and simulation to design clinical trials. While the utility of modeling PK/PD data is well known, few drug development programs actually go to the extent of using drug and disease models to simulate exposure-response and clinical trials to obtain estimates for risk management and decision making. Model robustness can be achieved by using and understanding prior data and carefully analyzing risk and uncertainty. Models must also be iteratively refined during each drug development phase, the number of iterations using data from clinical studies is a function of the quality of previous test data, risk, and associated costs a particular program may be willing to accept [523].

1) The Preclinical Phase: Empirical Dose Projection

Prior to initiating clinical studies, it is crucial to understand the PK/PD properties of drug candidates, and model drugs for dose, concentration, efficacy, and toxicity. Ultimately, the model and simulation approach should support dose selection to be used for first in human testing. The use of PK/PD based M&S prior to clinical testing is a function of the availability of preclinical study data of high quality plus data from the literature on comparisons between preclinical animal models and human beings. M&S can be used in preclinical development to suggest how a novel chemical entity may work quantitatively or M&S could be used to answer more limited and qualitative questions. For novel chemical entities that are similar to that already on market, a large body of data is available on comparator molecules, and such data can be used for M&S work to help plan for early clinical development. M&S can be used along with population PK data derived from preclinical animal studies coupled with allometric scaling of animal data to help predict an anticipated human dose. In the preclinical phase, modeling and simulation is used to help "learn" about properties of novel chemical entities, and these modeled parameters can then "confirmed" through data generated in early clinical development.

For an NCE, Phase 1 studies provide data on safety, tolerability, and PK over a broad array of possible doses to be used for efficacy testing. When Phase 1 testing is completed, dose selection data should be substantial in nature simply by using PK data to learn and confirm the knowledge obtained from modeling PK data obtained. In many cases, uncertainty over dose selection may remain after completion of Phase 1 if it is not possible to test completely the entire range of doses. In these cases, modeling and simulation provide tools to assess the likelihood of achieving treatment goals given drug exposures provided in a limited range of doses. Another potential use of modeling and simulation could be adding drug exposure data from toxicology studies. The overall body of data could determine the likelihood of obtaining clinical efficacy at a drug exposure level that is not toxic. As illustrated in this example, modeling and simulation can provide a tool to reduce dose uncertainty. It also potentially is used to evaluate the need for additional preclinical studies to estimate an efficacious human dose.

First in human data can then be used to confirm or update any predictions made based on preclinical modeling and simulation. PK models can then be updated with a wealth of human data, which can provide not only a comparison between predicted and achieved human exposure data but also biomarkers informing the relationship between drug exposure and response. Given the potential for utilization of preclinical data in modeling and simulation, gathering drug exposure data from preclinical PK studies is advantageous as the data can modeled along with clinical PK/PD data from similar comparator molecules of the same drug class.

2) Phase 1: Preliminary PK Modeling

First in human studies provides an opportunity to define the PK properties of a novel chemical entity and the concentration-response curve. Models derived from Phase 1 studies can be used to estimate dosing regimens for a Phase 2A study of initial efficacy and safety, and the data is of great value for designing any follow-on Phase 1 studies conducted to evaluate, for example, alternative drug delivery or drug formulation.

Population PK modeling can be conducted using Phase 1 data ideally pooled from multiple studies. Population PK modeling is an essential tool for characterizing PK of a new drug in various human population groups. PK variability in inpatient populations and critical covariates are not readily identifiable in most Phase 1 studies. Population PK modeling using data derived from much larger Phase 2 or 3 trials is necessary to obtain an in-depth understanding of inter-individual variability and a clear identification of the most important covariates. Preliminary population PK studies based only on Phase 1 data can be combined, however, with protein binding data, *in vitro* efficacy data, and other relevant information to help select the best doses for follow-on Phase 2 and 3 studies.

One good example of modeling and simulation is found in Phase 1 oncology studies, which are commonly conducted in cancer patients. Given the nature and extent of disease in cancer patients, a combination of therapeutic drugs is often used for treatment, which is a similar concept to the combination therapies embraced today for malaria treatment. The design of oncology Phase 1 studies is very well suited for population-based PK studies given the nature of the disease and the combination treatments being tested. Not only are safety objectives addressed in a Phase 1 oncology study, these studies also must define PK/PD interactions and inter-individual and inter-occasion variability. Similar to the malaria parasite, cancer cells are capable of developing resistance to drugs due to over-expression of transporter proteins of membrane efflux, and these membrane transporters have become new cancer targets of drug treatment. Using an interactive PK/PD model it is feasible to determine both PK interactions leading to possible clinical toxicity and assess the potential PD benefits associated with a cancer drug that targets a membrane transporter.

3) Phase 2/3: Drug-Disease Modeling and Study Designs

Early Phase 1 studies are focused on generating enough data on dose and safety to further design Phase 2 and 3 trials. As drug development approaches Phase 3, modeling and simulation become important tools to leverage data derived from past clinical trials to help design Phase 3 studies that will provide definitive data on the safety and efficacy of an NCE. To accomplish this goal, the objectives of PK/PD-based modeling and simulation are focused on helping to design clinical studies and facilitate rapid data analysis to help support a future regulatory filing. The overall aim of PK/PD modeling and simulation is to be able to compare the attributes of a novel chemical entity against a drug already on market and enable assessment of risks *versus* benefits to show an advantage of a new molecule over an existing one. Once developed, PK/PD models should be "validated" to insure the model is actually approximating reality.

There is a variety of validation methods, and a broad array of validation tools to include the posterior predictive check, which can be utilized to assess model performance. The extent of model validation assessment is dependent on the final use of a PK/PD model. There are a number of built in assumptions, which are required to estimate dose response curves, based on dose-response relationships. By properly identifying the target effect, modeling efforts should shift to optimizing the design of studies to show the desired effect. A study design should be picked that provides the highest likelihood of showing a final effect given model uncertainties and assumptions. Understanding a dose response after administration of a new drug can be accomplished through modeling alternative trial strategies (such as a factorial design) or by adding various dose groups with more subjects. For each simulation of a clinical study, the average response data can be altered from baseline commensurate with changes in dose, and this data can be fitted to two basic models to assess dose-response.

The first model one might make should assume all doses are the same, which yields a flat dose response, and the second should assume an E_{max} dose response. A dose response could be declared if the difference in the objective functions can be considered significant for one additional parameter. The percentage of trial replications among 200 different iterations where a dose response can be positively identified characterizes the power of the trial design. After completion of a Phase 2B trial, a number of analyses can be conducted in two ways. One way is to use population PK analysis to assess the variability of data, and the second is population PD analysis to understand response-time relationships between dose groups. The data obtained from a Phase 2B study is useful to extend the disease and drug model to enhance it to make further predictions. Understanding exposure-response relationships is an important part of defining the drug therapeutic index.

Further knowledge of the variability in PK/PD helps determine the proper dose adjustments necessary for special populations. Drug development programs that utilize PK/PD models incorporating all available knowledge on drug attributes, disease, and characteristics of patients can be used to make predictions of possible outcomes, and this approach is clearly a more effective use of knowledge and resources, which should empower and inform drug development decision making. Modeling and simulation are powerful tools to understand inter-individual and inter-occasion variability that is part of drug development. Simulations require appropriate disease and drug progression models, and these models can be structured using public domain data and built to explore drug characteristics. Development of PK/PD models should begin in advance of entry of a novel chemical entity into clinical development as model development requires refinement through each clinical study to gain power as a decision-making tool. PK/PD modeling and simulation are very useful tools that are being used more frequently to accelerate and streamline the drug development process.

8.3.4. Population PK/PD Modeling of Children

In order to develop guidelines for dosing children, population PK/PD modeling, and simulation can be used to optimize trial designs using preliminary data, develop and validate novel models derived from limited data, externally validate population PK/PD models by the use of independent data, and assess clinical trials prospectively. Dosing regimens that have been optimized provide both data and a model for creating dose guidelines for other drugs, existing or novel, with similar disposition profiles. Along with modeling drug disposition through PK studies, PD pathways that characterize drug effect should also be modeled and best practices for PK/PD modeling involves using a flexible data-sharing infrastructure [524].

1) Problem Definition for Use of Drugs in Children: Defining the Dose

Roughly, 93% of drugs that are administered to infants are prescribed off-label, and 70% of drugs given to children are prescribed off-label, despite the many differences in drug response and disposition that are known between adults and children. This sad statistic is a consequence of the dearth of clinical studies conducted in children. Accordingly, dosing regimens for children are generally calculated based on data either derived from healthy children or extrapolated from adult data based on body weight. Children of different ages are commonly dosed based on differences in body weight in a linear manner; higher weight, more drugs, less weight, less drug. The lack of clinical trial data in children is due to many constraints to include practical limitations on studies in children coupled with ethical and financial constraints.

The lack of data on drug efficacy and disposition presents an issue for both pharmaceutical companies and physicians. The European regulatory body, the EMEA, started requiring pediatric data beginning 2007 in Europe on drug efficacy and disposition in children. By the end of Phase 1 studies, a pediatric investigational plan (PIP) is required by the EMEA. This requirement does come with a benefit as the manufacturer gains a six month extension on their patent as an inducement for this study, and the new European Pediatric Law requires studies in children be conducted as a prerequisite to gain knowledge for effective drug labeling. All of this regulatory activity and the data derived from pediatric studies will ultimately be significant benefit to children and pediatric patient care will be enhanced worldwide.

2) Dosing Information for Children is Needed

Drug dosing of children should be derived from PK/PD data not extrapolated from adult data based on body weight. PD and PK responses may alter over time in children, and age-related PK differences, for example, can be due to changes in absorption, distribution, metabolism, and/ or excretion. In addition, developmental alterations in kidney function can radically change the elimination of drugs that are eliminated primarily through the kidneys.

There are also known differences in PD that can arise due to different progression of disease progression in children compared to adults. Differences in PD can occur as a consequence of age related alterations in the expression of receptors which can cause changes in the sensitivity of target tissues, and age-related changes can alter the nature of signal transduction and feedback mechanisms controlling drug responses. There are few well-validated PD study endpoints in children, but despite this deficiency, PD relationships still need to be studied in this population. One method of conducting studies in children is considering variability in age for both PK and PD at the same time to derive the data needed for developing dosing regimens [524]. Age-related changes in PD and PK must be evaluated along with other sources of variability including drug interactions, genetic factors, disease factors, and environmental variables. PD pathways should be modeled in a similar manner as PK pathways to help predict safety and efficacy in children of all ages.

3) PK/PD Information from Children Should Be Gathered and Analyzed

Conducting PK/PD studies in children is often difficult. A number of challenges exist to conducting PK/PD challenges in children including limitations in patient numbers as well as both practical and ethical restrictions on blood sampling and PD observations in young children, particularly infants. New technologies have been developed to provide the means for limited sampling in young children. LC-MS/MS, for example, is a very sensitive technique, which requires very small volumes of blood samples to quantitate drugs. In addition, the use of saliva and breath tests to monitor drug concentrations provides a non-invasive method of monitoring drug levels, and the innovation of using dried spots of blood obtained from heel stick sampling provides a minimally invasive method of acquiring small sample volumes for drug concentration studies. Most importantly, the innovation of population PK studies provides a method for conducting PK/PD studies in pregnant women and children. By the use of nonlinear mixed effects, modeling PD and PK parameters can be estimated at the same time for all participants in a study. The final outputs of these modeling efforts are well-defined population PD and PK parameters and estimates for inter-individual and inter-occasion variability.

After calculating PK/PD variability, the covariate analysis can be conducted to address the influence of, demographic and pathophysiologic variables (ex. age, weight, organ function, genetics, and disease severity) on PK/PD parameters. If any of these covariates exert a statistically significant effect on PK/PD parameters, these covariates may be the rationale for designing individual dosing regimens. Population PK based approaches permit sparse sample gathering at time points that are convenient for clinical care of patients rather than intensive sampling on a schedule driven by experimental need. This approach facilitates analysis of dense data, sparse data, and combinations of dense and sparse data derived from drug concentration levels and clinical observations. Given the evaluation is based on a population of data, PK/PD studies using this approach can readily be conducted in studies composed of children with a minimal burden to these patients [524].

4) The Role of Modeling and Simulation in Pediatric Clinical Dosing Studies

Validation is an important issue relevant to population PK/PD models, which are essential for conducting PK/PD studies in children. PK/PD models should be validated internally, externally, prospectively, and cross-validated where possible. Only 17% of pediatric PK/PD models have gone through a successful model validation process based on the published literature, however, it is essential to conduct, at a minimum, internal model validation. Internal validation involves the use of a number of standard diagnostic measures to include plotting model-predicted *versus* observed data with more advanced forms of validation, which include bootstrap re-sampling, visual predictive checks, or normalized prediction discrepancy errors (NPDE). Individual dosing regimens that are obtained from PK/PD models that have undergone rigorous external and internal validation are worthy of further clinical study which provides prospective validation. Cross validation is focused on testing the PK/PD models to examine predictions of drug effect and disposition by comparing the data to similar drugs sharing PK and PD pathways. After prospective trials, individualized dosing schemes for pediatric patients can be determined that provide a safe and effective dose for each child of a given genetic background, age, and weight [512-514].

5) Mechanism-Based PK-PD Modeling in Children

Applying this method to development of every drug that might be used in a pediatric population poses a problem given the costs and time to conduct population based PK studies to derive a dosing regimen. One possible alternative is the use of mechanism-based PK/PD models to model drugs that have not been studied based on data derived from other similar drugs that have been studied. Mechanism-based PK/PD models draw sharp contrasts between system parameters that are biological in nature and parameters that are drug-specific. Accordingly, the system specific parameters associated with receptor density, renal function, drug transporters, and metabolizing enzymes could be applied to another drug not studied that provides an example of how model cross-validation can be conducted. The use of system specific parameters from one drug to model another could provide a means to reduce the cost and time to develop drug-dosing schemes for other drugs. There are, however, potential limitations for this approach that must be considered.

Differences in receptor affinity of a new drug must be considered when using data derived from the example drug use to build a model. These differences must be considered when attempting to develop a drug-dosing regimen for a drug not studied using a model originally developed for another, similar drug. Cross validation studies as discussed here are still worthy examining to determine the feasibility of employing this approach to reduce the costs associated with drug dose estimation for special populations. Modeling and simulation provide important tools to develop dosing schemes for special populations such as children to improve both safety and efficacy given the empiric nature of drug dosing regimens derived today for children. Population PK/PD approaches will permit sparse sampling in children to allow for estimates of population PK/PD parameters without resorting to intensive blood sampling and observations [512-514, 516, 524].

8.3.5. Population PK/PD Modeling in Pregnant Patients

Pregnancy has a variety of effects on the PK characteristics of many antimalarial drugs. Previous studies have shown that dihydroartemisinin, artesunate, atovaquone, artemether, sulfadoxine, cycloguanil, proguanil, lumefantrine, and pyrimethamine, drug concentrations are reduced in pregnant women. This phenomenon may well be a factor in the cure rates noted in women that are pregnant and women that are not pregnant. Other studies have shown no PK changes in pregnant women compared to their non-pregnant counterparts for amodiaquine and pyrimethamine or the metabolite of amodiaquine, desethylamodiaquine. Reports on higher drug exposure in pregnant women treated with pyrimethamine during pregnancy have been published [524].

Amodiaquine has efficacy for treatment of blood-stage *vivax* malaria, however, very little published PK/PD data on the use of amodiaquine in women that are pregnant exists. To fill this gap, a study was conducted along the Thai-Myanmar border to evaluate the population PK/PD parameters of amodiaquine and, desethylamodiaquine, its metabolite, in women that were pregnant and infected with *vivax* malaria and in the same women again after delivery. Twenty-seven pregnant women infected with *vivax* malaria were administered amodiaquine monotherapy (10 mg/kg/day) every day for 3 days. Nineteen women who were infected with *vivax* malaria and without *vivax* malaria were dosed again with amodiaquine postpartum. A nonlinear mixed effects model was used to estimate the population PK/PD parameters of amodiaquine and its metabolite, desethylamodiaquine. In this study, amodiaquine drug concentrations were best-fitted using lagged first-order absorption with a two-compartment disposition model combined with a three- compartment disposition of desethylamodiaquine, which assumed the conversion of amodiaquine to desethylamodiaquine to be complete *in vivo*.

Nonlinear mixed-effects modeling provides a more in-depth evaluation of amodiaquine and desethylamodiaquine disposition and the patient population by modeling the parent drug and the metabolite simultaneously while other previous studies of amodiaquine simply used non-compartmental analyses of amodiaquine separately from desethylamodiaquine. A good mixed-effects model can be linked to PD endpoints to evaluate the clinical benefit of a drug, and the same model can be used to optimize a dose regimen and simulate clinical trials. Treatment of pregnant women with amodiaquine was evaluated using a time to event model incorporating a constant hazard function that included the antimalarial activity of desethylamodiaquine. Amodiaquine therapy was shown to reduce the probability from 22.2% to 7.4% by day 35. The results of this study showed that age and pregnancy status had an effect on the absorption lag time, however, neither variable impacted the other pharmacokinetic parameters. The authors concluded pregnancy was not associated with alterations in the PK parameters of amodiaquine or desethylamodiaquine beyond the decreased absorption lag time previously mentioned, and no dose adjustments were shown to be required for pregnant patients [525].

The PK parameters of dihydroartemisinin and piperaquine were evaluated in a study of pregnant and non-pregnant women along the Thai-Myanmar border infected with uncomplicated *falciparum* malaria. Twenty-four women who were pregnant and 24 women who were not pregnant were given a standard oral fixed dose of DHA-piperaquine daily for 3 days and drug concentrations for both DHA and piperaquine were obtained regularly for PK evaluation using a population PK approach using a nonlinear mixed-effects model. Piperaquine was fitted best using a three-compartment disposition model, and the modeled parameters showed a 45% increase in elimination clearance and a 47% rise in relative bioavailability in women who were pregnant compared with women who were not pregnant. The overall impact of pregnancy on piperaquine treatment amounted to a similar total exposure to piperaquine; however, piperaquine in pregnant women had a shorter half-life compared to non-pregnant women. Dihydroartemisinin was fitted best using a one-compartment disposition model, and the model parameters showed a

38% decrease in relative bioavailability in women who were pregnant compared to non-pregnant women.

The overall impact of pregnancy on DHA treatment was a diminished total exposure to DHA compared to non-pregnant patients. The results of this study showed pregnancy results in a lower exposure to DHA and a shorter piperaquine elimination half-life, which will likely decrease the post-treatment prophylactic effect of this drug treatment, which may affect cure rates in pregnant patients [524]. Further studies on the effects of pregnancy on artemisinin metabolism have been conducted. Two studies [181, 274], evaluated the pharmacokinetic parameters of treatment with artemether and artesunate in pregnant Thai women (second and third trimesters) with uncomplicated *falciparum* malaria. The data from these studies suggests the drug exposure of pregnant women to DHA is reduced substantially compared to exposure in women who are not pregnant.

In a different study using non-compartmental modeling, the clearance of DHA was found to be much more rapid in women who were pregnant compared to women who were not pregnant, however, clearance of DHA was not faster in the same women three months after giving birth. The mechanism behind the accelerated DHA clearance in pregnant women is unknown, as changes in PK processes associated with pregnancy have not been completely characterized. DHA is metabolized in the liver by glucuronidation by the enzymes UGT2B7 and UGT1A9. Enzyme induction could speed up the clearance of DHA and explain this data. Induction of these enzymes could occur through increased levels of sex hormones in pregnancy, and this could be the mechanism for the increases in glucuronidation known to take place for other drugs such as oxcarbazepine, lamotrigine, and lorazepam. As this study was conducted in women with uncomplicated *falciparum* malaria, it is not clear whether this data would describe the disposition of AS and DHA in patients with severe malaria. Decreased blood levels of DHA because of accelerated DHA clearance could result in reductions in efficacy for artemisinin compounds, and potential survival of parasites leading to increased risk of artemisinin [522].

8.4. POPULATION PK/PD EVALUATION OF CASES STUDIES OF ANTIMALARIAL COMBINATIONS

Modern anti-infective treatment regimens are frequently designed around drug combinations, and antimalarial drug combinations have been in use since the early 1970s [23]. As many of the drug regimens for antimalarial drug combinations were developed empirically, understanding the disposition of these drugs in combination when used to treat malaria provides a data driven process of optimizing drug combination dosing regimens, particularly for special populations. In this section, population PK/PD case studies for antimalarial combinations are reviewed and potential covariates of age and body weight are examined.

8.4.1. Population PK/PD Studies of Chlorproguanil/Dapsone, Artemisinin-Quinine, and Artemisinin-Mefloquine

1) The Antifolate Combination of Chlorproguanil/Dapsone

Chlorproguanil and dapsone or LapDap is an antifolate combination therapy, which has been proposed to replace sulfadoxine pyrimethamine. Chlorproguanil and dapsone are rapidly eliminated, which does aid in reducing the propensity for drug resistance albeit at the cost of a post-treatment prophylactic effect. Chlorproguanil combined with dapsone is much less expensive than other antimalarial drug combinations on market with a price of US $0.50 for a3 day treatment regimen for an adult. To assess the population PK parameters of chlorproguanil, its metabolite, chlorcycloguanil, and dapsone both rich and sparse PK data were prospectively collected from adults and children infected with uncomplicated *falciparum* malaria. All of the patients were treated with 2.0 mg/kg of chlorproguanil and 2.5 mg/kg of dapsone. Population PK parameter estimates for V/F and CL/F for dapsone were shown to correlate in a significant manner with weight. Infection with *falciparum* malaria, however, had no impact on the PK parameters of any of the three drugs tested [177].

2) Artemisinin-Quinine Combination Therapy

The combination of artemisinin and quinine has been examined for uncomplicated *falciparum* malaria treatment, and further studies have been conducted to understand the efficacy of this combination requires examination of the PK/PD properties of the two drugs to treat infected patients. A total of 268 patients infected with uncomplicated *falciparum* malaria were dosed with quinine at 10 mg/kg of three times per day for 7 days or administered artemisinin once at a dose of 20 mg/kg followed by treatment for 3 days with quinine (AQ3) or with quinine for 5 days (AQ5). Rates of recrudescence observed in this study were 16% for quinine (Q), 38% for the artemisinin quinine 3-day regimen (AQ3), and 15% for the artemisinin quinine 5-day regimen (AQ5) ($P < 0.001$). Recrudescent infections were shown to correlate with briefer parasite clearance times, and longer treatments to achieve complete parasite eradication. The population kinetics of parasitemia were calculated using nonlinear mixed-effect models, and after testing a number of models, the best fit featured a mono-exponential decline of parasitemia where the average parasite elimination half-life was decreased after artemisinin compared to the parasite half-life after administration of quinine. Simulation of an initial increase in parasitemia did not provide a superior model based on other biologically relevant assumptions.

Recrudescent infections were shown to correlate with longer parasite clearance times and an increase in the simulated terminal parasitemia, and assignment of patients into outcome groups based on terminal parasitemia was accurate in 78% of patients. The data supports the hypothesis that parasites with diminished sensitivity to quinine are widespread in Vietnam, and these parasites present clinical disease characterized by slower clearance of parasites and subsequent recrudescence. One dose of artemisinin was shown to induce rapid parasite reduction and a decreased terminal parasitemia; however, prevention of recrudescence after artemisinin treatment requires quinine treatment for a 3-day period after parasites were cleared for a treatment regimen of 5 days duration. The parasite elimination model used in this study demonstrates terminal parasitemia is a critical PD parameter, which predicts patient outcome, defined as either complete eradication of parasites or recrudescent infection.

The population kinetics model used in this study studied a number of pharmacodynamic variables associated with parasite kinetics in antimalarial treatment that are not commonly studied. These variables include the duration of treatment, terminal parasitemia, and eradication time. These variables could be studied, in this case, due to the short half-lives of artemisinin and quinine. When studying mefloquine, piperaquine, and chloroquine, the extremely long residence times result in an inability to estimate actually the eradication time. Parasite kinetics variables studied here could be used in studies of other drugs and may be useful tools to design novel antimalarial treatment regimens. Other studies of quinine treatment for 7 days in Vietnam have shown that quinine retains efficacy, however, the rates of recrudescent infections are high due to increases in quinine resistance. By adding one dose of artemisinin, the rate of parasite elimination is increased and cure rates improve [443].

Artemisinin influence on the PK parameters of mefloquine enantiomers were investigated in a study of these two drugs alone and in combination for treatment of uncomplicated malaria. Forty-two male and female patients were administered either 500 mg of orally dosed artemisinin over a 3 day period then followed by 750 mg of orally dose of mefloquine. Alternatively, 500 mg of oral artemisinin over a 3 day period plus 750 mg of orally dosed mefloquine on the first treatment day, or a single 750-mg dose of mefloquine administered orally on the first treatment day. The data derived from this study was modeled utilizing the nonlinear mixed-effects model software (NONMEM). Regardless of the treatment regimen, all of the patients in this study were treated successfully. The most rapid rates of parasite clearance were noted in patients who were administered artemisinin plus mefloquine on day 1 of treatment. A PD model derived from the *P. falciparum* life cycle was created, and this model was used to estimate the efficacy of both artemisinin and mefloquine and the artemisinin-mefloquine combination. Artemisinin was shown to maintain drug concentration above the minimum inhibitory concentration for an estimated period of 2.97 hours, and the mefloquine enantiomers were shown to have differences in PK parameters.

The RS-mefloquine enantiomer showed oral clearance of 3.5 l/h while the SR mefloquine enantiomer showed a clearance of 0.6 l/h. Patients treated with artemisinin only for 3 days exhibited clearance of artemisinin that was 6.9-times higher on the last treatment day compared to the first treatment day. No differences in the PK parameters of the two mefloquine enantiomers was noted when administered as monotherapy, when combined with artemisinin, or when administered after 3 days of artemisinin treatment. No significant PK interactions were noted when artemisinin and mefloquine were administered together. The *P. falciparum* malaria PD model described here was successfully used to describe the efficacy of artemisinin, mefloquine and the artemisinin-mefloquine combination. This data is contrary to other studies that have shown artemether or artesunate combined with mefloquine have been shown to decrease mefloquine concentrations in the plasma below those observed with mefloquine monotherapy.

In this study, the pharmacokinetic effects of mefloquine enantiomers were associated with mefloquine pharmacodynamic effects. As the CL/F of RS-mefloquine was shown to be six fold higher than the CL/F of SR-mefloquine, the enantiomeric ratios will become different over time. Given the two enantiomers have differences in potency, one question that arises is relating efficacy to the concentration of enantiomer as opposed to relating enantiomer efficacy against total drug concentration to establish an accurate PK/PD relationship. To answer this question, a model was created which fixed potency of RS-mefloquine to twice that of SR mefloquine, however, this model showed less efficacy than a model where the enantiomer potency was set to be equal. The authors concluded in this study that no PK interaction was present between artemisinin and mefloquine enantiomers and the combination of artemisinin and mefloquine had superior efficacy to monotherapy.

The artemisinin PK changes were presumed to be the consequence of auto-induction of liver enzymes associated with artemisinin metabolism, and auto-induction was observed after artemisinin was dosed the second time [503]. Understanding the PK and PD parameters of enantiomers of both established and novel antimalarial drugs may be of interest in the future if there are significant differences between enantiomeric forms and if there are commercial processes allowing purification of a more desirable enantiomer from the racemate.

8.4.2. Population PK/PD Analysis of Antimalarial Combinations Recommended by the WHO

1) Artemether-Lumefantrine (AL) Combination Therapy

The artemether-lumefantrine combination (AL) is the current treatment of choice in Tanzania for uncomplicated *falciparum* malaria. Lumefantrine exposure assists in providing an adequate parasitological and clinical cure, and the parasite clearance time has been shown to drop substantially with increased exposure to artemether and DHA, its metabolite. The basis for combining artemether with lumefantrine is to take advantage of the different PK parameters of these two drugs, improve treatment efficacy compared to monotherapy with either drug, and deter development of drug resistance. A PK/PD study was conducted in Tanzanian children infected with uncomplicated malaria to assess the PK and PD parameters of artemether, dihydroartemisinin, and lumefantrine. The parasite dynamics model constructed as part of this study utilized data showing drug concentrations and parasitemia from 50 Tanzanian children infected with *falciparum* malaria, and, in addition, peripheral parasite counts from 11 children who were asymptomatically infected. The combined data set of population PK and PD parameters for artemether, DHA, and lumefantrine were estimated using NONMEM.

Artemether distribution was fitted best using a two-compartment model where artemether is rapidly absorbed and cleared by its metabolism to DHA. Dihydroartemisinin concentrations were modeled best using a one-compartment model. The PK parameters of artemether were shown to be time dependent and oral clearance changed over time rising from 2.6 liters/h/kg on day 1 to 10 liters/h/kg on day 3. This may be due to the auto-induction of hepatic enzymes associated with metabolism. The PK parameters of lumefantrine were best fitted using a one-compartment model with an absorption lag time, and the oral clearance observed was calculated to be 77 ml/h/kg. The kinetics of artemether in this study is clearly time dependent, which has been previously, described in studies of adults. A semi-mechanistic model of parasite dynamics was derived to estimate the complex interactions between the malaria parasite and human host, and this model was found to an adequate description of the early effects of AM and DHA drug levels to reduce the density of malaria parasites in infected patients.

Some of the derived PD parameters, however, showed problems with precision, which outlines a requirement for additional data to enhance this model. Elimination of malaria parasites is commonly assessed by microscopy using peripheral blood smears, however, while this approach may be adequate for studies of *P. ovale*, *P. vivax*, or *P. malariae* infections, *falciparum* parasites sequester in the deep vasculature and the microscopist may not see a true reflection of the *falciparum* parasite burden or dominant stage. At certain stages of development, only a portion of *falciparum* parasites circulate in the blood at one time to be counted. Estimates of the total *falciparum* parasite burden would be of use given the lack of correlation between parasite count and disease severity in some cases. One of the biggest challenges faced when creating pharmacodynamic models of the effects of antimalarial drugs is to describe adequately parasite population dynamics when drugs are not present.

A number of semi-mechanistic pharmacodynamic models have been created to describe the blood stage life cycle of *falciparum*. These models all have a similar feature to describe the different stages of *falciparum* that are present and the relative composition of the parasite population divided into sequestered and circulating groups. This approach has been used to describe the PD effects of stage-specific drug action and provides a means to estimate the total parasite load comprised of both sequestering and circulating parasites rather than the visible parasite load comprised only of circulating parasites. A semi-mechanistic model of parasite dynamics was created to describe both the visible and sequestered parasite populations, which provides a means of assessing parasite cycle synchronization and the relation of parasite synchrony to treatment efficacy with a number of drugs to include DHA, AM, and lumefantrine [526].

2) Artesunate-Amodiaquine (AS-AQ) Combination Therapy

AS is commonly combined with amodiaquine (AQ) to treat uncomplicated *falciparum* malaria, and this ACT is on market as a fixed-dose combination. Surprisingly, the simultaneous PK parameters of AQ and desethylamodiaquine (DAQ), its active metabolite, in patients infected with *falciparum* malaria have not been adequately characterized in previous studies despite the use of amodiaquine for years for both monotherapy and in combination treatment. Accordingly, a clinical study was done using a population PK approach to estimate the PK parameters of amodiaquine and desethylamodiaquine in 54 adult patients with *falciparum* malaria who were treated with the AS-AQ drug combination. AQ was fitted best with a one-compartment model with first-order absorption and elimination and first-order and irreversible transformation of amodiaquine into desethylamodiaquine. Desethylamodiaquine in turn was best modeled using a two-compartment model with first-order elimination from a central compartment. The mean apparent clearance for AQ was estimated to be 3,410 liters/h, the distribution volume of AQ was estimated to be 39,200 liters, and the elimination half-life of desethylamodiaquine was estimated to be 211 hours. Significant inter-individual variability was shown in estimates of amodiaquine's volume of distribution and the elimination of desethylamodiaquine, and examination of coviarates showed body weight is a significant covariate. One of the objectives of this study was examining the PK parameters of a novel fixed-dose combination *versus* loose drugs. The fixed dose combination was found to yield similar PK parameters compared to the PK parameters noted in patients administered loose drug. All of the patients in these study-cleared parasites within 4 days after treatment was started which precluded investigating the effects of exposure to DAQ and efficacy.

This is the first study to conduct a simultaneous estimation of AQ and DAQ disposition, which provides a better model of the disposition of both drugs as other published population PK studies related the dose of AQ directly to concentrations of DAQ without modeling the metabolism of amodiaquine into desethylamodiaquine. The metabolism of AQ to DAQ should be estimated accurately as opposed to simply assuming 100% conversion without knowing the kinetics of conversion. One of the questions that could not be answered in this study was the relationship between fever which has been used as a surrogate to estimate disease severity to the volume of distribution. Fever has been shown to relate to variability in the estimates of volume of distribution of some antimalarials such as mefloquine, however, this covariate was not estimated in this AQ study, as acetaminophen self-medication was not controlled. Despite the findings that body weight is a significant covariate of AQ pharmacokinetics, the AS-AQ combination was so efficacious in this study that changes in AQ dosing based on body weight are not warranted.

Given the dose of AQ administered, there was sufficient drug on board to overcome any variability associated with body weight in these study patients, and likely, the dose of AQ administered also gave each patient sufficient exposure to DAQ to achieve efficacy. This study confirms the potential value AS-AQ administered as a fixed dose combination that provides efficacy similar to the loose drug form, which should improve adherence to treatment. Similar efficacy findings for the AS-AQ fixed dose combination in children and adults of different ages in other endemic area have been published. The results from this study also showed that a low percentage of patients would reach the efficacy threshold for desethylamodiaquine monotherapy previously established which does support the hypothesis that the efficacy of artesunate is compensating for the lower doses of AQ used in this study [527].

3) Artesunate-Mefloquine (AS-MQ) Combination Therapy

Given the impact of *falciparum* malaria in rural areas of Vietnam, prompt diagnosis of malaria coupled with rapid treatments with artemisinin combination therapy was implemented as a policy to enhance malaria control in the country. A number of comparative efficacy studies of both monotherapy and combination therapy using artemisinin compounds have been conducted in Vietnam to include studies of artemisinin derivative's combined with SP, quinine, mefloquine, and doxycycline. Single-dose combination regimens with mefloquine appeared to be a reasonable ACT regimen, and this became first line treatment. The Vietnamese policy on dosing mefloquine was conservative. In nearby Thailand, escalating drug resistance led to increases in the dose of mefloquine used which was increased to 25 mg/kg, however, a lower dose was applied in Vietnam as combination with artemisinin derivatives was assumed to delay development of resistance to mefloquine. Previous studies, however, showed that a single dose of artemisinin plus 10 mg/kg mefloquine did not prevent recrudescence, and a 15% recrudescence rate was noted with this regimen. In the absence of data on mefloquine drug resistance, the recommended dose of mefloquine was increased to 15 mg/kg, and this dose was originally used in Thailand for mefloquine monotherapy. The combination of mefloquine dosed at 15 mg/kg combined with a single dose of artesunate at 4 mg/kg was implemented as a standard treatment for *falciparum* malaria throughout Vietnam.

The efficacy of this drug combination was not assessed prior to its introduction, and possible interactions between artesunate and mefloquine were not assessed. To answer these questions, a study was conducted to examine drug efficacy, tolerability, and the population PK/PD of sequential administration of artesunate and mefloquine at different intervals in 360 patients infected with *falciparum* malaria. Patients were administered a single treatment regimen consisting of artesunate dosed initially at 4 mg/kg followed by treatment with mefloquine at 15 mg/kg administered at one time in one group, group A, after an 8 hour interval in another group, group B, and after a 24 hour interval in a third group, group C. The purpose of this study was to assess the efficacy of a combination treatment comprised of a single dose of artesunate combined with mefloquine to treat uncomplicated *falciparum* malaria in Vietnam. Other study objectives included assessing drug tolerability and estimating pharmacokinetic and pharmacodynamics parameters observed when mefloquine was dosed at different intervals. After treatment with single doses of artesunate and mefloquine administered at different intervals in the three study groups, follow-up was conducted on day 28. All patients recovered rapidly except one patient who failed therapy in the first 24 hours.

The pharmacokinetics of mefloquine was shown to be similar in all of the different treatment groups. Parasites were shown to reappear in 26% of the patients in the group A, 26% of the patients in group B, and 33% of the patients in group C. Recrudescence early in the course of treatment was shown to correlate with an initial high parasite count, slower clearance of parasites, rapid clearance of mefloquine, and decreased mefloquine plasma concentrations observed by day 28. Plasma concentrations of mefloquine were all shown to reach the target therapeutic levels that supports the hypothesis that efficacy was affected by reduced parasite drug sensitivity. There was no interaction shown between mefloquine and artesunate affecting drug tolerability, efficacy, or pharmacokinetics. Combination therapy with a single of artesunate combined with mefloquine at a dose of 15 mg/kg clearly did not prevent recrudescence and likely failed to diminish mefloquine resistance. The pharmacodynamics of this combination treatment could be separated into two periods, initial parasite elimination and complete parasite elimination.

The pharmacodynamics of artesunate observed in this study showed fast initial parasite killing and clinical recovery, which is similar to PD outcomes observed in other artemisinin studies. No synergy with mefloquine was observed. A high rate of incomplete parasite eradication was observed in this study, which is more complicated to explain. Artemisinin analogues are commonly combined with longer acting antimalarials in order to achieve initial rapid killing and long-term parasite eradication, which requires the presence of a longer-lived partner drug to provide a long period of parasite growth suppression.

Eradication of all parasites in this study was dependent on mefloquine exposure, however, the doses of mefloquine tested in this study were not sufficient to attain eradication of all parasites. The insufficient concentrations of mefloquine noted in this study may be a consequence of sub-therapeutic levels of mefloquine provided or the presence of drug resistant parasites. The plasma concentrations observed in this study were dependent on the dose, bioavailability, and disposition of drugs administered. The dose of mefloquine provided correlated well with the observed $AUC_{0\text{-}8}$ and the C_{max}, however, these parameters did not correlate with parasite recurrence. Variability in drug disposition was shown to be the cause of mefloquine plasma concentration variation observed on day 28. The lower levels of mefloquine observed in the plasma of patients on day 28 were correlated with parasite recurrence, which suggests that the length of drug exposure to parasiticidal plasma concentrations is a critical variable associated with long-term cures.

Incomplete eradication of parasites may be due to parasite resistance, and the formal definition of antimalarial drug resistance is derived from administration and absorption of an anti-malarial drug at a therapeutic but non-toxic dose, and not based on the actual plasma drug concentrations observed. The population pharmacokinetic model created in this study, however, provided very good descriptions of the individual curves relating drug concentration over time. The observed mefloquine plasma concentrations in this study were all beyond the drug levels required to suppress growth of a sensitive strain of *falciparum* malaria (500- 625 µg/L). This data suggests *falciparum* malaria parasites in southern Vietnam were demonstrating reduced drug sensitivity.

Mefloquine drug resistance had not been previously shown in Vietnam, and the consensus has been that resistance had not appeared in Vietnam because mefloquine was being used in combination with artemisinin compounds as opposed to monotherapy. The drug policy in Vietnam had restricted uncontrolled sales of antimalarial drugs in the private health sector to reduce drug resistance. Mefloquine was first utilized for treatment of *falciparum* malaria in Vietnam in 1992, and it has always been used combined with an artemisinin compound. This is a different circumstance than what has been observed in Thailand, where drug resistance to mefloquine emerged a few years after mefloquine monotherapy was initiated in endemic regions. Decreased sensitivity to mefloquine in Vietnam is concerning as it shows a policy of only using mefloquine in combination with artemisinin drugs is not sufficient to deter the emergence of drug resistant parasites.

This study shows a 15 mg/kg dose of mefloquine is insufficient even after rapid parasite killing after initial artesunate administration. This data can be used to guide the use of mefloquine and artesunate in other regions. The authors of this study concluded that different dosing times for mefloquine administered at 15 mg/kg in the first 24 hours after initial treatment with artesunate has no effect on efficacy. The pharmacodynamics of this combination are similar to the outcomes observed with artesunate monotherapy. Parasite recurrence was correlated with elevated initial parasite counts and delays in parasite clearance, and this finding confirms the link between decreased concentrations of mefloquine and parasite recurrence. The data also suggest *falciparum* parasites in Vietnam have reduced sensitivity to mefloquine. Accordingly, the authors recommended that the mefloquine dose for combination therapy should be boosted to 25 mg/kg and combined with artemisinin compounds, and the combination of the two should be given over a 3-day period [528].

4) Dihydroartemisinin-piperaquine (DP) Combination Therapy

The pharmacokinetic properties of DHA combined with piperaquine were assessed using a population PK approach in pregnant and non-pregnant women infected with uncomplicated malaria. Twenty-four pregnant and 24 matched non-pregnant women on the border of Thailand and Myanmar were administered DHA combined with piperaquine in a standard oral 3 day regimen, and PK evaluations of both drugs were assessed by obtaining frequent assessments of the plasma concentrations of both drugs. The pharmacokinetic parameters of the population were modeled using nonlinear mixed-effects modeling. The principal pharmacokinetic observation between the pregnant and non-pregnant women showed pregnant women had no change in piperaquine exposure over time; however, these women did show decreased exposure to DHA *versus* their non-pregnant female counterparts.

Piperaquine was modeled best using a three-compartment disposition model with a 45% higher elimination clearance and a 47% increase in relative bioavailability in pregnant women compared to non-pregnant women. The net effect of pregnancy on piperaquine disposition was an unchanged total exposure but a shorter elimination half-life. Dihydroartemisinin was best modeled using a one-compartment disposition model with a 38% lower relative bioavailability in pregnant women compared to non-pregnant women. The overall effect of pregnancy was decreased reduction in total exposure to dihydroartemisinin. The reduced piperaquine elimination half-life and diminished exposure to dihydroartemisinin is predicted to shorten the post-treatment prophylactic effect and may possibly affect rates of cure in pregnant women.

Piperaquine concentrations were shown to vary between doses, which might be explained by variations in mean transit time (45.8%) and in relative bioavailability (56.3%). Piperaquine is known to be a lipophilic compound with low oral bioavailability (50% bioavailability shown in rats), and thus, the absorption of piperaquine is variable and dependent on food consumption. Both of these factors will alter absorption and thus total drug exposure. Food intake was not a variable that was controlled in this study and differences in food consumption may explain the high intra-individual variability observed in drug absorption. A time-dependent increase in oral bioavailability that was observed in this study could be explained by cessation of symptoms during early treatment with increased intake of food in later treatment. Pregnant women dosed with piperaquine showed increased oral bioavailability (47% increase in pregnant women compared to non-pregnant women), which could be explained by reductions in intestinal motility, dietary differences, and extended periods of gastric emptying in pregnant women due to increases in concentrations of progesterone. Increased cardiac output in pregnant women (30 to 50% higher), translates into elevated blood flow to the small intestine, and stomach which may also help explain the increased bioavailability of piperaquine in pregnant women compared to non-pregnant women.

The elimination clearance of piperaquine was estimated to be 45% higher in pregnant women than in non-pregnant women in this study. The altered pharmacokinetic properties of piperaquine in pregnant women compared to non-pregnant women are not likely to affect clinical outcomes, as the total drug exposure of piperaquine was not changed. The effects of pregnancy on the oral bioavailability of piperaquine and the elimination of piperaquine yielded an overall effect of increases in the maximum drug concentration and a shorter half-life in pregnant women compared to non-pregnant women. A shorter elimination half-life would affect the period of post-treatment prophylaxis in these women and might affect the concentrations of piperaquine utilized for intermittent prophylaxis in pregnancy, which could result in piperaquine concentrations falling below the minimum inhibitory concentration of piperaquine required to inhibit the growth of parasites between doses. Simulated population mean profiles utilizing the derived model for this study estimated a 8.7% higher piperaquine concentration in non-pregnant women compared to pregnant women at 30 days post treatment, and a 45% higher piperaquine concentration in non-pregnant women compared to pregnant women 60 days post treatment.

This data suggests that administration of piperaquine once a month as intermittent prophylaxis should provide similar clinical efficacy in pregnant and non-pregnant women but administration at intervals beyond monthly should be studied further prior to implementation. Pregnant women in this study had a 38% lower dihydroartemisinin exposure resulting from reduced DHA bioavailability. This finding may affect clinical outcomes given the exposure to piperaquine is highly variable. A lower exposure to dihydroartemisinin would result in an increased number of residual parasites left alive to be killed by piperaquine, which could increase treatment failures and drive the emergence of drug resistance [521].

CHAPTER 9

Combination Therapy to Avoid Antimalarial Drug Toxicity

Abstract: The safety profiles of CTs and ACTs are a composite of the safety profiles of the partner drugs in combination. Overall, safety concerns of antimalarial combination therapies leading to serious adverse effects are focused on three known problem areas for these drugs: neurotoxicity, embryotoxicity, and cardiotoxicity. While neurotoxicity induced by artemisinin compounds in animal models has been thoroughly described in the literature, the current clinical treatment for ACTs for a 3-day period is likely too short a time for artemisinin drug exposure to induce neurotoxicity in man. Cardiotoxicity induced by antimalarial drugs such as halofantrine has been shown to result in serious adverse events when dosed to certain subpopulations of patients. Other antimalarial drugs of the quinoline class such as chloroquine and piperaquine have been shown to prolong the QT interval of treated patients, which does focus the attention of both medicinal chemists in early drug development and clinicians testing antimalarial drugs in the field. Early assessment of the potential for cardiotoxicity using hERG testing is an essential element in creating a drug that does not have overt potential for cardiotoxicity. While embryotoxicity induced by artemisinin compounds has been noted in various animal models, the period of concern is primarily in the first trimester where ACT administration to pregnant women has been contraindicated. The PK/PD data from pre-clinical studies has been very useful in establishing treatment parameters for artemisinin drugs to avoid potential embryotoxicity in man. A review of the literature on this subject will be provided in this chapter to assess the limitations of CTs and ACTs therapy to avoid triggering serious adverse events associated with neurotoxicity, cardiotoxicity, and embryotoxicity.

Keywords: Adverse effects, animals, artemether-lumefantrine, artemisinins, cardiotoxicity, embryotoxicity, halofantrine, neurotoxicity, pregnant women.

Early animal studies reviewing the potential of artemisinin-induced neurotoxicity conducted with high doses of artemisinin drugs have shown focal brain stem lesions associated with deficits in the auditory nerves, however, this data has not been shown in man [12]. Several studies of brain stem function in man including audiometry have not shown hearing abnormalities after repeated administration of artemisinins [529, 530]. To date, only one case-controlled study has shown hearing loss demonstrated by audiometric testing in factory workers who were administered artemether-lumefantrine for treatment of uncomplicated malaria [531]. This result should be cautiously interpreted given the design limitations of this work. A large body of research studies in animals have been conducted on artemisinin induced neurotoxicity, and the data does suggest the potential for neurotoxicity exists with longer dosing regimens.

Qigui Li and Mark R. Hickman

The potential cardiotoxicity of antimalarial drugs is best illustrated by the hERG signal and QT prolongation that observed in patients treated with halofantrine. Clinical studies of toxicity in normal patients did not elicit overt findings of cardiotoxicity, and serious adverse events, to include sudden death, were only observed in patients with underlying cardiac problems treated with elevated doses of halofantrine used to treat drug-resistant malaria. The structural similarity shown between halofantrine and lumefantrine, a partner drug for the artemether-lumefantrine ACT, also elicited concern that the combination of artemether-lumefantrine might have adverse cardiac effects. hERG testing conducted with lumefantrine showed this drug has minimal potential to adversely affect the hERG cardiac potassium channel. *In vivo* testing of lumefantrine was conducted using extensive animal testing to assess the potential for drug induced cardiotoxicity, and no significant induction of QTc prolongation have been noted [532, 533]. Extensive testing of lumefantrine in man has also not shown any propensity for this drug to trigger cardiotoxicity [534, 535]. In a review of AL trials, 6% of 291 children who received a six dose AL regimen showed prolongation of the QT interval longer than 60 milliseconds. In a large prospective study conducted in Thailand, no correlation shown between lumefantrine plasma concentrations range and changes in electrocardiograph results. These studies all suggest that lumefantrine has limited potential for adverse cardiac events [536].

Information on potential cardiotoxicity of the artemisinin compounds in man is limited. In animal studies conducted in beagle dogs, high intramuscular doses of the oil-soluble artemisinins, arteether and artemether, were shown to be associated with prolongation of the QT interval in electrocardiographic studies which does suggests this drug class has potential for inducing cardiotoxicity [537]. Clinical studies in man have reported modest QT interval prolongation after artemisinin administration, however, the specific contributions of artemisinin *versus* malaria to QT prolongation in these patients could not be separated, and malaria itself has been shown to be associated with prolongations in the QT interval [538]. Studies of QT prolongation in healthy volunteers, however, did not show artemisinin induced prolongation of the QT interval [534]. A recent study conducted in 21 adult patients in Bangladesh infected with severe *falciparum* malaria demonstrated that the QTc interval was not affected by bolus administration of intravenous artesunate at a dose of 2.4 mg/kg [539].

The artemisinin class of drugs has shown embryotoxicity in animal models early in gestation, which has elicited concerns over similar effects in man and recommendations for limited use of these drugs in man during the first trimester

[67]. Studies from Africa and Asia, including treatment of 44 pregnant women treated with artemisinin compounds during the first trimester have shown similar numbers of stillbirths, congenital abnormalities, and compared to pregnant women who did not receive artesunate therapy [540-542]. Overall, antimalarials used for clinical treatment are well tolerated and safe, and severe adverse drug reactions when administered to human patients are rare. In the majority of cases, the side effects of malaria disease itself cannot be differentiated from adverse effects from drugs. For patients receiving antimalarial drugs for prophylaxis, the adverse effects observed after drug administration is generally similar, however, the incidence of the adverse effects may be different. Many of the milder, common adverse drug reactions included vomiting, nausea, abdominal pain, diarrhea, and headache.

Treatment of malaria infected patients with quinine often results in cinchonism which is an array of symptoms, generally reversible, which include ringing in the ears (tinnitus), deafness, vomiting, and dizziness which is frequently noted patients receiving standard dose regimens. One of the more serious adverse effects noted after quinine administration is hypoglycemia. Artemisinin compound administration results in less frequent adverse effects and these compounds are generally considered safer than other antimalarial drugs. Rare cases of anaphylaxis have been noted after treatment with IV artesunate; however, the incidence of these adverse effects is very low. All of the serious adverse events illustrated here are related to the innate PK and PD properties of the antimalarial drugs, and appropriate testing and dosing regimens, particularly in combination, can be used to avoid these serious adverse effects.

Other antimalarial drugs such as the 8-aminoquinlines are well known to trigger extravascular hemolytic anemia and methemoglobinemia in G6PD deficient patients. Treatment and prophylaxis with mefloquine has been associated with dose dependent neurotoxicity, and administration of pyrimethamine-dapsone has been shown to be associated with agranulocytosis particularly in patients treated with higher doses. Administration of sulfadoxine-pyrimethamine (SP) and amodiaquine for prophylaxis has been reported to be associated with a variety of potentially fatal reactions, and neither drug is recommended for long term prophylaxis for malaria. Adverse effects associated with SP therapy include vomiting, nausea, photosensitivity, headache, and dizziness. Unusual adverse effects of SP therapy include Steven-Johnson syndrome, a serious condition of toxic epidermal necrolysis triggered by sulfadoxine, and other disorders of the blood to include anemia, low platelet counts, and low white blood cell counts. Atovaquone-proguanil is an efficacious antimalarial combination that is very well tolerated for both prophylaxis and treatment indications. Adverse effects associated with atovaquone-proguanil administration are rare, but nausea, abdominal pain, headache, and vomiting can occur. Administration of doxycycline has been associated with staining of permanent teeth in children fewer than eight, and doxycycline has also been shown to trigger photosensitivity and nausea after administration [65].

9.1. CARDIOTOXICITY INDUCED BY HIGH DOSES OF HALOFANTRINE IN HUMANS

There are consistent differences in electrographic QT data from patients infected with acute malaria, and patients who have recovered from acute malaria infection have been reported to show a prolonged QT interval. The prolongation of QT interval observed has often been misinterpreted because of antimalarial cardiotoxicity. Of the various antimalarial drug classes, only the quinolines and antimalarial drugs that are similar in structure have been shown to demonstrate cardiovascular effects that are clinically significant. Drugs in this class have been shown to have modest effects on delays in ventricular depolarization, which led to widening of the QRS complex. Only halofantrine and quinidine have been shown to have ventricular depolarization effects that are clinically significant (class 3 effects). Both drugs have the potential to cause potential QT prolongation effects that are problematic, and administration of halofantrine at high doses has been shown to be associated with *Torsade de pointes* (catastrophic cardiac blockade) and sudden death. The parenteral formulations of quinoline drugs (quinidine, quinine, and chloroquine) have been shown to inductive hypotension when rapidly injected, and cardiovascular collapse may occur consequently. At the current doses that are recommended, other antimalarial drugs have not been shown to have any cardiac effects that are clinically significant.

9.1.1. History of Cardiotoxicity Associated with Halofantrine (HF) Administration

Halofantrine (HF), a phenanthrenemethanol aminoalcohol compound was originally on market in 1988. Halofantrine was considered both safe and effective malaria treatment, to include treatment of infections caused by multidrug resistant *falciparum* malaria until 1993, when ter Kuile *et al.* showed a death was associated with HF cardiotoxicity [543]. This death was associated with HF administration at doses far higher than those recommended (72 mg/kg as opposed to the recommended dose of 25 mg/kg) to enhance antimalarial efficacy of HF for treatment of patients on the border of Burma and Thailand, which is an area known to possess high-level antimalarial drug resistance. This report of a sudden death in a patient treated with high dose HF led to a study utilizing prospective electrocardiographic measurements, which consistently showed treatment with HF lengthened the QT and PR intervals. Since then, a number of studies have shown the cardiotoxic potential of HF in both children and adults, and several cases of HF-induced cardiac toxicity or death have been presented. As a consequence of these side effects prescription of HF for malaria treatment dropped dramatically in spite of the rapid antimalarial efficacy of HF [532].

The first case of HF-induced cardiac toxicity was reported in 1993 after a Thai woman with an extensive history of tachyarrhythmia suddenly died. She was dosed with a dose of HF three times the standard dose (72 mg/kg *versus* the standard dose of 25 mg/kg) to treat a case of recrudescent *falciparum* malaria that had failed to respond to mefloquine treatment *falciparum* [543]. None of the safety studies of HF had indicated a potential for HF-induced cardiotoxicity, and no electrocardiograms were conducted in a study of this dose regimen conducted a year previously [543]. A new study conducted after the sentinel death showed high-dose HF treatment was shown to be associated with prolongation of the QTc interval. The lengthening of the QTc interval was correlated to the dose of HF administered, and the correlation between QTc prolongation and the plasma concentrations of HF metabolites were reported in another study. The extent of QTc prolongation was higher in patients who were treated with mefloquine prior to HF treatment. Several additional reports of HF-induced prolongation of the QTc interval, severe ventricular arrhythmias, and overt *Torsade de pointes* have been published involving patients who presented with QT prolongation from birth. Following the discovery of potential cardiac risks in 1993, the GSK and WHO recommended prescription changes for HF administration [532].

The HF cardiotoxicity studies showed that females represented 70% of cases, and gender appeared to be a predisposing factor. No data exists to examine the possible influence of body weight as a risk factor particularly in low body weight female patients. Within the general population, previous studies have shown that females have longer QT intervals, and the incidence of drug-induced QT prolongation and clinical cases of cardiac blockade (*Torsade de pointes*) is higher among females. There is no evidence, however, for an increased risk of dying among female patients, and the risk for sudden death among females is lower globally. HF associated side-effects were likely underreported given the elevated incidence of predisposing cardiac factors in patients from malaria endemic developing countries to include vitamin B1 deficiency secondary to nutritional insufficiency (which induces QT prolongation), electrolyte abnormalities or cardiac rheumatism observed in developing countries. Accordingly, HF toxicity may well be underreported in tropical areas.

In patients who died after administration of HF, death was reported to occur in 79% of cases during the first round of HF treatment. This finding is not surprising as a second round of HF treatment was suggested only for non-immune patients who represent a small fraction of the patients treated with HF. In electrocardiograms, significant changes have been shown elsewhere in the literature, however, occurring in the second round of HF treatment rather than the first, which is likely caused by elevated HF plasma concentrations, and this, in turn, likely predisposed non-immune patients who did receive a second course of HF treatment to an increased risk of cardiotoxicity. Pediatric HF-induced cardiotoxicity marked by asymptomatic electrocardiographic changes has been documented in half of the children treated. The risks of severe cardiotoxicity in children are low with the standard HF dosing recommendations as no children have shown cardiotoxicity in any of the HF studies that have been conducted when standard HF dosing recommendations were followed. In contrast, five fatal pediatric cases have been reported all of which occurred after administration of higher than recommended HF doses.

Thus, discerning how much of the cardiotoxicity liability of HF is due to the hERG blocking activity of this drug can be difficult in patients with existing predisposing factors. The first death from HF-induced cardiotoxicity is an excellent example as this patient had a known pre-existing cardiac condition, she was treated with HF at a dose almost three times the recommended amount, and she was also administered mefloquine, a drug with an extended half-life known to prolong the QTc interval, immediately prior to receiving HF. In one study, 53 cases of cardiotoxicity were noted (in the population of patients, however, the data were not analyzed due to variability in the data [543].

A published study of fatal HF cardiotoxicity was conducted using patient data derived from 35 cases documented in a review of the literature and the GSK Worldwide Global Clinical Safety and Pharmacovigilance database. The number of deaths (35) in this study is likely a severe underestimate of the total number of HF-induced cardiotoxicity deaths given the majority of these deaths occurred in the third world where reports of adverse events associated with drug treatment is the exception, not the rule. A comparison of fatalities associated with other quinolone drugs such as mefloquine would have been useful to expand this study, but at the time this study was published, the authors were unable to access the safety database of Hoffman-La Roche to obtain that information. In contrast to the deaths noted after HF administration, no deaths or other adverse cardiac effects have been published following treatment using lumefantrine, a drug that is structurally similar to HF [535, 536]. HF is a chiral compound, and the cardiotoxicity of HF is known to be stereoselective in nature, as the (+) HF enantiomer is the more cardiotoxic enantiomer. The significant differences in the potential to induce cardiotoxicity between two structurally similar compounds, HF and lumefantrine, are consistent with the decreased risk of cardiotoxicity associated with the (-) HF enantiomer and HF's principle metabolite, N-desbutyl HF [532].

The substantial risk of cardiotoxicity associated with HF has lead physicians to avoid the use of this drug in favor of safer alternative drugs. If there were no other alternative at hand, serious adverse outcomes could be avoided simply by dosing HF in accordance with the manufacturer recommendations. HF may be needed in the future if the limited number of antimalarial drugs available is inadequate in the future. Development of the N-desbutyl-metabolite of HF would be the best option, as it is significantly less cardiotoxic than HF. The development of pharmacogenetics tools could possibly permit safer use of HF and other drugs known to prolong the QT interval if patients could be prescreened to identify cardiotoxicity risks in advance [532].

9.1.2. Role of Halofantrine in Antimalarial Treatment

HF is effective against blood stage chloroquine-resistant *falciparum* and chloroquine-resistant *vivax* malaria. HF resistance and treatment failures in *falciparum* malaria were found on the Thai-Burma border and in Africa due to poor drug absorption. The treatment dose of HF in adults is three doses of 500 mg of HF dosed every 6 hours (total first course dose 1,500 mg), and in children weighing >10 kg, the recommended HF dose is 8 mg base/kg dosed every 6 hours for three doses. A second treatment regimen is suggested for non-immune patients one week after completion of initial treatment to ensure complete eradication of parasites. HF has several disadvantages when used for treatment including cross-resistance with mefloquine, variable bioavailability, and, most significantly, known risk of sudden death in certain patient populations from cardiotoxicity, along with a second course treatment requirement for non-immunes, which is problematic from a patient compliance perspective.

Clinical safety studies have shown that HF is well tolerated in most patients. Rare adverse effects include diarrhea, vomiting, nausea, and abdominal pain. Hepatic toxicity has been noted after HF administration characterized by temporary elevations in liver enzymes. A variety of other rare symptoms have been attributed to HF including cough, acute intravascular hemolysis, pruritis, convulsions, and skin rash. The most serious toxicity associated with HF administration is cardiac-related. HF administration has an effect on cardiac muscle similar to quinidine resulting in slower intra-cardiac conduction (increased QRS and PR intervals) and prolonged cardiac repolarization leading to an increase in the QTc interval. QTc prolongation is a well-recognized predisposing factor for ventricular arrhythmias, and QTc prolongation has been associated with cardiac blockade (*Torsade de pointes* syndrome) leading to sudden death. The cardiotoxicity associated with HF is unpredictable due to the wildly variable absorption of HF, which can be enhanced by co-administration with fatty food (similar to atovaquone-proguanil). Significant QTc prolongation has been shown to occur after HF administration at the standard dose (24 mg/kg/day for 3 days), and the degree of QTc prolongation has been shown to directly correlate with HF serum levels.

QTc prolongation is most likely to occur in patients who have been treated with mefloquine, and failed, and then retreated with high-dose HF. Over 20 sudden, unexpected deaths have occurred because of HF treatment, and cardiac blockade, both first and second-degree, has been documented. In a clinical study of 42 of HF-treated Nigerian children aged 1 to 11 years of age infected with uncomplicated *falciparum* malaria, treatment of two of these children with HF resulted in one patient developing Mobitz type I second-degree heart block and one patient developed first-degree heart block. These ECG changes took place within 48 hours after HF administration, the aberrant electrocardiogram readings resolved after 72 hours, and the ECG changes noted were associated with clinical symptoms. Interestingly, the principal metabolite of HF, N-desbutyl-HF, possesses antimalarial activity but it has far lower potential to induce cardiotoxicity than the parent molecule, HF [544].

HF should not be administered to any patients with prolonged QTc intervals or other cardiac arrhythmias. Contraindications for HF use include [544]:

1) HF allergy;

2) Cardiac disease (*e.g.* beriberi, ischemic heart disease);

3) Romano-Ward syndrome (congenital QTc interval prolongation);

4) History of sudden death of family members;

5) Concomitant administration of drugs that are also known to prolong the QTc interval such as erythromycin, tricyclic antidepressants, and antihistamines;

6) Recent treatment with mefloquine;

7) Pregnant women and breast-feeding women;

8) Children are under 1 year of age due to a lack of data.

Clinical use of HF is currently limited to patients infected with *falciparum* malaria that is drug resistant with no preexisting heart disease, who are not also being prescribed other drugs that can cause hypokalemia or QTc prolongation who do not have other treatment alternatives. While baseline QTc interval does not appear to correlate with HF-induced QTc prolongation, some have suggested the baseline QTc interval should be examined to determine if it is normal prior to initiating HF treatment. The WHO does not recommend HF as standby treatment for travelers. A prospective study conducted with high-dose HF therapy for treatment of patients with mild malaria demonstrated high-dose HF therapy correlated with prolongation of QTc intervals. The prolongation of the QTc interval in patients treated with HF has been shown to correlate with HF plasma concentrations. The degree of HF-induced QTc prolongation has been shown to be higher in patients whose treatment closely followed mefloquine.

9.1.3. Replacement of Halofantrine

With the introduction of ACT treatments for uncomplicated malaria, HF should not be routinely used as an antimalarial drug unless the emergence of drug resistant parasites leads to HF being the only possible alternative. Lumefantrine has proven to be a very good replacement for HF given its efficacy and good safety profile. HF is used in a few locations to include Pakistan and parts of Africa even in areas where drugs are available that are much safer. In some locations where HF is still used, physicians must examine all prospective patients for the previously discussed contraindications for HF treatment, in particular existing heart disease, or family history of heart disease, or treatment with other drugs known to enhance HF's propensity for cardiotoxicity such as mefloquine. HF should only be prescribed at the recommended dose of 25 mg/kg without food to avoid enhanced absorption, which may lead to cardiotoxic adverse events. In addition, HF treatment should only be used for treatment of drug resistant uncomplicated *falciparum* malaria inpatients with no risk of severe electrolyte imbalance. If these guidelines were adhered to, the risk of HF-induced cardiotoxicity would be minimized. In industrialized countries, other antimalarial drugs exist and there is no real need for HF other than for treatment of unusual cases.

9.2. TK/TD ANALYSES IN ANIMALS WITH NEUROTOXICITY INDUCED BY ARTEMISININS

Animal studies have shown fatal neurotoxicity associated with intramuscular administration of artemether (AE) and artemether (AM) or oral administration of an experimental artemisinin analogue, artelinic acid. Toxicokinetic studies have shown oil-soluble artemisinins when injected form a depot at the site of injection which leads to inflammation of the muscle fascia. Artelinic acid administered orally has been shown to induce gastrointestinal toxicity associated with delays in gastric emptying. This data suggests artemisinin exposure time in animals was prolonged due to drug accumulation in the blood, and, it is likely this extended exposure leads to neurotoxicity. Animal studies have shown that the neurotoxic exposure time, which describes the length of time drug exposure occurs above a threshold level neurotoxic exposure with a neurotoxic outcome, can be utilized as a prediction tool to evaluate the potential for induction of neurotoxicity *in vivo*. The threshold level for induction of neurotoxicity for defining neurotoxic exposure time is the lowest observed neurotoxic effect level (LONEL) in plasma associated with a neurotoxic outcome. The dose of AE, for example, associated with induction of minimal neurotoxicity is 6.0-12.5 mg/kg dosed daily for 7-28 days, which results in a 2-3 fold longer drug exposure in rhesus monkeys (179.5 hours) than in rats (67.1 hours) or dogs (103.7 hours). These results suggest that given neurotoxicity requires an exposure time of 179.5 hours in rhesus monkeys, dosing a man for up to 7 days or 168 hours should be safe.

In animal toxicity studies of artemether and artemether, which are oil-soluble compounds, the lowest dose of multiple intramuscular injections required to produce findings of neuropathology was 12. 5 mg/kg dosed for 7 days in rats, 6 mg/kg dosed for 28 days in dogs, and 8 mg/kg dosed for 14 days in rhesus monkeys. A similar finding was observed for oral artelinic acid, an experimental artemisinin analogue, where neurotoxicity was induced in rats after administration of oral artelinic acid at 160 mg/kg daily for 9 days. Very little neurotoxicity was demonstrated in mice administered oral artesunate, DHA, or artemether at doses of over 200 mg/kg/day for 28 days. All of the water-soluble artemisinin analogues such as artesunate or the experimental analogues, artelinic acid, were administered intravenously. No evidence of neurotoxicity, either behavioral or pathological, has been demonstrated in any animal species after intravenous administration of artesunate or artelinic acid up to the maximum tolerated dose (MTD). The MTD of AS, for example, in rats is 240 mg/kg and the MTD of artelinic acid in rats is 80 mg/kg based on IV injection for 3 days. Despite IV injection of elevated doses of both water-soluble artemisinin analogues, neurotoxicity was not induced in these animals [12].

In another study, administration of intravenous AS at dose of 120 mg/kg daily for 7 days showed no effect on neurotoxicity scores (unpublished data, WRAIR). Even after a single intramuscular injection of artesunate or artelinic acid at a dose of 420 mg/kg in rats, no neurotoxicity lesions were observed. Administration of oral AS at a dose of 200 mg/kg per day for 5-7 days also did not induce neurotoxicity or any specific clinical signs of neurotoxicity. The artemisinin neurotoxic exposure times is likely longer in man as monkeys are the better comparator to humans than dogs or rodents. Oral artelinic acid, an experimental artemisinin analogue, was shown to require an 8-fold longer exposure times than intramuscularly administered AE for induction of neurotoxicity which suggests water-soluble artemisinins are safer than oil-soluble artemisinins with regard to inducing neurotoxicity. As artemisinin drugs are administered in man at low doses (2- 4 mg/kg) and AE is rarely used for treatment of malaria in man, the safe dosing duration is likely even longer in humans. Accordingly, the current ACT regimens dosed for a period of 3-5 days are predicted not to induce neurotoxicity in man. These findings are consistent with a WHO guide for artemisinin treatment of patients with *falciparum* malaria, to avoid neurotoxicity [12].

9.2.1. Neurotoxicity Assessment of Artemisinins

Artemisinin compounds act quickly to kill drug-resistant *P. falciparum* parasites, and these drugs are the treatment of choice for uncomplicated *falciparum* malaria. While the neurotoxicity demonstrated from artemisinin treatment of animals is a concern, this effect is difficult to assess in man. No systematic toxicity has been shown in human patients, even in clinical trials with specific neurotoxicity endpoints such as impairments in hearing, movement, cerebral, or vestibular abnormalities. While it may be entirely reasonable to believe no neurotoxicity is being induced in man after artemisinin treatment, another possible explanation for the lack of reports of neurotoxicity symptoms observed in treated patients is due to the inability to distinguish between CNS events associated with disease and CNS events associated with drug treatment. Severe malarial infection, particularly cerebral malaria, can result in patients recovering with deficits in neural function.

This may make distinguishing between these two potentially causal factors very difficult even with the wide use of artemisinin drugs today. Five cases of neurotoxicity were reported in artemisinin-treated patients after multiple artemisinin treatment episodes. These reports may reflect true artemisinin-induced neurotoxicity that merits further investigation. Conceivably, repeat artemisinin administrations over time in areas endemic for malaria may lead to neurotoxicity given these drugs are sold over the counter without supervision. There is considerable disagreement regarding whether these putative episodes of neurotoxicity truly occurred, particularly given the confounder of concomitant infection. In the absence of definitive data, it is difficult to evaluate these reported episodes of neurotoxicity in man, and the arguments on whether these episodes have truly taken place will continue [12].

9.2.2. Accumulation of Artemisinins Leads to Prolonged Drug Exposure Times

Previous studies have shown artemisinin-induced neurotoxicity is not dependent on conversion of artemisinin to DHA, distribution of artemisinin compounds to the CNS, or to elevated exposure of artemisinins shown by the plasma C_{max} or AUC. Studies have shown that the artemisinin neurotoxicity is very dependent on the drug exposure time. These studies were conducted in rodents administered multiple doses of AE and AM administered intramuscularly and in animals administered multiple doses of oral artelinic acid. The drug concentration data demonstrated only the blood plasma showed accumulation of artemisinin drugs. As administration of artemisinin has been shown to induce drug metabolism, decreased plasma drug concentrations have been observed in both malaria-infected patients and healthy volunteers given repeat oral doses of artemisinins (QHS, AS, AM, and DHA). The C_{max} and AUC values derived from these individuals were markedly reduced on the last dose day by one-third to one-seventh compared with the C_{max} and AUC values observed on the first day. The reduction in levels of drug exposure observed during treatment is not a consequence of disease given the PK parameters of patients treated with artemisinin drugs is similar to the PK parameters observed in studies with healthy subjects. Animals treated with intravenous or intramuscular administered AS or AM showed a similar time-dependent decline blood concentration (Fig. **27**).

1) Accumulation of AM and AE after Intramuscular Injection

TK data derived from animals (rats, beagle dogs, rhesus monkeys) and human studies has shown that the lipid soluble artemisinins, AM and AE, accumulate in

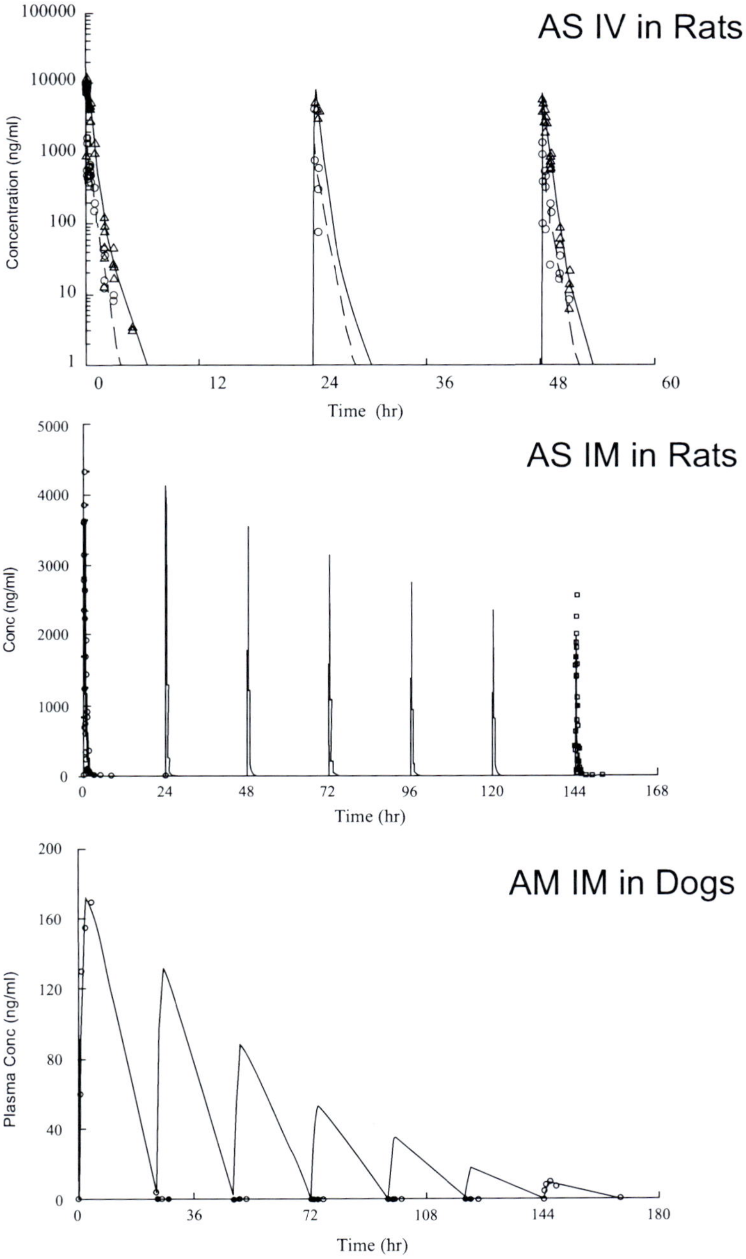

Figure 27: Pharmacokinetic profiles measured by HPLC-ECD (markers) and computer fitted curves of 36.7 mg/kg of intravenous artesunate (AS, top, dashed line), and its active metabolite DHA (top, solid line) once daily for 3 days [210]. Study of 25 mg/kg of intramuscular artemether (AM, middle) was dosed daily for 7 days in rats [311]. Another PK profiles after oral dose at 600 mg/kg of AM (bottom) daily for 7 days in beagle dogs [231].

plasma after multiple IM injections. Rats injected with AE intramuscularly showed plasma accumulation of AE is a consequence of slow absorption of drug from the site of injection. The elimination t½ of AE after 7 daily doses was prolonged from 13.7 hours observed on the first day of dosing to 31.2 hours on the last day of dosing (Fig. **28**, top). Accumulation of drug was also seen in beagle dogs administered AE at a daily IM dose of 15 mg/kg for 14 days, which induced severe neurotoxicity and death. The elimination t½ of AE in rats dosed for 14 days was extended from 11.9 hours on day 1 to 21.5 hours on day 14 (Fig. **28**, middle). Similar accumulation in the plasma of dogs was reported after daily IM injection of AM at a dose of 20, 40, and 80 mg/kg for 7 days. The toxicokinetic analysis from the data derived from animals dosed on days 2-7 was quite different from the data observed on day 1. After 7 daily doses, the elimination t½ of AM climbed from 9 hours on day 1 to 37 hours on day 7 which suggests exposure time for AM had also increased. In addition, the accumulation of AE in blood plasma of rhesus monkeys after daily IM dosing for 14 days at 16 mg/kg (see Fig. **28**, bottom) was also shown to increase. The elimination t½ of AE in these monkeys after 14 days of daily IM AE treatment increased from 22.6 hours on day 1 to 82.1 hours on day 14.

2) Accumulation of Artelinic Acid After Intragastric Administration

Oral administration of the experimental compound, artelinic acid, has been shown to induce gastrointestinal toxicity due to delayed gastric emptying. Rats administered artelinic acid at a dose of 160 mg/kg daily for 9 days also demonstrated moderate levels of neurotoxicity likely due to prolonged absorption of compound due to these delays in gastric emptying. When comparing the toxicokinetic parameters derived over time, the data on day 9 was shown to be very different from the data observed on day 1. On day 9, the half-life of artelinic acid was shown to be 3.82 times longer than the half-life observed on day 1 (10.7 hours *versus* 2.8 hours. The mean AUC of artelinic acid was increased on the last dosing day (168.01 μg·h/ml) compared to the AUC observed on day 1 (168.01 μg·h/ml *versus* 128. 38 μg·h/ml). The prolonged elimination of artelinic acid in this study is hypothesized to lead to accumulation of drug over time, and hence increased drug exposure.

3) Relationship of Drug Accumulation to Prolonged Drug Absorption

Intramuscular administration of AM and AE has been associated with slow absorption, and one of the reasons for this slow absorption involves administration of these drugs dissolved in sesame oil which forms a drug depot

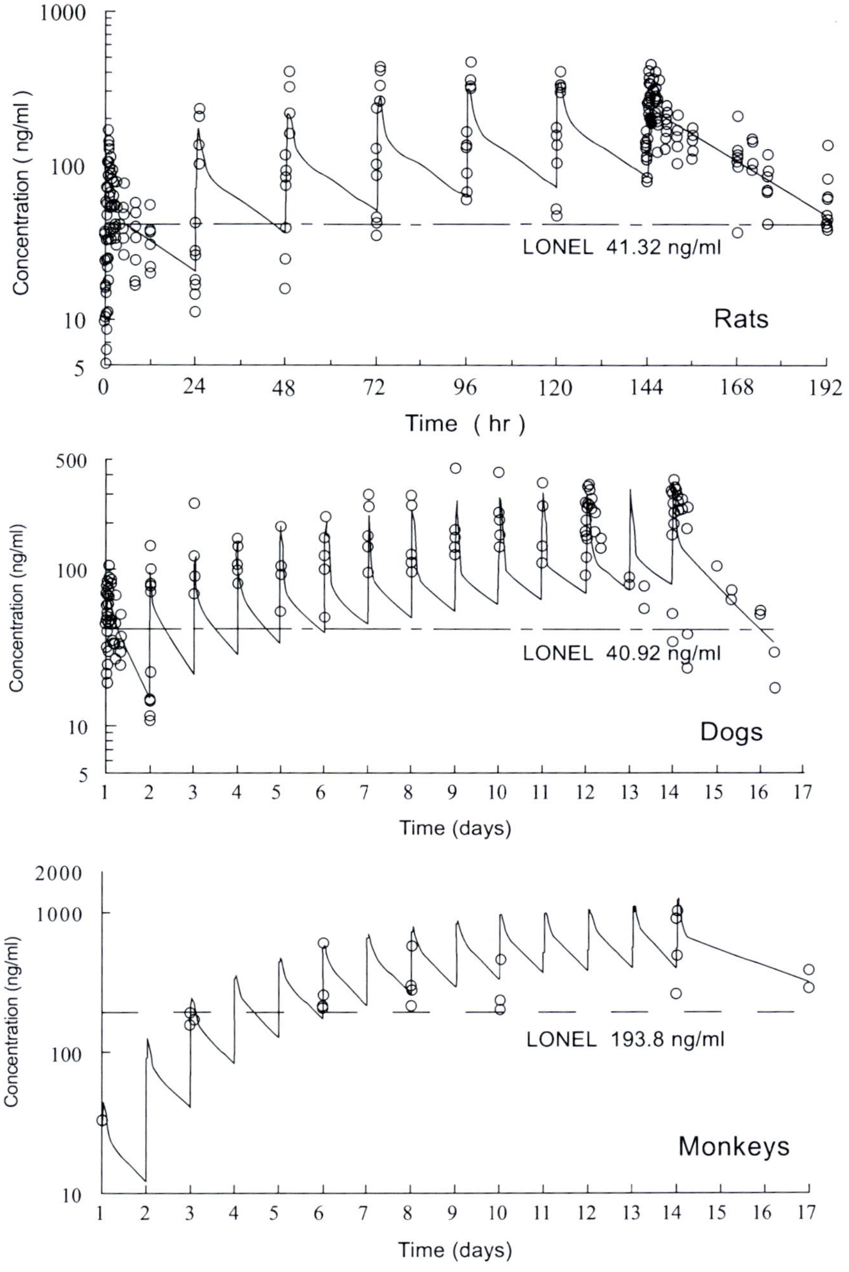

Figure 28: Pharmacokinetic profiles measured by HPLC-ECD (markers) and computer fitted curves (solid line) of arteether (AE) in sesame oil in rats at daily dose of 25 mg/kg for 7 days [219], in beagle dogs at daily dose of 15 mg/kg for 14 days [65], and in rhesus monkeys at daily dose of 16 mg/kg for 14 days [12]. The lowest observed neurotoxic effect level (LONEL, dashed line) from AE measurement was estimated 41.32 ng/ml in rats, 40.92 ng/ml in dogs, and 193.8 ng/ml in rhesus monkeys, respectively [12].

which releases these drugs slowly. The prolonged elimination of AE was shown in rats, and this prolonged release of drug led to accumulation of AE in the blood plasma. Daily intramuscular administration of AE at a dose of 25 mg/kg formulated in sesame oil for 7 days provided data consistent with other studies by showing absorption of AE from a muscle injection site was not complete. This study also showed up to 38% of an injected dose of AE can still be found at the site of injection 24 hours after injection, and 22% of an injected dose is still present in muscle tissue 48 hours after injection. After 7 days of multiple IM injections of AE at a dose of 25 mg/kg, 91.4% of a single injected dose was still present in muscle tissue at the sites of injection 24 hours after the last dose.

The histopathology data derived from this study demonstrated that the injections of AE were associated with muscle tissue damage at the site of injection (Table **27**). The extent of the damage to muscle where no injury was detected was scored. Sub-acute injury and mild inflammation was scored from 1-2. Sub-acute damage and chronic inflammation to connective tissues and between muscle bundles was scored from 2-3. Extensive inflammation involving muscle fibers was scored from 3-4. Significant damage to muscles with coagulative necrosis characterized by tissue repair shown through fibrosis, fibroplasia, atrophy of muscle tissue, and regeneration of muscle tissue was scored from 4-5. The distribution of damage observed involved major muscle bundles and occurred in linear tracts, and this damage is likely a consequence of the effects of the drug on the muscle.

Table 27: Muscle injury severity at injection site areas following repeated arteether (AE) and artemether (AM) injection with vehicle sesame oil by multiple daily intramuscular dosing at 25 mg/kg for 7 days (n = 3) in rats [65]

Date*	Findings	Sesame Oil Control	AE	AM	Student** T-Test
Day 7	fascial inflammation, pseudocysts, muscle necrosis, & hemorrhage	1.75 ± 0.43	3.17 ± 0.37	2.50 ± 0.50	P = 0.0019
Day 10	fascial inflammation, pseudocysts, & hemorrhage	1.50 ± 0.50	3.00 ± 0.58	2.00 ± 0.0	P = 0.0045

Finding severity were grading as 0 = no significant lesions, 1 = minimal, 2 = mild, 3 = moderate, 4 = marked, and 5 = severe.

*Day 7 and 10 are one and four days, respectively after last treatment of daily dose for 7 days. The date is given the dosing day as day 0. **The t-test was conducted between animals treated both with AE and AM in sesame oil.

Rats dosed with AE for 7 days showed more severe muscle lesions than those treated with AE for 10 days, and rats dosed with AE had showed more severe muscle lesions than animals treated with AM (Table **27**). The data showed chronic, moderately severe inflammation of muscle tissue at the sites of AE injection with a score ranging from 3.00 to 3.17 compared to mild inflammation observed at the AM injection sites, which showed a score ranging from 2.00-2.50. The muscle tissue inflammation observed after injection with AM and AE may play a role in extending drug absorption from muscle tissue.

Another study showing artemisinin drug accumulation was shown in rats dosed with 160 mg /kg of artelinic acid daily for 9 days, and these rats demonstrated moderate neurotoxicity associated with extended absorption of orally dosed artelinic acid in the stomach. This phenomenon is believed to be a reservoir effect similar to the drug depot observed after injection of the oil-soluble artemisinins, AE and AM, at sites of intramuscular injection. The stomach contents of these rats dosed with artelinic acid administered orally every day for 9 days at 160 mg/kg were measured at 8 and 24 hours post dosing at a number of time points. On day 3, 5, 7, and 9, artelinic acid was detected at concentrations of 0, 46.52, 178.59, and 486.21 µg of artelinic acid/g of stomach contents 8 hours after the last dose. The increased concentration of drug observed in the stomach over the treatment period demonstrated that gastric emptying of these animals was inhibited. The inhibition of gastric emptying observed in these animals started with mild inhibition of gastric emptying on day 5 to severe inhibition by day 9. Inhibition of gastric emptying in treated animals persisted at 24 hours post dosing. At twenty-four hours after dosing on days 5, 7, and 9, the contents of the stomach showed 5.74, 25.50, and 29.11 µg of artelinic acid/g of stomach contents, respectively. The authors hypothesize that the decrease in motility of the gastrointestinal tract may be due to a decrease in vagal tone because of diminished sympathetic outflow.

9.2.3. Lowest Observed Neurotoxic Effect Level (LONEL) of Artemisinins

Accumulation of drugs over time extends drug exposure times, which is likely a significant factor in artemisinin-induced neurotoxicity. The no observed adverse effect level or NOAEL is the highest concentration of drug or drug dose administered that does not lead to a biologically significant response to treatment compared to a control group. The lowest observed neurotoxic effect level (LONEL), by contrast, is the lowest plasma drug concentration obtained at the lowest dose associated with induction of a statistically significant neurological response to drug treatment compared to a control group. Accordingly, determining the drug exposure time above the LONEL or the neurotoxic exposure time is important, and the LONEL must be assessed prior to evaluating neurotoxic drug exposure times in different animal species.

1) LONEL of Intramuscular AE and Artelinic Acid in SD Rats

A neurotoxicity study conducted in rats to estimate the minimal daily dose of AE that could be administered without any neurotoxic histopathological effects (the NONED or no observed neurological effects dose) which was shown to be 6.25 mg/kg over a 7-day period. Neuropathology lesions in brain stem nuclei that were statistically significant were observed in AE treated rats at a dose of 12.5 mg/kg over a 7-day period. This data showed AE-induced brainstem neuropathology in rats can be observed at a dose of 12.5 mg/kg (double the NONED dose) over a 7-day period. Rats treated with AE at a dose of 12.5 mg/kg per day for 7 days show a minimal plasma drug concentration of 41.32 ng/ml. Given the no neurological effects dose of 6.25 mg/kg the drug level of 41.32 ng/ml was identified to be the minimal neurotoxic drug effect level. Given rats showed minimal neuropathological changes at this dose level, the 41.32 ng/ml value was therefore defined as the lowest neurotoxic exposure level (LONEL). Administration of drug above the LONEL concentration over a certain exposure time is predicted to result in neuropathological effects.

In a toxicokinetic or TK simulation, AE at a dose of 12.5 mg/kg was administered to rats daily for 7 days intramuscularly and a drug exposure time of 67.1 hours in plasma was calculated to be the minimum time these rats were exposed to AE above the LONEL concentration of 41.32 ng/ml. This treatment resulted in the formation of neurotoxicity lesions demonstrated by histopathological examination (Table **28**). These results showed AE-induced brainstem injury could be triggered at a dose of 12.5 mg/kg/day over 7 days, which yielded a drug exposure period of 67.1 hours where the drug plasma exposure was above the LONEL of 41.32 ng/ml.

A further study in rats showed that administration of artelinic acid resulted in moderate neurotoxicity shown by histopathology after treatment with artelinic acid at 160 mg /kg daily over a 9-day period, however, minimal neurotoxicity was observed after dosing with 5 doses at 288 mg/kg administered every other day in rats. The total dose of 1,440 mg/kg of artelinic acid and the 9-day length of administration were exactly the same [65]. The different neurotoxicity results shown in these two studies could be a consequence of prolonged drug exposure time of 186 hours in the 160 mg/kg group compared to the shorter time of 75 hours above the LONEL in the 288 mg/kg group (Fig. **29**). Given the data showing the inhibition of gastric emptying on day 5 and histopathology results from rodents administered oral artelinic acid daily for 9 days, the LONEL of artelinic acid was estimated to be 346.26 ng/ml (Fig. **29**). This study shows

Table 28: Drug accumulation, exposure level and neurotoxic exposure time of arteether (AE), Artemether (AM), artesunate (AS) and artelinic acid (AL) over the lowest observed neurotoxic effect level (LONEL) in rats, dogs, and rhesus monkeys concerning with histopathological neurotoxicity after various dose regimens [65, 255, 311]

Sprague-Dawley Rats	**Arteether, IM (Sesame Oil)**	**Arteether, IM (1:2CRM/Saline)**	**Arteether IM** (Sesame Oil)**	**Artesunate, IM (5%NaHCO$_3$)**
Neurotoxicity	Severe & death	Moderate	Minimal	No
Dose	25 mg/kg x 7	25 mg/kg x 7	12.5 mg/kg x 7	25 mg/kg x 7
AUC $_{1\text{-}7D}$ (μg·h/ml)	16.92 ± 4.04	46.29 ± 2.06	8.64 ± 4.11	8.57 ± 3.34
$C_{max\ Day\ 1}$ (ng/ml)	130 ± 39	1227 ± 171	56 ± 16	3981 ± 992
$C_{max\ Day\ 7}$ (ng/ml)	410 ± 91	1826 ± 118	173 ± 48	2078 ± 416
LONEL (ng/ml)	41.32	41.32	41.32	41.32 (from AE)
Exposure time (hr)*	164.3 ± 7.9	103.0 ± 5.3	67.1 ± 5.8	22.3 ± 4.9
Sprague-Dawley Rats		Artelinic acid Oral (Suspension)	Artelinic acid Oral (Suspension)	
Neurotoxicity		Moderate	Minimal	
Dose		160 mg/kg x 9	288 mg/kg x 5	
AUC $_{1\text{-}9D}$ (μg·h/ml)		1420 ± 454	1302 ± 905	
$C_{max\ Day\ 1}$ (ng/ml)		113 ± 83	149 ± 109	
$C_{max\ Day\ 9}$ (ng/ml)		122 ± 71	143 ± 93	
LONEL (ng/ml)		346.26	346.26	
Exposure time (hr)*		186.0 ± 28.0	75.0 ± 12.0	
Beagle Dogs	Arteether, IM (Sesame oil)	Artemether, IM (Peanut oil)	Arteether IM** (Sesame oil)	Artelinic acid Oral (Capsules)
Neurotoxicity	Severe & death	Moderate	Minimal	No
Dose	15 mg/kg x 14	20 mg/kg x 7	6 mg/kg x 28	25 mg/kg x 14
AUC $_{1\text{-}7,\ 14,\ or\ 28D}$ (μg·h/ml)	24.39 ± 18.04	32.13	9.86 ± 6.55	191.14 ± 90.80
$C_{max\ Day\ 1}$ (ng/ml)	90 ± 15	190	38 ± 5	6279 ± 2995
$C_{max\ Day\ 7,\ 14, or\ 28}$ (ng/ml)	352 ± 203	346	145 ± 83	7177 ± 6248
LONEL (ng/ml)	40.92	40.92	40.92	40.92 (from AE)
Exposure time (hr)*	277.6 ± 10.7	174.0	103.7 ± 8.6	47.4 ± 11.8
Rhesus monkeys***		Arteether, IM (Sesame oil)	Arteether IM** (Sesame oil)	
Neurotoxicity		Moderate	Minimal	
Dose		16 mg/kg x 14	8 mg/kg x 14	
AUC $_{1\text{-}14D}$ (μg·h/ml)		70962 ± 4588	31245 ± 2614	
$C_{max\ Day\ 1}$ (ng/ml)		63 ± 9	38 ± 5	
$C_{max\ Day\ 14}$ (ng/ml)		1038 ± 622	527 ± 306	
LONEL (ng/ml)		193.80	193.80	
Exposure time (hr)*		307.4	179.5	

*The exposure times above LONEL concentration were calculated with neurotoxic outcome. ** PK data were simulated from our previous studies. ***The monkey results are from our unpublished data.
DHA = Dihydroartemisinin; CRM = cremophor; AUC = area under the curve; IM = intramuscular

artelinic acid initiated moderate brainstem injury in rats at a severity of 3.25 during a neurotoxic exposure time of 186.0 hours. Administration of an artelinic acid regimen of 288 mg/kg dosed every other day for 5 days led to a reduction in exposure time from 186.0 to 75.0 hours, and the severity of the brainstem wound was reduced to 1.17.

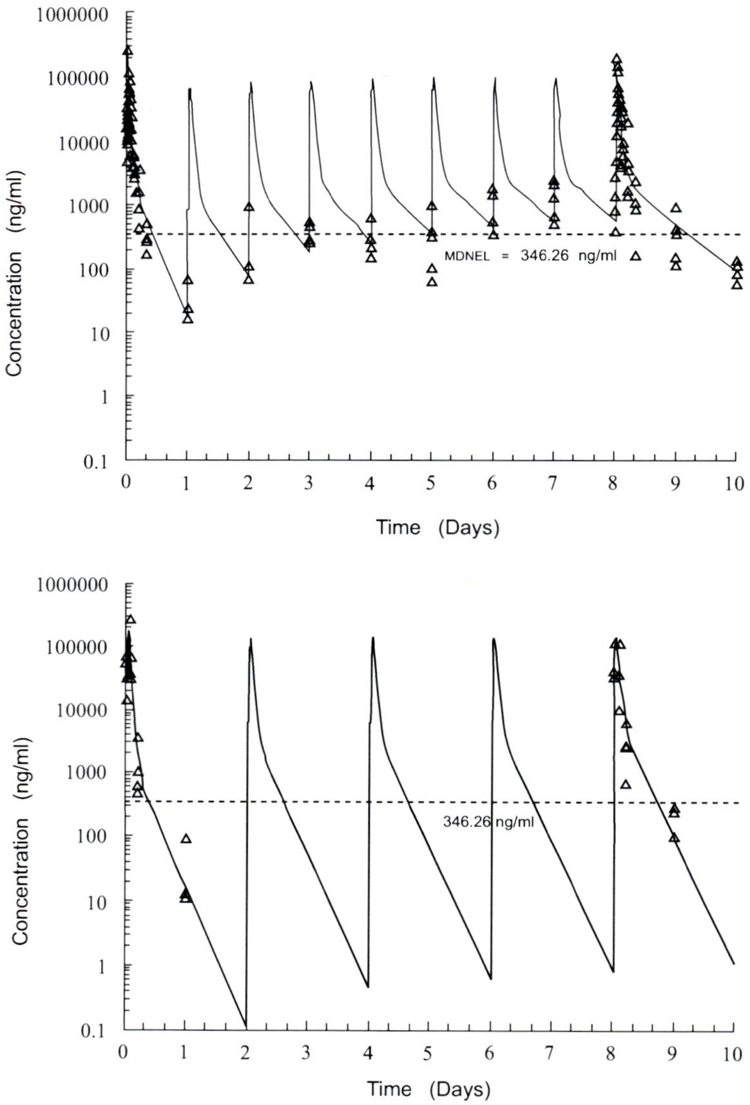

Figure 29: Pharmacokinetic profiles measured by HPLC-ECD (markers) and computer fitted curves (solid line) of oral artelinic acid (AL) in suspension at 160 mg/kg daily for 9 dosages (top, n = 5), and oral AL at 288 mg/kg every other daily for 5 dosages in rats (bottom, n = 4) [12]. The two regimens have same total dose with 1440 mg/kg and same treatment period for 9 days. The lowest observed neurotoxic effect level (LONEL) was defined as the plasma level of 346.26 ng/ml, at which anorectic and neuropathological toxicities were noted in daily dosing cohort of rats [12].

This study demonstrated the LONEL value for oral artelinic acid of 346.26 ng/ml is approximately 8 times higher than the LONEL of 41.32 ng/ml determined in rats after administration of intramuscular AE. IM injection of ^{14}C-arteether in rats was assessed compared to IV injection of ^{14}C-artelinic acid in rats, and the outcome of this study was 0.89% total radioactivity was noted in the brain after administration of ^{14}C-arteether while IV dosing of ^{14}C-artelinic acid in rats resulted in 0.1% of total brain radioactivity. This data supports the hypothesis that administration of ^{14}C-labeled artelinic acid is less capable of penetrating through the blood-brain barrier than ^{14}C-arteether.

2) LONEL of Intramuscular AE in Beagle Dogs

A neurotoxicity study conducted in beagle dogs demonstrated administration of a minimal daily dose of AE at 3 mg/kg for 28 days resulted in no clinical pathology or neurotoxicity which yielded a no observed neurotoxicity exposure dose or NONED. Brainstem neuropathology in beagle dogs induced by AE has been observed after administration of AE at a dose of 5 mg/kg/day, 6.25 mg/kg, and 6.75 mg/kg per day for 28 days. Given the data from these 3 studies, the average minimal dose of AE required to induce neurotoxicity by histopathology in dogs is 6 mg/kg dosed daily for 28 days. The minimal plasma concentration of AE observed in plasma after a dose of 6.0 mg/kg daily over a 28-day period has been measured at 40.92 ng/ml, and this result is lowest observed neurotoxic exposure level (LONEL). Accordingly, a LONEL of 40.92 ng/ml is the "at risk" level for causing neurotoxicity in dogs at a daily dose of 6 mg/kg for 28 days.

In a toxicokinetic simulation of AE administered intramuscularly to beagle dogs at 6 mg/kg conducted 28 times, an exposure time of 103.7 hours in plasma was calculated to be the minimum time above the LONEL (40.92 ng/ml) required to induce neurotoxicity. This simulation prediction was subsequently shown to be correct by the use of histopathological examination of the brains of the beagle dogs (Table **28**). The results showed AE-induced brainstem injury in dogs took place during a minimal period of 103.7 hours above the established LONEL of 40.92 ng/ml. Accordingly, the LONEL for AE induced neurotoxicity in beagle dogs was successfully simulated given the 100% findings of neuropathology findings following dosing of AE at a dose of 6 mg/kg daily for 28 days.

3) LONEL of Intramuscular AE in Rhesus Monkeys

As brainstem neuropathology in rhesus monkeys has been demonstrated to occur in monkeys at a minimal dose of 8 mg/kg administered daily for 14 days, the LONEL of AE was calculated to be 193.8 ng/ml. This calculation was derived from a toxicokinetic study performed in monkeys dosed with AE at 16 mg/kg daily over a 14-day period. The results of this TK study showed a neurotoxic exposure time of 179.5 hours in plasma was estimated to be the minimum time above the LONEL (193.8 ng/ml) necessary to induce pathology consistent with neurotoxicity. The outcome of this study demonstrated that AE-induced brainstem injury could occur during a minimal period of 179.5 hours of neurotoxic exposure time. The data from this study in rhesus monkeys of a LONEL for AE of 193.8 ng/ml is 4 times higher than the LONEL calculated for AE in dogs of 40.92 ng/ml and the LONEL calculated for rats of 41.3 ng/ml. This difference suggests dogs and rats may be more vulnerable than rhesus monkeys to artemisinin-induced neurotoxicity.

9.2.4. Artemisinin Exposure Times with Neurotoxic Effects

To assess the correlation between drug exposure time and neurotoxic outcomes after artemisinin dosing under various regimens, the neurotoxic exposure time above the LONEL was assessed in various animal species. While the LONEL is a minimum observed neurotoxic effect level, duration of exposure was required to assess the neurotoxic effects observed in studies documenting artemisinin-induced neurotoxicity. These kinds of studies provided an initial estimation of the LONEL and associated exposure times required to observe neurotoxicity in various species and facilitated correlation of these data with histopathology or observed neurotoxic effects.

1) TK/TD Analysis of AE and Artelinic Acid Dosing in Sprague-Dawley Rats

A neurotoxicity study was performed to assess the neurotoxicity of AE in two injection vehicles, sesame oil, and cremophore. The authors of this study estimated the exposure time of AE when AE formulated with sesame oil was dosed over the LONEL (41.32 ng /ml) in rats. For AE formulated in sesame oil, the exposure time above the LONEL yielding neurotoxicity was shown to be 164.3 hours for AE administered by intramuscular injection at 25 mg/kg administered daily for 7-days. The exposure time for AE formulated in a solution of cremophore and saline at the same dose level, which yielded neurotoxicity, was 103.0 hours, which is 1/3 of the time required to induce neurotoxicity for AE formulated in sesame oil. The neurotoxicity outcomes in those rats treated with AE formulated in cremophore: saline were demonstrated to drop from severe to moderate. A TK simulation was conducted for AE dosed daily at 12.5 mg/kg for 7 days, and the drug exposure time above the LONEL was only 67.1 hours, and neurotoxicity was reduced to a minimum. These data suggest duration of drug exposure is a critical variable for artemisinin-induced neurotoxicity (Table **28**).

The drug exposure periods of intramuscular artelinic acid and artesunate determined from animals administered at 25 mg/kg per day for 7 days were 42.48 and 22.3 hours above the LONEL calculated for intramuscular AE, respectively. These drug exposure times were 4-7 times shorter than that observed with intramuscular injections of AE (164.3 hours) without any neurotoxic outcomes. Exposure times of artelinic acid and AS were also shown to be much shorter than the minimal calculated exposure time of 67.1 hours (Table **28**). Animals administered artelinic acid and artesunate would have minimal risk of neurotoxicity because of the diminished drug exposure periods.

In a similar study, the neurotoxic exposure time for oral artelinic acid in rats was shown to be 186 hours, which defines a very prolonged period of exposure above the LONEL to induce neurotoxicity (Fig. **29**, top). The artelinic acid exposure time is related to artelinic acid accumulation in the plasma because of delays in gastric emptying, and these delays facilitate extended drug absorption from the stomach. Rats treated every other day with 5 doses of artelinic acid at 288 mg/kg for a 9 day period showed minimal levels of neuronal degeneration until day 7 after the last treatment (Table **28**). Given this data, the minimal drug exposure time above the LONEL necessary to induce neurotoxicity was estimated to be 75 hours (Fig. **29**, bottom). This data, suggests that limiting drug exposure time at the LONEL level can cut down the risk of neurotoxicity.

2) TK/TD Analysis of AE and Artelinic Acid in Beagle Dogs

Drug accumulation was shown in the plasma of beagle dogs after daily IM injection of AE at 15 mg/kg for 14 days. The AE concentration- time profile in beagle dogs is shown in Fig. **2** (middle). The most striking changes were shown to involve the AUC and the half-life of AE. The elimination $t_{½}$ of AE was extended from 11.9 hours on the first day of dosing to 22.5 hours on the last day of dosing which suggests the AE exposure time had almost doubled, and the LONEL (40.92 ng/ml) of AE in beagle dogs was reached on days 6-7. Therefore, the toxicokinetic data analysis suggested that neurotoxicity in beagles would be observed at the earliest the period from 6-7 days after drug administration of AE 15 mg/kg.

An exposure period of 277.59 hours above the LONEL of 40.92 ng/ml for induction of neurotoxicity was calculated for AE dosed in beagle dogs at 15 mg/kg over a 14-day period. The outcomes of this study included severe neurotoxicity and death. The neurotoxic exposure times for beagle dogs dosed orally with artelinic acid in suspension or in capsules, were estimated to be 57.9 hours for the artelinic acid suspension, and 47.4 hours for artelinic acid capsules.

Beagle dogs treated with oral artelinic acid showed no neurotoxic outcomes, which is likely due to the decreased drug exposures above the LONEL, which are much shorter than the minimal neurotoxic exposure time of 103.7 hours previously shown to be necessary for induction of even minimal evidence of histopathological (Table **28**).

3) TK/TD Analysis of AE in Rhesus Monkeys

Accumulation of AE in the plasma of rhesus monkeys after daily IM injection at a dose of 16 mg/kg per day over a 14-day period (Fig. **28**, bottom) was observed in a further study of AE induced neurotoxicity. Given previous data showing neurotoxicity induction in monkeys treated with AE at a dose of 8 mg/kg daily for 14 days, a LONEL of 193.8 ng/ml was estimated. The neurotoxic exposure period of AE in rhesus monkeys to achieve moderate neurotoxicity was calculated to be 307.4 hours for AE dosed intramuscularly at a dose of 16 mg/kg for 14 days (Table **28**). This longer time of neurotoxic exposure is likely to be an important element in induction of neurotoxicity in rhesus monkeys. Rhesus monkeys administered intramuscular AE at a dose of 8 mg/kg daily over a 14-day period-demonstrated drug exposure times above the LONEL estimated to be 179.5 hours. This period was significantly shorter than the drug exposure time of 307.4 hours derived from a prior study of AE administered IM at a dose of 16 mg/kg for 14 days [12].

9.3. PK/PD EVALUATION IN ANIMALS WITH EMBRYOLETHALITY RELATED TO ARTEMISININS

Preclinical experiments in rodents have shown that administration of artemisinins, particularly injectable artesunate, to pregnant animals can result in fetal death and congenital malformations at low doses. This embryotoxicity is induced in animals in a narrow window in early embryogenesis. Studies have shown the mechanism of embryotoxicity is believed to be through inhibition of angiogenesis in early developing erythrocytes, which may cause severe anemia in the embryo after higher drug peak concentrations. Clinical trials of artesunate from 1989 to 2009 to 1,837 women including 176 patients in the first trimester have not shown any evidence of embryotoxicity. In rodents, sensitive erythrocytes are produced synchronously over one day, and single or numerous exposures to an artemisinin have been associated with widespread cell death.

Primates require a much longer treatment period over 12 days to induce embryonic loss. In man limited data is available on this phase of erythrocyte development, however, early erythrocyte development has been shown to take place over an extended time, and it is likely the period of exposure to artemisinin compounds over a 2-3 day period required for ACT treatment is insufficient to result in embryotoxicity. In addition, oral administration, which is commonly used for ACT treatment in pregnant women, results in lower peak concentrations and shorter artemisinin exposure times, and it is unlikely a concentration-time profile of this nature is sufficient to trigger embryotoxicity. When comparing animal and human artemisinin toxicity profiles, the periods of drug sensitivity are different and the PK profiles reviewed here suggests there may be a greater margin of safety for dosing pregnant women with an ACT [12].

9.3.1. Background Data on Studies of Artemisinin-Induced Embryotoxicity in Animal Species

Treatment for both uncomplicated and severe malaria is commonly conducted today with ACTs and injectable artesunate, and over 100 million treatment regimens are administered every year. While both ACTs and injectable artesunate have been shown in a variety of studies to be both efficacious and well tolerated, neurotoxicity and embryotoxicity for artemisinin combinations and injectable artesunate have been reported in a variety of animal species. Generally, animal studies are valuable tools to reveal possible drug risks for humans. Artemisinin and artemisinin analogues are believed to be efficacious and safe for treatment of pregnant women in the last two trimesters of pregnancy, and a small number of pregnant women have administered artemisinin drugs in the first trimester of pregnancy. In clinical trials, none of these patients showed an increase in the incidence of stillbirth or miscarriage. A follow-up study of exposed babies showed no developmental delays in these children.

Recent studies have shown a potential correlation between administration of artemisinin compounds and adverse pregnancy outcomes. The authors of these studies, however, noted current data on this question are quite limited, and the studies that have been published are insufficiently powered to rule out rare adverse events, even in the second and third trimesters of pregnancy. Given the lack of data, there is not enough evidence to assess effectively the risks *versus* the benefits of administration of artemisinin compounds to pregnant women and particularly artemisinin exposure in the first trimester. Full knowledge of embryotoxicity mechanisms in animals is valuable when extrapolating the potential risks for humans. A non-clinical consultation meeting was organized in January 2006 to assess the published data of artemisinin animal studies conducted in rodents and primates to date and assess the potential implications for human treatment [1].

The WHO Guidelines for artemisinin use were altered in this meeting to recommend, "In uncomplicated malaria, ACT treatment should be used in the second and third trimester, but should be used in the first trimester only if it is the only effective treatment available [1]. For treatment of severe malaria, artemisinins are preferred over quinine in the second and third trimester because of the hypoglycemia associated with quinine administration, however, in the first trimester, until more evidence becomes available on the risk benefit ratio of artemisinins, both artesunate and quinine may be considered as options."

This new guideline was made based on published studies available at that time. Further studies of this phenomenon were inspired by anticancer studies of artesunate, and these studies demonstrated that the mechanism by which embryotoxicity was induced by artemisinin drugs was through an inhibition of angiogenesis in embryonic erythroblasts in very early developing erythrocytes causing severe anemia in the embryo. These sensitive early erythrocytes are only produced in a limited period, and a single exposure to an artemisinin drug can result in a high fraction of cell deaths. If the proportion of early red cell death is sufficiently severe, the embryos died, and in surviving embryos, embryo malformations were noted. Data acquired from primate experiments suggests artemisinin embryolethality may occur due to a similar mechanism of action beginning with anemia followed by embryo death. Treatment over 12 days of time were required to induce embryolethality in rhesus monkeys in this study, which is well beyond what is required for treatment of *falciparum* malaria in man. No embryo malformations were noted in this study, but these studies were limited in nature.

Given the significantly longer period of drug exposure required to induce embryolethality in monkeys compared to rodents, the exposure required in man for an artemisinin drug to induce embryotoxicity could be also longer as the comparison of data from monkey to human is more valid than the comparison of rodent to human. In addition, preclinical studies of artemisinin reproductive toxicity in animals (rats, mice, guinea pigs, rabbits, hamsters, and monkeys) have shown that of all the artemisinin drugs, injectable AS has the highest potential to induce animal embryotoxicity. After IV, IM, and subcutaneous administration, AS has been shown to have a 50% fetal re-sorption dose (FRD_{50}) of less than 1.0 mg/kg, which is far lower than the treatment dose of 2-4 mg/kg in humans. In other animal studies, oral artemisinins and IM injected AM were shown to be much safer than injectable AS as the 50% fetal re-sorption dose (FRD_{50}) for these drugs ranges from 6.1 to 51.0 mg/kg, which is well beyond the treatment dose of 2-4 mg/kg (Table **29**).

Table 29: Embryotoxic effects (NOAEL and $FRD_{50\ or\ 100}$) of artemisinin (QHS), dihydroartemisinin (DHA), artesunate (AS), artemether (AM) and arteether (AE), given intragastrically (Oral), intravenously (IV), intramuscularly (IM), and subcutaneously (SC) in pregnant mice, rats, hamster, guinea pig, rabbits, and monkeys [16]

Animal (Drugs)	Dose Duration	Dose regimens (Daily)	Dosing Route	No–Observed–Adverse–Effect–Level (NOAEL) on Fetus Resorption (mg/kg)				FRD_{100} (mg/kg)	FRD_{50} (95% CL) (mg/kg)
				Oral	IM	IV	SC		
Mice (AM)	GD 6–15	Multiple x 10	IM		5.4				11.3 (10.6 – 12.0)
(DHA)	GD 7	Single	SC				10		32.8 (27.7 – 38.9)
Rats (QHS)	GD 1–6	Multiple x 6	Oral	5.6					11.5 (10.5 – 12.2)
(QHS)	GD 7–13	Multiple x 7	Oral	7					≥ 35
(DHA)	GD 9.5, 10.5	Single	Oral	7.5					NA
(AM)	GD 6–15	Multiple x 10	Oral	2.5					14.4 (10.4 – 17.8)
(AS)	GD 6–17	Multiple x 12	Oral	5–7					7.74 (6.92 – 8.57)
(AS)	GD 10	Single	Oral					15.0	NA
(DHA)	GD 10	Single	Oral					11.1	NA
(AM)	GD10	Single	Oral					19.4	NA
(AE)	GD 10	Single	Oral					20.3	NA
(AS)	GD 11	Single	Oral					17.0	NA
(AS)	GD 6–15	Multiple x 10	SC				0.2		0.58 (0.55 – 0.61)*
(AM)	GD 6–15	Multiple x 10	IM		2.7				6.13 (4.52 – 8.26)
(AS)	GD 11	Single	IV			0.75		1.5	NA
(AS)	GD 6–13	Multiple x 13	IV, IM		0.5	0.4			0.60 – 0.61 (0.47–0.72)*
Hamster (DHA)	GD 7	Single	SC				4.2		6.06 (5.90 – 6.21)
(DHA)	GD 7	Single	Oral	20					51.0 (37.9 – 68.7)
(AS)	GD 5	Single	SC				0.35		1.0 (0.9 – 1.2)*
Guinea Pig (DHA)	GD 18	Single	IM		2.5				18.3 (13.9 – 24.2)
Rabbits (AM)	GD 7–18	Multiple x 12	IM		0.7				NA
(AS)	GD 7–19	Multiple x 13	Oral	5–7					NA
(DHA)	GD 9	Single	IM		5.0				7.57 (7.48 – 7.67)
Monkey (AS)	GD 20–50	Multiple x 12	Oral	4					≥ 12

FRD_{50} or $_{100}$ = drug dose induces 50% or 100% fetus re–absorbed; GD = gestation day (The day of mating was defined as day 0 of gestation.); * The severe toxic effects were detected in the animals treated with AS after single or multiple intramuscular, intravenous or subcutaneous injections. Values of ED_{50} are given as median (95% confidence limits). NA = not available.

The mechanism of how injectable AS can induce severe developmental embryotoxicity in animals was not published in 2006, and it was not known at that time that investigating the toxicokinetic (TK) profiles of injectable AS for induction of embryolethality would yield useful information. More recently, the primary anti-angiogenic effect of an artesunate metabolite, dihydroartemisinin, *in vitro* and *in vivo* has been shown in rat and frog embryos. More recent data on the mechanism of embryotoxicity of artemisinins in monkeys and rodents has been published which sheds new light on this issue. Studies have been conducted to explain the differences in the period of drug sensitivity between primates and rodents, the differences in PK profiles after administering artemisinin drugs *via* various routes, and the differences in the potential for embryotoxicity between different species of pregnant animals and pregnant human women [16].

9.3.2. Period of Drug Sensitivity in the Embryos of Rodents, Monkeys, and Humans

Rodent studies have shown artemisinins can trigger fetal death and congenital malformations at low dose levels, and the induction of embryotoxicity in rodents occurs in a narrow period during early embryogenesis. The fetus and neonate are very sensitive to drug mediated toxicity, and the window for induction of developmental embryotoxicity by artemisinins (dihydroartemisinin, artemether, artesunate, and arteether) in rodents ranges from the 10th gestation day to the 14th gestation day. Artemisinin-induced embryotoxicity has been demonstrated in rats after administration of oral artesunate at a dose of 17 mg/kg on single days between GD 10 and 14. Within this 4-day window period, GD 11 was shown to be the most sensitive day to induce embryolethality, and GD 10 was shown to be the most sensitive day for development of embryo malformations, which include cardiovascular defects and bone deformations. Developmental toxicity was not observed after administration of artesunate at the same dose on GD 9 or following administration of oral AS at a dose of 30 mg/kg on GD 16 or 17. These *in vivo* studies demonstrated AS, DHA, AE, and AM dosed orally to pregnant rats on GD 10 induced similar embryolethality and teratogenic outcomes. These findings suggest embryotoxicity is a class effect of the artemisinin compounds.

A recent study in cynomolgus monkeys found that AS treatment at doses of 12 mg/kg/day and 30 mg/kg/day given on GD 20 to 50 caused embryolethality between GD 30 and 40. The no adverse effect level or NOAEL level in this study was 4 mg/kg/day, which is the upper limit of therapeutic dosing in man. No embryo malformations were noted in the four fetuses that survived in the 12 mg/kg/day group, however, the sample size in this study was insufficient to draw any definitive conclusions that artesunate is not teratogenic in monkeys at that dose. All three live embryos in the group dose with artesunate at 30 mg/kg/day from GD 20 were removed by caesarean section on GD 26, 32 and 36 and all showed had marked reductions in erythroblasts. Treatments with artesunate at 12 mg/kg/day on for 3 days from GD 29 to 31 and for 7 days from GD 27 to 33 did not result in embryolethality or embryo malformation. This dose of artesunate was shown to result in marked embryolethality when dosed from GD 20 to GD 50 throughout the period of organogenesis. Given embryo death was observed after 12 days of treatment with artesunate at 12 mg/kg/day, the lack of developmental toxicity for shorter periods of time suggests decreased periods of treatment drops the risk of induction of embryotoxicity after AS administration in monkeys.

Rat primitive erythroblasts develop in the visceral yolk sac and these cells are released into embryonic circulation on GD 10, which is when the heart begins to beat. If primitive erythroblasts were also the principle target of AS in monkeys, the most sensitive period of time would correlate to when primitive erythroblasts are dominant in embryonic circulation. In the cynomolgus monkey, the heart begins beating at approximately GD 18. While no data exists to ascertain the period when monkeys switch production of primitive to mature erythroblasts in monkeys, greater than 90% of the visible erythroblasts in embryo sections taken at GD 26, 32, and 36 were nucleated, which suggests primitive erythroblasts predominate during GD 18 to 36. On GD 50, only 9% of erythrocytes were nucleated which suggests the transition from primitive to mature erythroblasts is mostly completed by GD 50. Given a 3-day or 7-day treatment with artesunate at a dose of 12 mg/kg/day did not result in embryo deaths in monkeys, the period of treatment may have been too brief to result in depletion of embryonic erythroblasts or the embryos of primates are capable of withstanding depletion of embryonic erythroblasts for brief periods.

The window of time for artemisinin-induced embryolethality observed in studies of animals corresponds in humans to the period from conception through week 13, which encompasses a critical period of organogenesis. Data on hand is not sufficient to define precisely the likely window of maximum artemisinin sensitivity in humans. Yolk sac hematopoiesis extends from GD 14 to GD 42 in humans, and circulation begins during the period from GD 21 to 23. In a woman, the mesoderm of the yolk sac shows localized thickening, which likely represents the primordial blood islands composed of hemangioblasts or erythrocyte precursors at approximately GD 16. The earliest primitive erythrocytes are found in the human yolk sac at GD 18.5. Circulation of blood starts when the embryonic heart begins beating, which is believed to begin between GD 19 and GD 21 in humans. The liver is the first organ colonized by the yolk sac, and it is the principal site of definitive erythropoiesis starting at week 5 through week 24 of gestation. Primitive erythrocytes are the dominant circulating form in the first 8 to 10 weeks of gestation. Liver-derived definitive erythrocytes enter circulation by week 8 of gestation, but definitive erythrocytes are not the dominate form of erythrocyte circulating until 11 to 12 weeks. All of the published studies agree yolk sac hematopoiesis in man disappears completely after GD 60.

In summary, the switchover from production of primitive to definitive erythroblasts is GD 10-14 for rats, GD 18-50 for monkeys, and GD 16-60 for humans. Given this data, if human embryos were sensitive to artesunate or dihydroartemisinin similar to rat or monkey embryos, the most sensitive window to induce development toxicity in humans could be predicted to begin at the onset of circulation beginning at GD 48 and ending at approximately GD 63 to GD 70. By GD 63 to 70, the primitive erythroblasts in human embryos are replaced by non-nucleated definitive erythroblasts, which appear to be less sensitive to artemisinin induce embryolethality. If primitive erythrocytes are formed in man for longer periods than in rats or monkeys, then a longer period of dosing beyond the 12 daily doses of an artemisinin required to induce embryotoxicity in monkeys could be necessary to induce primitive erythroblast death in humans. While no animal model is a perfect predictor of human biology, the comparison between man and non-human primate is the closest possible. With animal experiments, only a few aspects of systemic biology can be analyzed at one time.

In order to maximize the data extracted from each experiment, the choice of animal species used and the nature of the experiment must be carefully chosen to model human biology as closely as is possible. The more the animal model is different from human biology, the less value the results may have in predicting a human outcome. Today, more information is available than ever before describing the pharmacokinetic and toxicokinetic properties of artemisinins. The question of more closely defining the window of sensitivity for artemisinin induced embryotoxicity in man may not be readily addressed in patients undergoing routine ACT therapy as the duration of drug exposure to a three day course of ACT treatment for malaria infection is likely too brief to result in embryolethality. Further study of case reports of ACT treatment of women in the first trimester of pregnancy will be necessary to gather more definitive evidence for artemisinin induced embryotoxicity in man.

9.3.3. PK/PD Profiles of Oral and Injectable Artemisinins

There are a number of physiological changes in pregnancy, in which can affect plasma drug concentrations and areas under the curve (AUCs), which in turn can result in reduced antimalarial efficacy [23]. This loss of efficacy is likely due to enhanced drug clearance, larger volumes of distribution, and potentially changed drug absorption in pregnant women treated with orally administered antimalarials.

Oral antimalarial doses where necessary must be changed to maintain efficacy if significant differences are noted in PK parameters and PD outcomes when administered to malaria-infected pregnant patients compared to non-pregnant women [24]. The PK parameters for many antimalarial agents, however, do not how any significant differences between pregnant and non-pregnant women or any differences after administration to pregnant and non-pregnant animals.

Preclinical studies of artemisinin induced reproductive toxicity in pregnant rats showed that injectable AS at doses < 1 mg/kg induces severe embryotoxicity in animals after administration through various means to include IV, IM, and subcutaneous routes. Administration of oral artemisinins and intramuscular artemether (AM) to animals has been shown to be safer than injection with AS as doses of oral artemisinins and IM artemether ranging from 6.1-51.0 mg/kg have been shown to be necessary to induce embryotoxicity (Table **28**). Other studies have shown oral artesunate administered at 17 mg/kg and a single dose of intravenous AS at 1.5 mg/kg dosed on GD 11 both resulted in embryolethality in 100% of treated animals. These doses are close to the threshold for inducing embryotoxicity as a dose of oral AS at 10 mg/kg oral AS caused only 15% embryo re-sorption and a dose of intravenous AS at 0.75 mg/kg caused only 7% embryo re-sorption. Toxicokinetic data have shown that injectable AS induces severe embryotoxicity due to the following factors.

1) Injectable AS elicits elevated peak concentration (3-25 times higher) than either oral artemisinins or intramuscular AM in animals. *In vitro* embryo studies have shown the level of drug exposure and exposure time are critical variables for inducing embryotoxicity. *In vivo* studies have demonstrated, however, that drug exposure level is more significant than drug exposure time because DHA and AS both have very short half-lives (<1 hour) in animals and a similar half-life in man.

2) Artesunate is converted to dihydroartemisinin, and therefore AS is essentially a prodrug. In addition, DHA has been shown to be a more potent inhibitor of angiogenesis than AS *in vitro*. The embryotoxicity of artemisinins can be reduced by using artemisone, a new artemisinin analogue that is not metabolized to dihydroartemisinin, which has also been shown to have much less potency as an anti-angiogenic agent than DHA.

3) Artesunate has the highest rate of conversion than any artemisinins to DHA. The rate of conversion of AS to DHA has been demonstrated to

be 38.2-72.7% compared to the conversion activities of AE and AM which range from 12.4-14.2%.

4) The rate of conversion of artemisinin to dihydroartemisinin after multiple injections was shown to be elevated in pregnant animals compared to non-pregnant rats. The levels of dihydroartemisinin noted in pregnant rats given multiple injections of AS daily for three days were 2.2 times higher on the first dosing day and 4.5-times higher on the third dosing day compared to non-pregnant animals. The treatment resulted in a total AUC_{D1-3} (15,049 ng·h/ml) that was approximately 3.7 times higher in pregnant rats than the total AUC_{D1-3} (4,015 ng·h/ml) observed in non-pregnant rats. The ratios of AUC_{DHA}/AUC_{AS} were observed to be 0.99-1.02 for pregnant rats and 0.42-0.48 for non-pregnant animals, suggesting the total exposure in the treatment period of pregnant rats to dihydroartemisinin was increased compared to exposure of non -pregnant rats to dihydroartemisinin.

5) The total accumulation of artesunate and dihydroartemisinin observed in pregnant rats was much higher than the observed accumulation in non-pregnant animals after repeat administration. By contrast, studies of AS toxicokinetics have shown that the AS C_{max} or peak concentration observed in pregnant rats (16,545-14,927 ng/ml) was twice that observed in non-pregnant animals (8,668-5,037 ng/ml). The plasma concentration of AS were shown to increase from an AUC of 3,749 ng·h/ml on day 1 to 4,758 ng·h/ml on the third dosing day in pregnant rats, however, the AUC of AS in non-pregnant animals was shown to decrease from 3,984 ng·h/ml to 2,239 ng·h/ml from the first to the third dosing day. Similarly, the C_{max} of DHA in pregnant rats (10,335-9,087 ng/ml) was three fold higher compared to the AUC of non-pregnant animals (3,049-2,409 ng/ml) from the first to the third dosing day. Similar to the C_{max} values in this study, the mean AUC data for dihydroartemisinin were elevated in pregnant animals (3,681-4,821 ng·h/ml) compared to non-pregnant rats (1,636-1,049 ng·h/ml). The TK results observed also showed that the mean AUC of dihydroartemisinin was elevated on the first dosing day (3,681 ng·h/ml) to the third dosing day (4,821 ng·h/ml) in pregnant rats, but much lower on the first dosing day (1,636 ng·h/ml) to the third dosing day (1,049 ng·h/ml) in non-pregnant animals.

6) Injectable AS has been shown to provide elevated distribution of artesunate and dihydroartemisinin in fetal tissues of pregnant animals after repeat dosing. An *in vivo* tissue distribution experiment using ^{14}C-AS has shown total AUC_{0-192h} of radioactively labeled artesunate was 22,879 µg equivalents·h/g in all of the tissues of pregnant rats that were measured. Of the total radioactivity measured, 6.54% (1,480 µg equivalents·h/g). During the 192 hour treatment period of this study, the measured levels of radioactivity in the ovary was 555 µg equivalents·h/g, while 367 µg equivalents·h/g were noted in the placenta, and 216 µg equivalents·h/g were observed in the uterus. These values are 2 to 4 times higher than values noted in the blood where radioactivity of 134 µg equivalents·h/ml was observed. The tissue/blood partition coefficients ($K_{t:b}$) of radiolabeled artesunate were elevated in the uterus (1.61), placenta (2.75), and ovary (4.16). Toxicokinetic data demonstrated that the concentrations of artesunate and dihydroartemisinin in the blood of pregnant rats were elevated by 1.5 times to 3.7 times higher than non-pregnant animals. The radioactivity half-life of ^{14}C was 97.73 hours in the blood, while in the ovary the half-life of artesunate ^{14}C was 160 hours, in the placenta the half-life of artesunate ^{14}C was 201 hours, and the half-life of artesunate ^{14}C was 153 hours, which suggests that ^{14}C-AS in reproductive tissues for periods longer than in the blood.

While other research shows the pharmacokinetics of pregnant animals are altered resulting in decreased drug exposure levels of other antimalarials, this research demonstrates, in contrast, that artesunate and dihydroartemisinin levels in the reproductive tissues and plasma of pregnant rats administered multiple doses of injectable AS were elevated compared to non-pregnant animals. The elevations in the concentration of artesunate and dihydroartemisinin in animals may be a significant factor contributing to the severe embryotoxicity in pregnant animals undergoing injectable artesunate treatment even with low doses [16].

9.4. USE OF COMBINATION THERAPY TO MITIGATE TOXICITY ASSOCIATED WITH ANTIMALARIAL DRUGS

There is no data showing adverse drug interactions with the available or proposed drug combination treatments. Quinoline derivatives (halofantrine and piperaquine) have been shown to induce prolongation of the QT interval at treatment concentrations, and high dose halofantrine administration has been linked to sudden death, particularly in individuals with a history of cardiac arrhythmias. These compounds have also been shown to prolong the PR interval and have been shown to cause transient heart block at concentrations above the normal therapeutic range. Animal studies of artemisinins have shown data suggesting problems with embryolethality, fetal abnormality, and reports of occult brainstem neurotoxicity in dogs, rats, and monkeys. In view of these findings, the WHO has recommended against use of ACT treatment for children who weigh less than 5 kg or for women in the first trimester of pregnancy to avoid embryotoxicity, and 3-day dosing ACT regimens to prevent neurotoxicity.

9.4.1. ACT Combinations with Quinoline Partners that Avoid Cardiotoxicity

1) Artemether-Lumefantrine (AL)

Artemether-lumefantrine (AL) is a fixed-dose antimalarial drug combination containing lumefantrine, a compound that is structurally similar to mefloquine, quinine, and halofantrine. AL was innovated in China to treat *falciparum* malaria, and the fixed dose combination on market. Artemether is characterized by a rapid onset of schizonticidal action providing rapid fever relief and quick reduction and clearance of parasites. Recrudescence after artemether treatment is common when administered as monotherapy unless dosed for 5-7 days [65]. By contrast, lumefantrine as a monotherapy drug has been shown to have high cure rates when administered for duration of 2-3 days, however, fever and parasite clearance is much less rapid than with artemether. AL provides the advantages of both agents and provides a brief, simple, antimalarial therapy, which aids patient compliance. In areas of multidrug resistance, and in non- immune patients, the recommended treatment is 6 doses of 4 tablet each (80 mg artemether and 480 mg lumefantrine per dose) given over 60 hours. Otherwise, the recommended treatment is 4 doses of 4 tablets over 2 days.

Experience with AL administration is rapidly growing as use of this combination has quickly expanded around the world. In clinical trials, AL was well tolerated in all regimens tested. AL has better tolerated than mefloquine monotherapy or the combination of artesunate and mefloquine. The adverse effects of this combination that have been reported have been mild including gastrointestinal upset, dizziness, headache, fatigue, palpitations, sleep disturbance, arthralgia, myalgia, and rash (all of these symptoms may also be related to malaria infection). Given the structural similarities to other quinolines, one might expect that lumefantrine would have a cardiotoxicity liability; however, prospective clinical studies have not shown any evidence of cardiotoxicity. In healthy subjects, no changes in the QTc interval of significance were noted, and no link has been shown between QTc intervals and plasma levels of lumefantrine. In addition, there no clinically significant differences were noted in the QTc intervals between individuals administered mefloquine or AL administered as a combination or as separate for each component.

A number of other clinical studies have been conducted to examine the cardiotoxic potential for AL. In one trial, the potential cardiac effects of AL were evaluated and compared with those of halofantrine. Furthermore, the relationship between drug concentration in the plasma and the QTc interval concentration was explored for both compounds. The QTc interval effects in individuals administered single oral doses of 500 mg halofantrine or a combination of 80 mg artemether/480 mg lumefantrine were compared in a randomized crossover study of 13 healthy males. Electrocardiograms (ECGs) were obtained 48 hours before dosing until 48 hours after dosing. The highest QTc interval obtained before treatment, after treatment, and between treatments, and the data acquired along with drug levels was used to fit a linear model. After halofantrine administration, all participants demonstrated higher QTc intervals, and the average increase noted was 28 ms at maximum. The duration of the QTc interval correlated well to the level of halofantrine exposure. The QTc interval remained unchanged after AL treatments, and the difference between HF and AL treatments was statistically significant. It was clear that halofantrine induced clinically significant, exposure-related prolongations in the QTc interval while no increase was observed with AL [532].

In addition, other studies have shown that no QTc prolongation has been reported after oral treatment with artemether despite its wide use. Drug-induced QTc prolongation is usually concentration dependent. Halofantrine plasma concentrations in this study were well in the range of, or in a few subjects even somewhat higher than, halofantrine plasma concentrations reported in malaria patients undergoing treatment. As expected, the length of the QTc interval increased with increasing systemic exposure to halofantrine, however, even in those individuals with the lowest plasma concentrations (approximately C_{max} = 1,000 ng/ml), a clear prolongation in the QTc interval was observed. Likewise, increases in the QTc interval at halofantrine plasma concentrations of approximately 1,000 ng/ml or even lower can be found in the literature.

Plasma concentrations of lumefantrine in this study were comparable to those previously reported in Thai patients treated with four doses of AL but generally decreased compare to concentrations observed in Chinese patients treated with four doses of AL or subjects administered the six doses of AL regimen. Artemether concentrations were comparable to those found in clinical studies with AL, while dihydroartemisinin concentrations noted in the plasma of study volunteers were generally lower than in the clinical setting. Because the QTc interval duration is related to the magnitude of drug exposure, QTc prolongation cannot definitely be ruled out for patients with higher exposure to lumefantrine or dihydroartemisinin than observed in this study. In a drug interaction study, in which the QTc interval was studied in patients treated with a six-dose AL regimen with or without mefloquine pretreatment, no effects on the QTc interval were observed despite much higher exposure to AL. In that study, artemether and dihydroartemisinin exposure was similar, and lumefantrine exposure in some participants was even higher than the exposure observed in patients with malaria administered four to six doses of AL. The ECG data reported for malaria patients treated with AL are also highly reassuring. ECGs were recorded in more than 700 patients with *falciparum* malaria treated with AL in comparative studies with various other antimalarials [11].

In conclusion, AL was shown to have no relevant cardiac effects in any participants in this study. In contrast, halofantrine administered in a single dose of 500 mg orally caused a significant prolongation in the QTc interval above the normal range in all but one participant and produced nonspecific ST-T changes in some. The duration of the QTc interval correlated to plasma levels of halofantrine, and the maximum QTc prolongation correlated with the peak plasma concentration [11].

The frequency of QTc prolongation observed after AL treatment has been shown to be similar to or lower than the frequency of QTc prolongation observed after treatment with chloroquine, mefloquine, or the combination of artesunate and mefloquine; antimalarials that are not recognized to cause QTC prolongation. It is likely that the malaria disease itself contributes to the cardiac effects observed in these patients by causing changes in heart rate and electrolyte disturbances. In contrast, treatment of *falciparum* malaria with the comparators quinine and halofantrine, both of which are known to prolong the QTc interval, produced clearly more frequent episodes of QTc prolongation than AL. In QTc studies of malaria-infected patients treated with quinine, halofantrine, and AL, quinine was shown to cause QTc prolongation in 18.5% of patients while AL was shown to cause QTc prolongation in 3.5% of patients, and halofantrine was shown to cause QTc prolongation in 26% of patients while AL was shown to cause QTc prolongation in 8.3% of patients. As shown in healthy subjects, malaria infected patients showed a prolongation in the QTc interval, which correlated well to halofantrine plasma concentrations. On the other hand, no correlation was found between lumefantrine plasma concentrations and the duration of the QTc interval in subjects treated with AL, which also supports the hypothesis that AL has no significant prolongation of the QTc interval.

2) Dihydroartemisinin-Piperaquine (DP)

Dihydroartemisinin-piperaquine is administered over a 3-day period, and a number of clinical studies have demonstrated this combination treatment is both effective and safe. While DP is on market in some countries in Southeast Asia, detailed information on drug efficacy, pharmacokinetic parameters, and drug safety which is customarily provided to regulatory bodies prior to drug licensure in first world countries derived from clinical studies has not yet been carried out. Drugs licensed in the developed world require extensive preclinical potency, safety, and tolerability data in animals combined with Phase 1 trials using healthy volunteers to describe PK parameters of absorption, distribution, metabolism, and excretion, efficacy studies to relate drug concentrations in humans during treatment in Phase 2 studies, and large Phase 3 trials to evaluate efficacy and safety. Some data describing animal toxicity studies of piperaquine have been published, and the efficacy of piperaquine for treatment of malaria was shown in human studies conducted in the 1970s. Piperaquine's therapeutic index is not well defined and dose regimens for piperaquine (to include DP), have been approximated empirically based on clinical studies with no data driven approach to describe the relationship between toxicity and drug concentration.

The first formal Phase 2 study of DP was conducted in *falciparum* malaria-infected Cambodian patients, and DP was very efficacious with 100% cure rates by day 28 in children and 92.3% in adults. One child died during this trial unexpectedly, however, and while the root cause of this child's death is due to an illness not related to malaria, a reaction to the drug could not be ruled out. The most significant adverse effect noted in patients administered antimalarial quinoline drugs is cardiotoxicity manifested as QT interval prolongation on an electrocardiogram and postural changes in blood pressure. As artemisinin drugs are also known to increase the QT interval, a synergistic cardiotoxic effect is possible in patients treated with DP. The electrocardiographic effects of DP fixed combination therapy were studied in 62 patients with uncomplicated malaria.

A total of 30 Cambodian adults and 32 adults infected with *falciparum* or *vivax* malaria were administered DP orally dosed based on age over a 32-hour period. Blood pressure measurements were taken from patients in both the erect and supine positions, and the QT interval was measured prior to treatment and then regularly over a 4 day period of admission to monitor patients for efficacy and safety. All of the patients responded well to DP treatment, and DP treatment was well tolerated by all patients. The average clearance time of parasite was 19 hours, and the fever clearance time was 12 hours. The mean drop in systole blood pressure in patients prior to treatment after standing was 8 ± 6 mmHg, and follow-up assessments taken every 6 hours for the next 72 hours demonstrated no changes that were significant (P = 0.48). The mean QTc interval lengthened to a maximum of 11 ms (95% CI of 4-18 ms) compared to baseline at 24 hours (P = 0.003). The highest QTc prolongation noted in any patient was 53 ms. A mean reduction of 0.4 mmol/l in post-absorptive glucose levels in the first 48 hours was observed, but no episodes of hypoglycemia (defined as a plasma glucose level <3.0 mmol/ l) were noted. The conclusions reached from this study show that DP is a safe and effective combination therapy for treatment of uncomplicated blood stage malaria in adults and children. While piperaquine is structurally similar to other quinoline compounds, which are known to have cardiotoxic effects, such as quinine, no significant metabolic or cardiovascular effects were noted [145].

Eurartesim®, a new DP formulation, has been manufactured in accordance with international standards of good manufacturing practice has been introduced and achieved WHO recognition. Two pivotal, randomized, open-label, multicenter trials demonstrated the Eurartesim® formulation of DP to be non-inferior to artesunate plus mefloquine to treat *falciparum* malaria in adults and children in Asia and non-inferior to treat *falciparum* malaria compared to artemether-lumefantrine in children in Africa as shown by PCR corrected cure rates. In both trials, DP recipients were significantly less likely than patients administered artemether-lumefantrine or artesunate-mefloquine to experience re-infection. Gametocyte carriage was increased in patients receiving dihydroartemisinin-piperaquine compared to those receiving artesunate-mefloquine or artemether-lumefantrine. The Eurartesim® formulation of DP was well tolerated as a treatment agent for *falciparum* malaria, and this ACT elicited significantly less side effects of vomiting, nausea, and dizziness compared to treatment with the artesunate-mefloquine combination. While prolongation of the QTc interval in patients who have received DP treatment was observed, there are no published clinical data reporting clinically significant arrhythmias [388].

Additional *in vitro* studies of the cardiotoxicity properties of DP have been conducted and compared to *in vitro* testing of a large battery of known antimalarials. The *in vitro* antimalarial drug testing studies were structured to test the free therapeutic maximum concentration in plasma (C_{max}), derived from PK studies, and the cardiotoxicity data derived were compiled as the fold increase compared to their C_{max}. The following assessments were made to include hERG trafficking and blockade, drug treatment of rabbit heart ventricular preparations (used to assess the potential for cardiac blockade or *Torsade de pointes* syndrome), and interference of sodium and slow potassium ion currents (INa and IKs, respectively). Mefloquine, halofantrine, chloroquine, and lumefantrine were assessed in the hERG studies, but only chloroquine, lumefantrine, dofetilide (a positive control which acts to block the rapid element of the delayed rectifier outward potassium current), and the combination of artemether-lumefantrine (AL) were used in the hERG trafficking studies, rabbit heart ventricular preparations, and Ina and IKs analyses. Known hERG blockers and compounds that potentiate cardiac blockade or interfere with sodium and ion channels were used as positive controls for each test.

In the hERG channel studies, the 50% inhibitory concentration (IC_{50}) of halofantrine was assessed, and the hERG IC_{50} was shown to be lower than the C_{max} of halofantrine. All the other compounds tested were shown to block hERG, with IC_{50}s ranging from 3 fold to 30 times their C_{max}. In rabbit heart ventricular preparations, dofetilide, a positive control, showed a high probability of inducing *Torsade de pointes*, while chloroquine demonstrated a medium likelihood. Neither DP nor AL showed an *in vitro* signal suggesting a pro-arrhythmic risk. Only chloroquine blocked the Ina ion current and did so at approximately 30-fold the C_{max}. No effect of chloroquine on IKs was detected.

In summary, DP and AL do not appear to significantly affect hERG trafficking, or block slow potassium and sodium ion currents, or potentiate induction of *Torsade de pointes* effects. These results support the other *in vivo* studies suggesting that DHA has little cardiac toxicity. Piperaquine, which has been shown to prolong the QT interval clinically but has not been shown to correlate with *Torsade de pointes,* induced a block of the hERG channel not facilitated by trafficking. Piperaquine showed a low arrhythmogenic potential whether used alone or in combination with dihydroartemisinin in the rabbit ventricular preparation assay. In conclusion, the authors have shown *in vitro* data supporting the hypothesis that DP has limited cardiotoxic potential. DP is an excellent combination to use for treatment of drug resistant parasites, which cannot be treated with other antimalarials or even ACT treatment. There are many areas of Southeast Asia and Africa with endemic malaria resistant to artemether-lumefantrine where DP could be utilized (lumefantrine is cross-resistant to mefloquine which has been used widely in many endemic areas). AL treatment has shown failures in over 10% of treated patients in in Cambodia and clinical drug resistance to AL has been reported in Ghana and Burkina-Faso. DP administration has not been shown to sudden death in malaria patients and piperaquine monotherapy has not been shown to result in sudden death, which supports the data previously discussed regarding the cardiotoxic potential of DHA and piperaquine used for monotherapy, or in combination [545].

9.4.2. Administration of ACTs Will Avoid Induction of Embryotoxicity in Pregnant Women

The PK parameter of some, but not all, antimalarials is changed in pregnancy after oral administration, which causes decreased levels of drug exposure. As previously discussed, studies have shown that injection of AS has yielded significantly elevated reproductive tissue and plasma concentrations of DHA and AS and in pregnant rats compared to DHA and AS concentrations in the reproductive tissues and plasma of non-pregnant animals. The significant increases in DHA and AS concentrations in animals may be a significant contributor to severe embryotoxicity induced by administration of injectable AS even at low doses in pregnant animals [16].

Three factors support the argument that oral artemisinins can be safely used to treat pregnant women with malaria. 1) The pharmacokinetics of orally administered antimalarials is decreased in pregnancy, which, in turn, leads to diminished levels of drug exposure. 2) Administration of oral artemisinins produces only low peak concentrations when compared to injectable artemisinins. 3) 20 years of clinical trial data testing the potential impact of artemisinins on pregnancy have not resulted in findings of embryotoxicity in pregnant women treated with orally administered ACTs or monotherapy with oral artemisinins.

There are known changes in the physiology of pregnant women that affects the absorption, distribution, and clearance of drugs that begin in the first trimester and accelerate through the third trimester. Oral antimalarial pharmacokinetics are changed in pregnancy due to a variety of factors: increased volume of distribution, enhanced drug clearance, changes in drug binding to proteins, distribution of lipids, and drug absorption, as well as the impact of hormonal changes on the metabolism of drugs. These changes in physiology can induce decreases in drug exposure which results in decreased efficacy.

Few studies in pregnant women on the effects of artemisinins and other antimalarials have been published. For example, oral prophylaxis with chloroquine, mefloquine, proguanil, atovaquone, and oral DHA show different kinetics in pregnancy, and plasma levels have been shown to be significantly lower in pregnant women compared to non-pregnant women with malaria. This is a likely consequence of enhanced drug clearance, larger drug distribution volumes, and potentially changes in oral drug absorption. The AUC for DHA has been shown to be 1.8 times higher and the C_{max} values for DHA have been shown to be 4.2 times lower in pregnant Karen women than that in non-pregnant Thai women. A similar finding has been shown in animal studies of orally administered AS. Given published differences in pharmacokinetics and efficacy in some antimalarial drugs, the oral doses of these drugs must be changed when administered to pregnant malaria patients to maintain efficacy. Orally administered antimalarials appear to be safe because of reduced exposure to drugs combined with accelerated drug elimination in pregnant women [16].

The most significant impact of malaria on pregnant women is mostly caused by *P. falciparum*, and approximately 95% of cases are observed in sub-Saharan Africa and Asia. 50 million women become pregnant every year in in these malaria endemic regions. Artemisinins have been administered to pregnant women with malaria since 1989 (Table **30**), and a large body of evidence from 1,837 pregnant women who were administered artemisinin compounds from 1989 to 2009 and 176 of these pregnant women were in their first trimester. No significant drug associated adverse effects have been observed related to pregnancy outcome nor have any significant adverse effects been noted in the neurological and physical development of the infants, which does include 44 infants who were exposed to an artemisinin compound in the first trimester.

Recent data has been presented by the WHO [23] on exposure to artemisinin compounds in pregnancy in Zambia, Thailand, and Bangladesh. In Thailand, 1,530 women had first trimester exposures to a number of different antimalarial drugs to include 170 pregnant women who were treated with artemisinin compounds. Regardless of the antimalarial drug used, there was a correlation between the risks of spontaneous abortion and the number of *P. falciparum* infections treated in the first trimester. Furthermore, fever, older maternal age, and hyperparasitemia were shown to be risk factors for abortion in the first trimester, while antimalarial therapy was not shown to be a significant risk factor [16].

Table 30: Clinical trials and safety evaluation of oral and injectable artemisinins following monotherapy and artemisinin–based combination therapy (ACT) in pregnant women from 1989 to 2009 [16]

Author (Year)	Drugs	Regimen	No of Patients	Trimester (Patients)	Clinical Observation in Safety Pharmacology
Monotherapy					
Wang (1989)	QHS, AM	Oral, IM	6	2	none found evidence of drug toxicity
Guo (1990)	QHS, AS, AM	Oral, IV, IM	6, 2, 11	2, 3	no premature delivery or death–in–utero reported
Li (1994)	QHS, AS, AM	Oral, IV, IM	21	2	No side–effects
Sowunmi (1998)	AM	Oral	45	2, 3	do not produce undue deleterious effects
McGready (1998)	AS, AM	Oral, IM	83	1 (16), 2, 3 (67)	Caution: 20% abortions in first trimester group.
McGready (2001)	AS	Oral	64	2, 3	well–tolerated and safe for the mother and the fetus
McGready (2001)	AS, AM	Oral, IV	459, 2	1 (44), 2,3 (417)	well tolerated with no evidence of adverse effects
Adam (2004)	AM	IM	28	1 (1), 2,3 (27)	well tolerated with symptom–free within three days
McGready (2008)	AS	Oral	128	2, 3	well tolerated and safe.
Adam (2009)	AM	IM, Oral	48, 14	1	may be safe to use during early pregnancy (2 miscarriages)
ACTs					
McGready (2000)	AS+MQ	Oral	66	2, 3	AS–MQ was significantly better tolerated
Bounyasong (2001)	AS+MQ	Oral	60	2, 3	ACT might be the alternative treatment in pregnancy.
Deen (2001)	AS+SP	Oral	287	1 (50), 2, 3 (237)	well–tolerated and safe for the mother and the fetus.
McGready (2003)	AS+AP	Oral	27	1 (3), 2, 3 (24)	well tolerated and no toxicity for the mothers and fetus.
McGready (2005)	AS+AP	Oral	39	2, 3	AS–AP is a well–tolerated, and safe for the mother and the fetus.
Adam (2006)	AS+SP	Oral	32	2, 3	the drug was well tolerated, with symptom–free within 2 days.
Kalilani (2007)	AS+SP	Oral	47	2, 3	Safe, well tolerated and side–effects during pregnancy.
McGready (2008)	AL	Oral	125	2, 3	Well tolerated and safe.
Kaye (2008)	AL	Oral	110	2, 3	safe to use in treatment of uncomplicated malaria in pregnancy.
Rijken (2008)	DHA–PPQ	Oral	50	2, 3	well tolerated and no toxicity for the mothers or the fetus.
Mutabingwa (2009)	AS+AQ	Oral	77	2, 3	the combination tested was efficacious and appeared safe.

QHS = Artemisinin; AM = Artemether; AS = Artesunate; AS + MQ = Artesunate + Mefloquine; AS + SP = Artesunate + Sulfadoxine–Pyrimethamine;
AS + AP = artesunate + Atovaquone–Proguanil; AL = Artemether–Lumefantrine; AS + AQ = Artesunate + Amodiaquine; DHA–PPQ = Dihydroartemisinin–Piperaquine. IM = intramuscular; IV = intravenous; Refs. = References.

Given current WHO recommendations, the following are reasonable courses of action to minimize the risk of adverse outcomes when using artemisinin compounds to treat pregnant women. Exposure to injected AS should be minimized particularly during the early sensitive period of pregnancy ranging from GD 15 to GD 42 when embryo damage is most likely to occur. This is similar to the WHO recommendation precluding the use of artemisinin compounds in the first trimester. Second, WHO has recommended oral ACTs can be and should be used in later trimesters of pregnancy to treat uncomplicated malaria if other drugs are not well suited. Other authors feel that oral ACT regimens can be used to treat women who are pregnant in all three trimesters if other drugs are not available. The rationale for that recommendation is based on the lower peak artemisinin concentrations and shorter exposure times observed in patients treated with common oral ACT regimens. These two factors make oral ACTs a better choice to minimize the risk of embryotoxicity than administration of intramuscular or intravenous AS injection.

For treatment of severe malaria, WHO has recommended that artemisinins be used instead of quinine in the latter trimesters of pregnancy to minimize the potential for hypoglycemia which is linked with quinine treatment. Until more evidence is published on the risks *versus* benefits of first trimester artemisinin drug exposure, both injected quinine and artesunate can be considered as options with drawbacks for each treatment. Treatment of severe malaria should be initiated immediately with either antimalarial available. If it is possible, reliable pharmacovigilance and careful safety monitoring after drug exposure in the first trimester to either of these drugs are needed when treatment may be inadvertently administered or necessary to save human life.

It is not known how humans avoid the lethal embryotoxicity described in various animal species discussed previously. Therefore, further studies will be needed to define precisely mechanisms of drug damage in animal models for a number of reasons. 1) The critical period of embryo exposure to artemisinins in primates should be explored further along with the duration of drug exposure required to induce embryotoxicity. 2) Embryotoxicity studies should be performed on new artemisinins such as the modified artemisinins and the synthetic trioxanes and similar molecules to assess the likelihood of their inducing embryotoxicity. 3) Metabolic profile studies are needed in primates and rodents to correlate the metabolic profiles of these animals to humans. 4) *In vitro* whole embryo culture should be done to assess the impact of drug metabolites, reactive species, and oxygen on embryo development. Identification of drug metabolites should be conducted on human and animal plasma following administration of these new novel second-generation artemisinin drugs.

More research is needed to assess the safety of ACTs or artemisinins in pregnant women for these reasons. 1) Human primitive erythroblasts, which are very sensitive to artemisinin activity, may or may not be generated similarly to primitive erythroblasts found in rodents. Further research is necessary to research erythrocyte development in human embryos. 2) Safety reviews of all antimalarial medicines used to treat pregnant women are needed especially when these drugs are administered in the first trimester. One aspect, which is particularly needed, is a new review of pregnancy outcomes after artemisinin drug exposure in the first trimester. 3) Since 2002, studies of populations, which include pregnant women, have been conducted by the WHO and others in Kenya, Bangladesh, Tanzania, South Africa, and Zambia. These data are of use to the rest of the research world, and they should be published to assess the full body of data on first-trimester exposures.

Infection of pregnant women with *P. falciparum* is dangerous to both the child and the mother, and having safe, efficacious treatments available is very important. In animal studies, there is sufficient data on embryolethality after administration of artemisinins and some evidence of morphological abnormalities in rats, mice, guinea pigs, hamsters, guinea pig, monkeys, and rabbits in early pregnancy. The mechanisms and the pharmacokinetic profiles affecting embryotoxicity in animals are well described; however, it is not clear how this data can be translated into human beings. The data from 1,837 women exposed to artemisinin compounds in pregnancy, which included 176 cases of women exposed to artemisinin compounds in the first trimester, do not show increases in stillbirth or abortion nor do they show fetal abnormalities that have been observed in animals. Humans are clearly less sensitive than animals to artemisinin-induced embryotoxicity, and humans are known to have enhanced repair capabilities compared to animals. Other potential issues when considering the discrepancy in embryotoxicity between humans and animals include [16]:

1) Sensitive early erythrocytes are produced in a limited period, and these early erythrocytes are very vulnerable to cell death after administration of artemisinin drugs. In contrast, primates must be treated for far longer periods with artemisinin compounds to induce embryolethality. In humans, limited data on early erythrocyte development is available, but this period of development does take longer in man and a three-day treatment for malaria may not be long enough to induce embryotoxicity.

2) Animal data has shown that only injectable artesunate administered IM, IV or subcutaneously can induce embryotoxicity at lower doses (0.6-1.0 mg/kg) than the therapeutic treatment doses (2-4 mg/kg) used in man. Other doses of artemisinin compounds administered orally or intramuscularly, like IM artemether, have been shown to be safe at higher doses (6.1-51.0 mg/kg) than therapeutic doses used for human treatment. Oral administration, the most common route of drug administration of ACTs for treatment of pregnant women, provides lower peak concentration and shorter exposures, and this type of

concentration-time course is not likely to induce embryotoxicity. As 1,837 pregnant women have been treated with IM artemether or oral artemisinins with no observations of embryotoxicity, the lower concentrations resulting from oral ACT administration may explain the lack of embryotoxicity observed.

3) Many pregnant women become ill with malaria, and malaria is responsible for 5-12% of cases of low birth weight, 35% of cases of LBW that could be prevented during pregnancy, and contributes to 70,000-200,000 infant deaths every year. Given the impact of malaria on pregnant women, future studies should be conducted on whether reprotoxicity of pregnant women is associated with illness or from antimalarial drug(s).

4) Many publications on this subject have not considered the possible association of low birth weight, spontaneous abortion, or infant disorders in patients who were infected with malaria and treated with artemisinins. None of these publications had sufficient power to rule out rare serious adverse events, particularly in the second and third trimesters of pregnancy and there is insufficient data to assess effectively the risks *versus* the benefits of artemisinin administration to pregnant women, particularly first trimester exposures.

5) Post-marketing surveillance is limited in developing countries and potential reprotoxicity of ACTs or other antimalarials have not been well recorded.

In excess of 917 pregnant women (which include 23 patients in their first trimester) have received artemisinin monotherapy for malaria treatment, and more than 920 pregnant patients (which include 53 patients in their first trimester) have been treated with an ACT and no increase in adverse outcomes was observed (Table **30**). The authors of this study concluded there is not enough data now to make a recommendation to change WHO policy recommendations on ACT use to treat pregnant women with malaria. Current WHO Guidelines have recommended that ACTs be administered to pregnant patients with malaria only in the second and third trimesters, and the use of ACTs in the first trimester is only recommended if an ACT is the only effective treatment available. What constitutes the malaria treatment of choice in the first trimester of pregnancy differs due to variability in drug resistance of parasites in different areas. Immediate administration of artemisinins makes sense in cases where initial treatment is ineffective because of the dangers of repeat infections with malaria in pregnancy. In addition, oral ACTs may eventually be employed as the treatment of choice for pregnant women with malaria in all trimesters with further definitive safety studies [16].

CHAPTER 10

Efforts to Improve Antimalarial Combination Therapy

Abstract: Several drug development strategies for novel antimalarial drugs have been created to counter the rise of malaria drug resistance. These strategies include optimizing new antimalarial drug combinations through laboratory testing and clinical development. ACTs are the most successful drug combinations invented to date for treatment of malaria worldwide, however, the growing tide of malaria resistance, particularly in Southeast Asia, provides a compelling need to discover novel chemical entities to combine with artemisinin analogues or create new antimalarial combinations using existing drugs. Strategies to find novel chemical entities are outlined in this section ranging from irrational drug discovery with whole-cell phenotypic screening to target based screening against specific *Plasmodium* targets. Implementation of antimalarial drug combinations with diverse PK/PD profiles will likely require evaluation of multiple outcomes, which further complicates statistical modelling for factorial designs. Well- constructed, carefully conducted, and statistically rigorous clinical pharmacology studies are necessary for development of new malaria treatments and practical methods must be put in place for post licensure marketing surveillance to detect both emerging drug resistance and adverse effects. While a number of novel chemical entities are under development, bringing new, efficacious, safe, and well-tolerated antimalarial drugs to market is a quite a challenge particularly in today's regulatory environment. In addition, antimalarial treatment currently involves combinations of drugs with synergistic or additive properties, which makes drug discovery and development even more challenging.

Keywords: Clinical trial networks, drug combination, efficacy, long- acting medicines, long-acting formulations, molecular target, new mechanisms of action, novel antimalarials, novel chemical entities, parasite, resistance, safety.

Malaria takes a heavy toll in morbidity and mortality every year, and despite advances in drug discovery and development, treatment options are under pressure from a never-ending tide of malaria drug resistance. Developing new antimalarial drugs is a process that can take decades from start to finish. Mefloquine, for example, was developed at Walter Reed Army Institute of Research in the early 1970s and was not licensed by the FDA until 1989. One alternative approach, which is attractive, is to combine antimalarial drugs not used together and optimize their use for treatment. The rise of multidrug-resistant *P. falciparum* has made the choice of which drug to use for malaria prophylaxis and treatment all that more complicated particularly in areas like the Cambodian-Thai border or the Cambodian-Myanmar border that have a high incidence of

Qigui Li and Mark R. Hickman

resistance to most antimalarials on market. Furthermore, it is predicted that there will likely be increased incidence of malaria infections and subsequent deaths in the future due to the rapid spread of resistant parasites [1, 5-9]. ACTs are the most successful therapies for malaria treatment available today, however, predictions have been made that resistance to all of these combination treatments will almost certainly emerge. Evidence in support of this hypothesis is readily available in in Southeast Asia. Wongsrichanalai and others have reported the increase in treatment failures for artesunate-mefloquine for treatment of malaria on the border between Cambodia and Thailand [546]. Other reports of treatment failures with artemether- lumefantrine, DHA-piperaquine, and other ACTs in Southeast Asia are being published on a regular basis. Accordingly, novel antimalarial combinations using drugs already available or new drugs for treatment of uncomplicated malaria are desperately needed.

10.1. STRATEGIES TO OPTIMIZE EXISTED OR DEVELOP NEW ANTIMALARIAL COMBINATIONS

In this section, key strategies and research priorities have been summarized for development of new combination drugs for a number of therapeutic indications including malaria eradication. Close coordination with regulators will be required for use of antimalarial drugs for malaria eradication that have only been licensed for therapeutic indications.

10.1.1. Define Priorities to Contain and Prevent Artemisinin Resistance

Clinical treatment failures as a consequence of malaria drug resistance has been demonstrated against all of the existing antimalarial drug classes on market including newly emerging resistance to the artemisinins [5-8]. Artemisinin analogues are essential elements for *falciparum* malaria treatment, and if these drugs are lost to resistance, the world may be forced to deal with malaria that is virtually untreatable, which is currently the case in parts of Southeast Asia. The emergence of drug resistant parasites takes place in two stages: the first stage involves the initial mutation producing drug resistance and the second stage involves the subsequent process of selection where a malaria parasite gains an advantage to survive despite the activity of an antimalarial drug. The drug in turn leads to transmission of drug resistant parasites over drug sensitive ones and a corresponding spread of resistance. Policy changes to inhibit drug resistance, are focused on limiting drug pressure overall by selective use of antimalarials to improve clinical care, follow-up practices and enhanced patient compliance. The last method to reduce resistance is to use drugs or combinations of drugs less likely to encourage resistance or drugs with properties inhibiting emergence or spread of resistant parasites.

1) Strategies for Preventing the Spread and Emergence of Malaria Drug Resistance

After a drug resistant parasite has emerged, preventing the spread of a drug resistant parasite is difficult. The spread of resistant malaria parasites is aided by exposing parasites to sub-therapeutic concentrations of antimalarial drugs those results in the death of drug sensitive parasites but allows drug resistant parasites to survive and multiply. Compliance with dosing ensures drugs are taken at the proper dose for the proper duration, which reduces this risk.

Drug pressure is highest in regions where antimalarials with long half-lives are prescribed as the drug persists at sub-therapeutic concentrations in the blood of patients for extended periods of time, which selects for drug resistant parasites. This is prone to happen in high transmission regions where patients are infected more frequently and where patients take antimalarials regularly regardless of whether they are infected or not. In theory, drug pressure in high transmission areas could be reduced through the prescription of drugs with shorter half-lives and through restrictions on administration of first-line treatment drugs to those patients with confirmed, diagnosed cases of malaria. This strategy, however, reveals the conflict between the long-term needs of public health and the immediate needs for definitive patient care. Administration of ACTs with short-lived partner drugs that are rapidly eliminated results in having to take the drug combination for a longer period, which in turn results in poorer patient adherence and a reduced likelihood of achieving a cure. These kinds of combination therapies are not as convenient or efficacious when compared to partner drugs like mefloquine or SP that have longer half-lives and fit in to a three-day treatment regimen or single-dose treatment regimen. Due to the limited availability of diagnostic facilities available in third world countries, restricting the use of effective antimalarial drugs to only those patients who have a definitive diagnosis of malaria would reduce access to treatment for patients who in the most vulnerable and least served communities [9].

This type of restriction would lead to increases in morbidity and mortality due to a trade-off between trying to meet immediate patient treatment needs while still preserving drug treatments for the future. Broad implementation of reliable and simple malaria rapid diagnostic tests may be one way to decrease the misuse of antimalarial drugs to treat every fever encountered. The high levels of asymptomatic parasitemia found in endemic areas often leads to false-positive test results in high transmission areas, which unfortunately leads to limited use in lower transmission areas. Given the cost of rapid diagnostic tests at US $ 0.70 per test, the cost-effectiveness of RDTs is dependent on their cost compared to the costs of ACT treatment and the positive predictive value of an RDT assay to diagnose reliably malaria. If RDTs have a poor ability to diagnose clinical malaria, they will not be cost-effective tools to avoid indiscriminate prescription of antimalarials [494].

Given controlling antimalarial drug resistance is difficult once it has emerged, strategies are necessary to combat initial emergence of drug resistance before it spreads. Drug combinations with different targets may delay of the spread of drug resistance; however, this strategy imposes additional costs for malaria control, which do not yield a practical benefit until overt drug resistance is noted.

2) Reducing Overall Drug Pressure

The restrictions on prescriptions of antibiotics in first-world countries have been implemented to avoid the spread of drug resistant bacteria, and this strategy one of the few tools available for combating antibacterial drug resistance given the dearth of new drugs for treatment. As overall drug pressure is believed to be the most significant factor for development of malaria drug resistance, limiting malaria drug treatments through restrictive drug prescription practices would be useful to limit the spread of drug resistant parasites. That entails improving malaria diagnosis through better laboratory testing and clinical practice. The WHO's Integrated Management of Childhood Illness (IMCI) strives to enhance clinical diagnosis through implementation of well-designed clinical algorithms; however, many patients will still receive unnecessary antimalarial therapy particularly given the open availability of antimalarials in the marketplace.

One view that has been expressed is that drug resistance is less likely in areas of very low transmission, for example, in locations undergoing malaria elimination. Available evidence over time suggests otherwise, there are many examples of rapid spread of malaria drug resistance in low transmission settings, and the failed history of malaria elimination has shown it is not wise to believe that drugs will remain efficacious in areas where they are widely used. Even at "the last mile of malaria elimination," when only a few cases of malaria remain in an area, there is still a risk of malaria being reintroduced from another area or exported to another area. This risk at the "last mile" will only vanish in the final phases of global malaria eradication when foci of malaria infection are limited in number and geographically well separated. Development of new antimalarial drugs and combinations of drugs for eradication and elimination efforts should consider developing plans in advance to prevent the emergence and spread of drug resistance. These plans might include drug combinations with different targets or perhaps drugs with different mechanisms of resistance mechanisms.

3) Preventing Resistance with New Drug Combinations

The use of ACTs composed of an artemisinin analogue with a long-acting partner such as SP, amodiaquine, mefloquine, or piperaquine. The deployment of ACTs will yield two notable outcomes. First, artemisinin compounds are capable of rapid reductions in parasite biomass to very low levels at a time when the concentration of longer-lived partner drug is still at a high level. This outcome will significantly reduce the probability of parasites surviving the initial drug treatment and reduces the number of parasites that will be exposed to low levels of the longer acting partner drug [258]. Second, treatment of patients with artemisinin drugs has been shown to reduce gametocyte production by 8 to 18-fold [68]. This, in turn, reduces the probability that gametocytes carrying drug resistance genes will be transmitted, and, theoretically, artemisinin drug use may diminish malaria transmission rates. Use of artemisinin combination therapy has been shown to be associated with decreases in mefloquine drug resistance and reductions in malaria transmission rates in some parts of Thailand, and the combination of artesunate-mefloquine has therefore been suggested to use more widely in sub-Saharan Africa [123].

Artemisinin derivatives are particularly effective when combined with other antimalarial drug due to very high killing rates as artemisinin drugs have been shown to have parasite reduction rates of 10,000-fold per cycle [62]. Combination treatments have long been used to treat

HIV, leprosy, and tuberculosis and drug combination treatment has proven useful for malaria. When a combination of two drugs with dissimilar mechanisms of action and dissimilar mechanisms of drug resistance, are used for treatment, the per-parasite probability of drug resistant mutants developing for both drugs is calculated by multiplying the per parasite probabilities of mutation for each compound together. The probability for mutations to arise against one compound has been calculated to be 10^6 per asexual cycle and the probability of mutation against two compounds per asexual cycle would therefore be 10^{12}. The use of rapidly eliminated drugs will insure residual drug concentrations are not present to select for resistant parasites, but drugs with short half-lives must be administered for at least 7 days, and patient compliance with 7-day treatment regimens has been shown to be poor. For a 3-day drug treatment regimen, the elimination half-life of a drug must exceed 24 hours.

10.1.2. Novel Antimalarial Combination Therapies Not Based on Artemisinins

ACTs have been used worldwide successfully for years maintaining their treatment efficacy for malaria. The rising tide of artemisinin resistance in Southeast Asia, however, is reason for concern that these remarkable drug combinations may be at risk in the near future in a number of areas [5-8].Many factors have been cited as contributors to the rise of artemisinin resistance in Southeast Asia ranging from indiscriminate use of artemisinin monotherapy to poor prescribing practices. Current evidence does support the hypothesis that resistance to artemisinin drugs is the expected consequence of widespread artemisinin use in the region, which is similar to the rise of drug resistance to older antimalarials such as chloroquine, mefloquine, and SP. While efforts are under way to contain artemisinin resistance, it is entirely reasonable to believe that this effort will either be unsuccessful or that *Plasmodium* parasites in other regions of Southeast Asia are capable of developing *de novo* drug resistance without relying drug resistant parasites spreading geographically from the Thai border region. In the absence of ACT treatments, *falciparum* malaria treatment options for this region will be limited in nature. Given the disastrous implications of untreatable malaria, better strategies to make current antimalarials continue to be efficacious are needed along with efforts to innovate new drug combinations that do not involve artemisinin.

One alternative to artemisinin combination therapy that has been recommended by the WHO is the combination of clindamycin and quinine. The safety and efficacy the combination of quinine and clindamycin is not known, however, the use of these drugs in combination therapy is believed to improve malaria treatment and deter drug resistance to each partner drug in the combination [23].

Clindamycin is an antibiotic with intrinsic anti- malarial efficacy. It is also used to treat infections with gram positive and anaerobic bacteria, babesiosis, toxoplasmosis, and pneumonia from Pneumocystis carinii infections. Clindamycin is available in oral formulations as both a capsule and an oral suspension, and clindamycin is available formulated for intravenous administration. Clindamycin, like doxycycline or tetracycline, has efficacy against *falciparum* malaria, but the rate of killing is very slow with a parasite clearance time ranging from 4-6 days and a fever clearance time ranging from 3-5 days. Clindamycin administered as monotherapy for malaria treatment must be administered two times daily for 5 days. In general, clindamycin has been well tolerated, and the side effects observed have been shown to be minimal in nature. Quinine is the first antimalarial drug known to humankind, and it has been in use for malaria treatment for almost 400 years.

Quinine acts quickly and it is recommended for treating severe malaria, pregnant women with uncomplicated malaria, and for malaria that is resistant to other drugs. Quinine is formulated for oral, parenteral, intramuscular, or rectal administration and it is administered every eight hours for 7 days. Quinine treatment is associated with an array of side effects called cinchonism characterized by nausea, tinnitus, blurred vision, and headache. Quinine has historically been combined with a number of antibiotics to include clindamycin, tetracycline, doxycycline, and azithromycin, which significantly improves treatment efficacy. The use of quinine, however, is more challenging than other antimalarials given the complex dosing requirements, poor tolerability, and poor compliance over the 7-day treatment period [547].

The combination of clindamycin and quinine does qualify as an antimalarial drug combination as both drugs have independent antimalarial activity through different mechanisms of action. The combined efficacy is dependent on the rapid action of quinine to reduce the parasite biomass and the slower action of clindamycin to help kill the remaining parasites. When quinine is combined with clindamycin, the duration of treatment for the combination can be cut down to three days, which enhances patient compliance. This 3-day drug combination regimen is much more practical for treatment of uncomplicated malaria than quinine or clindamycin monotherapy. The combination of quinine-clindamycin can be given to pregnant women and children throughout the course of their pregnancy. A systematic review comparing clindamycin and quinine to other antimalarial drugs was conducted using data derived from seven trials with 929 patients to assess the comparative efficacy of this combination. The primary outcome measure utilized for this review was day 28-treatment failure.

The combination of clindamycin and quinine was shown to significantly reduce the probability of a treatment failure by day 28 *versus* quinine alone, quinine plus sulfadoxine-pyrimethamine, amodiaquine, or chloroquine, but had comparable efficacy to chloroquine combined with clindamycin, quinine combined with doxycycline, quinine combined with tetracycline, or artesunate combined with clindamycin. Adverse events of the combination of clindamycin and quinine were found to be the same in various groups; however, these adverse events were not broadly discussed. While the data is encouraging, the evidence for enhanced efficacy of the clindamycin-quinine combination to treat uncomplicated malaria is still not conclusive. Additional trials will be needed to provide a properly powered study to compare clindamycin-quinine to other ACTs [547]. In the absence of additional efficacy evidence, a consensus opinion of the WHO has recommended the use of clindamycin and quinine as the most appropriate drug for malaria treatment of pregnant women in their first trimester and for treatment when first-line, drugs have failed [23].

Given the recommendation against administration of artemisinin compounds to pregnant women in their first trimester, this provides a less risky option for treatment of these patients. Given the emergence of virtually untreatable malaria in Southeast Asia, this drug combination may be the only treatment option available for *falciparum* malaria. A similar literature review was conducted to compare the efficacy of amodiaquine combined with sulfadoxine-pyrimethamine (AQ-SP) to treat uncomplicated *falciparum* malaria *versus* a number of ACTs (artesunate-amodiaquine, artemether- lumefantrine, and artesunate-SP) in sub-Saharan Africa [548]. The primary outcome measure for this study was day 28-treatment failure. The outcome measures for seven randomized trials of 4,472 children were combined together utilizing a random effects model, and trial quality was found to be generally very good. The treatment failures of AQ-SP were significantly smaller compared to the treatment failures shown for AS-SP (relative risk (RR) = 0.56, 95% CI 0.42-0.75), however, the risk of treatment failure was increased *versus* AL (RR=2.80, 95% CI 2.32- 3.39). The overall AQ-SP treatment rate of failure was found to be on par with AQ- AS (RR=1.12, 95% CI 0.81-1.54). The authors concluded that the AQ-SP combination is a potential option for treatment of uncomplicated malaria in some settings [549]. These two systematic reviews show alternative combinations to ACTs are not only necessary but also effective and more studies should be conducted to assess novel combinations for safety and efficacy.

10.1.3. Pyronaridine, a Novel Antimalarial Combination Partner

The current set of five artemisinin combination drugs widely used for treatment is based on using existing antimalarial drugs that have been widely administered as monotherapy. The choice of long-lived partner drug has always been problematic given some of the drawbacks of these drugs, which include expense, side effects, absorption problems, or drug resistance. Both mefloquine and atovaquone-proguanil are relatively expensive (atovaquone-proguanil is also prone to failure when used for treatment rather than prophylaxis), mefloquine has unpleasant neurological side effects, lumefantrine has problems with drug absorption as well as cross-resistance to mefloquine, and chloroquine, amodiaquine, SP, and piperaquine have problems with high levels of pre-existing parasite resistance. Pyronaridine is another older antimalarial drug developed decades ago that is now under development to make a novel drug combination.

Pyronaridine was originally innovated in China as an antimalarial treatment at the Institute of Chinese Parasitic Disease in 1970. Pyronaridine, a benzonapthyridine compound, is very effective for treatment of *falciparum* malaria to include parasites resistant to chloroquine, and rodent malaria studies have demonstrated that pyronaridine is efficacious against parasite strains resistant to other antimalarials. Pyronaridine drug resistance has been shown to emerge slowly, and drug resistance to pyronaridine is diminished when pyronaridine is used as part of a drug combination with other antimalarial drugs such as artesunate. Pyronaridine toxicity studies have shown this drug is generally less toxic than chloroquine, and the most notable finding is transient elevations in liver enzymes. The manufacturer, Shin Poong Pharmaceuticals, recommends liver function testing when using pyronaridine for treatment, and they do not recommend this drug for malaria prophylaxis. Clinical pharmacokinetic data for patient has infected with uncomplicated *vivax* and *falciparum* malaria treated with an artemisinin-pyronaridine combination therapy showed an elimination $T_{1/2}$ for pyronaridine of 13.2 days for adults and 9.6 days for children. Clinical studies on malaria treatment with pyronaridine alone or in combination have demonstrated the drug is efficacious against both *vivax* and *falciparum* malaria.

1) Pyronaridine Plus Sulphadoxine-Pyrimethamine or Sulphadoxine-Primaquine

Preclinical potency and efficacy studies combined with a number of clinical studies, led to the approval of pyronaridine in China for its use as an antimalarial treatment combined with sulfadoxine-pyrimethamine and primaquine to treat chloroquine-resistant malaria. The clinical studies carried out in China tested the efficacy of pyronaridine-sulfadoxine-pyrimethamine and pyronaridine-sulfadoxine-primaquine. A study of 101 patients was carried out in Hainan province, China, which has endemic chloroquine-resistant malaria. Patients in this study were infected with *falciparum* malaria, and these patients were treated in sequence with orally administered pyronaridine combined with sulfadoxine-pyrimethamine using three different dosing regimens. The fever clearance times observed in patients treated with this combination ranged from 30.1-38.4 hours, and the mean parasitemia clearance time of these patients was within 41.9-48.7 hours. No recrudescence was noted in any of the patients in this study within four weeks after therapy was concluded.

2) Pyronaridine - Nitroquine

The combination of pyronaridine and nitroquine was assessed in Hainan, China, and the other drugs in the study for comparison included monotherapy treatment with piperaquine or pyronaridine. There was no improvement noted in patients treated with the pyronaridine-nitroquine combination based on the rates of recrudescence or the duration of parasite and fever clearance times compared to monotherapy with piperaquine or pyronaridine.

3) Pyronaridine - Dihydroartemisinin

The efficacy of antimalarial treatment using pyronaridine plus artesunate was investigated in a double-blind study in China. 25 patients with uncomplicated *falciparum* malaria were dosed with 1600 mg of pyronaridine, 24 patients were dosed with 640 mg of dihydroartemisinin alone, and 32 patients were dosed with a combination of 800 mg of pyronaridine combined with 300 mg of DHA. The rate of recrudescence observed by Day 28 was 0% for pyronaridine, 4.2% for DHA, and 0% for pyronaridine-DHA. The fever clearance time observed was much shorter with DHA combined with pyronaridine (35.7 hours) compared to DHA by itself (52.6 hours, $P < 0.01$). The parasite clearance time was significantly shorter with the drug combination (23.8 hours) compared to pyronaridine alone (49.4 hours, $P < 0.01$). The combination of pyronaridine and DHA showed gametocyte carriage prevalence of 20.0% while DHA alone demonstrated gametocyte carriage in 16.7% of cases and the prevalence of gametocytes was noted to be 60.9% in patients treated with pyronaridine by itself, which was much higher than the gametocyte carriage rate of the combination ($P < 0.01$). This data demonstrated the combination of pyronaridine-DHA is a promising alternative to current ACTs, and the data suggests lower doses of partner drugs can be efficacious compared to monotherapy with either compound at higher doses.

4) Pyronaridine - Artesunate Combination:

Pyronaridine has been further developed in combination by the innovation of a fixed dose combination treatment with artesunate to treat *falciparum* and *vivax* malaria under the trade name Pyramax®. This combination has been granted Positive Opinion by the European Medicines Agency (Article 58), which allows the EMA to provide scientific opinion on drugs intended for use in markets outside the European Union [550]. Pyramax® was developed by Shin Poong Pharmaceuticals and Medicines for Malaria Venture. This combination therapy is an oral treatment administered daily over a 3-day period for treatment of uncomplicated blood-stage *vivax* and *falciparum* malaria *vivax* in pediatric and adult patients. A Phase 2 study conducted in Gabon compared the efficacy of two formulations (granules and tablets) of pyronaridine-artesunate in a fixed-dose in children aged 2 to 14 years infected with uncomplicated *falciparum* malaria.

A dose escalation study was implemented, and 15 patients were recruited into four treatment arms. The combinations tested were dosed daily for a 3-day period as follows: 2 mg/kg artesunate/6 mg/kg pyronaridine, 3 mg/kg artesunate/ 9 mg/kg pyronaridine, and 4 mg/kg artesunate/12 mg/kg pyronaridine. In addition, a granular pediatric co- formulation was tested at 3 mg/kg artesunate/ 9 mg/kg pyronaridine in a fourth arm. The combination was well tolerated at all doses tested, and no serious adverse events were noted. Pharmacokinetic parameter analysis demonstrated a dose dependent rise in C_{max} and AUC values, and the tablets showed similar relative bioavailability to the co-formulated granular product. The efficacy of artesunate-pyronaridine was shown to be 100% at all doses tested by Day 28 after correction by PCR.

Four Phase 3 pivotal studies were conducted to compare the efficacy of pyronaridine- artesunate to other treatments on market. Two studies were conducted in adults and children to treat *falciparum* malaria comparing artesunate-pyronaridine to artemether-lumefantrine a study and mefloquine-artesunate in another. Another study assessed artesunate-pyronaridine efficacy *versus* artemether- lumefantrine to treat *falciparum* malaria in children using the granular co- formulation. In all four studies, 2,815 patients were administered pyronaridine-artesunate, to include 1,528 adults, 18,401 children aged 12-18 years, and 886 children under 12. Artesunate-pyronaridine was shown to be an excellent drug to treat malaria infections in both children and adults. The artesunate-pyronaridine combination was well tolerated, and the adverse events noted were mild in nature and similar between groups.

A pivotal, multicenter, study was carried out comparing the safety and efficacy of daily artesunate-pyronaridine with twice-daily treatment with artemether-lumefantrine to treat uncomplicated *falciparum* malaria infections in children and adults. In 1,272 patients, 15.1% from Asia and 84.9% from Africa were randomized into treatment groups. The primary endpoint of this study was an adequate Day-28 PCR-corrected parasitological and clinical response in the per protocol population. The results of the study showed artesunate-pyronaridine was to be similar in efficacy to artemether-lumefantrine. Both combination drugs were demonstrated to be have efficacy >99%, and no premature clinical failures were observed. The Day-28 and Day-42 PCR-corrected efficacy was shown to be the best in the cohort treated with artesunate-pyronaridine *versus* the cohort treated with artemether-lumefantrine. Kaplan-Meier analysis demonstrated one critical difference in the rates of re-infection observed in the different groups through Day 42 demonstrated by parasite clearance data was shown to be quicker in patients treated with pyronaridine-artesunate *versus* artemether-lumefantrine ($p < 0.001$) with the largest difference observed before Day 2. No differences in fever clearance times were noted between artesunate-pyronaridine and artemether-lumefantrine.

An additional multicenter study of patients infected with uncomplicated *falciparum* malaria was conducted comparing the efficacy of artesunate-mefloquine with artesunate-artesunate-pyronaridine. The PCR corrected cure rate by Day-28 was 99.2% for artesunate-pyronaridine and 98.1% for artesunate-mefloquine. The authors conclude that artesunate-pyronaridine is equivalent in efficacy to artesunate-mefloquine with a difference in treatment efficacy of only 1.1% (95% CI -0.2, 3.1; $p = 0.106$). Pyronaridine treatment efficacy as monotherapy against infections with other species of malaria was assessed in 10 patients infected with *P. ovale* and 16 patients infected with *P. malariae* in Cameroon. The average fever clearance time was 49.8 hours, and the average parasite clearance time was 33.5 hours. All of the treated patients had no fever by Day 4 and all demonstrated parasitological and clinical cures by Day 14 with no gametocytemia observed by Day 3.

Pyronaridine efficacy against *P. vivax* was tested using pyronaridine alone and combined with primaquine. In this study, 1,200 mg of pyronaridine monotherapy was administered in a three-day oral treatment regimen for blood stage of *vivax* malaria, and the treatment outcomes were similar to those obtained with chloroquine. Intramuscular pyronaridine has been shown to achieve slightly quicker clearance of parasites compared to orally administered or intravenous pyronaridine. Pyronaridine been tested in combination with a 3- or 4-day short-course primaquine for *vivax* malaria treatment. The combination showed acceptable efficacy though patients treated with primaquine for eight days showed the highest rate of radical cure and prevention of relapse. An orally administered fixed dose combination of artesunate-pyronaridine was administered in a three-day regimen for *vivax* blood stage of malaria infections in a pivotal Phase 3 multicenter trial. The objective of this study was to assess artesunate-pyronaridine efficacy artesunate-pyronaridine *versus* chloroquine for treatment of children and adults infected with *vivax* malaria.

Patients ranging in age from 3 to 60 with *vivax* malaria infections were assigned to receive either artesunate-pyronaridine (2.4 mg/kg artesunate and 7.2 mg/kg pyronaridine in one group, 4.6 mg/kg artesunate and 13.8 mg/kg pyronaridine in another group) *versus* a standard treatment dose of CQ administered daily for 3 days. Patients with normal levels of a critical enzyme, glucose-6-phosphate dehydrogenase (G6PD), necessary to provide reducing power to mediate detoxification of free radicals generated by primaquine metabolism were administered a 14-day primaquine treatment regimen at 15 mg/day beginning at Day 28 to eliminate the residual hypnozoite parasite forms in the liver. Day 14 cure rates were the principal endpoint in this study, and 99.5% cure rates were observed in patients treated with -artesunate-pyronaridine and a 100% cure rate was observed for patients treated with chloroquine. Pyronaridine was shown to be similar in efficacy to chloroquine with a difference in cure rates of 0.5%, and rates of cure at Days 21, 28, 35, and 42 were shown to be non-inferior to chloroquine. Parasite clearance times for artesunate-pyronaridine of 23 hours were decreased in the artesunate-pyronaridine treatment group compared to parasite clearance times for chloroquine of 32 hours. The fever clearance time of 15.9 hours for artesunate-pyronaridine was similarly reduced compared to the FCT of 23.8 hours for chloroquine, ($p = 0.0017$). The post-baseline infection incidence with either *falciparum* or *vivax* malaria up to Day 42 was 6.8% for artesunate-pyronaridine and 12.4% for chloroquine ($p = 0.022$, log rank test).

Pyronaridine tetra-phosphate-artesunate (PYRAMAX®) is a joint development project of Shin Poong Pharmaceuticals Company and the Medicines for Malaria Venture (MMV) focused on bringing a novel ACT in both granule and fixed dose formulation forward for treatment of *falciparum* and *vivax* malaria. Pivotal Phase 3 comparative clinical trials including treatment of over 3,000 adults, adolescents, and children in Sub-Saharan Africa and Southeast Asia 18 countries were completed in 2009. Positive Opinion was provided by the European Medicines Agency using Article 58, which provides a means for the EMA to render an opinion on a drug not destined for the EU in March 2012, and Shin Poong obtained drug approval from the Korean Federal Drug Agency for their new drug application in August 2011. New drug applications will be submitted to other national regulatory submissions and WHO review [550].

10.2. PK/PD BASED STRATEGIES TO OPTIMIZE AVAILABLE ANTIMALARIAL COMBINATIONS

The best drug for malaria eradication would possess a short elimination half-life and a long-term release from a drug depot coupled with rapid clearance. Such an ideal drug could be administered in combination with antimalarials possessing a similar PK profile to enhance efficacy and retard parasite drug resistance [422]. A combination of this nature would rapidly kill blood stage parasites and exist for an extended period allowing for administration infrequently in a single encounter and would rapidly clear parasites to avoid exposure of parasites to an extended period of sub-lethal drug levels facilitating selection of drug resistance. A drug treatment provided at a single encounter that cures malaria and provides four weeks or longer of prophylaxis afterward would be a worthy step along the way to obtaining the tools necessary for malaria eradication. Antimalarial drugs with half-lives as long as four weeks are available on market (ex. piperaquine) but no drug on market possesses the ideal PK/PD profile of periodic pulsed concentrations of drug at parasiticidal concentrations which is rapidly cleared to avoid selection for resistance. Prior work on vaccine polymers to achieve pulsatile antigen release was abandoned by the WHO despite initial promising results. Nanotechnology is an approach to develop drugs with a desirable PK/PD profile. Nanoparticle delivery of drugs is a promising but immature technology, and one technical barrier to deployment of nanotized drugs is the limitation on drug dose delivered. Drugs with high levels of potency to be administered at a low level are the best candidates for this drug delivery method. Implants administered subcutaneously similar to Norplant (low dose delivery of hormones for birth control) comprise another possible method that may provide the ideal PK/PD profile.

In some settings, administration of a drug with an ideal PK/PD profile may be less important particularly in areas with very low malaria transmission. On example of such a setting is mass drug administration to kill remaining infectious parasites at the lowest level of transmission in regions where malaria is seasonal rather than year-round. Given the diminished risk of parasites encountering sub-therapeutic levels of antimalarial drugs in such a setting, there may be no downside to administration of drug combinations possessing mismatched PK/PD profiles. This example illustrates why considering the epidemiology of malaria in a specific region is necessary to choose drugs with desired PK/PD profiles for malaria elimination. This example also supports the tailoring target product profiles (TPPs) to setting-specific therapeutic indications based on the resistance profile of circulating local parasites, local epidemiology, human populations, and the stage(s) of malaria control and eradication targeted [436].

10.2.1. Optimal Selection Criteria for a Novel Antimalarial Combination Treatment

A recent Medicines for Malaria Venture meeting reviewed questions of managing drug discovery and preclinical testing to achieve a robust pipeline of compounds under development to achieve novel combination therapies to meet key clinical needs for malaria treatment. Dose optimization of drug combination components was identified as a key element to achieve the best rates of cure and to preserve existing treatment drugs from emerging drug resistance. By 2001, the rise of *falciparum* malaria resistant to virtually all drugs on market in many countries was associated with having no effective, affordable drugs for malaria treatment available for use [23]. Along with the increased incidence of drug resistant parasites in 2001, there were concomitant increases in morbidity, mortality, and increases in the severity and frequency of epidemic malaria.

Artemisinin revolutionized antimalarial therapy and prevented a catastrophe by providing a drug with extraordinarily rapid rates of parasite killing. Combining artemisinin drugs with long-lived partners has resulted in high rates of sustained cures with a 3-day treatment schedule [284, 232]. Today, ACTs have been shown to be highly efficacious with cure rates by Day 28 in excess of 495% (adjusted for re- infection with PCR genotyping), and the cost of ACT treatment has dropped to less than $1 per adult treated [2-4, 23]. ACT driven improvements in treatment efficacy will not go on forever, as artemisinin resistant *falciparum* malaria has been observed in Southeast Asia, and the percentage of parasites isolated in Cambodia resistant to artemisinin as shown by the K13 propeller mutation has skyrocketed [5-8].

The specter of untreatable *falciparum* has energized research into antimalarial drug discovery and development, and today it is clear that ACTs are not the 'ultimate' antimalarial drug given the rise of artemisinin drug resistance in Southeast Asia, and post-artemisinin alternatives are needed. Transmission blocking drugs are a key element of many malaria eradication plans. While safety and efficacy are the most important drug development objectives, there is a new drugs must be protected against the emergence of parasite drug resistance. Thus, new antimalarials must be administered in combination with partners possessing different PK/PD profiles. To enhance drug compliance, drug combinations should be dosed as fixed-dose formulations, and the doses of these new combination drugs must be optimized for use in children given the increased risk of death in this non-immune population. Development of child-friendly formulations such as granules or dispersible tablets is needed to achieve treatment in this population.

This does leave the challenge of optimizing new antimalarial combinations and finding the proper doses for different patient populations and different treatment indications.

10.2.2. Challenges for Development of Novel Antimalarial Combination Treatments

While guidelines from regulatory bodies for development of antimalarial drug combination therapy are lacking, some guidance documents on fixed-dose combinations are pertinent references that include guidance on development of fixed-dose combinations. While experience has been gained with ACT drug development, this experience may not be sufficient to develop antimalarial drug combinations in the future (Table **31**). ACTs were needed quickly and initial dose- finding studies were empiric in nature with limited formal dose-finding studies. Development of HIV drugs involved extensive use of *in vitro* potency data and drug resistance data to inform the drug development pathway for choosing drug treatment regimens. In tuberculosis, murine models have been shown to be valuable tools for testing efficacy of potential drug combinations; however, there are no validated methods in rodent malaria models to choose combination partners or their relative doses [551].

Table 31: Challenges for novel antimalarial combination therapy drug development compared with the development of artemisinin-based combination therapies (ACTs)

Model Term*	ACT	Novel Combination Therapies
Combination components	Artemisinin plus an existing drug used previously as monotherapy	One or more combination partners are new chemical entities
Regulatory procedure	Safety and efficacy evaluated for the combination therapy	Stringent process. Proof of concept required for monotherapy and combination therapy. Safety and efficacy evaluated for the combination therapy
Clinical data	Initial evidence mostly from the Thailand border areas in adult populations	Clinical data required from multiple centers in Asia, Africa, and South America. Extensive clinical data from children required
Formulation	Loose or fixed combinations	Fixed combinations only
Pediatric formulation	Crushed adult formulation tablets used for pediatric administration. Pediatric formulations developed retrospectively in some cases.	Initial development of a pediatric formulation that can also be used in adults. Separate evaluation of dose and duration in children and adults
Dose finding	One dose fits all, empirically derived based on data from monotherapy studies	Rational and optimized within combination therapy

*The model terms are cited from reference [551].

In vitro studies have been shown to be cheap, useful tools to determine determining drug potency, but the results are dependent on the strain of parasite chosen for testing and the mix of parasites in different stages that is tested. Interactions between drugs can be tested *in vitro* using isobologram experiments, however, only the most profound examples of drug synergy *in vitro* have been shown to have clinical relevance *in vivo*, and *in vitro* data showing mild synergy or antagonism may not yield clinically relevant data. Rodent malaria models provide excellent data particularly during the optimization of a drug scaffold, and development of the humanized mouse model is another useful tool for drug development [552, 553]. Even with a number of useful pre-clinical study tools available for malaria drug development, there are still enormous uncertainties for clinical development of novel antimalarial drugs. New validated methods are also likely needed to test prospective drugs for transmission blocking potential and for stage specificity of action [436].

Clinical proof-of-concept studies can yield efficacy information on monotherapeutic agents, but these data might not be pertinent when describing dose response relationships of drugs in combination. Human PK studies are required by regulators, and these PK studies help select doses for combination therapies. These studies should be performed in both healthy and malaria infected patients Although PK/PD data help explain dosing to regulators, dose-ranging studies will be needed to provide data to derive a rational dosing decision. Unfortunately, until a drug combination is assessed for comparative efficacy in malaria- infected patients, the process for making dose choices is always challenging.

10.2.3. The Use of Factorial Study Designs and Dose-Response Plots as Tools for Making Dose Recommendations for Combination Treatment

Factorial study designs can aid in determining dosing levels of new combination drugs. A factorial design is an engineering tool for comparison of two or more components simultaneously. In drug development, factorial designs have been used in animal testing, but factorial designed studies have been limited in clinical development primarily focused on studies of hypertension drugs. A simple two by two-factorial design, which evaluates two drugs with each drug given at two different doses (2 x 2 matrixes), is a very useful tool to assess prospective malaria drug combinations.

Factorial design has not been used to develop dosing decisions for malaria drugs; however, recent advances in development of new antimalarial drugs and the rise of drug combination therapy for infectious disease made factorial design methods an attractive tool for drug development. Factorial studies utilize a model derived from statistics to interpolate the results of dose-response data. A quadratic model commonly used for designing factorial designs for clinical trials, and the quadratic model provides a means for study of non-linear dose-response relationships. Non-linear responses may only be observed when two or more drugs are used in combination. Factorial design models can be used to provide estimates of the best dose within the dose-response surface matrix, and such a model can inform the bets drug dose choice even when it has not been tested. One caveat for factorial study designs of malaria studies is a placebo comparison is ethically inappropriate in malaria trials given the risk of mortality after infection with *falciparum* malaria. In all cases, understanding what the lowest dose that is efficacious is required before creating the dosing matrix. Because factorial design models allow data comparisons across the whole matrix rather than simply by pair-wise comparisons, sample sizes can be quite low. This can cut back on the time to conduct studies, but the sample size requirement also affects the statistical power required to assess drug safety, and study sample sizes may be larger than larger than required for a factorial design to populate the safety database [551].

Factorial study designs have a number of advantages, which include:

- Simultaneous testing of monotherapy and combination therapy in one experiment;

- Factorial designs are typically cheaper than a dose-ranging study of individual combination drugs then a study of drugs in combination as only some dose combinations are required to establish the data required for interpretation;

- Unexpected outcomes associated with drug synergy or antagonism can be assessed in a factorial design as there is some flexibility to accommodate unexpected outcomes;

- Testing drug combinations composed of drugs with different PK/PD profiles is readily conducted with a factorial design as drug combination interactions may be hard to predict and compare across a range of doses;

- Factorial design calculations to establish the dose-response surface can preclude exposure of patients to either ineffective or toxic drug levels.

This is relevant to malaria as lower dose limits in dose ranging studies require interruption of an experiment should the patient require rescue with alternative treatments. *Falciparum* malaria can be deadly, particularly in non-immune subjects, and patients should not be given sub-therapeutic drug doses leading to adverse outcomes. Factorial study designs facilitate construction of a dose-response surface where the lowest number of patients might be given sub-therapeutic doses, which should be the most important element of a clinical trial design scheme to test antimalarial combination drugs in man. While the benefits of factorial design are many, there are requirements for statistical design work needed to design a factorial dose study. The initial design work includes both simulations and sensitivity analysis, and this initial design work requires specialized statistical resources.

In addition, conducting clinical trials designed with a number of combination drugs administered at a variety of doses can also be difficult. The choice of dose will likely be informed by the very real likelihood that candidate antimalarials may be efficacious across a broad array of doses. Another important question is picking appropriate outcome endpoints to choose when evaluating drug combinations and dose recommendations to address specific therapeutic application questions. Antimalarials that demonstrate rapid reduction in parasite burden, like the artemisinins, may not show an efficacy contribution when dosed in combination treatment. If the clinical endpoint is the outcome after Day 28, the testing of antimalarial drugs with long half-lives may not reveal recrudescence without an extended follow-up period. Evaluation of antimalarial combinations with varying PK/PD profiles may require evaluation of multiple endpoints. Assessing multiple endpoints makes a factorial design more complicated. As discussed previously, the minimally effective dose must be known, particularly for special population such as children, before any of these subjects can be included in a factorial design study to test dose optimization beyond this threshold.

Accordingly, initial dose data will be required from other groups such as adults with malaria, or with alternative endpoints such as data acquired from previously conducted clinical studies prior to going forward. Development of new antimalarial drugs provides assess different, new approaches to optimize doses for drug combinations, like factorial design. Factorial design is a tool that is worth consideration to optimize safety, efficacy, and long term use of future antimalarial combination therapies [551].

10.3. DEVELOPMENT OF COMBINATION THERAPIES WITH NEW MECHANISMS OF ACTION

In 1957 Wallace Peters wrote, "Development of an 8-aminoquinoline in depot form to give a safe and adequate blood level should be attempted as this would be an invaluable weapon against malaria if properly applied". After fifty years, this unmet need still exists for a safe drug with liver stage activity, anti-hypnozoite activity, schizonticidal activity, and gametocidal activity suitable for radical cure of both *falciparum* and *vivax* malaria. The only known antimalarial drugs that are capable of killing dormant liver stage hypnozoites and gametocytes are 8-aminoquinoline drugs such as primaquine and tafenoquine. All 8-aminoquinoline drugs tested in man are known to cause red blood cell hemolysis in patients with deficiencies in glucose 6-phosphate dehydrogenase, a genetic polymorphism commonly found in red cells of patients who reside in tropical regions, as the genetic deficiency itself is associated with protection against malaria.

Given that any malaria elimination drug in populations who are not ill must be very safe with low risks and increased benefits similar to the ratio of risk to benefit observed with routine immunizations. While an ideal TPP would specify a non-existing drug with all of the previously mentioned lead quality attributes, such a profile is the beginning of a discussion on what lead quality attributes are actually possible through drug development. Drugs that cannot meet an ideal standard for development may still be of use for malaria control and elimination depending on how close a developer can come to an ideal TPP *versus* an acceptable TPP. The best antimalarial drug would have activity against all species of malaria, but rejection of a drug that targeted only *falciparum* or *vivax* malaria would be shortsighted. Indeed, depending on the types of novel chemical entity leads identified, it is likely that different TPPs may be necessary for these two key species.

Given limited funding and laboratory capacity, conducting sufficient clinical malaria PK/PD studies can be very difficult, and consequently, the majority of antimalarial drugs are tested and used in populations where there is little to no data available for determining optimal dosing for safety and efficacy. Rigorously designed and carefully executed clinical trials are required to develop new drugs and drug combination chosen for malaria eradication, and innovative methods must be created for post licensure surveillance to detect adverse effects. This type of post-marketing surveillance will necessitate having the capacity to conduct drug quantitation, PK/PD studies, and pharmacovigilance. As the incidence of malaria drops at established malaria research sites, finding enough subjects to meet sample size requirements for new studies is becoming more difficult. Accordingly, clinical trial studies using mobile networks or new clinical trial designs must be implemented to enroll the numbers of subjects required. One possibility is conducting clinical studies of malaria incidence in malaria endemic regions to assess the prevalence of gametocytes to measure the performance of transmission blocking drugs. In addition, the dearth of malaria incidence at established sites, particularly for studies of non- immunes who have never been exposed to malaria may lead to increased use of human challenge studies to develop antimalarial drugs [436].

For many years, malaria treatment and prophylaxis needs have been met with a small family of drugs primarily from the quinoline class of compounds, but the emergence of endemic drug resistant parasites has led to increases in failures in malaria treatment and associated adverse effects in malarious regions. The rising tide of malaria drug resistance has focused researchers to create new drugs and new drug targets, and to accurately characterize the molecular basis of drug resistance to compounds now in use as a means of facilitating detection of resistance and also to help develop novel approaches to overcome resistance. Additionally, antimalarial drugs rely on interfering with parasite metabolism without affecting the metabolism of the human host for their efficacy and specificity. The mechanisms of action of new drugs such as the artemisinins differs from the mechanisms of older drugs which inhibit malaria growth largely by inhibiting formation of hemazoin, a bio-mineralized form of hemoglobin metabolized by the malaria parasite.

Plasmodium infects host erythrocytes during the blood stage portion of their life cycle, and the replication and release of blood stage parasites leads to the symptoms of malaria. Parasite survival in the human host requires a number of metabolic adaptations that make vulnerable to chemotherapeutic attack. This is shown both in the mechanisms of action of existing antimalarials and in the many potential drug targets, which are being identified through sequencing the malaria genome. A number of drug targets are related to distinct malaria organelles. There are three malaria organelles which are excellent drug targets including: the lysosomal food vacuole where degradation of hemoglobin and formation of hemozoin takes place, the apicoplast, a plastid organelle which provides critical lipid synthesis required for cell metabolism, and an acrystate mitochondrion possessing a limited electron transport system.

10.3.1. Targeting Drug Resistance Markers for Discovery of Novel Drugs

A number of research studies have illustrated the central role that *pfcrt*, the chloroquine resistance transporter to *P. falciparum*, plays in mediating chloroquine resistance (CQR). The mechanism of how *pfcrt* mutations lead to CQ resistance has been an area of ongoing research. Chloroquine sequesters in the parasite's digestive vacuole (DV) which is acidic in nature because of the weakly basic properties of the chloroquine structure. Inside the DV, CQ is believed to inhibit the formation of hemazoin, which renders toxic hemoglobin waste products inert. The CQR phenotype is characterized by decreased CQ uptake in the DV. Transfection of the mutant *pfcrt* gene into a CQ sensitive parasite has been shown to lead to CQ resistance, and the K76T *pfcrt* mutation has been shown to be required for this phenotype. Further studies have shown that *pfcrt*-mediated CQR phenotype results from increased efflux of CQ out of the DV through mechanisms involving a carrier or a channel [554].

CQ translocation across the *pfcrt* transporter can be influenced by verapamil. CQ can cause a verapamil sensitive increase in alkalization of the DV, which suggests the efflux of CQ is dependent on the protonation of CQ. Bioinformatic comparisons to other drug metabolite transporters and studies in Xenopus laevis oocytes expressing *pfcrt* have shown that the K76T mutation leads to a loss of positive charge enabling protonated CQ to cross the transporter, which leads to CQ moving out of the DV and into the cytoplasm of the parasite. As the DV, not the cytoplasm, is the site of CQ action, CQ no longer has a biological effect to inhibit hemozoin formation [555]. Using a transfection-based approach, further studies have shown the overall parasite genome drives the CQR phenotype mediated by mutations in *pfcrt*. This finding supports previous data obtained studying genetically diverse parasite isolates and culture-adapted lines [556].

The most unusual findings for *pfcrt* were observed with a transfected parasite clone, D10, which was engineered to express mutant *pfcrt*. The transfected parasite showed decreased CQ susceptibility, and this susceptibility was most notable at the IC_{90} level, the concentration of CQ inhibiting 90% growth, but not at the IC_{50} level. Further experiments showed that other genes were involves in this phenotype as expression of mutant *pfcrt* could lead to either parasite drug resistance or tolerance. Single base pair mutations or changes in gene expression of the *pfmdr1*1 gene (*Plasmodium falciparum* multidrug resistance gene) which encodes a protein, Pgh1, can affect the CQR phenotype in certain strains. Other studies have demonstrated that Pgh1 expression increases after parasite exposure to the anticonvulsant phenobarbitone, and this, in turn, leads to higher IC_{50} values *in vitro* in both CQR and CQS parasites. The mechanism of phenobarbital-induced over-expression of Pgh1 is likely related to the binding of phenobarbital to nuclear-receptor- binding sites homologous to mammalian sequences in the *pfmdr1*1 and *pfcrt* promoter regions. These findings lead to a further hypothesis suggesting responses to drug exposure by nuclear receptor may be one means by which genes are regulated in *falciparum* malaria [555].

CQ-resistant strains of *falciparum* malaria have been noted in all malaria-endemic areas; however, *vivax* chloroquine resistance is rare and is limited to certain geographic regions in Indonesia and the Pacific region. The genetic basis of *vivax* resistance to chloroquine is not known, and chloroquine resistance is not dependent on mutations in *pvcg10*, the *vivax* ortholog of *pfcrt*. A review was conducted of variations in 36 microsatellite markers in nineteen *vivax* parasite strains that were chloroquine resistant and twenty-one *vivax* parasite strains that were chloroquine sensitive obtained from Indonesian patients. The authors examined the data to detect the presence of a selective sweep, which is a reduction in DNA sequence variation in sequences neighboring sites of mutation which is a consequence of strong positive selection. The data did not support a selective sweep and their studies revealed an overall low level of genetic diversity. Another study on *P. vivax* samples derived from Southeast Asia involved genotyping the *pvmdr1* gene, which showed a linkage between resistance to chloroquine and a mutation, Y976F [557]. The data from this study also suggested an association between the copy number of the *pvmdr1* gene and mefloquine drug resistance shown by increases in mefloquine IC_{50}s, which is similar to the well-established relationship association between *pfmdr1*1 copy number and increased drug resistance and mefloquine IC_{50} values [558].

Another study found no association of chloroquine resistance with the ortholog of *pfcrt* or *pfmdr1*1, but one unexpected finding was mutations in *UBP-1*, a deubiquitinating enzyme, which were observed in parasites placed under chloroquine or artesunate drug pressure. Understanding alternate mechanisms of chloroquine resistance present in other *Plasmodium* species will be important to understand acquisition and mechanisms of drug resistance. A study conducted in Guinea-Bissau recently reported findings that chloroquine administered at twice the normal dose was still effective demonstrating cures in 78% of uncomplicated malaria patients harboring parasites with the *K76T pfcrt* chloroquine resistance mutation. Many questions regarding chloroquine resistance and chloroquine treatment failures are still relevant today given the reduced incidence of chloroquine resistance observed in Malawi. With reduced usage of chloroquine in this African country, chloroquine can now be used for drug treatment.

Antimalarial drug resistance has been observed to arise, however, drug resistance has been noted to produce a less fit parasite, and with the removal of drug pressure, in theory, less fit drug resistant parasites should be less competitive for survival than wild-type parasites. While Malawi noted a significant drop in chloroquine resistance with the removal of chloroquine as a drug treatment, mutant parasites with the *pfcrt* mutation persisted far longer in Hainan Island, China after the removal of chloroquine treatment as an option. This does raise many questions about relationships between drug pressure and parasite fitness, and this does suggest that while removal of drug pressure in areas with established drug resistance should decrease the prevalence of resistant parasites, the rates of decrease in the prevalence of mutant parasites may well be quite different. Research efforts to define the molecular contribution of resistance markers have been greatly enhanced by the sequencing of the *Plasmodium* genome. Sequencing and microarray studies have shown thousands of polymorphisms in the genome of *P. falciparum*, and linkage disequilibrium analyses have been used to identify known and unknown loci associated with phenotypes of drug resistance to a number of existing antimalarials such as quinine, chloroquine, and sulfadoxine-pyrimethamine. Increased research into the mechanisms of antimalarial drug resistance is crucial to understand the potential mechanisms for resistance to new antimalarial drugs in the pipeline. This knowledge can be leveraged to develop more drugs that are efficient, more efficacious combinations, surveillance of parasite drug resistance, and comparative efficacy treatment studies [559].

10.3.2. Screening New Drug Targets with Small Molecule Inhibitors

Strategies to find novel chemical entities are outlined in this section ranging from irrational drug discovery with whole-cell phenotypic screening to target based screening against specific *Plasmodium* targets.

1) Irrational Drug Discovery through Whole Cell In Vitro Phenotypic Screening

Target-based drug discovery has generated many possibilities for drug screening to find parasite specific targets to inhibit growth. To date, however, target based approaches have not yielded much fruit with actual compounds moving forward into clinical testing. Historically, antimalarial compounds have been discovered in nature (quinine, artemisinin), or they have been discovered through irrational drug discovery through large scale animal screening (mefloquine), or they have created synthetically through analogue campaigns around existing scaffolds (tafenoquine, amodiaquine, ferroquine, atovaquone), or they have been discovered in the modern era through whole cell *in vitro* phenotypic screening (spirindolones).

Whole cell phenotypic screening for growth inhibition has two intrinsic advantages over target-based approaches. One advantage is the growth inhibition test is conducted against an intact parasite inside a red blood cell. Any growth inhibitory compound must be capable of penetrating multiple membranes to get inside the malaria parasite to inhibit growth. Target based screens only find compounds capable of binding to the target, and these compounds may be wholly incapable of crossing multiple membranes to reach the same target in an intact cell. The second advantage of whole cell phenotypic screening is no knowledge of a target is required to screen compounds. Target based approaches require in-depth knowledge of the target to be screened in the malaria parasite in terms of the protein sequence of the target, any post- translational modifications that are made to the protein, and whether the target to be inhibited is actually essential. The secondary, tertiary, and quaternary structures of the target protein and any requirements for protein folding may be needed to achieve the final structure observed in the parasite. An *in vitro* protein synthesis strategy is necessary to express any recombinant target protein to be screened against along with insuring any essential post-translational modifications and protein-folding requirements can actually be made *in vitro*.

High throughput screening methods have been innovated to rapidly screen target libraries through whole cell screening campaigns. The most popular screening technique used today is the Malaria SYBR Green I fluorescence assay. The Malaria SYBR Green I-Based Fluorescence assay is micro titer plate in drug sensitivity used to assess the potency of antimalarial drugs based on the intercalation of SBYR green, an intercalating dye, which binds to the DNA of malaria parasites. SYBR Green dye fluorescence is a measure of parasite growth, and test compounds with malaria inhibitory activity will lead to reduced parasite DNA associated fluorescence [560].

One example of the use of whole-cell screening campaigns is the discovery of the spirindolones, a new class of potent drugs with schizonticidal activity against *falciparum* and *vivax* parasites. The profile compound of this class was identified through whole-cell phenotypic screening against a 12,000 compound library composed of both synthetic compounds with natural product features and natural products After a medicinal chemistry analogue campaign that created and analyzed 200 derivatives, a final lead compound, NITD609, was selected for further clinical evaluation [571].

2) Targeting Chromatin-Modifying Enzymes

The sequencing of the malaria genome has provided tools to understand the mechanisms of gene regulation in *Plasmodium*. Studies investigating the allelic exclusion in the *var* gene family have shown an important role for the *falciparum* histone deacetylase Sir2 that serves an important role in dynamic chromatin modeling [561]. The genes have been silenced through chromatin remodeling triggered by the activity of HDAC enzymes. Drug discovery efforts have shown HDAC inhibitors with *in vitro* potency against cultured *falciparum* parasites and efficacy against rodent malaria parasites *in vivo*. In 2008, a study reported highly selective, potent HDAC inhibitors with IC_{50} values as low as 3 nM, whose action on the *falciparum* parasite leads to hyper acetylation of parasite histone proteins and altered expression of a number of *P. falciparum* genes [555].

3) Targeting the Apicoplast Organelle

As previously discussed, a number of *Plasmodium* drug targets are believed to be associated with a plastid organelle, the apicoplast, which produces critical lipids needed for malaria metabolism. A number of studies have shown the apicoplast has a mevalonate-independent isoprenoid synthesis pathway and a Type II fatty acid biosynthesis, which are very different from synthetic pathways for fatty acids in humans and other eukaryotes lacking a plastid organelle such as the apicoplast. Recent research has been conducted into the type II fatty acid biosynthesis pathway used in the apicoplast hypothesized to be a drug target for a number of compounds with antimalarial activity including triclosan and thiolactomycin [562].

Isoprenoid biosynthesis is another apicoplast pathway, which may also serve as a target for antimalarial drug development. One compound, fosmidomycin, has known inhibitory activity directed against the isoprenoid enzyme 1-deoxy-D-xylulose 5- phosphate (DOXP) reductase. Fosmidomycin monotherapy and combination treatment is efficacious against *falciparum* malaria infections in human patients. While fosmidomycin has shown efficacy as an antimalarial drug, fosmidomycin does not have the best PK profile, and analogue development will be necessary to create a fosmidomycin analogue with a suitable PK profile. The most widely used antimalarials whose mode of action involves the apicoplast include a number of antibiotics such as doxycycline, clindamycin, and azithromycin, which target translation in the apicoplast. These antibacterial drugs produce a well-characterized 'delayed death' phenotype against *Plasmodium* parasites, and they have been used for malaria prophylaxis as monotherapy and as part of drug combination therapy [562]. *In vitro* resistance to azithromycin, however, has been shown to be rapidly induced *in vitro* which renders this antibiotic more prone to drug resistance. Combinations of azithromycin and chloroquine have been shown to have synergy against *P. falciparum* parasites, and this combination may prove to be an alternate combination therapy for prophylaxis of malaria in man [563].

Unique plasmodial pathways provide an opportunity for target based drug development, and apicoplast enzyme such as Acetyl-CoA carboxylase (ACC), ketoacyl-ACP synthase, and enoyl- ACP reductase are examples of unique enzymes that might be drug development targets. In the apicomplexan non-mevalonate pathway, 1-Deoxy-D- xyluose-5-phosphate (DOXP) reductoisomerase has inhibited by fosmidomycin, and this enzyme may be another potential target for antimalarial drug development. Another potential target in this same biosynthetic pathway is 2C-methyl- D-erythritol 2, 4-cyclodiphosphate synthase (*1spF*). Complexes of this synthase enzyme with inhibitor compounds have been discussed which may provide an opportunity for target based drug development through structure-based design.

4) Targeting Parasite Metabolism

Targeting parasite metabolism inhibitors capable of inhibiting parasite-specific metabolic pathways or transport processes is another area of interest for drug discovery. One target that has been discussed is vitamin biosynthesis, which occurs in *Plasmodium* parasites but not in man. One drug development effort is focused on creating prodrugs activated by pyridoxine kinase that capable of inhibiting pyridoxal phosphate, one of the natural forms of Vitamin B6. Another vitamin synthesis pathway that is a potential target is the synthesis of coenzyme A from Vitamin B5 or pantothenate. Pantothenate analogues have been identified, which have potency against *falciparum* malaria [564].

5) Targeting Parasite Transporters

Nutrient transport proteins that acquire nutrients from the human host are unique targets that have been investigated. One study reported inhibition of the parasite specific biopterin-folate transporters, *PfFBT1* and *PfFBT2*, by methotrexate, a dihydrofolate reductase inhibitor, and probenecid, an organic anion transporter inhibitor. Folic acid transport has also been inhibited by para-aminobenzoic acid, a folate precursor, suggesting these two parasite transporters can be targeted by a wide spectrum of substrates. Another drug development program targeting parasite-specific metabolic pathways is focused on inhibiting *de novo* phosphatidylcholine biosynthesis. This research has identified choline analogs capable of inhibiting *falciparum* malaria growth *in vitro* at nano-molar concentrations. Animal testing in malaria infected rodents and non-human primates have shown cures *in vivo*. These types of compounds are believed to inhibit transport of choline and inhibit parasite phospholipid biosynthesis [555].

6) Inhibition of Mitochondrial Enzymes

One of the major strengths of these choline inhibitors is their multiple modes of action, which may help delay the emergence of drug resistance. The pyrimidine biosynthetic pathway has been a fruitful target of drug discovery. *Plasmodium* parasites are not capable of recycling pyrimidines and must create all of their pyrimidine by *de novo* synthesis. Inhibitors of dihydroorotate dehydrogenase (DHODH) which is an essential enzyme required to synthesize pyrimidines have been created, and a lead compound has progressed to Phase 1 and 2 trials. Other studies have identified a class of compounds called the dihydroacridinediones that act to inhibit plasmodial mitochondrial processes. These compounds bind to the quinol oxidation site (Q_o) of the mitochondrial bc1 complex of the parasite resulting in membrane potential collapse in the mitochondria and subsequent cell death [565].

Red cell invasion by parasites could be inhibited by a small molecule, and one known means by which the parasite invades a red blood cell involves a microneme protein, EBA-175, which recognizes the sialic acid residues of the host red blood cell glycophorin A [566]. Using NMR techniques and molecular modeling, a recently published study explored the hypothesis that neuraminic acid derivatives could outcompete the parasite to bind to the sialic acid residues on EBA-17.

7) Targeting Parasite Proteases

In theory, interrupting the interaction between sialic acid and EBA-175 could potentially inhibit the parasite's invasion of host red blood cells. Another approach is focused on inhibiting protease enzyme of *Plasmodium*. Falcipain, a family of *Plasmodium* cysteine protease enzymes, and plasmepsin, a family of *Plasmodium* aspartate protease enzymes, play an important role in the DV of the malaria parasite digesting hemoglobin, and these two-enzyme families have previously identified as potential drug targets. Scientists at GlaxoSmithKline have identified falcipain 2 and 3 inhibitors that halt *falciparum* growth at nanomolar concentrations. These inhibitors have been shown to have efficacy *in vivo* by curing *falciparum* malaria infections in a novel humanized SCID mouse model of blood stage efficacy of malaria. Plasmepsin drug discovery has waned given the identification of 10 plasmepsin paralogs in the malaria genome, and the additional finding of functional redundancy among the plasmepsin proteins. Recent studies have shown redundancy in in these two families of hemoglobinases, and studies have shown that plasmepsin zymogens are activated by falcipains or autoactivated when falcipain is inhibited. HIV protease inhibitors, which also target parasite aspartate proteases, have been demonstrated to have antimalarial activity. A study has been published showing the efficacy of HIV protease inhibitors tested against *falciparum* malaria *in vitro* and against *Plasmodium chabaudi in vivo*. Given many patients present with HIV and malaria co-infections, this data is quite interesting. HIV protease inhibitors are widely used for treatment of HIV in malaria-endemic regions [555].

8) Novel Folate Inhibitors

Methotrexate and aminopterin, which are both cancer drugs, have been shown to inhibit all of the dihydrofolate reductase (DHFR) enzymes, including the DHFR enzymes of humans. *In vitro* studies have shown that methotrexate and aminopterin inhibit the growth of *falciparum* malaria, and methotrexate has been shown to inhibit cancer cell division and the growth of parasites at similar concentrations. Given their toxicity to man and the narrow therapeutic index for treatment use, these drugs are not good choices for malaria treatment. A prodrug approach may be one way to provide antimalarial efficacy with an adequate therapeutic index. 2, 4-diamino-6-hydroxymethyl-pteridine (DAP), 2, 4-diaminopteroic acid (DAPA), and 2, 4 diamino- N10-methyl-pteroic acid (DAMPA) could be created by converting aminopterin (from DAP and DAPA), and methotrexate could be converted from DAMPA. DAP, DAPA, and DAMPA have been shown to inhibit parasite growth with micromolar IC_{50} values. DAMPA was shown to be the most active compound with IC_{50} values *in vitro* of 446 ng/ml tested with a parasite strain sensitive to antifolate compounds and 812 ng/ml against a parasite strain with high levels of anti-folate drug resistance. The authors of this study hypothesized DAMPA is metabolized to methotrexate by the activity of *falciparum* DHFR synthase, and if this is true, parasite specific toxic compounds converted by the malaria parasite from non-toxic precursors might be used as a paradigm for drug discovery efforts with other novel potent antimalarial compounds [569].

9) Emerging Technologies

Powerful new ‘omic’ methods are under development to determine drug mechanisms of action and mechanisms of drug resistance. A quantitative proteomics method is also under development to find malaria proteins with levels of expression that change after parasite treatment with chloroquine or artemisinin.

Another study has been published showing a high-throughput platform for selecting *falciparum* parasites with drug resistance mutations, and this platform is being used to screen for sequence or transcriptional using microarrays and high-throughput Solexa DNA sequencing technology. This technology has been used to develop extensive genome map of *falciparum* malaria. The study demonstrated over 93,000 single nucleotide polymorphisms, and this technology can be used to show selective sweeps associated with mutations associated with drug resistance (to include *pfcrt*); this technology can be used to characterize populations of parasites [59]. These studies on genomics created a genomic "barcode" comprised of 24 PCR primers, which can be used to identify a given strain with a unique genotype. This technology has great potential to provide the means to find drug resistance genes [59].

10.3.3. New Studies of the Mechanism of Action of Artemisinin

Drugs studies of the killing effects of artemisinin compounds have suggested the activity of this class may result from endoperoxide bridge interactions with heme associated iron derived from degradation of hemoglobin inside the digestive vacuole [567]. This hypothesis suggests that the interaction of heme iron reduces the endoperoxide bridge of artemisinin generating free radicals capable of parasite protein and lipid oxidation and alkylation. This hypothesis is supported by other data showing artemisinin potency is enhanced by oxidizing agents and by oxygen and decreased by reducing agents. Another proposed mechanism of action for artemisinin revolves around activation of artemisinins *via* endoperoxide bond cleavage driven by redox centers of intracellular iron and sulfur commonly found in the enzymes of *Plasmodium*. Enzyme alkylation results in parasite death, and other data has shown that incubation of radiolabeled artemisinin with parasite lysates led to the identification of several interacting proteins, which further suggests artemisinin activity may be the result of protein alkylation and inactivation.

One finding that argues against the heme iron hypothesis is the well-known efficacy of artemisinins against ring-stage parasites that have low heme concentrations. Artemisinin target proteins that have been hypothesized include electron transport proteins, cysteine proteases, and *pfatp6*, a SERCA-type Ca^{2-} ATPase. The potential interaction between pfatp6 and artemisinin is supported by experimental data showing the activity of this enzyme in transfected *Xenopus laevis* oocytes is inhibited by artemisinin, however, the activity of this enzyme is not affected by inactive artemisinin compounds such as desoxy-artemisinin, which does not have the characteristic endoperoxide bridge. Additional work using *Xenopus laevis* oocytes have shown a point mutation in *pfatp6* (L263E) can abolish growth inhibition by artemisinins. Additional studies investigating the artemisinin mechanism of action suggest artemisinin compounds may disrupt the digestive vacuole, but they do not affect the endoplasmic reticulum structure where PfATP6 is likely located. A proteomics based, study was published showing artemisinin compounds may be involved in disrupting parasite endocytosis of host proteins [555].

A very recent publication has shown a close association of artemisinin resistance in patients in a multicenter study of 1,241 adults and children at 15 sites in 10 countries. Patients were treated with artesunate administered at either 2 mg/kg or 4 mg/kg over a three-day period with another three days of treatment with an ACT. Patients infected with malaria in the Congo showed a median parasite clearance time of 1.9 hours while patients from the border region of Thailand and Cambodia showed a parasite clearance time of 7 hours. Parasites obtained from patients with the extended parasite clearance time which is the phenotypic hallmark of artemisinin drug resistance associated with point mutations in the kelch protein gene of *P. falciparum* located on chromosome 13 (kelch 13). Ultimately, the extended treatment with a three-day artemisinin treatment with another three days of ACT treatment showed a cure rate of 97.7% at day 42. This study demonstrates both a promising means of identifying patients with artemisinin resistant parasites by using molecular testing, and it shows a means of treating patients infected with artemisinin resistant *falciparum* malaria [128].

Over the last ten years, many have been optimistic that ACT treatment would provide a long-term solution for reducing malaria morbidity and mortality. This is similar to the optimism observed in earlier malaria eradication campaigns conducted years ago with CQ, which many believed would remain efficacious for many years. As we now know no drug is immune from development of drug resistance, identification of emerging drug resistance remains very important. The Worldwide Antimalarial Drug Resistance Network is a new network of laboratories testing isolated parasites for drug resistance, and this coordinated effort is an important initiative to define malaria drug resistance [568].

10.4. DEVELOPMENT OF NOVEL NON-ARTEMISININ-BASED COMBINATION THERAPIES

With the rising prevalence of artemisinin resistant, parasites in Southeast Asia observed over the last decade, there is new treatments are needed for drug-resistant malaria. While a number of potential candidate antimalarial drugs are under development, creating antimalarial drugs that are safe, well tolerated, and efficacious is not easy particularly in today's regulatory environment [570-572]. The new method of dosing antimalarial drugs in combinations with either additive or synergistic properties makes drug discovery more difficult.

10.4.1. Azithromycin-Chloroquine

Given the failures of ACT therapy in Southeast Asia, new antimalarial combinations must be discovered and developed clinically. With recent reports of a high prevalence of CQ sensitive *falciparum* parasites in Malawi because of the government's enforcement of no chloroquine sales, chloroquine-based combinations may be feasible in this country. Accordingly, studies were conducted to further characterize a combination of chloroquine and azithromycin to characterize this combination. *In vitro* studies of the chloroquine-azithromycin combination conducted over a 96-hour period, showed additive interactions against P. *falciparum* parasites. Synergistic interactions were noted at the 90% inhibitory concentration level. Further *in vitro* testing demonstrated the ability of amlodipine to reverse resistance against both quinine and chloroquine. *In vivo* rodent efficacy testing using the *P. yoelii* parasite in a 4 day Peters suppressive test showed suppression of 99.9% of parasitemia after treatment with a combination comprised of azithromycin, chloroquine, and the R enantiomer of amlodipine (the R enantiomer of amlodipine is devoid of the cardiotoxic liabilities observed when dosing the racemate or the S enantiomer of amlodipine).

PK/PD analyses conducted in this rodent model extrapolated to a 65 kg human adult suggests a dose of 1.8 g of R-amlodipine per day would be necessary to provide efficacy in a human, however, this is not a safe drug dose. While this study rules amlodipine out as part of a CQ-AZ combination treatment, the data does support the hypothesis that azithromycin (AZ) as both safe and efficacious as an antimalarial combination partner. AZ is attractive for antimalarial treatment as it is safe, well tolerated, and efficacious against malaria and other diseases. Clinical evaluations of a chloroquine-azithromycin combination treatment for intermittent prophylaxis treatment for pregnant women showed this combination was equally efficacious to SP, the previously used product. Given the emergence of growing resistance to SP treatment, a CQ-AZ combination may be useful for both intermittent preventive treatment and for malaria prophylaxis [115].

The CQ-AZ combination was tested to treat uncomplicated *falciparum* malaria in non-pregnant adults and consistent efficacy was achieved using a 3-day regimen composed of 1 g of azithromycin and 600 mg chloroquine dosed daily. Mass trachoma treatment campaigns have shown that azithromycin monotherapy selects for macrolide resistance in S. pneumonia bacteria, but this induced drug resistance reverses after therapy is completed. Azithromycin-chloroquine could be used in place of SP, and this combination has shown efficacy in clinical trials for treatment of chloroquine- resistant *falciparum* malaria in non-pregnant adults in sub-Saharan Africa, India, and Colombia. The CQ-AZ combination can be administered throughout pregnancy. This combination provides the added benefit of treating a number of STDs and other infections of the reproductive tract at the same time. Dose adjustment based on pharmacokinetic studies in pregnant women suggests that no adjustment to the AZ dose is necessary; however, the daily chloroquine dose should be adjusted to 600 mg for 3 days [573].

10.4.2. Clindamycin-Quinine

Clindamycin plus quinine is an antimalarial drug combination whose partner drugs have potent antimalarial properties when used as monotherapy with dissimilar modes of action. The rapid activity of quinine can provide efficacy immediately while the slower clindamycin will take more time to achieve killing of malaria parasites. When quinine is combined with clindamycin, quinine treatment can be cut down to 3 days which, given the unpleasant side effects of quinine (cinchonism) may improve patient compliance, and this 3 day regimen is much more practical as a treatment option. The clindamycin-quinine combination has the added benefit of safe administration to pregnant women, in all 3 trimesters, and children.

A systematic study was done including data from a number of randomized, controlled trials, which compared the clindamycin-quinine combination against other anti-malarial compounds for to treat uncomplicated malaria. The primary endpoint of this study was Day 28 treatment failure. Seven trials with 929 participants were utilized for this systematic review. The combination of clindamycin and quinine was shown to significantly reduce the Day 28 treatment failures compared to monotherapy with quinine (relative risk or RR of 0.14), the combination of quinine-sulfadoxine-pyrimethamine (RR 0.17), amodiaquine monotherapy (RR 0.11), or chloroquine monotherapy (RR 0.11). Similar efficacy was shown when the combination of clindamycin-quinine was compared to the combination of quinine-tetracycline (RR 0.33 [95% CI 0.01 to 8.04]), quinine-doxycycline (RR 1.00), artesunate-clindamycin (RR 0.57), or chloroquine-clindamycin (RR 0.38).

Adverse events in this review were poorly reported, but those that were reported were similar among treatment groups. While this data is encouraging, additional trials with more power are needed to compare quinine-clindamycin to existing artemisinin combination treatments such as artesunate-mefloquine or DHA-piperaquine or artemether-lumefantrine to treat pregnant women with uncomplicated malaria. Additional studies are also needed to determine the utility of clindamycin-quinine to treat pregnant women with malaria [547].

10.4.3. Fosmidomycin and Clindamycin

A study was conducted to investigate the PK profile of fosmidomycin administered as monotherapy or combined with clindamycin to treat Thai patients infected with uncomplicated *falciparum* malaria in Tak Province. Patients were treated with1,200 mg of fosmidomycin administered every 8 hours over a 7 day period (n = 15) or a drug combination comprised of 900 mg of fosmidomycin and 600 mg of clindamycin administered every 12 hours over a 7 day period (n = 18). Samples of both blood and urine were taken for PK studies of fosmidomycin and clindamycin. The efficacy endpoints for this study included parasitological and clinical evaluations, and safety measures were made based on laboratory and clinical data. No fosmidomycin or combination therapy associated adverse events were noted in this study.

The fosmidomycin-clindamycin combination treatment was very efficacious with cure rates of 100%, while the cure rate of fosmidomycin monotherapy was shown to be only 22% at day 28-day. The pharmacokinetic parameters of fosmidomycin monotherapy and combination treatment were comparable with the exception of Vd/F and CL/F, which declined in patients dosed with fosmidomycin and clindamycin in combination. The profiles of fosmidomycin and clindamycin over time were best modeled using a one-compartment open model comprised of first-order absorption and elimination including absorption lag time. Steady state concentrations of both drugs were achieved at approximately the second or third dose. Dose accumulation was not noted during administration of multiple doses, and recovery of fosmidomycin in the urine was shown to be 18.7% following monotherapy and 20% after combination treatment.

This PK study was the first published work that characterized the PK profiles of clindamycin and fosmidomycin to optimize the dose for fosmidomycin by itself or combined with clindamycin to treat uncomplicated *falciparum* malaria. These studies showed treatment regimen of fosmidomycin-clindamycin in combination for 3 days is needed to achieve 100% cures of multidrug-resistant *P. falciparum*, and this dosing regimen was shown to be not only efficacious but also well tolerated. Further study in other geographic locations will be needed for further confirmation of this dose and the ratio of one partner drug to the other over a 3-

day dosing interval to achieve similar results of safety and efficacy for treatment of drug resistant *falciparum* [574].

10.5. DEVELOPMENT OF NEW LONG-ACTING MEDICINES AND FORMULATIONS

10.5.1. The Challenges of Maintaining ACT Efficacy for Treatment of Uncomplicated Malaria

All current ACTs on market contain partner drugs whose efficacy is affected by endemic parasite drug resistance in many parts of the world. Retaining the use of artemisinin combination therapies and other combination treatments will require clinical trials to provide adequate data to pick the right combination comprised of the right partner drugs to be used in the right geographic setting, and such studies must consider the potential issues associated with using various treatments. These issues can only be understood by conducting longitudinal trials, which are conducted over an extended period to get patient follow up data by treating patients with the same drug for every malaria infection they present with over a one-year period. Longitudinal trials have the advantage of not only assessing initial treatment efficacy but also assessing the loss of efficacy or emergence of drug resistant parasites after repeated drug administration. Some African studies have already indicated a significant failure rate [5-8] in combination therapies that include amodiaquine due to amodiaquine drug resistance in the local parasite population. Amodiaquine resistance is likely to spread more rapidly as amodiaquine combinations are being adopted the treatment of choice for uncomplicated *falciparum* malaria [74].

Because new malaria control policies are being made based on sound, well-conducted clinical studies, the goal of replacing antimalarials that are failing with more efficacious combination treatments is being achieved. To enhance the benefits and extend the longevity of existing combination treatments, will require learning from past mistakes to avoid making future mistakes. New strategies are required to inhibit current combination treatments that are working from going down the same drug resistance pathways of drugs like chloroquine, which have failed due to overuse, and lack of good partner drugs. It is an open question whether increased knowledge of how drugs work, the PK/PK profiles of existing and new candidate drugs, and innovative clinical study design can create or sustain new or existing combination drugs. Given the data on renewed efficacy of chloroquine in Malawi, new questions arise regarding whether it is possible to rotate drugs in and out of use to preserve efficacy over time.

Another question that has arisen is whether drug resistance can be diminished by using a number of combination treatments in parallel rather than simply replacing one failed therapy with another. Looking beyond drug treatment policy, a further question arises regarding the use of combination drugs along with other control measures like indoor residual spraying, insecticide-treated bed nets, vector control, and potentially malaria vaccine treatment will lead to reductions in malaria transmission and decreases in drug resistance. The answers to these kinds of questions will be useful in understanding the best policies for implementation of all antimalarial interventions in the most efficacious manner possible to avoid emergence of drug resistance.

Given the cost of implementing new antimalarial combination treatments and other antimalarial interventions, funding must be provided through outside donors and policy interventions in endemic countries must be instituted to make sure that funds provided are used wisely. While the safety and efficacy of combination treatments have been shown through many studies and clinical use in endemic regions, special population studies of young children, pregnant women, and breast-feeding mothers with babies are lacking. Many comparative efficacy studies on combination treatments have been published illustrating the advantages and disadvantages of those drugs compared, but none of the studies has compared all combinations and the study methodologies chosen are variable. Thus, finding clear answers to all questions posed given the vast quantity of data accumulated is not easy. Accordingly, a multi-treatment random- effects meta-analysis was conducted to create a tool for comparing the efficacy of various ACT drugs [238].

With this method, clinical efficacy by day 28 was assessed between arrays of commonly used artemisinin combination drugs. Total 32 studies provided the data for this meta-analysis; 4 of these studies were conducted in Asia, 2 were conducted in South America, and the remaining 26 studies were conducted in Africa. The drugs compared included AS-SP, AQ-SP, AS-MQ, AS-CQ, CQ-SP, and AL. The percentages of treatment success for each antimalarial combination therapy corrected by PCR at day 28 are shown in Table **32**. The meta-analysis showed artemether-lumefantrine has increased clinical efficacy as shown by the Day 28 cure rates corrected by PCR over all other combinations assessed followed closely by the combination of AS-MQ. AS-AQ and AS-SP were not necessarily found to be inferior, but their percentage of success corrected by PCR at day 28 is lower and close to the 90% threshold. The lowest percentage of success was shown in patients treated with CQ-AS (45.8%), and the highest percentage of success was show in patients treated with AL (97.4%) [575].

Regardless of the study methods used to assess clinical treatment failure, prevention of drug resistance using combination treatment is an essential requirement of every malaria control program.

Table 32: Percentages of success for each antimalarial combination therapy at day 28 PCR corrected [575]

Treatment Combination(s)	Percentage Success (%)
Amodiaquine + Artesunate (AQ-AS)	88.5
Amodiaquine + Sulfadoxine-pyrimethamine (AQ-SP)	85.7
Chloroquine + Artesunate (CQ-AS)	45.8
Chloroquine + Sulfadoxine-pyrimethamine (CQ-SP)	72.1
Mefloquine + Artesunate (MQ-AS)	96.9
Sulfadoxine-pyrimethamine + Artesunate (SP-AS)	82.6
Artemether-lumefantrine (AL)	97.4

The data was also cited from a WHO guideline [1].

10.5.2. Other ACT Combinations in Development

Parasite resistance to sulfadoxine-pyrimethamine and chloroquine led to the implementation of ACTs for first-line malaria treatment. Unlike other antimalarial drugs, artemisinins are exceptionally potent against early ring stage of malaria parasites and have been shown to reduce malaria transmission. Maintaining the efficacy of current ACTs is a worthy goal, and ultimately, the spread of drug resistance to either artemisinin derivatives or drug partners will require innovation of new artemisinin combination therapies for malaria treatment.

1) Artesunate-Chlorproguanil-Dapsone

One combination that has been studied is artesunate combined with chlorproguanil and dapsone. Chlorproguanil-dapsone is an antifolate-sulfonamide combination with a similar mechanism of action to SP and synergistic properties similar to SP. Chlorproguanil can be considered as a pro-drug for the active antifolate drug chlorcycloguanil, as chlorproguanil is readily metabolized to chlorcycloguanil by CYP 2C19. The activity of CYP 2C19 is reduced in 20% of Asians, and enzyme activity is also reduced by increased concentration of estrogen hormones found in pregnant women and women using oral contraceptives. The advantages of this combination include good tolerability, increased activity against moderately resistant *falciparum* parasites compared to SP, and more rapid drug elimination, which provides less selective pressure and helps avoid emergence of drug resistance.

Both chlorproguanil and SP are ineffective against *falciparum* parasites with a specific folate enzyme mutation (the Ile164Leu mutation) which is commonly found in parasites in South America, Asia, and in parts of Africa. The disadvantages of this drug combination include cross-resistance to SP and safety concerns regarding administration of dapsone, which causes hemolytic anemia in G6PD deficient patients who are quite common in malaria endemic areas, and the lack of a post-treatment prophylactic effect. This ACT was developed by a collaboration of GSK, UNICEF, the World Bank, Medicines for Malaria Venture, and WHO. Unfortunately, this combination was withdrawn in 2008 from development because of significant reductions in hemoglobin of patients treated with both combinations of chlorproguanil-dapsone and artesunate-chlorproguanil-dapsone [375].

2) Artesunate-Atovaquone-Proguanil (AAP)

Another novel combination under clinical development is artesunate combined with atovaquone-proguanil (AAP). The combination of atovaquone-proguanil has a different and synergistic mechanism of action from other antimalarials as it affects parasite respiration. Proguanil has antimalarial activity in this combination, and the mechanism of action is not *via* its triazine metabolite, the antifolate drug cycloguanil, so it remains efficacious against antifolate resistant parasites. One point mutation in the binding site of atovaquone in the cyt b protein provides high levels of resistance to atovaquone, which is reduced by the drug synergism provided by proguanil. Atovaquone absorption, similar to halofantrine and lumefantrine, is enhanced by co-administration with fats. The elimination half-life of atovaquone (1-2 days) is consistent with a daily dosed drug being used for 3-day treatment. Pregnant women have reduced plasma concentrations of atovaquone and proguanil in pregnancy, which is quite commonly observed in pregnant women dosed with other antimalarials. Atovaquone-proguanil is very well tolerated with no serious adverse effects. The principal barrier to its use has been the high cost of atovaquone synthesis, and this combination drug is unaffordable for patients in malaria endemic areas [347].

In 2005, a study of 81 pregnant Karen women with uncomplicated *falciparum* malaria reported less treatment failures by day 63 after administration of artesunate- atovaquone-proguanil administered as part of a study comparing the efficacy of supervised quinine administration over a 7-day period *versus* 3 days of artesunate combined with atovaquone-proguanil. Eighty -one pregnant women were enrolled in this study, and 42 were administered SQ7while 39 were administered AAP. There were no differences observed in the duration of pregnancy, the weight of babies borne, or the rates of genetic abnormalities of babies, or the development and growth of infants who were monitored for 1 year. AAP has been demonstrated to be a safe, effective, and well-tolerated treatment for *falciparum* malaria in pregnant women, but the cost of this combination is high. While the number of patients in this study was small, these results support the hypothesis AAP is both efficacious and safe for both the fetus and the mother [576, 577].

3) Artemisinin-Napthoquine (ART-NQ)

Artemisinin-napthoquine (ART-NQ) is a co-formulated single dose antimalarial drug under clinical development. Given the limited PK data on the two drug components, a study was conducted on the disposition of ART-NQ in children living in Papua New Guinea aged 5 to12 years infected with uncomplicated malaria. A single dose combination dose of 22 mg of artemisinin and 9 mg/kg of Napthoquine administered with milk were administered to 17 children and 2 daily combination doses of 22 mg of artemisinin and 9 mg/kg of napthoquine administered with water to 16 children. The plasma NQ concentrations were assayed by HPLC, and the plasma ART concentration was assayed using LC-MS. A set of population-based, multi-compartment PK models for ART and NQ were created to analyze the data derived from this study.

The disposition of NQ was best modeled using a three-compartment model comprised of a mean absorption half-life of 1.0 hour, and the predicted C_{max} was shown to range as high as 57 μg/liter after administration of a second dose in patients administered 9 mg/kg of napthoquine with water. The mean NQ biological half-life was shown to be 22.8 days, the clearance relative to bioavailability (CL/F) was shown to be 1.1 liters/h/kg, and the drug volume at steady state relative to bioavailability (V(ss)/F) was shown to be 710 liters /kg. When NQ was administered with fat *versus* water, and increase in bioavailability of 25% was observed. The disposition of artemisinin was best modeled using a two-compartment model with a mean CL/F of 4.1 liters/h/kg and a V(ss)/F of 21 liters/kg, which is similar to what has been observed in previous artemisinin PK studies. A decrease of 77% in bioavailability of artemisinin was noted in the treatment group administered 22 mg of artesunate after the second artemisinin dose which may be a consequence of auto-induction of CYP-mediated artemisinin metabolism. The results of this study show NQ has PK properties consistent with a role as part of an artemisinin combination treatment for uncomplicated pediatric malaria [578].

These studies of NQ were reported in China, and both NQ and artesunate have been shown to be safe, well tolerated, and efficacious as monotherapy and in combination for treatment of patients suffering from malaria. The combination of artemisinin and napthoquine phosphate is under development as an oral fixed dose combination tablet called Co-napthoquine. Artemisinin monotherapy over a seven-day period has been shown to be associated with reduced patient compliance, and there is an increased risk associated with artemisinin neurotoxicity associated with seven-day treatment duration. Napthoquine phosphate has a longer half-life than artesunate, and monotherapy has been shown to provide efficacy with a low rate of recrudescence. The two elements of this combination have been shown to act synergistically in animal models of malaria, and clinically the combination provides enhanced relief of malaria symptoms and better rates of cure than either component administered as monotherapy [579].

4) Artesunate -Azithromycin (AS-AZ)

The combination of artesunate and azithromycin (AS-AZ) has been tested in a number of comparative efficacy trials. One such trial was conducted in 261 children in Tanzania infected with uncomplicated malaria. Total 129 of the children were randomized to the AS-AZ arm (artesunate at 4 mg/kg and azithromycin at 20 mg/kg of azithromycin administered daily for 3 days). A total of 132 children were randomized to the AL arm of the study (1 fixed dose tablet of AL dosed every day over a 3 day period for children under 15 kg and 2 fixed dose tablets of AL dosed every day over a 3 day period for children greater 15 kg. The results of this study showed parasitological treatment failure rates by Day 28 of 32% in the AS-AZ treatment group and 9% in the AL treatment group. Similar findings were observed by Day 42, and the authors concluded that the AS and AZ in combination is not recommended for malaria treatment [580, 581].

A second trial of this combination was conducted in a Phase 2/3 clinical trial of 228 patients aged 8 to 65 in Bangladesh who were randomized in a 2:1 ratio into treatment with daily treatment with AS-AZ for 3 days or artemether-lumefantrine administered orally twice daily for 3 days. The results of this study were at odds with the study conducted in Tanzania as the 42 day cure rate for the AS-AZ arm was shown to be 94.6% (95% CI 89.38%-97.44%) and 97% for the AL arm (95% CI 89.45%-99.4%). The authors of this study concluded that AS-AZ was efficacious and recommended for treatment of uncomplicated malaria. The only difference between the two studies was the dose of AZ used, 20 mg/kg of AZ in the Tanzanian study in 2009 and 30 mg/kg of AZ used for the Bangladesh study in 2010 (the dose of AS administered was 4 mg/kg in both studies). Clearly, the dose of AZ used is important to achieve efficacy for the AS-AZ combination [580, 582].

5) Artemisinin-Piperaquine

To determine the best dose of the combination therapy of artemisinin-piperaquine to treat uncomplicated *falciparum* malaria, a comparative efficacy study was undertaken to test seven candidate regimens in 411 patients infected with uncomplicated malaria in Bangkok. Studies of the various candidate regimens were performed from May 2005 to June 2006. The authors of this study compared three-day treatment regimens artemether-lumefantrine compared to artesunate-mefloquine, dihydroartemisinin-piperaquine (Artekin) to compare with candidate regimens of artemisinin-piperaquine (Artequick) administered over a 2-3 day period. Initially, patients administered each of the drug regimens had a rapid parasitological and clinical response. All of the various regimens tested were safe and well tolerated and no serious adverse effects were noted. The 28-Day rates of cure for artemisinin-piperaquine dosed at 2.4 mg/kg of artemisinin and 14.4 mg/kg of piperaquine administered daily for two days were <80%, and the cure rates for artemisinin-piperaquine dosed at 3.2 mg/kg of artemisinin and 16.0 mg/kg of piperaquine dosed daily for two days as also <80%. The cure rates of both of these candidate regimens administered for 3 days were >98%.

The 2-day courses of artemisinin combined with piperaquine were associated with late recrudescence within the 28 days of hospital observation in approximately 25% of the patients treated. In contrast, both candidate artemisinin-piperaquine (Artequick®) 3-day regimens and dihydroartemisinin-piperaquine (Artekin®) dosed for 3 days, resulted in cure rates >98% and were as well tolerated as the reference treatments. Both Artequick and Artekin combinations represent potential alternatives to artesunate-mefloquine and artemether-lumefantrine and merit further evaluation, including better pharmacokinetic characterizations of these combinations, additional studies in children and pregnant women, and carefully conducted field trials [583].

10.5.3. The Future of ACTs

The future for ACT treatment looks promising barring any increase in artemisinin derivative resistance. The majority of the novel artemisinin combination treatments discussed here have potential, and the challenge going forward is the development of an array of new combination treatments that are safe, efficacious, cheap, and easy to administer to provide alternatives when existing ACTs are lost to emerging drug resistance or must be retired to avoid the onset of treatment failure. Ultimately, all of these efforts will be needed to develop the necessary means to control, contain, and eventually eradicate malaria [347].

CONCLUSION

Artemisinin drugs are an essential element to treat drug-resistant *falciparum* malaria, and if these drugs are lost to resistance, the world may be faced with malaria that cannot be treated. Antimalarial drug resistance involves an initial mutation producing a drug resistant parasite, and the second stage involves the selection of malaria parasites which now have a survival advantage when exposed to an antimalarial drug leading to parasite transmission and spread of resistant parasites. To protect existing ACTs and novel drug combinations devised in the future, worldwide efforts are needed to monitor resistance, come up with new plans to decrease the impact of drug resistance, and characterize the molecular basis of drug resistance. PK/PD evaluations and other TK/TD studies that we will discuss in depth in other chapters will outline the advantages and disadvantages of leading prospective drug combinations that are the most effective and most sustainable in the populations of malaria endemic countries. We also discuss the pros and cons of developing novel CT drugs with new mechanisms of action not based on current ACTs, and the strategies by which it may be possible to optimize the use of currently available combination therapy drugs for years to come.

Maintaining the efficacy of current ACTs is a worthy goal, and ultimately, the spread of drug resistance to either artemisinin derivatives or drug partners will require innovation of new artemisinin combination therapies for malaria treatment. ACTs on market rely on partner drugs subject to drug resistance. The long-term utility of an ACT is dependent on finding the best partner drugs to be used in the right setting, and such studies must consider what the different impacts may be when various treatments are assessed. Simply conducting a study and not following up long-term does not provide the necessary data to assess an operational impact, which extends many months after studies, are normally completed. Longitudinal trials extending over a year's time can identify emergence of drug resistant parasites and a loss of treatment efficacy when regiments are used repeatedly. Some African studies have already indicated a significant failure rate in combination therapies that include amodiaquine likely due to amodiaquine drug resistance in the local parasite population. Amodiaquine resistance is predicted to spread more rapidly as amodiaquine combinations are being adopted for first-line treatment in several African countries.

Innovative CQ-like molecules such as pyronaridine and napthoquine have been studied, and clinical trial data for both show promise. The novel combination of

Qigui Li and Mark R. Hickman

two older antimalarial drugs, chlorproguanil, and dapsone, with artesunate is another promising non-artemisinin combination under development. Atovaquone–proguanil combined with artesunate has been shown to be efficacious against drug resistant *falciparum* malaria. Synthetic trioxolanes may be cheaper than the artemisinin compounds currently in use, and traditional derivatives may be displaced as part of an ACT. Future ACT development should also include safety evaluation particularly of underserved populations at risk such as children and pregnant women. Efficacy and safety are always the most important elements of antimalarial drug combination development, but development of parasite resistance is a third imperative that must be considered.

New drug combinations should be administered as fixed-dose formulations to avoid problems with compliance, and fixed dose combinations must be tested carefully for use in children. Child friendly drug formulations such as granules or dispersible tablets must be researched as part of the effort to create treatments optimized for this special population group. New techniques are required to preclude ACTs from being lost to drug resistance similar to chloroquine, which failed due to overuse and a lack of good partner drugs. As new malaria control policies are made based on good clinical research, the goal of replacing malaria monotherapy drugs with better ACTs is being accomplished. In order to enhance the benefits and prolong the use of ACTs, we must learn from past mistakes to avoid making future mistakes.

Drug combinations must be composed of drugs with shorter half-lives ideally providing steady release of drug, which is quickly cleared combined with a second drug with a similar PK/PD profile. Such a combination treatment would provide enhanced efficacy with decreased probability of selecting for drug resistance. This type of combination therapy would provide rapid killing of parasites with a long enough half-life to facilitate administration over a limited period of time, which will enhance compliance. Rapid elimination of a combination therapy precludes parasite exposure to sub-therapeutic drug levels, which are well known to select for drug resistant parasites.

Nanotechnology may offer another approach for developing drugs with the ideal PK/PD profile. Innovative drug development approaches will be needed to create novel antimalarials or extend the use of existing drugs. Setting-specific criteria must also be employed to determine the right choice of drug for the right epidemiologic setting. One example where the use of long-duration drugs with sub-therapeutic levels may be appropriate is mass drug administration to eradicate malaria in areas with seasonal transmission. This example shows why setting-specific epidemiology criteria are needed for tailored target product profiles for drug use based on the local parasites, populations, epidemiological settings, and the proposed use of a drug to reach a population eradication goal.

With some experience gained in developing the first-generation ACTs, there are examples of empiric drug development that show what was done, however, these examples may not be the best method for the future to enhance treatment efficacy and achieve reductions in morbidity and mortality and malaria transmission in endemic countries. Assessment of the use of first generation ACTs also suggest that drug combination therapies (*e.g.* ACTs) can affect malaria transmission similar to use of insecticide treated bednets in regions with low malaria transmission. Because new malaria control policies are being made on the basis of good clinical research, the goal of replacing monotherapeutic treatments that are failing with better combination drugs is being reached. Future development of novel antimalarials and drug combinations will be a challenging task requiring the best practices of the modern era to achieve success.

REFERENCES

REFERENCES

[1] WHO, Guidelines for the treatment of malaria. Second edition March 2010. Geneva, Switzerland, WHO. Available from: http://www.who.int/malaria/publications/atoz/9789241547925/en/; or http://whqlibdoc.who.int/publications/2010/9789241547925_eng.pdf

[2] WHO, Global Report on Antimalarial Drug Efficacy and Drug Resistance: 2000-2010. Geneva: World Health Organization; 2010.

[3] WHO Marketing of Oral Artemisinin-Based Monotherapy Medicines at Country Level 2010; Available from: http://www.who.int/malaria/monotherapy_NDRAs.pdf.

[4] WHO, Global Fund proposal development: WHO policy brief on malaria WHO/GMP July 2011. Available from: http://www.who.int/malaria/publications/atoz/malaria_gf_proposal_dev_who_policy_brief/en/index.html; or http://www.who.int/malaria/publications/atoz/malaria_gf_proposal_dev_who_policy_brief_201106.pdf

[5] Dondorp AM, Nosten F, Yi P, Das D, Phyo AP, Tarning J, Lwin KM, Ariey F, Hanpithakpong W, Lee SJ, Ringwald P, Silamut K, Imwong M, Chotivanich K, Lim P, Herdman T, An SS, Yeung S, Singhasivanon P, Day NP, Lindegardh N, Socheat D, White NJ. Artemisinin resistance in *Plasmodium falciparum* malaria. N Engl J Med. 2009;361: 455-467.

[6] Ariey F, Witkowski B, Amaratunga C, Beghain J, Langlois AC, Khim N, Kim S, Duru V, Bouchier C, Ma L, Lim P, Leang R, Duong S, Sreng S, Suon S, Chuor CM, Bout DM, Ménard S, Rogers WO, Genton B, Fandeur T, Miotto O, Ringwald P, Le Bras J, Berry A, Barale JC, Fairhurst RM, Benoit-Vical F, Mercereau-Puijalon O, Ménard D. A molecular marker of artemisinin-resistant *Plasmodium falciparum* malaria. Nature 2014 Jan 2;505(7481):50-5.

[7] Fairhurst RM, Nayyar GM, Breman JG, Hallett R, Vennerstrom JL, Duong S, Ringwald P, Wellems TE, Plowe CV, Dondorp AM. Artemisinin-resistant malaria: research challenges, opportunities, and public health implications. Am J Trop Med Hyg. 2012; 87: 231-41.

[8] WHO, Global Plan for Artemisinin Resistance Containment (GPARC) Geneva: World Health Organization; 2011.

[9] White NJ. Delaying antimalarial drug resistance with combination chemotherapy. Parasitologia. 1999; 41: 301-8.

[10] Li Q, Weina P. Artesunate: the best drug in the treatments of severe and complicated malaria. Pharmaceuticals. 2010; 3: 2322-2332.

[11] Bindschedler M, Lefèvre G, Degen P, Sioufi A. Comparison of the cardiac effects of the antimalarials co-artemether and halofantrine in healthy participants. Am J Trop Med Hyg. 2002; 66: 293-8.

[12] Li Q, Hickman M. Toxicokinetic and toxicodynamic (TK/TD) evaluation to determine and predict the neurotoxicity of artemisinins. Toxicology. 2011; 279: 1-9.

[13] Li Q, Hickman M. Chapter 17: Pharmacokinetic (PK) and Pharmacodynamic Profiles of Artemisinin Derivatives Influence Drug Neurotoxicity in Animals. Ed. By Ayman Noreddin in "Advanced Pharmacokinetics - Theory, Methods and Applications". InTech Open Access Publisher, Rijeka (April 20, 2012) Page: 323- 356.

[14] Gautam A, Ahmed T, Batra V, Paliwal J. Pharmacokinetics and pharmacodynamics of endoperoxide antimalarials. Curr Drug Metab. 2009;10: 289-306.

[15] Li Q, Si Y, Xie L, Zhang J, Weina P. Severe embryolethality of artesunate related to pharmacokinetics following intravenous and intramuscular doses in pregnant rats. Birth Defects Res B Dev Reprod Toxicol. 2009; 86: 385-393.

[16] Li Q, Weina P. Severe embryotoxicity of artemisinin derivatives in experimental animals, but possibly safe in pregnant women. Molecules. 2010; 15: 40-57.

[17] Gordi T, Xie R, Jusko WJ. Semi-mechanistic pharmacokinetic/pharmacodynamic modelling of the antimalarial effect of artemisinin. Br J Clin Pharmacol. 2005; 60: 594-604.

[18] Pongtavornpinyo W, Yeung S, Hastings IM, Dondorp AM, Day NP, White NJ. Spread of anti-malarial drug resistance: mathematical model with implications for ACT drug policies. Malar J. 2008; 7: 229.

[19] Wongsrichanalai C, Pickard AL, Wernsdorfer WH, Meshnick SR. Epidemiology of drug-resistant malaria. Lancet Infect Dis. 2002; 2: 209-18.

[20] WHO, Update on artemisinin resistance - April 2012, Geneva: World Health Organization; 2012.

Qigui Li and Mark R. Hickman

[21] Sá JM, Twu O, Hayton K, Reyes S, Fay MP, Ringwald P, Wellems TE. Geographic patterns of *Plasmodium falciparum* drug resistance distinguished by differential responses to amodiaquine and chloroquine. Proceedings of the National Academy o Sciences of the United States of America, 2009; 106: 18883-18889.

[22] Malisa AL, Pearce RJ, Abdulla S, Mshinda H, Kachur PS, Bloland P, Roper C. Drug coverage in treatment of malaria and the consequences for resistance evolution evidence from the use of sulphadoxine/pyrimethamine. Malaria Journal, 2010; 9: 190.

[23] WHO. Guidelines for the treatment of malaria. 2nd Ed. Geneva, World Health Organization. 2010.

[24] White NJ. Antimalarial drug resistance. J Clin Invest. 2004; 113: 1084-1092.

[25] Noedl H, Se Y, Schaecher K, Smith BL, Socheat D, Fukuda MM. Artemisinin Resistance in Cambodia 1 (ARC1) study consortium: Evidence of artemisinin-resistant malaria in western Cambodia. N Engl J Med. 2008; 359: 2619-2620.

[26] Uhlemann AC, Cameron A, Eckstein-Ludwig U, Fischbarg J, Iserovich P, Zuniga FA, East M, Lee A, Brady L, Haynes RK, Krishna S. A single amino acid residue can determine the sensitivity of SERCAs to artemisinins. Nat Struct Mol Biol. 2005; 12: 628-629.

[27] Chretien JP, Fukuda M, Noedl H. Improving surveillance for antimalarial drug resistance. JAMA.,2007; 297: 2278-2281.

[28] WHO. Susceptibility of *Plasmodium falciparum* to antimalarial drugs. Report on global monitoring 1996-2004. Geneva, World Health Organization. 2005.

[29] Huong NM, Hewitt S, Davis TM, Dao LD, Toan TQ, Kim TB, Hanh NT, Phuong VN, Nhan DH, Cong LD. Resistance of *Plasmodium falciparum* to antimalarial drugs in a highly endemic area of southern Viet Nam: a study *in vivo* and *in vitro*. Transactions of the Royal Society of Tropical Medicine and Hygiene, 2001; 95: 325-329.

[30] Yang H, Liu D, Yang Y, Fan B, Yang P, Li X, Li C, Dong Y, Yang C. Changes in susceptibility of *Plasmodium falciparum* to artesunate *in vitro* in Yunnan Province, China. Transactions of the Royal Society of Tropical Medicine and Hygiene, 2003; 97: 226-228.

[31] Noedl H, Socheat D, Satimai W. Artemisinin-resistant malaria in Asia. New England Journal of Medicine, 2009; 361: 540-541.

[32] Lim P, Wongsrichanalai C, Chim P, Khim N, Kim S, Chy S, Sem R, Nhem S, Yi P, Duong S, Bouth DM, Genton B, Beck HP, Gobert JG, Rogers WO, Coppee JY, Fandeur T, Mercereau-Puijalon O, Ringwald P, Le Bras J, Ariey F. Decreased *in vitro* susceptibility of *Plasmodium falciparum* isolates to artesunate, mefloquine, chloroquine, and quinine in Cambodia from 2001 to 2007. Antimicrobial Agents and Chemotherapy, 2010; 54: 2135-2142.

[33] Luxemburger C, Brockman A, Silamut K, Nosten F, van Vugt M, Gimenez F, Chongsuphajaisiddhi T, White NJ. Two patients with *falciparum* malaria and poor *in vivo* responses to artesunate. Transactions of the Royal Society of Tropical Medicine and Hygiene, 1998; 92: 668-669.

[34] Satimai W, Sudathip P, Vijaykadga S, Khamsiriwatchara A, Sawang S, Potithavoranan T, Sangvichean A, Delacollette C, Singhasivanon P, Kaewkungwal J, Lawpoolsri S. Artemisinin resistance containment project in Thailand. II: responses to mefloquine-artesunate combination therapy among *falciparum* malaria patients in provinces bordering Cambodia. Malar J. 2012; 11: 300.

[35] Miller LH, Ackerman HC, Su XZ, Wellems TE. Malaria biology and disease pathogenesis: insights for new treatments. Nat Med. 2013; 19: 156-67.

[36] WWARN, 2011. Asia Regional Center Activities: Tracking Resistance to Artemisinin Collaboration (TRAC). Available at: http://www.wwarn.org/about-us/regional-centres/asia-regionalcentre.

[37] Dondorp AM, Yeung S, White L, *et al*. Artemisinin resistance: current status and scenarios for containment. Nat Rev Microbiol. 2010; 8: 272-280.

[38] Anderson TJ, Nair S, Nkhoma S, *et al*. High heritability of malaria parasite clearance rate indicates a genetic basis for artemisinin resistance in western Cambodia. J Infect Dis. 2010; 201: 1326-1330.

[39] O'Brien C, Henrich PP, Passi N, Fidock DA. Recent clinical and molecular insights into emerging artemisinin resistance in *Plasmodium falciparum*. Curr Opin Infect Dis. 2011; 24: 570-7.

[40] Adjuik M, Babiker A, Garner P, Olliaro P, Taylor W, White N. International Artemisinin Study Group. Artesunate combinations for treatment of malaria: Meta-analysis. Lancet. 2004; 363: 9-17.

[41] Carrara VI, Zwang J, Ashley EA, Price RN, Stepniewska K, Barends M, Brockman A, Anderson T, McGready R, Phaiphun L, Proux S, van Vugt M, Hutagalung R, Lwin KM, Phyo AP, Preechapornkul P, Imwong M, Pukrittayakamee S, Singhasivanon P, White NJ, Nosten F. Changes in the treatment

responses to artesunate-mefloquine on the northwestern border of Thailand during 13 years of continuous deployment. PLoS ONE. 2009; 4: e4551.

[42] Plowe CV, Roper C, Barnwell JW, Happi CT, Joshi HH, Mbacham W, Meshnick SR, Mugittu K, Naidoo I, Price RN, Shafer RW, Sibley CH, Sutherland CJ, Zimmerman PA Rosenthal PJ. World Antimalarial Resistance Network (WARN) III: molecular markers for drug resistant malaria. Malar J 2007; 6: 121.

[43] Deplaine G, Lavazec C, Bischoff E, Natalang O, Perrot S, Guillotte-Blisnick M, Coppe'e JY, Pradines B, Mercereau-Puijalon O, David PH. Artesunate tolerance in transgenic *Plasmodium falciparum* parasites over-expressing a tryptophan rich protein. Antimicrob Agents Chemother 2011; 55: 2576-2584.

[44] Mok S, Imwong M, Mackinnon M, Sim J, Ramadoss R, Yi P, Mayxay M, Chotivanich K, Liong KY, Russell B, Socheat D, Newton PN, Day NP, White NJ, Preiser PR, Nosten F, Dondorp AM, Bozdech Z. Artemisinin resistance in *Plasmodium falciparum* is associated with an altered temporal pattern of transcription. BMC Genomics. 2011; 12: 391.

[45] Imwong M, Dondorp AM, Nosten F, Yi P, Mungthin M, Hanchana S, Das D, Phyo AP, Lwin KM, Pukrittayakamee S, Lee SJ, Saisung S, Koecharoen K, Nguon C, Day NP, Socheat D, White NJ, 2010. Exploring the contribution of candidate genes to artemisinin resistance in *Plasmodium falciparum*. Antimicrob Agents Chemother 2010; 54: 2886-2892.

[46] Teuscher F, Gatton ML, Chen N, *et al.* Artemisinin-induced dormancy in *Plasmodium falciparum*: duration, recovery rates, and implications in treatment failure. J Infect Dis. 2010; 202: 1362-1368.

[47] Witkowski B, Lelievre J, Barragan MJ, *et al.* Increased tolerance to artemisinin in *Plasmodium falciparum* is mediated by a quiescence mechanism. Anti-microb Agents Chemother. 2010; 54: 1872-1877.

[48] Klonis N, Crespo-Ortiz MP, Bottova I, *et al.* Artemisinin activity against *Plasmodium falciparum* requires hemoglobin uptake and digestion. Proc Natl Acad Sci U S A. 2011; 108: 11405-11410.

[49] Codd A, Teuscher F, Kyle DE, *et al.* Artemisinin-induced parasite dormancy: a plausible mechanism for treatment failure. Malar J. 2011; 10: 56.

[50] Saralamba S, Pan-Ngum W, Maude RJ, *et al.* Intrahost modeling of artemisinin resistance in *Plasmodium falciparum*. Proc Natl Acad Sci U S A. 2010; 108: 397-402.

[51] WHO. Methods for surveillance of antimalarial drug efficacy. Geneva, World Health Organization. 2009.

[52] Vestergaard LS, Ringwald P. Responding to the challenge of antimalarial drug resistance by routine monitoring to update national malaria treatment policies. Am J Trop Med Hyg 2007; 77(Suppl. 6): 153-159.

[53] Stepniewska K, White NJ. Some considerations in the design and interpretation of antimalarial drug trials in uncomplicated *falciparum* malaria. Malar J 2006; 5: 127.

[54] Price RN, Dorsey G, Ashley EA, Barnes KI, Baird JK, d'Alessandro U, Guerin PJ, Laufer MK, Naidoo I, Nosten F, Olliaro P, Plowe CV, Ringwald P, Sibley CH, Stepniewska K, White NJ. World Antimalarial Resistance Network I: Clinical efficacy of antimalarial drugs. Malar J 2007; 6:119.

[55] Bacon DJ, Jambou R, Fandeur T, Le Bras J, Wongsrichanalai C, Fukuda MM, Ringwald P, Sibley CH, Kyle DE. World Antimalarial Resistance Network (WARN) II: *In vitro* antimalarial drug susceptibility. Malar J 2007; 6: 120.

[56] Denis MB, Tsuyuoka R, Lim P, Lindegardh N, Yi P, Top SN, Socheat D, Fandeur T, Annerberg A, Christophel EM, Ringwald P. Efficacy of artemether-lumefantrine for the treatment of uncomplicated *falciparum* malaria in northwest Cambodia. Trop Med Int Health 2006; 11: 1800-1807.

[57] Barnes KI, Lindegardh N, Ogundahunsi O, Olliaro P, Plowe CV, Randrianarivelojosia M, Gbotosho GO, Watkins WM, Sibley CH, White NJ. World Antimalarial Resistance Network (WARN) IV: Clinical pharmacology. Malar J 2007; 6: 122.

[58] Nair S, Nash D, Sudimack D, Jaidee A, Barends M, Uhlemann AC, Krishna S, Nosten F, Anderson TJ. Recurrent gene amplification and soft selective sweeps during evolution of multidrug resistance in malaria parasites. Mol Biol Evol 2007; 24: 562-573.

[59] Volkman SK, Sabeti PC, DeCaprio D, Neafsey DE, Schaffner SF, Milner DA Jr, Daily JP, Sarr O, Ndiaye D, Ndir O, Mboup S, Duraisingh MT, Lukens A, Derr A, Stange-Thomann N, Waggoner S, Onofrio R, Ziaugra L, Mauceli E, Gnerre S, Jaffe DB, Zainoun J, Wiegand RC, Birren BW, Hartl DL,

Galagan JE, Lander ES, Wirth DF. A genome-wide map of diversity in *Plasmodium falciparum*. Nat Genet. 2007; 39: 113-119.

[60] Plowe CV, Roper C, Barnwell JW, *et al.* World Antimalarial Resistance Network (WARN) III: Molecular markers for drug resistant malaria. Malar J. 2007; 6: 121.

[61] White NJ, van Vugt M, Ezzet F. Clinical pharmacokinetics and pharmacodynamics of artemether-lumefantrine. Clin Pharmacokinet. 1999; 37:105-25.

[62] White N. Antimalarial drug resistance and combination chemotherapy. Philos Trans R Soc Lond B Biol Sci. 1999; 354(1384): 739-49.

[63] Vinetz JM, Clain J, Bounkeua V, *et al.* Chemotherapy of malaria. In: Brunton L, Chabner B, Knollman B, editors. Goodman & Gilman's the pharmacological basis of therapeutics. 12. New York, NY: McGraw Hill Medical; 2011. pp. 1383-1418.

[64] Hastings I. How artemisinin-containing combination therapies slow the spread of antimalarial drug resistance. Trends Parasitol. 2011; 27: 67-72.

[65] Li Q. Weina P. Antimalarial in Drugs: Age of the Artemisinins. Edited by Qigui Li & Peter Weina. Nova Science Publishers Inc, New York; 1st edition, August 2011. pp. 1-645.

[66] Li Q, Hickman M. Toxicokinetic and toxicodynamic (TK/TD) evaluation to determine and predict the neurotoxicity of artemisinins. Toxicology. 2011; 279(1-3): 1-9.

[67] Li Q, Weina P. Severe embryotoxicity of artemisinin derivatives in experimental animals, but possibly safe in pregnant women. Molecules. 2010; 15: 40-57.

[68] Price RN, Nosten F, Luxemburger C, ter Kuile FO, Paiphun L, Chongsuphajaisiddhi T, White NJ. Effects of artemisinin derivatives on malaria transmissibility. Lancet. 1996; 347: 1654-1658.

[69] WHO. Antimalarial Drug Combination Therapy: Report of a Technical Consultation. 2001, World Health Organization, Geneva.

[70] Woodrow CJ, Krishna S. Antimalarial drugs: Recent advances in molecular determinants of resistance and their clinical significance. Cell Mol Life Sci. 2006; 63: 1586-1596.

[71] de Vries PJ, Dien TK. Clinical pharmacology and therapeutic potential of artemisinin and its derivatives in the treatment of malaria. Drugs. 1996; 52: 818-836.

[72] Price R, van Vugt M, Phaipun L, Luxemburger C, Simpson J, McGready R, ter Kuile F, Kham A, Chongsuphajaisiddhi T, White NJ, Nosten F. Adverse effects in patients with acute *falciparum* malaria treated with artemisinin derivatives. Am J Trop Med Hyg 1999; 60: 547-555.

[73] Hastings IM, Watkins WM. Tolerance is the key to understanding antimalarial drug resistance. Trends Parasitol. 2006; 22: 71-77.

[74] Martinelli A, Moreira R, Ravo PV. Malaria combination therapies: Advantages and shortcomings. Mini Rev Med Chem. 2008; 8: 201-212.

[75] Vijaykadga S, Rojanawatsirivej C, Cholpol S, Phoungmanee D, Nakavej A, Wongsrichanalai C. *In vivo* sensitivity monitoring of mefloquine monotherapy and artesunate-mefloquine combinations for the treatment of uncomplicated *falciparum* malaria in Thailand in 2003. Trop Med Int Health. 2006; 11: 211-219.

[76] van Vugt M, Looareesuwan S, Wilairatana P, McGready R, Villegas L, Gathmann I, Mull R, Brockman A, White NJ, Nosten F. Artemether-lumefantrine for the treatment of multidrug-resistant *falciparum* malaria. Trans R Soc Trop Med Hyg. 2000; 94: 545-548.

[77] Krishna S, White NJ. Pharmacokinetics of quinine, chloroquine and amodiaquine. Clinical implications. Clin Pharmacokinet. 1996; 30: 263-299.

[78] Nosten F, Luxemburger C, ter Kuile FO, Woodrow C, Eh JP, Chongsuphajaisiddhi T, White NJ. Treatment of multidrug-resistant *Plasmodium falciparum* malaria with 3-day artesunate-mefloquine combination. J Infect Dis. 1994; 170: 971-977.

[79] Hutagalung R, Paiphun L, Ashley EA, McGready R, Brockman A, Thwai KL, Singhasivanon P, Jelinek T, White NJ, Nosten FH. A randomized trial of artemether-lumefantrine *versus* mefloquine-artesunate for the treatment of uncomplicated multi-drug resistant *Plasmodium falciparum* on the western border of Thailand. Malar J. 2005); 4: 46.

[80] Karema C, Aregawi MW, Rukundo A, Kabayiza A, Mulindahabi M, Fall IS, Gausi K, Williams RO, Lynch M, Cibulskis R, Fidele N, Nyemazi JP, Ngamije D, Umulisa I, Newman R, Binagwaho A. Trends in malaria cases, hospital admissions and deaths following scale-up of anti-malarial interventions, 2000-2010, Rwanda. Malar J. 2012; 11: 236.

[81] Attaran A, Barnes KI, Curtis C, d'Alessandro U, Fanello CI, Galinski MR, Kokwaro G, Looareesuwan S, Makanga M, Mutabingwa TK, Talisuna A, Trape JF, Watkins WM. WHO, the Global Fund, and medical malpractice in malaria treatment. Lancet. 2004; 363: 237-240.

[82] WHO, World Malaria Report, 2012, World Health Organization, Geneva. http://www.who.int/malaria/publications/world_malaria_report_2012/en/.

[83] Malenga G, Palmer A, Staedke S, Kazadi W, Mutabingwa T, Ansah E, Barnes KI, Whitty CJ. Antimalarial treatment with artemisinin combination therapy in Africa. *BMJ* 2005; *331*: 706-707.

[84] Das D, Price RN, Bethell D, Guerin PJ, Stepniewska K. Early parasitological response following artemisinin-containing regimens: a critical review of the literature. Malar J. 2013; 12:125

[85] WHO. Facts on ACTs (artemisinin-based combination therapies), World Health Organization. January 2006.

[86] Ogbonna A, Uneke CJ. Artemisinin-based combination therapy for uncomplicated malaria in sub-Saharan Africa: The efficacy, safety, resistance and policy implementation since Abuja 2000. Trans R Soc Trop Med Hyg. 2008; 102: 621-627.

[87] Chou TC. Theoretical basis, experimental design, and computerized simulation of synergism and antagonism in drug combination studies. Pharmacol Rev. 2006; 58: 621-81.

[88] Bell A. Antimalarial drug synergism and antagonism: mechanistic and clinical significance. FEMS Microbiol Lett. 2005; 253: 171-84.

[89] Sponer U, Prajakwong S, Wiedermann G, Kollaritsch H, Wernsdorfer G, Wernsdorfer WH. Pharmacodynamics interaction of doxycycline and artemisinin in *Plasmodium falciparum*. Animicrob. Agents Chemorther. 2002; 46: 262-264.

[90] Fivelman QL, Walden JC, Smith PJ, Folb PI, Barnes KI. The effect of artesunate combined with standard antimalarials against chloroquine-sensitive and chloroquine-resistant strains of *Plasmodium falciparum in vitro*. Trans. R. Soc. Trop. Med. Hyg. 1999; 93: 429-432.

[91] Alin MH, Björkman A, Wernsdorfer WH. Synergism of benflumetol and artemether in *Plasmodium falciparum*. Am. J. Trop. Med. Hyg. 1999; 61: 439-445.

[92] Vivas L, Rattray L, Stewart L, Bongard E, Robinson BL, Peters W, Croft SL. Anti-malarial efficacy of pyronaridine and artesunate in combination *in vitro* and *in vivo*. Acta Trop. 2008; 105: 222-228.

[93] Noedl H, Krudsood S, Leowattana W, Tangpukdee N, Thanachartwet W, Looareesuwan S, Miller RS, Fukuda M, Jongsakul K, Yingyuen K, Sriwichai S, Ohrt C, Knirsch C. *In vitro* antimalarial activity of azithromycin, artesunate, and quinine in combination and correlation with clinical outcome. Antimicrob.Agents. Chemother. 2007; 51: 651-656.

[94] Gupta S, Thapar MM, Wernsdorfer WH, Björkman A. *In vitro* interactions of artemisinin with atovaquone, quinine, and mefloquine against *Plasmodium falciparum*. Antimicrob. Agents Chemother. 2002; 46: 1510-1515.

[95] Lutgendrof C, Rojanawatsirivet C, Wernsdorfer G, Sirichaisinthop J, Kollaritsch H, Wernsdorfer WH. Pharmacodynamic interaction between atovaquone and other antimalarial compounds against *Plasmodium falciparum in vitro*. Wein. Klion. Wochenscher, 2006; 118: 70-76.

[96] Akompong T, Eksi S, Williamson K, Haldari K. Gametocytocidal activity and synergistic interactions of riboflavin with standard antimalarial drugs against growth of *Plasmodium falciparum in vitro*. Antimicrob. Agents Chemother., 2000; 44: 3107-3111.

[97] Mishra LC, Bhattacharya A, Bhasin VK. Antiplasmodial interactions between artemisinin and triclosan or ketoconazole combinations against blood stages of *Plasmodium falciparum in vitro*. Am. J. Trop. Med. Hyg. 2007; 76: 497-501.

[98] Purfield AE, Tidwell RR, Meshnick SR. Interaction of DB75, a novel antimalarial agent, with other antimalarial drugs *in vitro*. Antimicrob. Agents Chemother. 2008; 52: 2253-2255.

[99] Fivelman QL, Adagu IS, Warhurst DC. Effects of piperaquine, chloroquine, and amodiaquine on drug uptake and of these in combination with dihydroartemisinin against drugsensitive and-resistant *Plasmodium falciparum* strains. Antmicrob. Agents Chemother. 2007; 51: 2265-2267.

[100] Thriemer K, Wernsdorfer G, Rojanawatsirivet C, Kollaeitsch H, Sirichainsinthop J, Wernsdorfer WH. *In vitro* activity of artemisinin alone and in combination with retinol against *Plasmodium falciparum*. Wien Klin Wochenschr, 2005; 117: 45-48.

[101] Davis TME, Hamzah J, Ilett KF, Karunajeewa HA, Reeder JC, Batty KT, Hackett S, Barrett PH. *In vitro* interactions between piperaquine, dihydroartemisinin, and other conventional and novel antimalarial drugs. Antimicrob. Agents Chemother. 2006; 50: 2883-2885.

[102] Noedl H, Krudsood S, Leowattana W, Tangpukdee N, Thanachartwet W, Looareesuwan S, Scott Miller R, Fukuda M, Jongsakul K, Yingyuen K, Sriwichai S, Ohrt C, Knirsch C. *In vitro* Antimalarial Activity of Azithromycin, Artesunate, and Quinine in Combination and Correlation with Clinical Outcome. Antimicrob Agents Chemother. 2007; 51: 651-656.

[103] Zaloumis S, Humberstone A, Charman SA, Price RN, Moehrle J, Gamo-Benito J, McCaw J, Jamsen KM, Smith K, Simpson JA. Assessing the utility of an anti-malarial pharmacokinetic-pharmacodynamic model for aiding drug clinical development. Malar J. 2012; 11: 303.

[104] Price RN, Nosten F, Luxemburger C, van Vugt M, Phaipun L, Chongsuphajaisiddhi T, White NJ. Artesunate/mefloquine treatment of multi-drug resistant *falciparum* malaria. Trans. R. Soc. Trop. Med. Hyg., 1997; 91: 574-577.

[105] Suputtamongkol Y, Chindarat S, Silpasakorn S, Chaikachonpatd S, Lim K, Chanthapakajee K, Kaewkaukul N, Thamlikitkul V. The efficacy of combined mefloquine-artesunate *versus* mefloquine-primaquine on subsequent development of *Plasmodium falciparum* gametocytemia. Am. J. Trop. Med. Hyg. 2003; 68: 620-623.

[106] Vivas L, Rattray L, Stewart LB, Robinson BL, Fugmann B, Haynes RK, Peters W, Croft SL. Antimalarial efficacy and drug interactions of the novel semi-synthetic endoperoxide artemisone *in vitro* and *in vivo*. J. Antimicrob. Chemother. 2007; 59: 658-665.

[107] Batty KT, Law ASF, Stirling V, Moore BR. Pharmacodynamics of doxycycline in a murine malaria model. Antimicrob. Agents Chemother. 2007; 51: 4477-4479.

[108] Fleck SL, Robinson BL, Peters W. The chemotherapy of rodent malaria. LIV. Combinations of "Fenozan B07" (Fenozan-50F), a difluorinated 3,30-spirocyclopentane 1,2,4-trioxane, with other drugs against drug-sensitive and drug-resistant parasites. Ann. Trop. Med. Parasitol. 1997; 91: 33-39.

[109] Vennerstrom JL, Ager Jr AL, Andersen SL, Grace JM, Wongpanich V, Angerhofer CK, Hu JK, Wesche DL. Assessment of the antimalarial potential of tetraoxane WR148999. Am. J. Trop. Med. Hyg. 2000; 62: 573-578.

[110] Snynder C, Chollet J, Santo-Thomas J, Scheurer C, Wittlin S. *In vitro* and *in vivo* interaction of synthetic peroxide RBx11160 (OZ277) with piperaquine in *Plasmodium* models. Exp. Parasitol., 2007; 115: 296-300.

[111] Jaquet C, Stohler HR, Chollet J, Peters W. Antimalarial activity of the bicyclic peroxide Ro 42-1611 (arteflene) in experimental models. Trop. Med. Parasitol. 1994; 45: 266-271.

[112] Peters W, Robinson BL, Milhous WK. The chemotherapy of rodent malaria. LI. Studies on a new 8-aminoquinoline, WR 238,605. Ann. Trop. Med. Parasitol. 1993; 87: 547-552.

[113] Neerja J, Puri SK. *Plasmodium yoelii*: activity of azithromycin in combination with pyrimethamine or sulfadoxine against blood and sporozoite induced infections in Swiss mice. Exp. Parasitol. 2004; 107: 120-124.

[114] Lundgren JD, Dragsted UB. Atovaquone/proguanil. Prophylaxis and treatment of malaria. Ugeskr Laeger. 2000; 162: 4177-81.

[115] Pereira MR, Henrich PP, Sidhu AS, Johnson D, Hardink J, Van Deusen J, Lin J, Gore K, O'Brien C, Wele M, Djimde A, Chandra R, Fidock DA. *In vivo* and *In vitro* Antimalarial Properties of Azithromycin-Chloroquine Combinations That Include the Resistance Reversal Agent Amlodipine. Antimicrob Agents Chemother. 2011; 55: 3115-3124.

[116] Croft SL, Duparc S, Arbe-Barnes SJ, Craft JC, Shin C, Fleckenstein L, Borghini-Fuhrer I, Rim H. Review of pyronaridine anti-malarial properties and product characteristics Malar J. 2012; 11: 270.

[117] Landau I, Chabaud A, Cambie G, Ginsburg H. Chronotherapy of malaria: An approach to malaria chemotherapy. Parasitol Today. 1991; 7: 350-352.

[118] White NJ. The assessment of antimalarial drug efficacy. Trends Parasitol. 2002; 18: 458-464.

[119] Volkman SK, Sabeti PC, DeCaprio D, Neafsey DE, Schaffner SF, Milner DA Jr, Daily JP, Sarr O, Ndiaye D, Ndir O, Mboup S, Duraisingh MT, Lukens A, Derr A, Stange-Thomann N, Waggoner S, Onofrio R, Ziaugra L, Mauceli E, Gnerre S, Jaffe DB, Zainoun J, Wiegand RC, Birren BW, Hartl DL, Galagan JE, Lander ES, Wirth DF. A genome-wide map of diversity in *Plasmodium falciparum*. Nat Genet. 2007; 39: 113-119.

[120] Mårtensson A, Strömberg J, Sisowath C, Msellem MI, Gil JP, Montgomery SM, Olliaro P, Ali AS, Björkman A. Efficacy of artesunate plus amodiaquine *versus* that of artemether-lumefantrine for the treatment of uncomplicated childhood *Plasmodium falciparum* malaria in Zanzibar, Tanzania. Clin Infect Dis. 2005; 41: 1079-1086.

[121] Adjei GO, Kurtzhals JA, Rodrigues OP, Alifrangis M, Hoegberg LC, Kitcher ED, Badoe EV, Lamptey R, Goka BQ. Amodiaquine-artesunate *vs.* artemether-lumefantrine for uncomplicated malaria in Ghanaian children: A randomized efficacy and safety trial with one year follow-up. Malar J. 2008; 7: 127.

[122] Ashley EA, Pinoges L, Turyakira E, Dorsey G, Checchi F, Bukirwa H, van den Broek I, Zongo I, Urruta PP, van Herp M, Balkan S, Taylor WR, Olliaro P, Guthmann JP. Different methodological approaches to the assessment of *in vivo* efficacy of three artemisinin-based combination antimalarial treatments for the treatment of uncomplicated *falciparum* malaria in African children. Malar J. 2008; 7: 154.

[123] Olliaro PO, Pinoges L, Checchi F, Vaillant M, Guthmann JP. Risk associated with asymptomatic parasitemia occurring post-antimalarial treatment. Trop Med Int Health. 2008; 13: 83-90.

[124] Karunajeewa H, Lim C, Hung TY, Ilett KF, Denis MB, Socheat D, Davis TM. Safety evaluation of fixed combination piperaquine plus dihydroartemisinin (Artekin) in Cambodian children and adults with malaria. Br J Clin Pharmacol. 2004; 57: 93-99.

[125] Denis MB, Davis TM, Hewitt S, Incardona S, Nimol K, Fandeur T, Poravuth Y, Lim C, Socheat D. Efficacy and safety of dihydroartemisinin-piperaquine (Artekin) in Cambodian children and adults with uncomplicated *falciparum* malaria. Clin Infect Dis. 2002; 35: 1469-1476.

126] Tran TH, Dolecek C, Pham PM, Nguyen TD, Nguyen TT, Le HT, Dong TH, Tran TT, Stepniewska K, White NJ, Farrar J. Dihydroartemisinin-piperaquine against multidrug-resistant *Plasmodium falciparum* malaria in Vietnam: Randomized clinical trial. Lancet. 2004; 363: 18-22.

[127] Wilairatana P, Krudsood S, Chalermrut K, Pengruksa C, Srivilairit S, Silachamroon U, Treeprasertsuk S, Looareesuwan S, An open randomized clinical trial of Artecom *vs.* artesunate-mefloquine in the treatment of acute uncomplicated *falciparum* malaria in Thailand. Southeast Asian J Trop Med Public Health. 2002; 33: 519-524.

[128] Ashley EA, Krudsood S, Phaiphun L, Srivilairit S, McGready R, Leowattana W, Hutagalung R, Wilairatana P, Brockman A, Looareesuwan S, Nosten F, White NJ. Randomized, controlled dose-optimization studies of dihydroartemisinin-piperaquine for the treatment of uncomplicated multidrug-resistant *falciparum* malaria in Thailand. J Infect Dis. 2004; 190: 1773-1782.

[129] Tjitra E, Hasugian AR, Siswantoro H, Prasetyorini B, Ekowatiningsih R, Yusnita EA, Purnamasari T, Driyah S, Salwati E; Nurhayati, Yuwarni E, Januar L, Labora J, Wijayanto B, Amansyah F, Dedang TA, Purnama A; Trihono. Efficacy and safety of artemisinin-naphthoquine *versus* dihydroartemisinin-piperaquine in adult patients with uncomplicated malaria: a multi-centre study in Indonesia. Malar J. 2012; 11: 153.

[130] Adam I, Ali DM, Abdalla MA. Artesunate plus sulfadoxine-pyrimethamine in the treatment of uncomplicated *Plasmodium falciparum* malaria during pregnancy in eastern Sudan. Trans R Soc Trop Med Hyg. 2006; 100: 632-635.

[131] Dorsey G, Njama D, Kamya MR, Cattamanchi A, Kyabayinze D, Staedke SG, Gasasira A, Rosenthal PJ. Sulfadoxine/pyrimethamine alone or with amodiaquine or artesunate for treatment of uncomplicated malaria: a longitudinal randomised trial. Lancet. 2002; 360: 2031-2038.

[132] Bosman A, Mendis KN. A major transition in malaria treatment: The adoption and deployment of artemisinin-based combination therapies. Am J Trop Med Hyg. 2007; 77(Suppl. 6): 193-197.

[133] van den Broek I, Amsalu R, Balasegaram M, Hepple P, Alemu E, Hussein el B, Al-Faith M, Montgomery J, Checchi F. Efficacy of two artemisinin combination therapies for uncomplicated *falciparum* malaria in children under 5 years, Malakal, Upper Nile, Sudan. Malar J. 2005; 4: 14.

[134] Yeka A, Banek K, Bakyaita N, Staedke SG, Kamya MR, Talisuna A, Kironde F, Nsobya SL, Kilian A, Slater M, Reingold A, Rosenthal PJ, Wabwire-Mangen F, Dorsey G. Artemisinin *versus* nonartemisinin combination therapy for uncomplicated malaria: Randomized clinical trials from four sites in Uganda. PLoS Med. 2005; 2: e190.

[135] Rwagacondo CE, Karema C, Mugisha V, Erhart A, Dujardin JC, Van Overmeir C, Ringwald P, D'Alessandro U. Is amodiaquine failing in Rwanda? Efficacy of amodiaquine alone and combined with artesunate in children with uncomplicated malaria. Trop Med Int Health. 2004; 9: 1091-1098.

[136] Abacassamo F, Enosse S, Aponte JJ, Gómez-Olivé FX, Quintó L, Mabunda S, Barreto A, Magnussen P, Rønn AM, Thompson R, Alonso PL. Efficacy of chloroquine, amodiaquine, sulphadoxine-pyrimethamine and combination therapy with artesunate in Mozambican children with non-complicated malaria. Trop Med Int Health. 2004; 9: 200-208.

[137] Swarthout TD, van den Broek IV, Kayembe G, Montgomery J, Pota H, Roper C. Artesunate + amodiaquine and artesunate + sulphadoxine-pyrimethamine for treatment of uncomplicated malaria in Democratic Republic of Congo: A clinical trial with determination of sulphadoxine and pyrimethamine-resistant haplotypes. Trop Med Int Health. 2006; 11: 1503-1511.

[138] Sutherland CJ, Ord R, Dunyo S, Jawara M, Drakeley CJ, Alexander N, Coleman R, Pinder M, Walraven G, Targett GA. Reduction of malaria transmission to Anopheles mosquitoes with a six-dose regimen of co-artemether. PLoS Med. 2005; 2: e92.

[139] Faye B, Ndiaye JL, Ndiaye D, Dieng Y, Faye O, Gaye O. Efficacy and tolerability of four antimalarial combinations in the treatment of uncomplicated *Plasmodium falciparum* malaria in Senegal. Malar J. 2007; 6: 80.

[140] Ibrahium AM, Kheir MM, Osman ME, Khalil IF, Alifrangis M, Elmardi KA, Malik EM, Adam I. Efficacies of artesunate plus either sulfadoxine-pyrimethamine or amodiaquine, for the treatment of uncomplicated, *Plasmodium falciparum* malaria in eastern Sudan. Ann Trop Med Parasitol. 2007; 101: 15-21.

[141] Mockenhaupt FP, Ehrhardt S, Dzisi SY, Teun Bousema J, Wassilew N, Schreiber J, Anemana SD, Cramer JP, Otchwemah RN, Sauerwein RW, Eggelte TA, Bienzle U. A randomized, placebo-controlled, double-blind trial on sulfadoxine-pyrimethamine alone or combined with artesunate or amodiaquine in uncomplicated malaria. Trop Med Int Health 2005; 10: 512-520.

[142] Gargano N, Cenci F, Bassat Q. Antimalarial efficacy of piperaquine-based antimalarial combination therapies: facts and uncertainties. Trop Med Int Health 2011; 16: 1466-73.

[143] Rijken MJ, McGready R, Boel ME, Barends M, Proux S, Pimanpanarak M, Singhasivanon P, Nosten F. Dihydroartemisinin-piperaquine rescue treatment of multidrug-resistant *Plasmodium falciparum* malaria in pregnancy: a preliminary report. Am J Trop Med Hyg. 2008; 78: 543-5.

[144] Manyando C, Kayentao K, D'Alessandro U, Okafor HU, Juma E, Hamed K. A systematic review of the safety and efficacy of artemether-lumefantrine against uncomplicated *Plasmodium falciparum* malaria during pregnancy. Malar J. 2012; 11: 141.

[145] Pécoul B Interview with Dr Bernard Pécoul, Executive Director of the Drugs for Neglected Diseases Initiative. Future Med Chem. 2009, 1(2):243-8.

[146] Rowland M, Peck C, Tucker G. Physiologically-based pharmacokinetics in drug development and regulatory science. Annu Rev Pharmacol Toxicol. 2011; 51: 45-73.

[147] WHO. World Health Organization and United Nations Children Fund, 2005. World Malaria Report III. Global Financing and Service Delivery.

[148] Pincock S. Drug company to offer new malaria drug cheaply in Africa. BMJ. 2003; 327: 360.

[149] Mutabingwa TK, Anthony D, Heller A, Hallett R, Ahmed J, Drakeley C, Greenwood BM, Whitty CJ. Amodiaquine alone, amodiaquine+sulfadoxine-pyrimethamine, amodiaquine+artesunate, and artemether-lumefantrine for outpatient treatment of malaria in Tanzanian children: A four-arm randomised effectiveness trial. Lancet. 2005; 365: 1474-1480.

[150] Mutabingwa TK. Artemisinin-based combination therapies (ACTs): Best hope for malaria treatment but inaccessible to the needy! Acta Trop. 2005; 95: 305-315.

[151] Hale V, Keasling JD, Renninger N, Diagana TT. Microbially derived artemisinin: a biotechnology solution to the global problem of access to affordable antimalarial drugs. Am J Trop Med Hyg. 2007; 77(6 Suppl): 198-202.

[152] Watkins WM, Mosobo M. Treatment of *Plasmodium falciparum* malaria with pyrimethamine-sulfadoxine: Selective pressure for resistance is a function of long elimination half-life. Trans R Soc Trop Med Hyg. 1993; 87: 75-78.

[153] Hastings IM, Watkins WM, White NJ. The evolution of drug-resistant malaria: The role of drug elimination half-life. Philos Trans R Soc Lond B Biol Sci. 2002; 357: 505-519.

[154] White NJ. Preventing antimalarial drug resistance through combinations. Drug Resist Updat. 1998; 1: 3-9.

[155] Dye C, Williams BG. Multigenic drug resistance among inbred malaria parasites. Proc Biol Sci. 1997; 264: 61-67.

[156] Hastings IM, D'Alessandro U. Modeling a predictable disaster: The rise and spread of drug-resistant malaria. Parasitol Today. 2000; 16: 340-347.

[157] Cross AP, Singer B. Modeling the development of resistance of *Plasmodium falciparum* to anti-malarial drugs. Trans R Soc Trop Med Hyg. 1991; 85: 349-355.

[158] Myint HY, Ashley EA, Day NP, Nosten F, White NJ. Efficacy and safety of dihydroartemisinin-piperaquine. Trans R Soc Trop Med Hyg. 2007; 101: 858-866.
[159] Austin DJ, White NJ, Anderson RM. The dynamics of drug action on the within-host population growth of infectious agents: Melding pharmacokinetics with pathogen population dynamics. J Theor Biol. 1998; 194: 313-339.
[160] White NJ. Assessment of the pharmacodynamic properties of antimalarial drugs *in vivo*. Antimicrob Agents Chemother. 1997; 41: 1413-1422.
[161] White NJ. Antimalarial drug resistance: The pace quickens. J Antimicrob Chemother. 1992; 30: 571-585.
[162] Peters W, Robinson BL. The chemotherapy of rodent malaria XXXV. Further studies on the retardation of drug resistance by the use of a triple combination of mefloquine, pyrimethamine and sulfadoxine in mice infected with *P. berghei* and '*P. berghei* NS'. Ann Trop Med Parasitol. 1984; 78: 459-466.
[163] Barnes KI, Watkins WM, White NJ. Antimalarial dosing regimens and drug resistance. Trends Parasitol. 2008; 24: 127-134.
[164] ter Kuile F, White NJ, Holloway P, Pasvol G, Krishna S. *Plasmodium falciparum*: *In vitro* studies of the pharmacodynamic properties of drugs used for the treatment of severe malaria. Exp Parasitol. 1993; 76: 85-95.
[165] Landau I, Chabaud A, Cambie G, Ginsburg H. Chronotherapy of malaria: An approach to malaria chemotherapy. Parasitol Today. 1991; 7: 350-352.
[166] Jiang JB, Li GQ, Guo XB, Kong YC, Arnold K. Antimalarial activity of mefloquine and qinghaosu. Lancet. 1982; 2: 285-288.
[167] A-Elbasit IE, Alifrangis M, Khalil IF, Bygbjerg IC, Masuadi EM, Elbashir MI, Giha HA. The implication of dihydrofolate reductase and dihydropteroate synthetase gene mutations in modification of *Plasmodium falciparum* characteristics. Malar J. 2007; 6: 108.
[168] Pukrittayakamee S, Wanwimolruk S, Stepniewska K, Jantra A, Huyakorn S, Looareesuwan S, White NJ. Quinine pharmacokinetic-pharmacodynamic relationships in uncomplicated *falciparum* malaria. Antimicrob Agents Chemother. 2003; 47: 3458-3463.
[169] Gordi T, Xie R, Jusko WJ. Semi-mechanistic pharmacokinetic/pharmacodynamic modeling of the antimalarial effect of artemisinin. Br J Clin Pharmacol. 2005; 60: 594-604.
[170] Hietala SF, Bhattarai A, Msellem M, Röshammar D, Ali AS, Strömberg J, Hombhanje FW, Kaneko A, Björkman A, Ashton M. Population pharmacokinetics of amodiaquine and desethylamodiaquine in pediatric patients with uncomplicated *falciparum* malaria. J Pharmacokinet Pharmacodyn. 2007; 34: 669-686.
[171] Hien TT, Davis TM, Chuong LV, Ilett KF, Sinh DX, Phu NH, Agus C, Chiswell GM, White NJ, Farrar J. Comparative pharmacokinetics of intramuscular artesunate and artemether in patients with severe *falciparum* malaria. Antimicrob Agents Chemother. 2004; 48: 4234-4239.
[172] Newton, PN; Ward, S; Angus, BJ; Chierakul, W; Dondorp, A; Ruangveerayuth, R; Silamut, K; Teerapong, P; Suputtamongkol, Y; Looareesuwan, S; White, NJ; Early treatment failure in severe malaria resulting from abnormally low plasma quinine concentrations. Trans R Soc Trop Med Hyg. (2006). 100, 184-186.
[173] Barnes KI, Little F, Smith PJ, Evans A, Watkins WM, White NJ. Sulfadoxine-pyrimethamine pharmacokinetics in malaria: Pediatric dosing implications. Clin Pharmacol Ther. 2006; 80: 582-596.
[174] Ringwald P, Same Ekobo A, Keundjian A, Kedy Mangamba D, Basco LK. Chemoresistance of P. *falciparum* in urban areas of Yaounde, Cameroon. Part 1: Surveillance of *in vitro* and *in vivo* resistance of *Plasmodium falciparum* to chloroquine from 1994 to 1999 in Yaounde, Cameroon. Trop Med Int Health. 2000; 5: 612-619.
[175] Checchi F, Piola P, Fogg C, Bajunirwe F, Biraro S, Grandesso F, Ruzagira E, Babigumira J, Kigozi I, Kiguli J, Kyomuhendo J, Ferradini L, Taylor WR, Guthmann JP. Supervised *versus* unsupervised antimalarial treatment with six-dose artemether-lumefantrine: Pharmacokinetic and dosage-related findings from a clinical trial in Uganda. Malar J. 2006; 5: 59.
[176] Li Q, Lugt CB, Looareesuwan S, Krudsood S, Wilairatana P, Vannaphan S, Chalearmrult K, Milhous WK. Pharmacokinetic investigation on the therapeutic potential of artemotil (beta-arteether) in Thai patients with severe *Plasmodium falciparum* malaria. Am J Trop Med Hyg. 2004; 71: 723-731.

[177] Simpson JA, Hughes D, Manyando C, Bojang K, Aarons L, Winstanley P, Edwards G, Watkins WA, Ward S. Population pharmacokinetic and pharmacodynamic modeling of the antimalarial chemotherapy chlorproguanil/dapsone. Br J Clin Pharmacol. 2006; 61: 289-300.
[178] Price RN, Hasugian AR, Ratcliff A, Siswantoro H, Purba HL, Kenangalem E, Lindegardh N, Penttinen P, Laihad F, Ebsworth EP, Anstey NM, Tjitra E. Clinical and pharmacological determinants of the therapeutic response to dihydroartemisinin-piperaquine for drug-resistant malaria. Antimicrob Agents Chemother. 2007; 51: 4090-4097.
[179] Desai M, ter Kuile FO, Nosten F, McGready R, Asamoa K, Brabin B, Newman RD. Epidemiology and burden of malaria in pregnancy. Lancet Infect Dis. 2007; 7: 93-104.
[180] Lee SJ, McGready R, Fernandez C, Stepniewska K, Paw MK, Viladpai-nguen SJ, Thwai KL, Villegas L, Singhasivanon P, Greenwood BM, White NJ, Nosten F. Chloroquine pharmacokinetics in pregnant and nonpregnant women with *vivax* malaria. Eur J Clin Pharmacol. 2008; 64: 987-992.
[181] McGready R, Stepniewska K, Ward SA, Cho T, Gilveray G, Looareesuwan S, White NJ, Nosten F. Pharmacokinetics of dihydroartemisinin following oral artesunate treatment of pregnant women with acute uncomplicated *falciparum* malaria. Eur J Clin Pharmacol. 2006; 62: 367-371.
[182] Newton P, Suputtamongkol, Y, Teja-Isavadharm P, Pukrittayakamee S, Navaratnam V, Bates I, White N. Antimalarial bioavailability and disposition of artesunate in acute *falciparum* malaria. Antimicrob Agents Chemother. 2000; 44: 972-977.
[183] Menendez C. Malaria during pregnancy. Curr Mol Med. 2006; 6: 269-273.
[184] Abdelrahim II, Adam I, Elghazali G, Gustafsson LL, Elbashir MI, Mirghani RA. Pharmacokinetics of quinine and its metabolites in pregnant Sudanese women with uncomplicated *Plasmodium falciparum* malaria. J Clin Pharm Ther. 2007; 32: 15-19.
[185] Ward SA, Sevene EJ, Hastings IM, Nosten F, McGready R. Antimalarial drugs and pregnancy: Safety, pharmacokinetics, and pharmacovigilance. Lancet Infect Dis. 2007; 7: 136-144.
[186] Green MD, van Eijk AM, van Ter Kuile FO, Ayisi JG, Parise ME, Kager PA, Nahlen BL, Steketee R, Nettey H. Pharmacokinetics of sulfadoxine-pyrimethamine in HIV-infected and uninfected pregnant women in Western Kenya. J Infect Dis. 2007; 196: 1403-1408.
[187] WHO. Regional Office for Africa. A strategic framework for malaria prevention and control during pregnancy in the African region. Brazzaville: World Health Organization, 2004.
[188] White NJ. Intermittent presumptive treatment for malaria. PLoS Med. 2005; 2: e3.
[189] O'Meara WP, Smith DL, McKenzie FE. Potential impact of intermittent preventive treatment (IPT) on spread of drug-resistant malaria. PLoS Med. 2006; 3: e141.
[190] Alexander N, Sutherland C, Roper C, Cissé B, Schellenberg D. Modeling the impact of intermittent preventive treatment for malaria on selection pressure for drug resistance. Malar J. 2007; 6: 9.
[191] van Eijk AM, De Cock KM, Ayisi JG, Rosen DH, Otieno JA, Nahlen BL, Steketee RW. Pregnancy interval and delivery outcome among HIV-seropositive and HIV-seronegative women in Kisumu, Kenya. Trop Med Int Health. 2004; 9: 15-24.
[192] Cohen C, Karstaedt A, Frean J, Thomas J, Govender N, Prentice E, Dini L, Galpin J, Crewe-Brown H. Increased prevalence of severe malaria in HIV-infected adults in South Africa. Clin Infect Dis. 2005; 41: 1631-1637.
[193] Shah SN, Smith EE, Obonyo CO, Kain KC, Bloland PB, Slutsker L, Hamel MJ. HIV immunosuppression and antimalarial efficacy: sulfadoxine-pyrimethamine for the treatment of uncomplicated malaria in HIV-infected adults in Siaya, Kenya. J Infect Dis. 2006; 194: 1519-1528.
[194] Khoo S, Back D, Winstanley P. The potential for interactions between antimalarial and antiretroviral drugs. AIDS. 2005; 19: 995-1005.
[195] German P, Greenhouse B, Coates C, Dorsey G, Rosenthal PJ, Charlebois E, Lindegardh N, Havlir D, Aweeka FT. Hepatotoxicity due to a drug interaction between amodiaquine plus artesunate and efavirenz. Clin Infect Dis. 2007; 44: 889-891.
[196] Barradell LB, Fitton A, Artesunate. A review of its pharmacology and therapeutic efficacy in the treatment of malaria. Drugs 1995; 50: 714-741.
[197] van Hensbroek MB, Onyiorah E, Jaffar S. A trial of artemether or quinine in children with cerebral malaria. N Engl J Med. 1996; 335: 69-75.
[198] Tran TH, Day NP, Nguyen HP, Nguyen TH, Tran TH, Pham PL, Dinh XS, Ly VC, Ha V, Waller D, Peto TE, White NJ. A controlled trial of artemether or quinine in Vietnamese adults with severe *falciparum* malaria. N Engl J Med. 1996; 335: 76-83.

[199] Meshnick, SR; Taylor, TE; Kamchonwongpaisan, S; Artemisinin and the antimalarial endoperoxides: From herbal remedy to targeted chemotherapy. Microbiol Rev. (1996). 60, 301-315.

[200] Dondorp A, Nosten F, Stepniewska K, Day N, White N. Artesunate *versus* quinine for treatment of severe *falciparum* malaria: a randomised trial. Lancet 2005; 366: 717-725.

[201] Dondorp AM, Fanello CI, Hendriksen IC, Gomes E, Seni A, Chhaganlal KD, Bojang K, Olaosebikan R, Anunobi N, Maitland K, Kivaya E, Agbenyega T, Nguah SB, Evans J, Gesase S, Kahabuka C, Mtove G, Nadjm B, Deen J, Mwanga-Amumpaire J, Nansumba M, Karema C, Umulisa N, Uwimana A, Mokuolu OA, Adedoyin OT, Johnson WB, Tshefu AK, Onyamboko MA, Sakulthaew T, Ngum WP, Silamut K, Stepniewska K, Woodrow CJ, Bethell D, Wills B, Oneko M, Peto TE, von Seidlein L, Day NP, White NJ; AQUAMAT group. Artesunate *versus* quinine in the treatment of severe *falciparum* malaria in African children (AQUAMAT): an open-label, randomised trial. Lancet. 2010; 376(9753):1647-57.

[202] Artemether-Quinine Meta-analysis Study Group. A meta-analysis using individual patient data of trials comparing artemether with quinine in the treatment of severe *falciparum* malaria. Trans R Soc Trop Med Hyg 2001; 95: 637-650.

[203] Xie LH, Johnson TO, Weina PJ, Si Y, Haeberle A, Upadhyay R, Wong E, Li Q. Risk assessment and therapeutic indices of artesunate and artelinic acid in *Plasmodium* berghei-infected and uninfected rats. Int J Toxicol. 2005; 24: 251-264.

[204] Li Q, Gerena L, Xie L, Zhang J, Kyle D, Milhous W. Development and validation of flow cytometric measurement for parasitemia in cultures of P. *falciparum* vitally stained with YOYO-1. Cytometry A. 2007; 71: 297-307.

[205] Park BK, O'Neill PN, Maggs JL, Pirmohamed M. Safety assessment of peroxide antimalarials: Clinical and chemical perspectives. Br J Clin Pharmacol 1998; 46: 521-529.

[206] Ashton M, Hai TN, Sy ND, Huong DX, Van Huong N, Nieu NT, Cong LD. Artemisinin pharmacokinetics is time-dependent during repeated oral administration in healthy male adults. Drug Metab Dispos. 1998; 26: 25-27.

[207] Ashton M, Sy ND, Gordi T, Hai TN, Thach DC, Huong, NV, Johansson M, Coeng LD. Evidence for time-dependence artemisinin kinetics in adults with uncomplicated malaria. Pharm Pharmacol Lett. 1996; 6: 127-130.

[208] van Agtmael MA, Cheng-Qi S, Qing JX, Mull R, van Boxtel CJ. Multiple dose pharmacokinetics of artemether in Chinese patients with uncomplicated *falciparum* malaria. Int J Antimicrob Agents. 1999; 12: 151-158.

[209] Khanh NX, de Vries PJ, Ha LD, van Boxtel CJ, Koopmans R, Kager PA. Declining concentrations of dihydroartemisinin in plasma during 5-day oral treatment with artesunate for *falciparum* malaria. Antimicrob Agents Chemother. 1999; 43: 690-692.

[210] Li Q, Xie LH, Si Y, Wong E, Upadhyay R, Yanez D, Weina PJ. Toxicokinetics and hydrolysis of artelinic acid and artesunate in malaria-infected rats. Int J Toxicol. 2005; 24: 241-250.

[211] Salako LA. Pharmacokinetics of antimalarial drugs: Their therapeutic and toxicological implications. Ann Ist Super Sanita. 1985; 21: 315-325.

[212] Li QG, Peggins JO, Brewer TG. Comparative anoretic toxicity of im arteether in rats using sesame oil or cremophor as vehicle. AM J Trop Med Hyg. 1996; 55: 182.

[213] Alin MH, Bjorkman A. Concentration and time dependence of artemisinin efficacy against *Plasmodium falciparum in vitro*. Am J Trop Med Hyg. 1994; 50: 771-776.

[214] White NJ, Krishna S. Treatment of malaria: Some considerations and limitations of the current methods of assessment. Trans Roy Soc Trop Med Hyg. 1989; 83: 767-777.

[215] Skinner TS, Manning LS, Johnston WA, Davis TM. *In vitro* stage-specific sensitivity of *Plasmodium falciparum* to quinine and artemisinin drugs. Int J Parasit. 1996; 26: 519-525.

[216] Karbwang J, Na-Bangchang K, Thanavibul A, Molunto P. Plasma concentrations of artemether and its major plasma metabolite, dihydroartemisinin, following a 5-day regimen of oral artemether, in patients with uncomplicated *falciparum* malaria. Ann Trop Med Parasit. 1998; 92: 31-36.

[217] Sharma P, Swarup D, Saxena GN, Bhandari S, Sharma UB, Tuteja R. An open study to evaluate the efficacy of artemether in severe *falciparum* malaria. J Assoc Physicians India. 1999; 47: 883-885.

[218] Gachot B, Eliaszewicz M, Dupont B. Artesunate and cerebellar dysfunction in *falciparum* malaria. N Engl J Med. 1997; 337: 792-793.

[219] Li QG, Brueckner RP, Peggins JO, Trotman KM, Brewer TG. Arteether toxicokinetics and pharmacokinetics in rats after 25 mg/kg/day single and multiple doses. Eur J Drug Metab Pharmacokinet. 1999; 24: 213-223.
[220] Li Q, Lugt CB, Looareesuwan S, Krudsood S, Wilairatana P, Vannaphan S, Chalearmrult K, Milhous WK. Pharmacokinetic investigation on the therapeutic potential of artemotil (beta-arteether) in Thai patients with severe *Plasmodium falciparum* malaria. Am J Trop Med Hyg. 2004; 71: 723-731.
[221] Suputtamongkol Y, Newton PN, Angus B, Teja-Isavadharm P, Keeratithakul D, Rasameesoraj M, Pukrittayakamee S, White NJ. A comparison of oral artesunate and artemether antimalarial bioactivities in acute *falciparum* malaria. Br J Clin Pharmacol. 2001; 52: 655-661.
[222] Marsh K, Forster D, Waruiru C, Mwangi I, Winstanley M, Marsh V, Newton C, Winstanley P, Warn P, Peshu N. *et al.* Indicators of life-threatening malaria in African children. N Engl J Med 1995; 332: 1399-1404.
[223] Jung M, Lee K, Kim H, Park M. Recent advances in artemisinin and its derivatives as antimalarial and antitumor agents. Curr Med Chem. 2004; 11: 1265-1284.
[224] Li Q, Milhous WK, Weina PJ. Fatal neurotoxicity of the artemisinin derivatives is related to drug pharmacokinetic profiles in animal species. Curr. Topics Toxicol 2006; 3: 1-16.
[225] White NJ. Antimalarial pharmacokinetics and treatment regimens. Br J Clin Pharmacol. 1992; 34: 1-10.
[226] Bustos MD, Gay F, Diquet B. *In vitro* tests on Philippine isolates of *Plasmodium falciparum* against four standard antimalarials and four qinghaosu derivatives. Bull World Health Organ, 1994; 72: 729-735.
[227] Ittarat W, Pickard AL, Rattanasinganchan P, Wilairatana P, Looareesuwan S, Emery K, Low J, Udomsangpetch R, Meshnick SR. Recrudescence in artesunate-treated patients with *falciparum* malaria is dependent on parasite burden not on parasite factors. Am J Trop Med Hyg. 2003; 68: 147-152.
[228] Li Q, Xie LH, Haeberle A, Zhang J, Weina P. The evaluation of radiolabeled artesunate on tissue distribution in rats and protein binding in humans. Am J Trop Med Hyg. 2006; 75: 817-826.
[229] Li QG, Peggins JO, Lin AJ, Masonic K, Trotman KM, Brewer TG. Pharmacology and toxicology of artelinic acid: Preclinical investigation on pharmacokinetics, metabolism, protein and RBC binding, acute and anorectic toxicities. Trans R Soc Trop Med Hyg. 1998; 92: 332-340.
[230] Gu HM, Warhurst DC, Peters W. Uptake of [^{3}H]-dihydroartemisinin by erythrocytes infected with *Plasmodium falciparum in vitro*. Trans. R. Soc. Trop. Med. Hyg. 1984; 78: 265-270.
[231] Classen W, Altmann B, Gretener P, Souppart C, Skelton-Stroud P, Krinke G. Differental effects of orally *versus* parenterally administered qinghaosu derivatives artemether in dogs. Exp Toxicol Pathol 1999; 51: 507-516.
[232] Giao PT, de Vries PJ. Pharmacokinetic interactions of antimalarial agents. Clin Pharmacokinet. 2001; 40: 343-373.
[233] Looareesuwan S. Overview of clinical studies on artemisinin derivatives in Thailand. Trans Roy Soc Trop Med Hyg. 1994; 88(Suppl. 1): S9-11.
[234] White NJ. Why is it that antimalarial drug treatments do not always work? Ann Trop Med Parasitol. 1998; 92: 449-458.
[235] Ambroise-Thomas P. Intra-muscular artemether in the treatment of severe malaria: synthesis of current results. Med Trop (Mars). 1997; 57: 289-293.
[236] McLean WG, Ward SA. *In vitro* neurotoxicity of artemisinin derivatives. Med Trop (Mars). 1998; 58(Suppl. 3): 28-31.
[237] Bhatt KM, Samia BM, Bhatt SM, Wasunna KM. Efficacy and safety of an artesunate/mefloquine combination, (artequin) in the treatment of uncomplicated P. *falciparum* malaria in Kenya. East Afr Med J. 2006; 83: 236-242.
[238] Horton RJ, Parr SN, Bokor LC. Clinical experience with halofantrine in the treatment of malaria. Drugs Exp Clin Res. 1990; 16: 497-503.
[239] Hussein Z, Eaves J, Hutchinson DB, Canfield CJ. Population pharmacokinetics of atovaquone in patients with acute malaria caused by *Plasmodium falciparum*. Clin Pharmacol Ther. 1997; 61: 518-530.
[240] Milton KA, Edwards G, Ward SA, Orme ML, Breckenridge AM. Pharmacokinetics of halofantrine in man: Effects of food and dose size. Br J Clin Pharmacol. 1989; 28: 71-77.

[241] ter Kuile FO, Dolan G, Nosten F, Edstein MD, Luxemburger C, Phaipun L, Chongsuphajaisiddhi T, Webster HK, White NJ. Halofantrine *versus* mefloquine in treatment of multidrug-resistant *falciparum* malaria. Lancet. 1993; 341: 1044-1049.

[242] Bunnag D, Viravan C, Looareesuwan S, Karbwang J, Harinasuta T. Double blind randomized clinical trial of oral artesunate at once or twice daily dose in *falciparum* malaria. Southeast Asian J Trop Med Public Health. 1991; 22: 539-543.

[243] White NJ. Antimalarial pharmacokinetics and treatment regimens. Br J Clin Pharmacol. 1992; 34: 1-10.

[244] Rehwagen C. WHO ultimatum on artemisinin monotherapy is showing results. BMJ. 2006); 332: 1176.

[245] Yeates RA. Artemotil Artecef. Curr Opin Investig Drugs. 2002; 3: 545-549.

[246] Kyle DE. Teja-Isavadharm, P; Li, Q; Leo, K. Pharmacokinetics and pharmacodynamics of qinghaosu derivatives: How do they impact on the choice of drug and the dosage regimens? Med Trop (Mars). 1998; 58(Suppl. 3): 38-44.

[247] Li QG, Peggins JO, Fleckenstein LL, Masonic K, Heiffer MH, Brewer TG. The pharmacokinetics and bioavailability of dihydroartemisinin, arteether, artemether, artesunic acid and artelinic acid in rats. J Pharm Pharmacol. 1998; 50: 173-182.

[248] Dayan AD. Neurotoxicity and artemisinin compounds do the observations in animals justify limitation of clinical use? Med Trop (Mars). 1998; 58(Suppl. 3): 32-37.

[249] Genovese RF, Newman DB. Understanding artemisinin-induced brainstem neurotoxicity. Arch Toxicol. 2008; 82: 379-385.

[250] Li QG, Mog SR, Si YZ, Kyle DE, Gettayacamin M, Milhous WK. Neurotoxicity and efficacy of arteether related to its exposure times and exposure levels in rodents. Am J Trop Med Hyg. 2002; 66: 516-525.

[251] Navaratnam V, Mansor SM, Sit NW, Grace J, Li QG, Olliaro P. Pharmacokinetics of artemisinin-type compounds. Clin Pharmacokinet. 2000; 39: 255-270.

[252] Angus BJ, Thaiaporn I, Chanthapadith K, Suputtamongkol Y, White NJ. Oral artesunate dose-response relationship in acute *falciparum* malaria. Antimicrob Agents Chemother. 2002; 46: 778-782.

[253] Li Q, Louis R. Cantilena, Kevin J. Leary, George A. Saviolakis, R. Scott Miller, Victor Melendez, and, Weina PJ. Pharmacokinetic profiles of artesunate following single intravenous dose are 0.5, 1, 2, 4, and 8 mg/kg in healthy volunteers: Phase I study. Am J Trop Med Hyg 2009; 81: 615-621.

[254] Miller RS, Li Q, Cantilena LR, Leary KJ, Saviolakis GA, Melendez V, Smith B, Weina PJ. Pharmacokinetic profiles of artesunate following multiple intravenous doses of 2, 4, and 8 mg/kg in healthy volunteers: Phase 1b study. Malar J. 2012;11: 255.

[255] Li Q, Xie LH, Johnson TO, Si Y, Haeberle AS, Weina PJ. Toxicity evaluation of artesunate and artelinic acid in *Plasmodium* berghei-infected and uninfected rats. Trans R Soc Trop Med Hyg. 2007; 101: 104-112.

[256] Mehta SR, Das S. Management of malaria: Recent trends. J Commun Dis. 2006; 38: 130-138.

[257] Newton PN, Barnes KI, Smith PJ, Evans AC, Chierakul W, Ruangveerayuth R, White NJ. The pharmacokinetics of intravenous artesunate in adults with severe *falciparum* malaria. Eur J Clin Pharmacol. 2006; 62: 1003-1009.

[258] White NJ, Nosten F, Looareesuwan S, Watkins WM, Marsh K, Snow RW, Kokwaro G, Ouma J, Hien TT, Molyneux ME, Taylor TE, Newbold CI, Ruebush TK 2nd, Danis M, Greenwood BM, Anderson RM, Olliaro P. Averting a malaria disaster. Lancet. 1999; 353: 1965-1967.

[259] Luxemburger C, ter Kuile FO, Nosten F, Dolan G, Bradol JH, Phaipun L, Chongsuphajaisiddhi T, White NJ. Single day mefloquine- artesunate combination in the treatment of multi-drug resistant *falciparum* malaria. Trans R Soc Trop Med Hyg. 1994; 88: 213-217.

[260] Dieckmann A, Jung A. Stage-specific sensitivity of *Plasmodium falciparum* to antifolates. Z Parasitenkd. 1986; 72: 591-594.

[261] Geary TG, Divo AA, Jensen JB. Stage specific actions of antimalarial drugs on *Plasmodium falciparum* in culture. Am J Trop Med Hyg. 1989; 40: 240-244.

[262] Rieckmann K, Suebsaeng L, Rooney W. Response of *Plasmodium falciparum* infections to pyrimethamine-sulfadoxine in Thailand. Am J Trop Med Hyg. 1987; 37: 211-216.

[263] White NJ, Chapman D, Watt G. The effects of multiplication and synchronicity on the vascular distribution of parasites in *falciparum* malaria. Trans R Soc Trop Med Hyg. 1992; 86: 590-597.

[264] Yayon A, Vande Waa JA, Yayon M, Geary TG, Jensen JB. Stage-dependent effects of chloroquine on *Plasmodium falciparum in vitro*. J Protozool. 1983; 30: 642-647.
[265] Zhang Y, Asante KS, Jung A. Stage-dependent inhibition of chloroquine on *Plasmodium falciparum in vitro*. J Parasitol. 1986; 72: 830-836.
[266] Hien TT, White NJ, Qinghaosu. Lancet. 1993; 341: 603-608.
[267] White NJ. Clinical pharmacokinetics and pharmacodynamics of artemisinin and derivatives. Trans R Soc Trop Med Hyg. 1994; 88(Suppl. 1): S41-43.
[268] Drusano GL. Role of pharmacokinetics in the outcome of infections. Antimicrob Agents Chemother. (1988). 32, 289-297.
[269] Nosten F, ter Kuile F, Chongsuphajaisiddhi T, Luxemburger C, Webster HK, Edstein M, Phaipun L, Thew KL, White NJ. Mefloquine-resistant *falciparum* malaria on the Thai-Burmese border. Lancet. 1991; 337: 1140-1143.
[270] Ilett KF, Batty KT, Powell SM, Binh TQ, Thu le TA, Phuong HL, Hung NC, Davis TM. The pharmacokinetic properties of intramuscular artesunate and rectal dihydroartemisinin in uncomplicated *falciparum* malaria. Br J Clin Pharmacol. 2002; 53: 23-30.
[271] Nealon C, Dzeing A, Müller-Römer U, Planche T, Sinou V, Kombila M, Kremsner, PG, Parzy D, Krishna S. Intramuscular bioavailability and clinical efficacy of artesunate in gabonese children with severe malaria. Antimicrob Agents Chemother. 2002; 46: 3933-3939.
[272] Jelinek T. Intravenous artesunate recommended for patients with severe malaria: Position statement from TropNetEurop. Euro Surveill. 2005; 10: E051124.5.
[273] Luxemburger C, Nosten F, Raimond SD, Chongsuphajaisiddhi T, White NJ. Oral artesunate in the treatment of uncomplicated hyperparasitemic *falciparum* malaria. Am J Trop Med Hyg. 1995; 53: 522-525.
[274] McGready R, Cho T, Keo NK, Thwai KL, Villegas L, Looareesuwan S, White NJ, Nosten F. Artemisinin antimalarials in pregnancy: A prospective treatment study of 539 episodes of multidrug-resistant *Plasmodium falciparum*. Clin Infect Dis. 2001; 33: 2009-2016.
[275] Dellicour S, Hall S, Chandramohan D, Greenwood B. The safety of artemisinins during pregnancy: A pressing question. Malar J. 2007; 6: 15.
[276] Nosten F, Ashley E, McGready R, Price R. We still need artesunate monotherapy. BMJ. 2006; 333: 45.
[277] Weina PJ, Haeberle AS, Lowe MC, Cantilena L, Milhous WK. Intravenous artesunate: New product for the treatment of severe and complicated malaria. Am J Trop Med Hyg. 2005; 73: 32.
[278] Hastings IM. A model for the origins and spread of drug-resistant malaria. Parasitology. 1997; 115: 133-141.
[279] Chongsuphajaisiddhi T, Sabcharoen A, Attanath P. *In vivo* and *in vitro* sensitivity of *Falciparum* malaria to quinine in Thai children. Ann Trop Paediatr. 1981; 1: 21-26.
[280] Hellgren U, Kihamia CM, Mahikwano LF, Björkman A, Eriksson O, Rombo L. Response of *Plasmodium falciparum* to chloroquine treatment: Relation to whole blood concentrations of chloroquine and desethylchloroquine.Bull World Health Organ. 1989; 67: 197-202.
[281] Slutsker LM, Khoromana CO, Payne D, Allen CR, Wirima JJ, Heymann DL, Patchen L, Steketee RW. Mefloquine therapy for *Plasmodium falciparum* malaria in children under 5 years of age in Malawi: *In vivo*/*in vitro* efficacy and correlation of drug concentration with parasitological outcome. Bull World Health Organ. 1990; 68: 53-59.
[282] Thu LTA, Davis TME, Binh TQ, van Phuong, N; Anh, TK; Delayed parasite clearance in a Splenectomized patients with *falciparum* malaria who was treated with artemisinin derivatives. Clin Infect Dis. (1997). 25, 923-925.
[283] Batty KT, Le AT, Ilett KF, Nguyen PT, Powell SM, Nguyen CH, Truong XM, Vuong VC, Huynh VT, Tran QB, Nguyen VM, Davis TM. A pharmacokinetic and pharmacodynamic study of artesunate for *vivax* malaria. Am J Trop Med Hyg. 1998; 59: 823-827.
[284] Hassan Alin M, Ashton M, Kihamia CM, Mtey GJ, Bjorkman A. Multiple dose pharmacokinetics of oral artemisinin and comparison of its efficacy with that of oral artesunate in *falciparum* malaria patients. Trans R Soc Trop Med Hyg. 1996; 90: 61-65.
[285] Wilairatana P, Chanthavanich P, Singhasivanon P, Treeprasertsuk S, Krudsood S, Chalermrut K, Phisalaphong C, Kraisintu K, Looareesuwan S. A comparison of three different dihydroartemisinin

formulations for the treatment of acute uncomplicated *falciparum* malaria in Thailand. Int J Parasitol. 1998; 28: 1213-1218.

[286] Titulaer HA, Zuidema J, Lugt CB. Formulation and pharmacokinetics of artemisinin and its derivatives. Int J Pharmaceui. 1991; 69: 83-92.

[287] Murphy S, Watkins WM, Bray PG, Lowe B, Winstanley PA, Peshu N, Marsh K. Parasite viability during treatment of severe *falciparum* malaria: Differential effects of artemether and quinine. Am J Trop Med Hyg. 1995; 53: 303-305.

[288] Ashton M, Nguyen DS, Nguyen VH, Gordi T, Trinh NH, Dinh XH, Nguyen TN, Le DC. Artemisinin kinetics and dynamics during oral and rectal treatment of uncomplicated malaria. Clin Pharmacol Ther. 1998; 63: 482-93.

[289] Wise R. Maximizing efficacy and reducing the emergence of resistance. J Antimicrob Chemother. 2003; 51(Suppl.): 37-42.

[290] Zhao KC, Song ZY. Pharmacokinetics of dihydroqinghaosu in human volunteers and comparison with qinghaosu. Yao Xue Xue Bao. 1993; 28: 342-346.

[291] Koopmans R, Ha LD, Duc DD, Dien TK, Kager PA, Khanh NX, van Boxtel CJ, De Vries PJ. The pharmacokinetics of artemisinin after administration of two different suppositories to healthy Vietnamese subjects. Am J Trop Med Hyg. 1999; 60: 244-247.

[292] Looareesuwan S, Oosterhuis B, Schilizzi BM, Sollie FA, Wilairatana P, Krudsood S, Lugt CB, Peeters PA, Peggins JO. Dose-finding and efficacy study for i.m. artemotil (beta-arteether) and comparison with i.m. artemether in acute uncomplicated P. *falciparum* malaria. Br. J. Clin. Pharmacol. 2002; 53: 492-500.

[293] Singh N, Shukla MM, Asthana OP, Sharma VP. Effectiveness of alpha-beta arteether in clearing *Plasmodium falciparum* parasitemia in central India (Madhya Pradesh). Southeast Asian J. Trop. Med. Public Health. 1998; 29: 225-227.

[294] Sinclair D, Donegan S, Isba R, Lalloo DG. Artesunate *versus* quinine for treating severe malaria. Cochrane Database Syst Rev. 2012; 6: CD005967.

[295] Olupot-Olupot P, Maitland K. Management of severe malaria: results from recent trials. Adv Exp Med Biol. 2013; 764: 241-50.

[296] Nosten F, Ashley E, McGready R, Price R. We still need artesunate monotherapy. BMJ. 2006; 333: 45.

[297] Li Q, Cantilena LR, Leary KJ, Saviolakis GA, Miller RS, Melendez V, Weina PJ. Pharmacokinetic profiles of artesunate following single intravenous dose are 0.5, 1, 2, 4, and 8 mg/kg in healthy volunteers: Phase I study. Am J Trop Med Hyg 2009; 81: 615-621.

[298] Meshnick SR, Thomas A, Ranz A, Xu CM, Pan HZ. Artemisinin (qinghaosu): The role of intracellular hemin in its mechanism of antimalarial action. Mol Biochem Parasitol. 1991; 49: 181-189.

[299] Li ZL, Gu HM, Warhurst DC, Peters W. Effects of qinghaosu and related compounds on incorporation of [G-3H] hypoxanthine by *Plasmodium falciparum in vitro*. Trans R Soc Trop Med Hyg. 1983; 77: 522-523.

[300] Brand VB, Sandu CD, Duranton C, Tanneur V, Lang KS, Huber SM, Lang F. Dependence of *Plasmodium falciparum in vitro* growth on the cation permeability of the human host erythrocyte. Cell Physiol Biochem. 2003; 13: 347-356.

[301] Schrier SL. Red cell membrane biology--introduction. Clin Haematol. 1985; 14: 1-12.

[302] Asawamahasakda W, Benakis A, Meshnick SR. The interaction of artemisinin with red cell membranes. J Lab Clin Med. 1994; 123: 757-762.

[303] Maguire PA, Sherman IW. Phospholipid composition, cholesterol content and cholesterol exchange in *Plasmodium falciparum*-infected red cells. Mol Biochem Parasitol. 1990; 38: 105-112.

[304] Fujioka H, Aikawa M. Morphological changes of clefts in *Plasmodium*-infected erythrocytes under adverse conditions. Exp Parasitol. 1993; 76: 302-307.

[305] Pouvelle B, Spiegel R, Hsiao L, Howard RJ, Morris RL, Thomas AP, Taraschi TF. Direct access to serum macromolecules by intraerythrocytic malaria parasites. Nature. 1991; 353: 73-75.

[306] Ginsburg H, Kutner S, Zangwil M, Cabantchik ZI. Selectivity properties of pores induced in host erythrocyte membrane by *Plasmodium falciparum*. Effect of parasite maturation. Biochim Biophys Acta. 1986; 861: 194-196.

[307] Barnwell JW. Vesicle-mediated transport of membrane and proteins in malaria-infected erythrocytes. Blood Cells. 1990; 16: 379-395.

[308] Yuthavong Y, Wilairat P, Panijpan B, Potiwan C, Beale GH. Alterations in membrane proteins of mouse erythrocytes infected with different species and strains of malaria parasites. Comp Biochem Physiol B. 1979; 63: 83-85.
[309] Asawamahasakda W, Ittarat I, Pu YM, Ziffer H, Meshnick SR. Reaction of antimalarial endoperoxides with specific parasite proteins. Antimicrob Agents Chemother. 1994; 38: 1854-1858.
[310] Cofresi A, Milhous WK, Komisar J. Increasing parasitemia modulates *in vitro* concentration response to artemisinin drugs: Can parasite burden alter treatment outcomes in severe and complicated malaria? (our unpublished data)
[311] Li Q, Weina P, Milhous W. Pharmacokinetic and pharmacodynamic profiles of rapid-acting artemisinins in the antimalarial therapy. Current Drug Therapy. 2007; 2: 210-223.
[312] Navaratnam V, Mordi MN, Mansor SM. Simultaneous determination of artesunic acid and dihydroartemisinin in blood plasma by high-performance liquid chromatography for application in clinical pharmacological studies. J Chromatogr B Biomed Sci Appl. 1997; 692: 157-162.
[313] Li GQ, Guo XB, Fu LC, Jian HX, Wang XH. Clinical trials of artemisinin and its derivatives in the treatment of malaria in China. Trans R Soc Trop Med Hyg. 1994; 88(Suppl. 1): S5-6.
[314] White NJ. Artemisinin: Current status. Trans R Soc Trop Med Hyg. 1994; 88(Suppl. 1): S3-4.
[315] Anstey NM, Price RN, White NJ. Improving the availability of artesunate for treatment of severe malaria. Artesunate reduces mortality and should now be the treatment of choice in severe malaria in adults: Good news for countries in our region, but registration in Australia must wait. Med J Aust. 2006; 184: 3-4.
[316] WHO. Severe *falciparum* malaria. World Health Organization, Communicable Diseases Cluster. Trans R Soc Trop Med Hyg. 2000; 94 (Suppl 1): 1-90.
[317] Jones KL, Donegan S, Lalloo DG. Artesunate *versus* quinine for treating severe malaria. Cochrane Database Syst Rev. 2007; 17: CD005967.
[318] White NJ, Looareesuwan S, Warrell DA, Warrell MJ, Bunnag D, Harinasuta T. Quinine pharmacokinetics and toxicity in cerebral and uncomplicated *falciparum* malaria. Am J Med. 1982; 73: 564-572.
[319] Lesi A, Meremikwu M. High first dose quinine regimen for treating severe malaria. Cochrane Database Syst Rev. 2004; CD003341.
[320] Barennes H, Kailou D, Pussard E, Munjakazi JM, Fernan M, Sherouat H, Sanda A, Clavier F, Verdier F. Intrarectal administration of quinine: an early treatment for severe malaria in children? Sante. 2001; 11: 145-153.
[321] Woodrow CJ, Haynes RK, Krishna S. Artemisinins. Postgrad Med J. 2005; 81: 71-78.
[322] Pukrittayakamee S, Supanaranond W, Looareesuwan S, Vanijanonta S, White NJ. Quinine in severe *falciparum* malaria: evidence of declining efficacy in Thailand. Trans R Soc Trop Med Hyg. 1994; 88: 324-327.
[323] Miller KD, Greenberg AE, Campbell CC. Treatment of severe malaria in the United States with a continuous infusion of quinidine gluconate and exchange transfusion. N Engl J Med. 1989; 321: 65-70.
[324] White NJ, Looareesuwan S, Warrell DA, Chongsuphajaisiddhi T, Bunnag D, Harinasuta T. Quinidine in *falciparum* malaria. Lancet. 1981; 2: 1069-1071.
[325] Pe Than Myint, Tin Shwe. A controlled clinical trial of artemether (qinghaosu derivative) *versus* quinine in complicated and severe *falciparum* malaria. Trans R Soc Trop Med Hyg. 1987; 81: 559-561.
[326] Seaton RA. Trevett AJ, Wembri JP, Nwokolo N, Naraqi S, Black J, Laurenson IF, Kevau I, Saweri A, Lalloo DG, Warrell DA. Randomized comparison of intramuscular artemether and intravenous quinine in adult, Melanesian patients with severe or complicated, *Plasmodium falciparum* malaria in Papua New Guinea. Ann Trop Med Parasitol. 1998; 92: 133-139.
[327] Newton PN, Angus BJ, Chierakul W, Dondorp A, Ruangveerayuth R, Silamut K, Teerapong P, Suputtamongkol Y, Looareesuwan S, White NJ. Randomized comparison of artesunate and quinine in the treatment of severe *falciparum* malaria. Clin Infect Dis. 2003; 37: 7-16.
[328] Checkley AM, Whitty CJ. Artesunate, artemether or quinine in severe *Plasmodium falciparum* malaria. Expert Rev Anti Infect Ther. 2007; 5: 199-204.
[329] Barnes KI, Mwenechanya J, Tembo M, McIlleron H, Folb PI, Ribeiro I, Little F, Gomes M, Molyneux ME. Efficacy of rectal artesunate compared with parenteral quinine in initial treatment of

moderately severe malaria in African children and adults: a randomised study. Lancet. 2004; 363: 1598-1605.

[330] Arguin PM, Weina PJ, Dougherty CP. Artesunate for malaria. N Engl J Med. 2008; 359: 313.

[331] Cao XT, Bethell DB, Pham TP, Ta TT, Tran TN, Nguyen TT, Pham TT, Nguyen TT, Day NP, White NJ. Comparison of artemisinin suppositories, intramuscular artesunate and intravenous quinine for the treatment of severe childhood malaria. Trans R Soc Trop Med Hyg. 1997; 91: 335-342.

[332] Aceng JR, Byarugaba JS, Tumwine JK. Rectal artemether *versus* intravenous quinine for the treatment of cerebral malaria in children in Uganda: randomised clinical trial. BMJ. 2005; 330: 334.

[333] Gomes MF, Faiz MA, Gyapong JO, Warsame M, Agbenyega T, Babiker A, Baiden F, Yunus EB, Binka F, Clerk C, Folb P, Hassan R, Hossain MA, Kimbute O, Kitua A, Krishna S, Makasi C, Mensah N, Mrango Z, Olliaro P, Peto R, Peto TJ, Rahman R, Ribeiro I, Samad R, White NJ. Study 13 Research Group. Pre-referral rectal artesunate to prevent death and disability in severe malaria: a placebo-controlled trial. Lancet. 2009; 373(9663): 557-566.

[334] Gomes M, Ribeiro I, Warsame M, Karunajeewa H, Petzold M. Rectal artemisinins for malaria: a review of efficacy and safety from individual patient data in clinical studies. BMC Infect Dis. 2008; 8: 39.

[335] Karunajeewa HA, Manning L, Mueller I, Ilett KF, Davis TM. Rectal administration of artemisinin derivatives for the treatment of malaria. JAMA. 2007; 297: 2381-2390.

[336] Simpson JA, Agbenyega T, Barnes KI, Di Perri G, Folb P, Gomes M, Krishna S, Krudsood S, Looareesuwan S, Mansor S, McIlleron H, Miller R, Molyneux M, Mwenechanya J, Navaratnam V, Nosten F, Olliaro P, Pang L, Ribeiro I, Tembo M, van Vugt M, Ward S, Weerasuriya K, Win K, White NJ. Population pharmacokinetics of artesunate and dihydroartemisinin following intra-rectal dosing of artesunate in malaria patients. PLoS Med. 2006; 3: e444.

[337] Ashley EA, White NJ. Artemisinin-based combinations. Curr Opin Infect Dis. 2005; 18: 531-536.

[338] D'Alessandro U. Treating severe and complicated malaria. BMJ. 2004; 328: 155.

[339] Rosenthal PJ. Artesunate for the treatment of severe *falciparum* malaria. N Engl J Med. 2008; 358: 1829-1836.

[340] Silamut K, Newton PN, Teja-Isavadharm P, Suputtamongkol Y, Siriyanonda D, Rasameesoraj M, Pukrittayakamee S, White NJ. Artemether bioavailability after oral or intramuscular administration in uncomplicated *falciparum* malaria. Antimicrob. Agents Chemother. 2003; 47: 3795-3798.

[341] Karbwang J, Na-Bangchang K, Congpuong K, Molunto P, Thanavibul A. Pharmacokinetics and bioavailability of oral and intramuscular artemether. Eur. J. Clin. Pharmacol. 1997; 52: 307-310.

[342] Newton PN, van Vugt M, Teja-Isavadharm P, Siriyanonda D, Rasameesoroj M, Teerapong P, Ruangveerayuth R, Slight T, Nosten F, Suputtamongkol Y, Looareesuwan S, White NJ. Comparison of oral artesunate and dihydroartemisinin antimalarial bioavailabilities in acute *falciparum* malaria. Antimicrob. Agents Chemother. 2002; 46: 1125-1127.

[343] Na-Bangchang K, Thanavibul A, Tippawangkosol P, Karbwang J. Pharmacokinetics of the four combination regimens of dihydroartemisinin/mefloquine in acute uncomplicated *falciparum* malaria. Southeast Asian J. Trop. Med. Public Health. 2005; 36: 23-33.

[344] Omari AA, Gamble C, Garner P. Artemether-lumefantrine for uncomplicated malaria: a systematic review. Trop. Med. Int. Health. 2004; 9: 192-199.

[345] Poravuth Y, Socheat D, Fandeur T *et al.* Efficacy and safety of six dose regimen of Coartem® in the treatment of acute uncomplicated *falciparum* malaria in Cambodia. In: Gay F, editor. Proceedings of Mekong Malaria Symposium, 2002, Siem Reap, Angkor Wat, Kingdom of Cambodia. (Mekong Malaria Forum, RMCP-EC): 2002; 54-133.

[346] Khim N, Bouchier C, Ekala MT, Incardona S, Lim P, Legrand E, Jambou R, Doung S, Puijalon OM, Fandeur T. Countrywide survey shows very high prevalence of *Plasmodium falciparum* multilocus resistance genotypes in Cambodia. Antimicrob. Agents Chemother. 2005; 49: 3147-3152.

[347] Davis TM, Karunajeewa HA, Ilett KF. Artemisinin-based combination therapies for uncomplicated malaria. Med. J. Aust. 2005; 182: 181-185.

[348] Le Bras J, Musset L, Clain J. Antimalarial drug resistance. Med. Mal. Infect. 2006; 36: 401-405.

[349] Luxemburger C, ter Kuile FO, Nosten F, Dolan G, Bradol JH, Phaipun L, Chongsuphajaisiddhi T, White NJ. Single day mefloquine- artesunate combination in the treatment of multi-drug resistant *falciparum* malaria. Trans. R. Soc. Trop. Med. Hyg. 1994; 88: 213-217.

[350] Smithuis F, Kyaw MK, Phe O, Aye KZ, Htet L, Barends M, Lindegardh N, Singtoroj T, Ashley E, Lwin S, Stepniewska K, White NJ. Efficacy and effectiveness of dihydroartemisinin-piperaquine *versus* artesunate-mefloquine in *falciparum* malaria: an open-label randomised comparison. Lancet. 2006; 367(9528): 2075-2085.

[351] Janssens B, van Herp M, Goubert L, Chan S, Uong S, Nong S, Socheat D, Brockman A, Ashley EA, Van Damme W. A randomized open study to assess the efficacy and tolerability of dihydroartemisinin-piperaquine for the treatment of uncomplicated *falciparum* malaria in Cambodia. Trop. Med. Int. Health. 2007; 12: 251-259.

[352] Kawai S, Kano S, Suzuki M. Morphologic effects of artemether on *Plasmodium falciparum* in Aotus trivirgatus. Am. J. Trop. Med. Hyg. 1993; 49: 812-818.

[353] Maeno Y, Brown AE, Smith CD, Tegoshi T, Toyoshima T, Ockenhouse CF, Corcoran KD, Ngampochjana M, Kyle DE, Webster HK. A nonhuman primate model for human cerebral malaria: effects of artesunate (qinghaosu derivative) on rhesus monkeys experimentally infected with *Plasmodium* coatneyi. Am. J. Trop. Med. Hyg. 1993; 49: 726-734.

[354] Na-Bangchang K, Tippawangkosol P, Thanavibul A, Ubalee R, Karbwang J. Pharmacokinetic and pharmacodynamic interactions of mefloquine and dihydroartemisinin. Int J Clin Pharmacol Res. 1999; 19: 9-17.

[355] Giboda M, Denis MB. Response of Kampuchean strains of *Plasmodium falciparum* to antimalarials: *In vivo* assessment of quinine and quinine plus tetracycline; multiple drug resistance *in vitro*. J Trop Med Hyg. 1988; 91: 205-211.

[356] van Vugt M, Brockman A, Gemperli B, Luxemburger C, Gathmann I, Royce C, Slight T, Looareesuwan S, White NJ, Nosten F. Randomized comparison of artemether-benflumetol and artesunate-mefloquine in treatment of multidrug-resistant *falciparum* malaria. Antimicrob Agents Chemother. 1998; 42: 135-139.

[357] Vugt MV, Wilairatana P, Gemperli B, Gathmann I, Phaipun L, Brockman A, Luxemburger C, White NJ, Nosten F, Looareesuwan S. Efficacy of six doses of artemether-lumefantrine (benflumetol) in multidrug-resistant *Plasmodium falciparum* malaria. Am J Trop Med Hyg. 1999; 60: 936-942.

[358] Price RN. Artemisinin drugs: novel antimalarial agents. Expert Opin. Investig. Drugs. 2000; 9: 1815-1827.

[359] White NJ. Delaying antimalarial drug resistance with combination chemotherapy. Parasitologia. 1999; 41, 301-308.

[360] White NJ, Olliaro P. Artemisinin and derivatives in the treatment of uncomplicated malaria. Med. Trop. (Mars.) 1998; 58 (3 Suppl.3): 54-56.

[361] Nosten F, vanVugt M, Price RN, Luxemburger C, Thway KL, Brockman A, McGready R, ter Kuile F, Looareesuwan S, White NJ. Effects of artesunate-mefloquine combination on incidence of *Plasmodium falciparum* malaria and mefloquine resistance in western Thailand: a prospective study. Lancet. 2000; 356(9226): 297-302.

[362] Haynes RK. From artemisinin to new artemisinin antimalarials: biosynthesis, extraction, old and new derivatives, stereochemistry and medicinal chemistry requirements. Curr. Top. Med. Chem. 2006; 6: 509-537.

[363] White NJ, van Vugt M, Ezzet F. Clinical pharmacokinetics and pharmacodynamics of artemether lumefantrine. Clin. Pharmacokinet. 1999; 37: 105-125.

[364] Mayxay M, Thongpraseuth V, Khanthavong M, Lindegardh N, Barends M, Keola S, Pongvongsa T, Phompida S, Phetsouvanh R, Stepniewska K, White NJ, Newton PN. An open, randomized comparison of artesunate plus mefloquine *vs.* dihydroartemisinin-piperaquine for the treatment of uncomplicated *Plasmodium falciparum* malaria in the Lao People's Democratic Republic (Laos). Trop. Med. Int. Health. 2006; 11: 1157-1165.

[365] Schlitzer M. Antimalarial drugs - what is in use and what is in the pipeline. Arch Pharm (Weinheim). 2008; 341: 149-163.

[366] Hobbs C, Duffy P. Drugs for malaria: something old, something new, something borrowed. F1000 Biol Rep. 2011; 3: 24.

[367] Edwards G, Winstanley PA, Ward SA. Clinical pharmacokinetics in the treatment of tropical diseases. Some applications and limitations. Clin Pharmacokinet. 1994; 27(2): 150-65.

[368] Winstanley PA, Newton CR, Watkins WM, el al. Towards optimal parenteral quinine regimens for young children with cerebral malaria: importance of unbound quinine concentration. Trans R Soc Trop Med Hyg 1993; 87: 201-6.

[369] Omari AA, Gamble C, Garner P. Artemether-lumefantrine for uncomplicated malaria: a systematic review. Trop Med Int Health. 2004; 9: 192-9.

[370] Makanga M, Krudsood S. The clinical efficacy of artemether/lumefantrine (Coartem). Malar J. 2009; 8 (Suppl 1): S5.

[371] O'Neill PM, Ward SA, Berry NG, Jeyadevan JP, Biagini GA, Asadollaly E, Park BK, Bray PG. A medicinal chemistry perspective on 4-aminoquinoline antimalarial drugs. Curr Top Med Chem. 2006; 6: 479-507.

[372] Chen L, Qu FY, Zhou YC. Field observations on the antimalarial piperaquine. Chin Med J (Engl), 1982; 95: 281-286.

[373] Davis TM, Hung TY, Sim IK, Karunajeewa HA, Ilett KF. Piperaquine: a resurgent antimalarial drug. Drugs. 2005; 65: 75-87.

[374] Nzila A. The past, present and future of antifolates in the treatment of *Plasmodium falciparum* infection. J Antimicrob Chemother. 2006; 57: 1043-1054.

[375] Nosten F, White NJ. Artemisinin-based combination treatment of *falciparum* malaria. Am J Trop Med Hyg. 2007; 77(6 Suppl): 181-92.

[376] Denis MB, Tsuyuoka R, Poravuth Y, *et al.* Surveillance of the efficacy of artesunate and mefloquine combination for the treatment of uncomplicated *falciparum* malaria in Cambodia. Trop Med Int Health. 2006; 11: 1360-1366.

[377] Noedl H, Se Y, Sriwichai S, *et al.* Artemisinin resistance in Cambodia: a clinical trial designed to address an emerging problem in Southeast Asia. Clin Infect Dis. 2010; 51: e82-e89.

[378] Kamya MR, Yeka A, Bukirwa H, Lugemwa M, Rwakimari JB, Staedke SG, Talisuna AO, Greenhouse B, Nosten F, Rosenthal PJ, Wabwire-Mangen F, Dorsey G. Artemether-lumefantrine *versus* dihydroartemisinin-piperaquine for treatment of malaria: a randomized trial. PLoS Clin Trials. 2007; 2: e20.

[379] Yeka A, Dorsey G, Kamya MR, Talisuna A, Lugemwa M, Rwakimari JB, Staedke SG, Rosenthal PJ, Wabwire-Mangen F, Bukirwa H. Artemether-lumefantrine *versus* dihydroartemisinin-piperaquine for treating uncomplicated malaria: a randomized trial to guide policy in Uganda. PLoS One. 2008; 3: e2390.

[380] Arinaitwe E, Sandison TG, Wanzira H, Kakuru A, Homsy J, Kalamya J, Kamya MR, Vora N, Greenhouse B, Rosenthal PJ, Tappero J, Dorsey G. Artemether-lumefantrine *versus* dihydroartemisinin-piperaquine for *falciparum* malaria: a longitudinal, randomized trial in young Ugandan children. Clin Infect Dis. 2009; 49: 1629-37.

[381] Song J, Socheat D, Tan B, Seila S, Xu Y, Ou F, Sokunthea S, Sophorn L, Zhou C, Deng C, Wang Q, Li G. Randomized trials of artemisinin-piperaquine, dihydroartemisinin-piperaquine phosphate and artemether-lumefantrine for the treatment of multi-drug resistant *falciparum* malaria in Cambodia-Thailand border area. Malar J. 2011; 10: 231.

[382] Wang SQ, Christophel E, Lin SG, Meng F, Hu XM, Wang GZ, Liu J, Zeng LH. Efficacy of dihydroartemisinin-piperaquine and artemether-lumefantrine in the treatment of uncomplicated *falciparum* malaria in Hainan, China. Zhongguo Ji Sheng Chong Xue Yu Ji Sheng Chong Bing Za Zhi. 2008; 26: 50-2.

[383] Bassat Q, Mulenga M, Tinto H, Piola P, Borrmann S, Menéndez C, Nambozi M, Valéa I, Nabasumba C, Sasi P, Bacchieri A, Corsi M, Ubben D, Talisuna A, D'Alessandro U. Dihydroartemisinin-piperaquine and artemether-lumefantrine for treating uncomplicated malaria in African children: a randomised, non-inferiority trial. PLoS One. 2009; 4: e7871.

[384] Thanh NX, Trung TN, Phong NC, Quang HH, Dai B, Shanks GD, Chavchich M, Edstein MD. The efficacy and tolerability of artemisinin-piperaquine (Artequick®) *versus* artesunate-amodiaquine (Coarsucam™) for the treatment of uncomplicated *Plasmodium falciparum* malaria in south-central Vietnam. Malar J. 2012; 11: 217.

[385] Gargano N, Ubben D, Tommasini S, Bacchieri A, Corsi M, Bhattacharyya PC, Rao BH, Dubashi N, Dev V, Ghosh SK, Kumar A, Srivastava B, Valecha N. Therapeutic efficacy and safety of dihydroartemisinin-piperaquine *versus* artesunate-mefloquine in uncomplicated *Plasmodium falciparum* malaria in India. Malar J. 2012; 11: 233.

[386] Sigma-tau, Application for inclusion of dihydroartemisinin plus piperaquine (DHA/PPQ) fixed dose combination tablets in the 17th edition of the WHO model lists of essential medicines. http://www.who.int/selection_medicines/committees/expert/18/applications/D_Piperaquine.pdf.

[387] Valecha N, Phyo AP, Mayxay M, Newton PN, Krudsood S, Keomany S, Khanthavong M, Pongvongsa T, Ruangveerayuth R, Uthaisil C, Ubben D, Duparc S, Bacchieri A, Corsi M, Rao BH, Bhattacharya PC, Dubhashi N, Ghosh SK, Dev V, Kumar A, Pukrittayakamee S. An open-label, randomised study of dihydroartemisinin-piperaquine *versus* artesunate-mefloquine for *falciparum* malaria in Asia. PLoS One. 2010; 5: e11880.

[388] Keating GM. Dihydroartemisinin/Piperaquine: a review of its use in the treatment of uncomplicated *Plasmodium falciparum* malaria. Drugs. 2012; 72: 937-61.

[389] Hasugian AR, Purba HL, Kenangalem E, Wuwung RM, Ebsworth EP, Maristela R, Penttinen PM, Laihad F, Anstey NM, Tjitra E, Price RN. Dihydroartemisinin-piperaquine *versus* artesunate-amodiaquine: superior efficacy and posttreatment prophylaxis against multidrug-resistant *Plasmodium falciparum* and *Plasmodium vivax* malaria. Clin Infect Dis. 2007; 44: 1067-74.

[390] Karunajeewa HA, Mueller I, Senn M, Lin E, Law I, Gomorrai PS, Oa O, Griffin S, Kotab K, Suano P, Tarongka N, Ura A, Lautu D, Page-Sharp M, Wong R, Salman S, Siba P, Ilett KF, Davis TM. A trial of combination antimalarial therapies in children from Papua New Guinea. N Engl J Med. 2008; 359: 2545-57.

[391] Sinclair D, Gogtay N, Brand F, Olliaro P. Artemisinin-based combination therapy for treating uncomplicated *Plasmodium vivax* malaria. Cochrane Database Syst Rev. 2011; (7):CD008492.

[392] Bassat Q. The use of artemether-lumefantrine for the treatment of uncomplicated *Plasmodium vivax* malaria. PLoS Negl Trop Dis. 2011; 5: e1325.

[393] Douglas NM, Anstey NM, Angus BJ, Nosten F, Price RN. Artemisinin combination therapy for *vivax* malaria. Lancet Infect Dis. 2010; 10: 405-16.

[394] van Steeg TJ, Boralli VB, Krekels EH, Slijkerman P, Freijer J, Danhof M, de Lange EC. Influence of plasma protein binding on pharmacodynamics: Estimation of *in vivo* receptor affinities of beta blockers using a new mechanism-based PK-PD modelling approach. J Pharm Sci. 2009; 98: 3816-28.

[395] Rogers WO, Sem R, Tero T, Chim P, Lim P, Muth S, Socheat D, Ariey F, Wongsrichanalai C. Failure of artesunate-mefloquine combination therapy for uncomplicated *Plasmodium falciparum* malaria in southern Cambodia. Malar J. 2009; 8: 10.

[396] Na-Bangchang K, Ruengweerayut R, Mahamad P, Ruengweerayut K, Chaijaroenkul W. Declining in efficacy of a three-day combination regimen of mefloquine-artesunate in a multi-drug resistance area along the Thai-Myanmar border. Malar J. 2010; 9: 273.

[397] Vijaykadga S, Alker AP, Satimai W, MacArthur JR, Meshnick SR, Wongsrichanalai C. Delayed *Plasmodium falciparum* clearance following artesunate-mefloquine combination therapy in Thailand, 1997-2007. Malar J. 2012; 11: 296.

[398] Borrmann S, Sasi P, Mwai L, Bashraheil M, Abdallah A, Muriithi S, Frühauf H, Schaub B, Pfeil J, Peshu J, Hanpithakpong W, Rippert A, Juma E, Tsofa B, Mosobo M, Lowe B, Osier F, Fegan G, Lindegårdh N, Nzila A, Peshu N, Mackinnon M, Marsh K. Declining responsiveness of *Plasmodium falciparum* infections to artemisinin-based combination treatments on the Kenyan coast. PLoS One. 2011; 6: e26005.

[399] Rueangweerayut R, Phyo AP, Uthaisin C, Poravuth Y, Binh TQ, Tinto H, Pénali LK, Valecha N, Tien NT, Abdulla S, Borghini-Fuhrer I, Duparc S, Shin CS, Fleckenstein L; Pyronaridine-Artesunate Study Team. Pyronaridine-artesunate *versus* mefloquine plus artesunate for malaria. N Engl J Med. 2012; 366: 1298-309.

[400] Piyaphanee W, Krudsood S, Tangpukdee N, Thanachartwet W, Silachamroon U, *et al.* Emergence and clearance of gametocytes in uncomplicated *Plasmodium falciparum* malaria. Am J Trop Med Hyg. 2006; 74: 432-435.

[401] Stepniewska K, Price RN, Sutherland CJ, Drakeley CJ, von Seidlein L, *et al. Plasmodium falciparum* gametocyte dynamics in areas of different malaria endemicity. Malar J. 2008; 7: 249.

[402] Bousema T, Okell L, Shekalaghe S, Griffin JT, Omar S, *et al.* Revisiting the circulation time of *Plasmodium falciparum* gametocytes: molecular detection methods to estimate the duration of gametocyte carriage and the effect of gametocytocidal drugs. Malar J. 2010; 9: 136.

[403] Coulibaly B, Zoungrana A, Mockenhaupt FP, Schirmer RH, Klose C, *et al.* Strong gametocytocidal effect of methylene blue-based combination therapy against *falciparum* malaria: a randomised controlled trial. PLoS One. 2009; 4: e5318.

[404] Shekalaghe S, Drakeley C, Gosling R, Ndaro A, van Meegeren M, *et al.* Primaquine clears submicroscopic *Plasmodium falciparum* gametocytes that persist after treatment with sulphadoxine-pyrimethamine and artesunate. PLoS One. 2007; 2: e1023.

[405] D'Alessandro U. Progress in the development of piperaquine combinations for the treatment of malaria. Curr Opin Infect Dis. 2009; 22: 588-92.

[406] van den Broek I, Kitz C, Al Attas S, Libama F, Balasegaram M, Guthmann JP. Efficacy of three artemisinin combination therapies for the treatment of uncomplicated *Plasmodium falciparum* malaria in the Republic of Congo. Malar J. 2006; 5: 113.

[407] Zwang J, Ashley EA, Karema C, D'Alessandro U, Smithuis F, Dorsey G, Janssens B, Mayxay M, Newton P, Singhasivanon P, Stepniewska K, White NJ, Nosten F. Safety and efficacy of dihydroartemisinin-piperaquine in *falciparum* malaria: a prospective multi-centre individual patient data analysis. PLoS One. 2009; 4: e6358.

[408] Awab GR, Pukrittayakamee S, Imwong M, Dondorp AM, Woodrow CJ, Lee SJ, Day NP, Singhasivanon P, White NJ, Kaker F. Dihydroartemisinin-piperaquine *versus* chloroquine to treat *vivax* malaria in Afghanistan: an open randomized, non-inferiority, trial. Malar J. 2010; 9: 105.

[409] Ratcliff A, Siswantoro H, Kenangalem E, Maristela R, Wuwung RM, Laihad F, Ebsworth EP, Anstey NM, Tjitra E, Price RN. Two fixed-dose artemisinin combinations for drug-resistant *falciparum* and *vivax* malaria in Papua, Indonesia: an open-label randomised comparison. Lancet. 2007; 369(9563): 757-65.

[410] Grande T, Bernasconi A, Erhart A, Gamboa D, Casapia M, Delgado C, Torres K, Fanello C, Llanos-Cuentas A, D'Alessandro U. A randomised controlled trial to assess the efficacy of dihydroartemisinin-piperaquine for the treatment of uncomplicated *falciparum* malaria in Peru. PLoS One. 2007; 2: e1101.

[411] van Vugt M, van Beest A, Sicuri E, van Tulder M, Grobusch MP. Malaria treatment and prophylaxis in endemic and nonendemic countries: evidence on strategies and their cost-effectiveness. Future Microbiol. 2011; 6: 1485-500.

[412] Sousa M, Pozniak A, Boffito M. Pharmacokinetics and pharmacodynamics of drug interactions involving rifampicin, rifabutin and antimalarial drugs. J Antimicrob Chemother. 2008; 62: 872-8.

[413] Yeka A, Harris JC. Treating uncomplicated malaria in children: comparing artemisinin-based combination therapies. Curr Opin Pediatr. 2010; 22: 798-803.

[414] Lefevre G, Looareesuwan S, Treeprasertsuk S, Krudsood S, Silachamroon U, Gathmann I, Mull R, Bakshi R. A clinical and pharmacokinetic trial of six doses of artemether-lumefantrine for multidrug-resistant *Plasmodium falciparum* malaria in Thailand. Am J Trop Med Hyg. 2001; 64: 247-256.

[415] Falade CO, Ogundele AO, Yusuf BO, Ademowo OG, Ladipo SM. High efficacy of two artemisinin-based combinations (artemether-lumefantrine and artesunate plus amodiaquine) for acute uncomplicated malaria in Ibadan, Nigeria. Trop Med Int Health. 2008; 13: 635-643.

[416] Ndayiragije A, Niyungeko D, Karenzo J, Niyungeko E, Barutwanayo M, Ciza A, Bosman A, Moyou-Somo R, Nahimana A, Nyarushatsi JP, Barihuta T, Mizero L, Ndaruhutse J, Delacollette C, Ringwald P, Kamana J. Efficacy of therapeutic combinations with artemisinin derivatives in the treatment of non complicated malaria in Burundi. Trop Med Int Health. 2004; 9: 673-679.

[417] Plowe CV. Combination therapy for malaria: Mission accomplished? Clin Infect Dis. 2007; 44: 1075-1077.

[418] Zongo I, Dorsey G, Rouamba N, Dokomajilar C, Séré Y, Rosenthal PJ, Ouédraogo JB. Randomized comparison of amodiaquine plus sulfadoxine-pyrimethamine, artemether-lumefantrine, and dihydroartemisinin-piperaquine for the treatment of uncomplicated *Plasmodium falciparum* malaria in Burkina Faso. Clin Infect Dis. 2007; 45: 1453-1461.

[419] Piedade R, Gil JP. The pharmacogenetics of antimalaria artemisinin combination therapy. Expert Opin Drug Metab Toxicol. 2011; 7: 1185-200.

[420] German PI, Aweeka FT. Clinical pharmacology of artemisinin-based combination therapies. Clin Pharmacokinet. 2008; 47: 91-102. Review. Erratum in: Clin Pharmacokinet. 2008; 47: 152.

[421] Brockman A, Price RN, van Vugt M, Heppner DG, Walsh D, Sookto P, Wimonwattrawatee T, Looareesuwan S, White NJ, Nosten F. *Plasmodium falciparum* antimalarial drug susceptibility on the

north-western border of Thailand during five years of extensive use of artesunate-mefloquine. Trans R Soc Trop Med Hyg. 2000; 94: 537-544.

[422] Nyunt MM, Plowe CV. Pharmacologic advances in the global control and treatment of malaria: Combination therapy and resistance. Clin Pharmacol Ther. 2007; 82: 601-605.

[423] Meshnick SR, Alker AP. Amodiaquine and combination chemotherapy for malaria. Am J Trop Med Hyg. 2005; 73: 821-823.

[424] Grandesso F, Hagerman A, Kamara S, Lam E, Checchi F, Balkan S, Scollo G, Durand R, Guthmann JP. Low efficacy of the combination artesunate plus amodiaquine for uncomplicated *falciparum* malaria among children under 5 years in Kailahun, Sierra Leone. Trop Med Int Health. 2006; 11: 1017-1021.

[425] Ramharter M, Oyakhirome S, Klein Klouwenberg P, Adégnika AA, Agnandji ST, Missinou MA, Matsiégui PB, Mordmüller B, Borrmann S, Kun JF, Lell B, Krishna S, Graninger W, Issifou S, Kremsner PG. Artesunate-clindamycin *versus* quinine-clindamycin in the treatment of *Plasmodium falciparum* malaria: A randomized controlled trial. Clin Infect Dis. 2005; 40: 1777-1784.

[426] Sisowath C, Strömberg J, Mårtensson A, Msellem M, Obondo C, Björkman A, Gil JP. *In vivo* selection of *Plasmodium falciparum* pfmdr1 86N coding alleles by artemether-lumefantrine (Coartem). J Infect Dis. 2005; 191: 1014-1017.

[427] Hastings IM, Ward SA. Coartem (artemether-lumefantrine) in Africa: The beginning of the end? J Infect Dis. 2005; 192: 1303-1304.

[428] Palmer KJ, Holliday SM, Brogden RN, Mefloquine. A review of its antimalarial activity, pharmacokinetic properties and therapeutic efficacy. Drugs. 1993; 45: 430-475.

[429] Wells TN, Alonso PL, Gutteridge WE. New medicines to improve control and contribute to the eradication of malaria. Nat Rev Drug Discov. 2009; 8: 879-91.

[430] Srivastava S, Sherman C, Meek C, Leff R, Gumbo T. Pharmacokinetic mismatch does not lead to emergence of isoniazid- or rifampin-resistant Mycobacterium tuberculosis but to better antimicrobial effect: a new paradigm for antituberculosis drug scheduling. Antimicrob Agents Chemother. 2011; 55: 5085-9.

[431] Brockman A, Price RN, van Vugt M, Heppner DG, Walsh D, Sookto P, Wimonwattrawatee T, Looareesuwan S, White NJ, Nosten F. *Plasmodium falciparum* antimalarial drug susceptibility on the north-western border of Thailand during five years of extensive use of artesunate-mefloquine. Trans R Soc Trop Med Hyg. 2000; 94: 537-44.

[432] Foley M, Tilley L. Quinoline antimalarials: mechanisms of action and resistance and prospects for new agents. Pharmacol. Ther. 1998; 79: 55-87.

[433] Famin O, Ginsburg H. Differential effects of 4-aminoquinoline-containing antimalarial drugs on hemoglobin digestion in *Plasmodium falciparum*-infected erythrocytes. Biochem. Pharmacol. 2002; 63: 393-398.

[434] Looareesuwan S, Chulay JD, Canfield CJ, Hutchinson DB. Malarone (atovaquone and proguanil hydrochloride): a review of its clinical development for treatment of malaria. Malarone Clinical Trials Study Group. Am. J. Trop. Med. Hyg. 1999; 60: 533-541.

[435] Srivastava IK, Vaidya AB. A mechanism for the synergistic antimalarial action of atovaquone and proguanil. Antimicrob. Agents Chemother. 1999; 43: 1334-1339.

[436] malERA Consultative Group on Drugs, Alonso PL, Djimde A, Kremsner P, Magill A, *et al.* A research agenda for malaria eradication: drugs. PLoS Med 2011; 8: e1000402.

[437] Ding XC, Beck HP, Raso G. *Plasmodium* sensitivity to artemisinins: magic bullets hit elusive targets. Trends Parasitol 2011; 27: 73-81.

[438] White NJ. Artemisinin resistance-the clock is ticking. Lancet 2010; 376: 2051-2052.

[439] Painter HJ, Morrisey JM, Vaidya AB. Mitochondrial electron transport inhibition and viability of intraerythrocytic *Plasmodium falciparum*. Antimicrobial Agents and Chemotherapy 2010; 54: 5281-5287.

[440] Sanz LM, Crespo B, De-Cózar C, Ding XC, Llergo JL, Burrows JN, García-Bustos JF, Gamo FJ. P. *falciparum in vitro* killing rates allow to discriminate between different antimalarial mode-of-action. PLoS One. 2012; 7: e30949.

[441] O'Neill PM, Barton VE, Ward SA. The molecular mechanism of action of artemisinin-the debate continues. Molecules 2010; 15: 1705-1721.

[442] Laufer MK. *et al.* Return of chloroquine antimalarial efficacy in Malawi. N. Engl. J. Med. 2006; 355: 1959-1966.

[443] de Vries PJ, Bich NN, Van Thien H, Hung LN, Anh TK, Kager PA, Heisterkamp SH. Combinations of artemisinin and quinine for uncomplicated *falciparum* malaria: efficacy and pharmacodynamics. Antimicrob Agents Chemother. 2000; 44: 1302-8.

[444] Hoshen MB, Stein WD, Ginsburg H. Mathematical modelling of malaria chemotherapy: combining artesunate and mefloquine. Parasitology. 2002; 124(Pt 1): 9-15.

[445] Brocks DR, Mehvar R. Stereoselectivity in the pharmacodynamics and pharmacokinetics of the chiral antimalarial drugs. Clin Pharmacokinet. 2003; 42:1359-1382.

[446] Tett SE, McLachlan AJ, Cutler DJ, Day RO. Pharmacokinetics and pharmacodynamics of hydroxychloroquine enantiomers in patients with rheumatoid arthritis receiving multiple doses of racemate. Chirality. 1994; 6: 355-359.

[447] Miler DR, Fiechtner JJ, Carpenter JR, Brown RR, Stroshane RM, Stecher VJ. Plasma hydroxychloroquine concentrations and efficacy in rheumatoid arthritis.Arthritis Rheum. 1987; 30: 567-571.

[448] Brocks DR, Skeith KJ, Johnston C, Emamibafrani J, Davis P, Russell AS, Jamali F. Hematologic disposition of hydroxychloroquine enantiomers. J Clin Pharmacol. 1994; 34: 1088-1097.

[449] Wesche DL, Schuster BG, Wang WX, Woosley RL. Mechanism of cardiotoxicity of halofantrine. Clin Pharmacol Ther. 2000; 67: 521-529.

[450] Abernethy DR, Wesche DL, Barbey JT, Ohrt C, Mohanty S, Pezzullo JC, Schuster BG. Stereoselective halofantrine disposition and effect: Concentration-related QTc prolongation. Br J Clin Pharmacol. 2001; 51: 231-237.

[451] Ghavami G, Kazemali MR, Sardari S. Informatics of drug synergism in naturally occurring anticancer agents. Recent Pat Anticancer Drug Discov. 2011; 6: 26-44.

[452] Ahmad AM. Recent advances in pharmacokinetic modeling. Biopharm Drug Dispos. 2007; 28: 135-43.

[453] Suttle AB, Pollack GM, Brouwer KLR. Use of a pharmacokinetic model incorporating discontinuous gastrointestinal absorption to examine the occurrence of double peaks in oral concentration-time profiles. Pharm Res 1992; 9: 350-355.

[454] Wright JD, MA T, Chu CK, Boudinot FD. Discontinuous oral absorption pharmacokinetic model and bioavailability of 1-(2-flouro-5-methyl-b-l-arabinofuranosyl)uracil (L-FMAU) in rats. Biopharm Drug Dispos 1996; 17: 197-207.

[455] International Neoral Renal Transplantation Study Group. Cyclosporine micro emulsion (Neoral) absorption profiling and sparse-sample predictors during the first three months after renal transplantation. Am J Transplant 2002; 2: 148-156.

[456] Debord J, Risco E, Harel M, *et al.* Application of a gamma model of absorption to oral cyclosporin. Clin Pharmacokinet 2001; 40: 375-382.

[457] Rousseau A, Leger F, Le Meur Y, *et al.* Population pharmacokinetic modeling of oral cyclosporine using NONMEM. Ther Drug Monit 2004; 26: 23-30.

[458] Gallo JM, Vicini P, Orlansky A, *et al.* Pharmacokinetic model-predicted anti-cancer drug concentrations in human tumors. Clin Cancer Res 2004; 10: 8048-8058.

[459] Huang CS-H, Boudinot FD, Feldman S. Maternal-fetal pharmacokinetics of Zidovudine in rats. J Pharm Sci 1996; 85: 965-970.

[460] Sakanaka K, Kawazu K, Tomonari M, *et al.* Ocular pharmacokinetic/pharmacodynamic modeling for bunazosin after instillation into rabbits. Pharm Res 2004; 21: 770-776.

[461] Ranta V-P, Laavola M, Toropainen E, Vellonen K-S, Talvitie A, Urtii A. Ocular pharmacokinetic modeling using corneal sorption and desorption rates from *in vitro* permeation experiments with cultured corneal epithelial cells. Pharm Res 2003; 20: 1409-1416.

[462] Ezzet F, Krishna G, Wexler DB, *et al.* A population pharmacokinetic model that describes multiple peaks due to enterohepatic recirculation of ezetimibe. Clin Ther 2001; 23: 871-885.

[463] Yamano K, Yamamoto K, Katashima M, *et al.* Prediction of midazolam-CYP3A inhibitors interaction in the human liver from *in vivo/in vitro* absorption, distribution and metabolism data. Drug Metab Dispos 2001; 29 (part 1): 443-452.

[464] Ward ES, Pollack GM, Brouwer KLR. Probenecid-associated alterations in valproate glucuronide hepatobiliary disposition: mechanistic assessment using mathematical modeling. J Pharmacol Exp Ther 2001; 297: 141-147.

[465] Svensson USH, Maki-Jouppila M, Hoffmann K-J, Ashton M. Characterization of the human liver *in vitro* metabolic pattern of artemisinin and auto-induction in the rat by the use of non-linear mixed effects modeling. Biopharm Drug Dispos 2003; 24: 71-85.
[466] Elsherbiny DA, Asimus SA, Karlsson MO, Ashton M, Simonsson US. A model based assessment of the CYP2B6 and CYP2C19 inductive properties by artemisinin antimalarials: implications for combination regimens. J Pharmacokinet Pharmacodyn. 2008; 35: 203-17.
[467] Ni L, Boudinot FD. Non-linear renal and biliary clearances of antiviral polyoxometalates in rats. Eur J Drug Metab Pharmacokinet 1995; 20: 209-217.
[468] Hansen RJ, Balthasar JP. Pharmacokinetic/pharmacodynamic modeling of the effects of intravenous immunoglobulin on the disposition of antiplatelet antibodies in a rat model of immune thrombocytopenia. J Pharm Sci 2003; 92: 1206-1215.
[469] Mager DE, Neuteboom B, Efthymiopoulos C, *et al.* Receptor-mediated pharmacokinetics and pharmacodynamics of interferon-b1a in monkeys. J Pharmacol Exp Ther 2003; 306: 262-270.
[470] Wang B, Ludden TM, Cheung EN, *et al.* Population pharmacokinetic pharmacodynamic modeling of filgrastim (r-metHuG-CSF) in healthy volunteers. J Pharmacokinet Pharmacodyn 2001; 28: 321-342.
[471] Rowland M, Peck C, Tucker G. Physiologically-based pharmacokinetics in drug development and regulatory science. Annu Rev Pharmacol Toxicol. 2011; 51: 45-73.
[472] Peters SA, Ungell AL, Dolgos H. Physiologically based pharmacokinetic (PBPK) modeling and simulation: applications in lead optimization. Curr Opin Drug Discov Devel. 2009; 12: 509-18.
[473] Yang RSH, Andersen ME, Dennison JE, Ou YC, Liao KH, Reisfeld B. Physiologically based pharmacokinetic and pharmacodynamic modeling. Chapter 23. In: Mouse Models of Cancer, E.C. Holland, Ed. Wiley Inc., New York, NY. 2004; p. 391-405.
[474] Lazarou J, Pomeranz BH, Corey PN. Incidence of adverse drug reactions in hospitalized patients: a meta-analysis of prospective studies. JAMA. 1998; 279: 1200-5.
[475] Kanamitsu S, Ito K, Green CE, Tyson CA, Shimada N, Sugiyama Y. Prediction of *in vivo* interaction between triazolam and erythromycin based on *in vitro* studies using human liver microsomes and recombinant human CYP3A4. Pharm Res. 2000; 17: 419-26.
[476] Blesch KS, Gieschke R, Tsukamoto Y, Reigner BG, Burger HU, Steimer JL. Clinical pharmacokinetic/pharmacodynamic and physiologically based pharmacokinetic modeling in new drug development: the capecitabine experience. Invest New Drugs 2003; 21: 195-223.
[477] Ploeger BA, van der Graaf PH, Danhof M. Incorporating receptor theory in mechanism-based pharmacokinetic-pharmacodynamic (PK-PD) modeling. Drug Metab Pharmacokinet. 2009; 24: 3-15.
[478] Rang HP. The receptor concept: pharmacology's big idea. Br. J. Pharmacol. 2006; 147: S9-16.
[479] Black JW, Leff P. Operational models of pharmacological agonism. Proc. R Soc. Lond. B. Biol. Sci., 1983; 220: 141-162.
[480] de Lange EC, Ravenstijn PG, Groenendaal D, van Steeg TJ. Toward the prediction of CNS drug-effect profiles in physiological and pathological conditions using microdialysis and mechanism-based pharmacokinetic-pharmacodynamic modeling. Aaps J. 2005; 7: E532-543.
[481] Tuk B, van Oostenbruggen MF, Herben VM, Mandema JW, Danhof M. Characterization of the pharmacodynamic interaction between parent drug and active metabolite *in vivo*: midazolam and alpha-OH-midazolam. J. Pharmacol. Exp. Ther. 1999; 289:1067-1074.
[482] Danhof M, de Jongh J, De Lange EC, Della Pasqua O, Ploeger BA, Voskuyl RA. Mechanism-based pharmacokinetic- pharmacodynamic modeling: biophase distribution, receptor theory, and dynamical systems analysis. Annu. Rev. Pharmacol. Toxicol. 2007; 47: 357-400.
[483] Visser SA, Smulders CJ, Reijers BP, Van der Graaf PH, Peletier LA, Danhof M. Mechanism-based pharmacokinetic- pharmacodynamic modeling of concentrationdependent hysteresis and biphasic electroencephalogram effects of alphaxalone in rats. J. Pharmacol. Exp. Ther. 2002; 302: 1158-1167.
[484] Frigyesi A, Hossjer O. Estimating the parameters of the operational model of pharmacological agonism. Stat. Med.2006; 25: 2932-2945.
[485] Leff P, Prentice DJ, Giles H, Martin GR, Wood J. Estimation of agonist affinity and efficacy by direct, operational model-fitting. J. Pharmacol. Methods. 1990; 23: 225-237.
[486] Van der Graaf PH, Danhof M. On the reliability of affinity and efficacy estimates obtained by direct operational model fitting of agonist concentration-effect curves following irreversible receptor inactivation. J. Pharmacol. Toxicol. Methods. 1997; 38: 81-85.

[487] Van der Graaf PH, Stam WB. Analysis of receptor inactivation experiments with the operational model of agonism yields correlated estimates of agonist affinity and efficacy. J. Pharmacol. Toxicol. Methods. 1999; 41: 117-125.

[488] Garrido M, Gubbens-Stibbe J, Tukker E, Cox E, von Frijtag J, Kunzel D, IJzerman AP, Danhof M, van der Graaf PH. Pharmacokinetic-pharmacodynamic analysis of the EEG effect of alfentanil in rats following beta-funaltrexamine-induced mu-opioid receptor ``knockdown" *in vivo*. Pharm. Res. 2000; 17: 653-659.

[489] Leff P, Dougall IG, Harper D. Estimation of partial agonist affinity by interaction with a full agonist: a direct operational model-fitting approach. Br. J. Pharmacol. 1993; 110: 239-244.

[490] Jonker DM, Visser SA, van der Graaf PH, Voskuyl RA, Danhof M. Towards a mechanism-based analysis of pharmacodynamic drug-drug interactions *in vivo*. Pharmacol. Ther. 2005; 106: 1-18.

[491] FDA, Guidance for Industry: End-of-Phase 2A Meetings. U.S. Department of Health and Human Services Food and Drug Administration, Center for Drug Evaluation and Research (CDER), September 2009 Procedural. www.fda.gov/downloads/Drugs/GuidanceComplianceRegulatoryInformation/Guidances/UCM079690.pdf

[492] Krishna R, Schaefer HG, Bjerrum OJ. Effective integration of systems biology, biomarkers, biosimulation, and modeling in streamlining drug development. J Clin Pharmacol. 2007; 47: 738-43.

[493] Gobburu JV, Marroum PJ. Utilisation of pharmacokinetic-pharmacodynamic modelling and simulation in regulatory decision-making. Clin Pharmacokinet. 2001; 40: 883-92.

[494] Yeung S, Pongtavornpinyo W, Hastings IM, Mills AJ, White NJ. Antimalarial drug resistance, artemisinin-based combination therapy, and the contribution of modeling to elucidating policy choices. Am J Trop Med Hyg. 2004; 71(2 Suppl): 179-86.

[495] Escalante AA, Smith DL, Kim Y. The dynamics of mutations associated with anti-malarial drug resistance in *Plasmodium falciparum*. Trends Parasitol. 2009; 25: 557-63.

[496] Pongtavornpinyo W, Yeung S, Hastings IM, Dondorp AM, Day NP, White NJ. Spread of anti-malarial drug resistance: Mathematical model with implications for ACT drug policies Malar J. 2008; 7: 229.

[497] Meagher AK, Forrest A, Dalhoff A, Stass H, Schentag JJ. Novel pharmacokinetic-pharmacodynamic model for prediction of outcomes with an extended-release formulation of ciprofloxacin. Antimicrob Agents Chemother. 2004; 48: 2061-8.

[498] Czock D, Keller F. Mechanism-based pharmacokinetic-pharmacodynamic modeling of antimicrobial drug effects. J Pharmacokinet Pharmacodyn. 2007; 34: 727-51.

[499] Simpson JA, Watkins ER, Price RN, Aarons L, Kyle DE, White NJ. Mefloquine Pharmacokinetic-Pharmacodynamic Models: Implications for Dosing and Resistance Antimicrob Agents Chemother. 2000; 44: 3414-3424.

[500] Mackinnon MJ. Drug resistance models for malaria. Acta Trop. 2005; 94: 207-17.

[501] Martini C, Olofsen E, Yassen A, Aarts L, Dahan A. Pharmacokinetic-pharmacodynamic modeling in acute and chronic pain: an overview of the recent literature. Expert Rev Clin Pharmacol. 2011; 4: 719-28.

[502] Hoshen MB, Na-Bangchang K, Stein WD, Ginsburg H. Mathematical modeling of the chemotherapy of *Plasmodium falciparum* malaria with artesunate: postulation of 'dormancy', a partial cytostatic effect of the drug, and its implication for treatment regimens. Parasitology. 2000; 121 (Pt 3): 237-46.

[503] Svensson US, Alin H, Karlsson MO, Bergqvist Y, Ashton M. Population pharmacokinetic and pharmacodynamic modelling of artemisinin and mefloquine enantiomers in patients with *falciparum* malaria. Eur J Clin Pharmacol. 2002; 58: 339-51.

[504] Hoshen MB, Stein WD, Ginsburg H. Mathematical modelling of malaria chemotherapy: combining artesunate and mefloquine. Parasitology. 2002; 124(Pt 1): 9-15.

[505] Okell LC, Drakeley CJ, Bousema T, Whitty CJ, Ghani AC. Modelling the impact of artemisinin combination therapy and long-acting treatments on malaria transmission intensity. PLoS Med. 2008; 5: e226.

[506] Aarons L. Sparse data analysis. Eur J Drug Metab Pharmacokinet. 1993; 18: 97-100.

[507] Vozeh S, Steimer JL, Rowland M, Morselli P, Mentre F, Balant LP, Aarons L. The use of population pharmacokinetics in drug development. Clin Pharmacokinet. 1996; 30: 81-93.

[508] Simpson JA, Aarons L, White NJ. How can we do pharmacokinetic studies in the tropics? Trans R Soc Trop Med Hyg. 2001; 95: 347-51.
[509] Ezzet F, Mull R, Karbwang J. Population pharmacokinetics and therapeutic response of CGP 56697 (artemether + benflumetol) in malaria patients. Br J Clin Pharmacol 1998; 46: 553-62.
[510] Simpson JA, Price R, ter Kuile F, Teja-Isavatharm P, Nosten F, Chongsuphajaisiddhi T, Looareesuwan S, Aarons L, White NJ. Population pharmacokinetics of mefloquine in patients with acute *falciparum* malaria. Clin Pharmacol Ther. 1999; 66: 472-84.
[511] Ezzet F, van Vugt M, Nosten F, Looareesuwan S, White NJ. Pharmacokinetics and pharmacodynamics of lumefantrine (benflumetol) in acute *falciparum* malaria. Antimicrob Agents Chemother. 2000; 44: 697-704.
[512] Sidhu JS, Ashton M, Huong NV, Hai TN, Karlsson MO, Sy ND, Jonsson EN, Cong LD. Artemisinin population pharmacokinetics in children and adults with uncomplicated *falciparum* malaria. Br J Clin Pharmacol. 1998; 45: 347-54.
[513] Hendriksen IC, Maiga D, Lemnge MM, Mtove G, Gesase S, Reyburn H, Lindegardh N, Day NP, von Seidlein L, Dondorp AM, Tarning J, White NJ. Population pharmacokinetic and pharmacodynamic properties of intramuscular quinine in Tanzanian children with severe *Falciparum* malaria. Antimicrob Agents Chemother. 2013; 57: 775-83.
[514] Tarning J, Zongo I, Somé FA, Rouamba N, Parikh S, Rosenthal PJ, Hanpithakpong W, Jongrak N, Day NP, White NJ, Nosten F, Ouedraogo JB, Lindegardh N. Population pharmacokinetics and pharmacodynamics of piperaquine in children with uncomplicated *falciparum* malaria. Clin Pharmacol Ther. 2012; 91: 497-505.
[515] Charles BG, Miller AK, Nasveld PE, Reid MG, Harris IE, Edstein MD. Population pharmacokinetics of tafenoquine during malaria prophylaxis in healthy subjects. Antimicrob Agents Chemother. 2007; 51: 2709-15.
[516] Stepniewska K, Taylor W, Sirima SB, Ouedraogo EB, Ouedraogo A, Gansané A, Simpson JA, Morgan CC, White NJ, Kiechel JR. Population pharmacokinetics of artesunate and amodiaquine in African children. Malar J. 2009; 8: 200.
[517] Hennig S, Waterhouse TH, Bell SC, France M, Wainwright CE, Miller H, Charles BG, Duffull SB. A D-Optimal designed population pharmacokinetic study of oral itraconazole in adult cystic fibrosis patients. Br J Clin Pharmacol. 2007; 63: 438-450.
[518] Kris M Jamsen, Stephen B Duffull, Joel Tarning, Niklas Lindegardh, Nicholas J White, Julie A Simpson. Optimal designs for population pharmacokinetic studies of oral artesunate in patients with uncomplicated *falciparum* malaria. Malar J. 2011; 10: 181.
[519] WHO. Methods and techniques for assessing exposure to antimalarial drugs in clinical field studies. Geneva, Switzerland; 2011.
[520] Jamsen KM, Duffull SB, Tarning J, Lindegardh N, White NJ, Simpson JA. Optimal designs for population pharmacokinetic studies of the partner drugs co-administered with artemisinin derivatives in patients with uncomplicated *falciparum* malaria. Malar J. 2012; 11: 143.
[521] Tarning J, Rijken MJ, McGready R, Phyo AP, Hanpithakpong W, Day NPJ, WhiteNJ, Nosten F, Lindegardh N. Population Pharmacokinetics of Dihydroartemisinin and Piperaquine in Pregnant and Nonpregnant Women with Uncomplicated Malaria Antimicrob Agents Chemother. 2012; 56: 1997-2007.
[522] Morris CA, Onyamboko MA, Capparelli E, Koch MA, Atibu J, Lokomba V, Douoguih M, Hemingway-Foday J, Wesche D, Ryder RW, Bose C, Wright L, Tshefu AK, Meshnick S, Fleckenstein L. Population pharmacokinetics of artesunate and dihydroartemisinin in pregnant and non-pregnant women with malaria. Malar J. 2011; 10: 114.
[523] Chien JY, Friedrich S, Heathman MA, de Alwis DP, Sinha V. Pharmacokinetics/Pharmacodynamics and the stages of drug development: role of modeling and simulation. AAPS J. 2005; 7: E544-59.
[524] Ince I, de Wildt SN, Tibboel D, Danhof M, Knibbe CA. Tailor-made drug treatment for children: creation of an infrastructure for data-sharing and population PK-PD modeling. Drug Discov Today. 2009; 14: 316-20.
[525] Tarning J, Chotsiri P, Jullien V, Rijken MJ, Bergstrand M, Cammas M, McGready R, Singhasivanon P, Day NPJ, White NJ, Nosten F, Lindegardh N. Population Pharmacokinetic and Pharmacodynamic Modeling of Amodiaquine and Desethylamodiaquine in Women with *Plasmodium vivax* Malaria during and after Pregnancy. Antimicrob Agents Chemother. 2012; 56: 5764-5773.

[526] Hietala SF, Mårtensson A, Ngasala B, Dahlström S, Lindegårdh N, Annerberg A, Premji Z, Färnert A, Gil P, Björkman A, Ashton M. Population pharmacokinetics and pharmacodynamics of artemether and lumefantrine during combination treatment in children with uncomplicated *falciparum* malaria in Tanzania. Antimicrob Agents Chemother. 2010; 54: 4780-8.
[527] Jullien V, Ogutu B, Juma E, Carn G, Obonyo C, Kiechel JR. Population pharmacokinetics and pharmacodynamic considerations of amodiaquine and desethylamodiaquine in Kenyan adults with uncomplicated malaria receiving artesunate-amodiaquine combination therapy. Antimicrob Agents Chemother. 2010; 54: 2611-7.
[528] Hung le Q, de Vries PJ, Binh TQ, Giao PT, Nam NV, Holman R, Kager PA. Artesunate with mefloquine at various intervals for non-severe *Plasmodium falciparum* malaria. Am J Trop Med Hyg. 2004; 71: 160-6.
[529] Ribeiro IR, 0lliaro P. Safety of artemisinin and its derivatives. A review of published and unpublished clinical trials. Med. Trap. (Mars) 1998; 58(3 Suppl.): 50-53.
[530] Kissinger E, Hien TT, Hung NT *et al.* Clinical and neurophysiological study of the effects of multiple doses of artemisinin on brain-stem function in Vietnamese patients. Am. J. Trap. Med. Hyg. 2000; 63: 48-65.
[531] Toovey S, Jamieson A. Audiometric changes associated with the treatment of uncomplicated *falciparum* malaria with co-artemether. Trans. R. Soc. Trop. Med. Hyg. 2004; 98: 261-367.
[532] Bouchaud O, Imbert P, Touze JE, Dodoo AN, Danis M, Legros F. Fatal cardiotoxicity related to halofantrine: a review based on a worldwide safety data base. Malar J. 2009; 8: 289.
[533] Na-Bangchang K. Pharmacodynamics of antimalarial chemotherapy. Expert Rev Clin Pharmacol. 2009; 2: 491-515.
[534] Lefevre 0, Carpenter P, Souppart C *et al.* Interaction trial between artemether-lumefantrine (Riamet) and quinine in healthy subjects. J. Clin. Pharmacol. 2002; 42: 1147-1158.
[535] van Vuge M, Ezzet F, Nosten F, Gathrnann 1, Wilairatana P, Looareesuwan S, White NJ. No evidence of cardiotoxicity during antimalarial treatment with artemether—lumefantrine. Am. J. Trap. Med. Hyg. 1999; 61: 964-967.
[536] White NJ. Cardiotoxicity of antimalarial drugs. Lancet Infect Dis. 2007; 7: 549-58.
[537] Davidson DE Jr. Role of arreether in the treatment of malaria and plans for further development. Trans. R. Soc. Trap. Med. Hyg. 1994; 88(Suppl. 1): S51—S52.
[538] Traebert M, Dumotier B. Antimalarial drugs: QT prolongation and cardiac arrhythmias. Expert Opin. Drug Saf 2006; 4: 421-431.
[539] Maude RJ, Plewes K, Faiz MA *et al.* Does arresunate prolong the electrocardiograph QT interval in patients with severe malaria? Am. J. Trop. Med. Hyg. 2009; 80: 126-132.
[540] Dellicour S, Hall S, Chandramohan D, Greenwood B. The safety of artemisinins during pregnancy: a pressing question. Maiar. J. 2007; 6:15.
[541] Kalilani L, Mofolo I, Chaponda M *et al.* A randomized controlled pilot trial of azithromycin or artesunate added to sulfadoxine-pyrimethamine as treatment for malaria in pregnant women. PLoS ONE 2007; 2: e116.
[542] Rijken MJ, McGready R, Boel ME *et al.* Dihydroartemisinin-piperaquine rescue trearment of multidrug-resistant *Plasmodium falciparum* malaria in pregnancy: a preliminary report. Am. J. Trap. Med. Hyg. 2008; 78: 543-545.
[543] ter Kuile FO, Dolan G, Nosten F, Edstein MD, Luxemburger C, Phaipun L, Chongsuphajaisiddhi T, Webster HK, White NJ. Halofantrine *versus* mefloquine in treatment of multidrug-resistant *falciparum* malaria. Lancet. 1993; 341(8852): 1044-9.
[544] Taylor WR, White NJ. Antimalarial drug toxicity: a review. Drug Saf. 2004; 27: 25-61.
[545] Borsini F, Crumb W, Pace S, Ubben D, Wible B, Yan GX, Funck-Brentano C. *In vitro* Cardiovascular Effects of Dihydroartemisin-Piperaquine Combination Compared with Other Antimalarials. Antimicrob Agents Chemother. 2012; 56: 3261-3270.
[546] Wongsrichanalai C, Meshnick SR. Declining artesunate-mefloquine efficacy against *falciparum* malaria on the Cambodia-Thailand border. Emerg. Infect. Dis. 2008; 14: 716-719.
[547] Obonyo CO, Juma EA. Clindamycin plus quinine for treating uncomplicated *falciparum* malaria: a systematic review and meta-analysis. Malar J. 2012; 11: 2.
[548] Whitty CJ, Chandler C, Ansah E, Leslie T, Staedke SG. Deployment of ACT antimalarials for treatment of malaria: challenges and opportunities. Malar J. 2008; 7(Suppl 1): S7.

[549] Obonyo CO, Juma EA, Ogutu BR, Vulule JM, Lau J. Amodiaquine combined with sulfadoxine/pyrimethamine *versus* artemisinin-based combinations for the treatment of uncomplicated *falciparum* malaria in Africa: a meta-analysis. Trans R Soc Trop Med Hyg. 2007; 101: 117-26.

[550] Croft SL, Duparc S, Arbe-Barnes SJ, Craft JC, Shin CS, Fleckenstein L, Borghini-Fuhrer I, Rim HJ. Review of pyronaridine anti-malarial properties and product characteristics. Malar J. 2012; 11: 270.

[551] Duparc S, Lanza C, Ubben D, Borghini-Fuhrer I, Kellam L. Optimal dose finding for novel antimalarial combination therapy. Trop Med Int Health. 2012; 17: 409-13.

[552] Langhorne J, Buffet P, Galinski M, Good M, Harty J, Leroy D, Mota MM, Pasini E, Renia L, Riley E, Stins M, Duffy P. The relevance of non-human primate and rodent malaria models for humans. Malar J. 2011; 10: 23.

[553] Arnold L, Tyagi RK, Meija P, Swetman C, Gleeson J, Pérignon JL, Druilhe P. Further Improvements of the *P. falciparum* Humanized Mouse Model. PLoS One. 2011; 6: e18045.

[554] Klonis N, Tan O, Jackson K, Goldberg D, Klemba M, Tilley L. Evaluation of pH during cytostomal endocytosis and vacuolar catabolism of hemoglobin in *Plasmodium falciparum*. Biochem J. 2007; 407: 343-354.

[555] Fidock DA, Eastman RT, Ward SA, Meshnick SR. Recent highlights in antimalarial drug resistance and chemotherapy research. Trends Parasitol. 2008; 24: 537-544.

[556] Cooper RA, Hartwig CL, Ferdig MT. *pfcrt* is more than the *Plasmodium falciparum* chloroquine resistance gene: A functional and evolutionary perspective. Acta Trop. 2005; 94: 170-180.

[557] Russell B, Chalfein F, Prasetyorini B, Kenangalem E, Piera K, Suwanarusk R, Brockman A, Prayoga P, Sugiarto P, Cheng Q, Tjitra E, Anstey NM, Price RN. Determinants of *in vitro* drug susceptibility testing of *Plasmodium vivax*. Antimicrob Agents Chemother. 2008; 52: 1040-1045.

[558] Lim P, Alker AP, Khim N, Shah NK, Incardona S, Doung S, Yi P, Bouth DM, Bouchier C, Puijalon OM, Meshnick SR, Wongsrichanalai C, Fandeur T, Le Bras J, Ringwald P, Ariey F. *Pfmdr1* copy number and arteminisin derivatives combination therapy failure in *falciparum* malaria in Cambodia. Malar J. 2009; 8: 11.

[559] Ekland EH, Fidock DA. Advances in understanding the genetic basis of antimalarial drug resistance. Curr Opin Microbiol. 2007; 10: 363-370.

[560] Johnson JD, Dennull RA, Gerena L, Lopez-Sanchez M, Roncal NE, Waters NC. Assessment and continued validation of the malaria SYBR green I-based fluorescence assay for use in malaria drug screening. Antimicrob Agents Chemother. 2007; 51: 1926-1633.

[561] Scherf A, Rivière L, Lopez-Rubio JJ. SnapShot: var. gene expression in the malaria parasite. Cell. 2008; 134: 190.

[562] Ralph SA, van Dooren GG, Waller RF, Crawford MJ, Fraunholz MJ, Foth BJ, Tonkin CJ, Roos DS, McFadden GI. Tropical infectious diseases: Metabolic maps and functions of the *Plasmodium falciparum* apicoplast. Nat Rev Microbiol. 2004; 2: 203-216.

[563] Sidhu AB, Sun Q, Nkrumah LJ, Dunne MW, Sacchettini JC, Fidock DA. *In vitro* efficacy, resistance selection, and structural modeling studies implicate the malarial parasite apicoplast as the target of azithromycin. J Biol Chem. 2007; 282: 2494-2504.

[564] Spry C, Chai CL, Kirk K, Saliba KJ. A class of pantothenic acid analogs inhibits *Plasmodium falciparum* pantothenate kinase and represses the proliferation of malaria parasites. Antimicrob Agents Chemother. 2005; 49: 4649-4657.

[565] Biagini GA, Fisher N, Berry N, Stocks PA, Meunier B, Williams DP, Bonar-Law R, Bray PG, Owen A, O'Neill PM, Ward SA. Acridinediones: Selective and potent inhibitors of the malaria parasite mitochondrial bc1 complex. Mol Pharmacol. 2008; 73: 1347-1355.

[566] von Itzstein M, Plebanski M, Cooke BM, Coppel RL. Hot, sweet and sticky: The glycobiology of *Plasmodium falciparum*. Trends Parasitol. 2008; 24: 210-218.

[567] Hartwig CL, Rosenthal AS, D'Angelo J, Griffin CE, Posner GH, Cooper RA. Accumulation of artemisinin trioxane derivatives within neutral lipids of *Plasmodium falciparum* malaria parasites is endoperoxide-dependent. Biochem Pharmacol. 2009; 77: 322-336.

[568] Sibley CH, Barnes KI, Watkins WM, Plowe CV. A network to monitor antimalarial drug resistance: A plan for moving forward. Trends Parasitol. 2008; 24: 43-48.

[569] Nduati E, Hunt S, Kamau EM, Nzila A. 2,4-Diaminopteridine-Based Compounds as Precursors for *De Novo* Synthesis of Antifolates: a Novel Class of Antimalarials. Antimicrob Agents Chemother. 2005; 49: 3652-3657.

[570] Ben Mamoun C, Prigge ST, Vial H. Targeting the lipid metabolic pathways for the treatment of malaria. Drug Dev. Res. 2010; 71: 44-55.

[571] Rottmann M, Yeung BK, Lee MC, Zou B. *et al.* Spiroindolones, a potent compound class for the treatment of malaria. Science 2010; 329: 1175-1180.

[572] Wells TN, Alonso PL, Gutteridge WE. New medicines to improve control and contribute to the eradication of malaria. Nat. Rev. Drug Discov. 2009; 8: 879-891.

[573] Chico RM, Chandramohan D. Azithromycin plus chloroquine: combination therapy for protection against malaria and sexually transmitted infections in pregnancy. Expert Opin Drug Metab Toxicol. 2011; 7: 1153-67.

[574] Na-Bangchang K, Ruengweerayut R, Karbwang J, Chauemung A, Hutchinson D. Pharmacokinetics and pharmacodynamics of fosmidomycin monotherapy and combination therapy with clindamycin in the treatment of multidrug resistant *falciparum* malaria. Malar J. 2007; 6: 70.

[575] Jansen FH, Lesaffre E, Penali LK, Zattera MJ, Die-Kakou H, Bissagnene E. Assessment of the relative advantage of various artesunate-based combination therapies by a multi-treatment Bayesian random-effects meta-analysis. Am J Trop Med Hyg. 2007; 77: 1005-1009.

[576] Ramharter M, Kurth F, Schreier AC, Nemeth J, Glasenapp Iv, Bélard S, Schlie M, Kammer J, Koumba PK, Cisse B, Mordmüller B, Lell B, Issifou S, Oeuvray C, Fleckenstein L, Kremsner PG. Fixed-dose pyronaridine-artesunate combination for treatment of uncomplicated *falciparum* malaria in pediatric patients in Gabon. J Infect Dis. 2008; 198: 911-9.

[577] McGready R, Ashley EA, Moo E, Cho T, Barends M, Hutagalung R, Looareesuwan S, White NJ, Nosten F. A randomized comparison of artesunate-atovaquone-proguanil *versus* quinine in treatment for uncomplicated *falciparum* malaria during pregnancy. J Infect Dis. 2005; 192: 846-853.

[578] Batty KT, Salman S, Moore BR, Benjamin J, Lee ST, Page-Sharp M, Pitus N, Ilett KF, Mueller I, Hombhanje FW, Siba P, Davis TM. Artemisinin-naphthoquine combination therapy for uncomplicated pediatric malaria: a pharmacokinetic study. Antimicrob Agents Chemother. 2012; 56: 2472-84.

[579] Wang JY, Cao WC, Shan CQ, Zhang M, Li GF, Ding DB, Shi YL, Wu BA.Naphthoquine phosphate and its combination with artemisinine. Acta Trop. 2004; 89: 375-81.

[580] Gaudin K, Millet P, Fawaz F, Olliaro P, White NJ, Cassus-Coussère C, Agbahoungha U, Dubost JP. Investigation of porous graphitic carbon at high-temperature liquid chromatography with evaporative light scattering detection for the analysis of the drug combination artesunate--azithromycin for the treatment of severe malaria. J Chromatogr A. 2010; 1217: 75-81.

[581] Sykes A, Hendriksen I, Mtove G, Mandea V, Mrema H, Rutta B, Mapunda E, Manjurano A, Amos B, Reyburn H, Whitty CJ. Azithromycin plus artesunate *versus* artemether-lumefantrine for treatment of uncomplicated malaria in Tanzanian children: a randomized, controlled trial. Clin Infect Dis. 2009; 49:1195-1201.

[582] Thriemer K, Starzengruber P, Khan WA, Haque R, Marma AS, Ley B, Vossen MG, Swoboda P, Akter J, Noedl H. Azithromycin combination therapy for the treatment of uncomplicated *falciparum* malaria in Bangladesh: an open-label randomized, controlled clinical trial. J Infect Dis. 2010; 202: 392-398.

[583] Krudsood S, Tangpukdee N, Thanchatwet V, Wilairatana P, Srivilairit S, Pothipak N, Jianping S, Guoqiao L, Brittenham GM, Looareesuwan S. Dose ranging studies of new artemisinin-piperaquine fixed combinations compared to standard regimens of artemisisnin combination therapies for acute uncomplicated *falciparum* malaria. Southeast Asian J Trop Med Public Health. 2007; 38: 971-8.

Subject Index

Subject Index

A

Qigui Li and Mark R. Hickman

B

D

E

F

G

H

I

K

L

M

Q

R

S

Made in United States
North Haven, CT
04 November 2026

21743226R10299